# Physiology of the CSF and Blood Brain Barriers

# Physiology of the CSF and Blood Brain Barriers

Edited by Katherine Stokes

hayle
medical

New York

Hayle Medical,
750 Third Avenue, 9th Floor,
New York, NY 10017, USA

Visit us on the World Wide Web at:
www.haylemedical.com

This book contains information obtained from authentic and highly regarded sources. Copyright for all individual chapters remain with the respective authors as indicated. All chapters are published with permission under the Creative Commons Attribution License or equivalent. A wide variety of references are listed. Permission and sources are indicated; for detailed attributions, please refer to the permissions page and list of contributors. Reasonable efforts have been made to publish reliable data and information, but the authors, editors and publisher cannot assume any responsibility for the validity of all materials or the consequences of their use.

ISBN: 978-1-63241-674-2

**Trademark Notice:** Registered trademark of products or corporate names are used only for explanation and identification without intent to infringe.

**Cataloging-in-Publication Data**

Physiology of the CSF and blood brain barriers / edited by Katherine Stokes.
p. cm.
Includes bibliographical references and index.
ISBN 978-1-63241-674-2
1. Cerebrospinal fluid--Physiology. 2. Blood-brain barrier--Physiology.
3. Cerebrospinal fluid. 4. Blood-brain barrier. I. Stokes, Katherine.
QP372 .P48 2019
612.804 2--dc23

# Table of Contents

**Permissions**

**List of Contributors**

**Index**

# Preface

The cerebrospinal fluid (CSF) is a clear colorless fluid found in the brain and the spinal cord. It acts as a cushion for the brain, providing basic immunological and mechanical protection to the brain inside the skull. It serves an important role in cerebral autoregulation of cerebral blood flow. The brain produces approximately 500 ml of cerebrospinal fluid everyday. The blood brain barrier (BBB) is a selective semipermeable boundary separating the circulating blood from the brain and the extracellular fluid of the central nervous system. It restricts the diffusion of solutes in the blood and hydrophilic molecules into the CSF but allows the diffusion of hormones, oxygen, carbon dioxide and other polar molecules. The blood brain barrier acts to protect the brain from circulating pathogens. In cases where an infection occurs, a drug has to be administered directly into the CSF such that it can cross over into the blood-cerebrospinal fluid barrier. This book contains some path-breaking studies in the physiology of the cerebrospinal fluid and blood brain barriers. It will also provide interesting topics for research, which interested readers can take up. Coherent flow of topics, student-friendly language and extensive use of examples make this book an invaluable source of knowledge.

This book is the end result of constructive efforts and intensive research done by experts in this field. The aim of this book is to enlighten the readers with recent information in this area of research. The information provided in this profound book would serve as a valuable reference to students and researchers in this field.

At the end, I would like to thank all the authors for devoting their precious time and providing their valuable contribution to this book. I would also like to express my gratitude to my fellow colleagues who encouraged me throughout the process.

**Editor**

# MicroRNA-155 contributes to shear-resistant leukocyte adhesion to human brain endothelium in vitro

Camilla Cerutti[1,3]*, Patricia Soblechero-Martin[1], Dongsheng Wu[1,4], Miguel Alejandro Lopez-Ramirez[1,5], Helga de Vries[6], Basil Sharrack[2], David Kingsley Male[1] and Ignacio Andres Romero[1]

## Abstract

**Background:** Increased leukocyte adhesion to brain endothelial cells forming the blood–brain barrier (BBB) precedes extravasation into the central nervous system (CNS) in neuroinflammatory diseases such as multiple sclerosis (MS). Previously, we reported that microRNA-155 (miR-155) is up-regulated in MS and by inflammatory cytokines in human brain endothelium, with consequent modulation of endothelial paracellular permeability. Here, we investigated the role of endothelial miR-155 in leukocyte adhesion to the human cerebral microvascular endothelial cell line, hCMEC/D3, under shear forces mimicking blood flow in vivo.

**Results:** Using a gain- and loss-of-function approach, we show that miR-155 up-regulation increases leukocyte firm adhesion of both monocyte and T cells to hCMEC/D3 cells. Inhibition of endogenous endothelial miR-155 reduced monocytic and T cell firm adhesion to naïve and cytokines-induced human brain endothelium. Furthermore, this effect is partially associated with modulation of the endothelial cell adhesion molecules VCAM1 and ICAM1 by miR-155.

**Conclusions:** Our results suggest that endothelial miR-155 contribute to the regulation of leukocyte adhesion at the inflamed BBB. Taken together with previous observations, brain endothelial miR-155 may constitute a potential molecular target for treatment of neuroinflammation diseases.

**Keywords:** Blood–brain barrier, Cell adhesion molecules, Flow shear stress, Leukocyte adhesion, microRNA-155, Neuroinflammation

## Background

Leukocyte recruitment from blood into tissues is a crucial event in both physiological and pathological conditions and is described as a multistep process involving leukocyte rolling, adhesion, crawling and diapedesis [1] under hemodynamic shear stress. In the central nervous system (CNS), firm leukocyte adhesion to the highly specialized brain endothelial cells forming the blood–brain barrier (BBB) is important in immunosurveillance and plays a critical role in the pathogenesis of neuroinflammatory diseases such as multiple sclerosis (MS) [2].

Leukocyte adhesion occurs in postcapillary venules [3] as a result of specific interactions between leukocyte integrins, α4β1 (VLA-4) and αLβ2-integrin (LFA-1), and endothelial adhesion molecules, VCAM1 and ICAM1, respectively [4]. In MS, chemokines and proinflammatory cytokines such as TNFα and IFNγ are secreted in the inflammatory loci thereby leading to VCAM1 and ICAM1 overexpression on activated brain endothelial cells [2]. Furthermore, it has been observed that both monocytes and T cells are present in the perivascular inflammatory infiltrates [5]. Despite numerous studies, the endothelial molecular controls on leukocyte firm adhesion to brain endothelium have not been fully elucidated.

MicroRNAs (miRs) are a class of highly conserved, single-stranded, non-coding RNA molecules (20–25

*Correspondence: Camilla.cerutti@kcl.ac.uk
[3] Randall Division of Cell and Molecular Biophysics, King's College London, New Hunt's House, Guy's Campus, London SE1 1UL, UK
Full list of author information is available at the end of the article

nucleotides), that modulate gene expression by repression of their target genes at the post-transcriptional level [6]. Recent studies have identified miRs as key regulators of a vast number of biological processes and disorders, including MS [7] and those regulating neurovascular function in inflammation [8], such as regulation of cell adhesion molecules and leukocyte trafficking across brain endothelium [9, 10].

MiR-155 is a multifunctional miR which plays a crucial role in physiological and pathological processes including inflammation [11, 12]. MiR-155 expression is increased in brain endothelium in MS active lesions and proinflammatory cytokines, TNFα and IFNγ, up-regulate miR-155 expression in the human cerebral microvascular endothelial cell line, hCMEC/D3 [13]. Furthermore, miR-155 overexpression in hCMEC/D3 cells increases endothelial permeability and negatively affects expression of tight junctional molecules, whereas miR-155 inhibition is associated with decreased microvascular permeability [13]. In this study, we determined the role of human brain endothelial miR-155 in controlling T cell and monocyte firm adhesion to hCMEC/D3 cells, an in vitro model of human brain endothelium [14], when subjected to shear forces mimicking blood flow at the venular vessel level in vivo. In addition, the effect of miR-155 on the expression of the cell adhesion molecules VCAM1 and ICAM1 in hCMEC/D3 cells was also investigated.

## Methods
### Cell culture
The hCMEC/D3 cell line [14] was used at passages 26–34 and cultured in endothelial cell basal medium-2 (EGM-2) medium (Lonza, Walkersville, USA) and supplemented with the following components obtained from the manufacturer: 0.025 % (v/v) rhEGF, 0.025 % (v/v) VEGF, 0.025 % (v/v) IGF, 0.1 % (v/v) rhFGF, 0.1 % (v/v) gentamycin, 0.1 % (v/v) ascorbic acid, 0.04 % (v/v) hydrocortisone and 2.5 % (v/v) foetal bovine serum (FBS), hereafter referred to as endothelial complete medium. hCMEC/D3 cells were grown to confluence (~$1 \times 10^5$ cells/cm$^2$) on tissue culture flasks coated with collagen from calf skin (Sigma, St. Louis, USA). The T cell line Jurkat from acute T cell leukaemia and the monocytic line THP1 from acute monocytic leukaemia were a kind gift from Dr. V Male (Cambridge University). Jurkat and THP1 cells were grown in suspension in RPMI 1640 W/GLUTAMAX I (Gibco®Invitrogen, Paisley,UK) culture medium (containing 10 % FBS and 100 µg/ml streptomycin + 100 units/ml penicillin). All cell lines were maintained in a 95 % humidified air and 5 % CO$_2$ incubator at 37 °C.

### MicroRNA transfection
hCMEC/D3 cells were grown to ~70 % confluence and transfected in antibiotic-free endothelial media. To introduce miR-155 precursor, hCMEC/D3 cells were transfected with 30 nM of pre-miR-155 or its control, scrambled-pre-miR (Ambion, Fischer Scientific UK), using Siport™ Polyamine Transfection Agent (Ambion) in Opti-mem®I (Gibco®) media for 24 h. For inhibition studies, 60 nM of anti-miR-155 or its control, scrambled-anti-miR (Dharmacon, Waltham, USA) was transfected using Lipofectamine® 2000 (Thermo Fisher Scientific, Carlsbad, USA) for 6 h, media was then changed with endothelial complete medium for 18 h. siGENOME SMARTpool siRNAs for human VCAM1 or siRNA control pool (ThermoFisher Scientific) were transfected into hCMEC/D3 cells using Lipofectamine 2000® (Thermo Fisher Scientific).

### Flow-based leukocyte adhesion assay: live cell adhesion imaging under flow conditions
A flow-based adhesion assay previously described in Wu et al. was used [10]. hCMEC/D3 cells were grown in Ibidi® µ-Slide VI$^{0.4}$ (Ibidi® GmbH, Martinstreid, Germany), transfected, treated or not with 1 ng/ml TNFα and IFNα for 24 h in static conditions and washed before flow adhesion assay. THP-1 and Jurkat cells ($2 \times 10^6$ cells/ml) were labelled with CMFDA (5–chloromethylfluoresceindiacetate, Life Technologies, Eugene, USA) and were allowed to flow through the channel with endothelial monolayers and accumulate at 0.5 dyn/cm$^2$ for 5 min. Then, the flow was increased to 1.5 dyn/cm$^2$ (venular vessel wall shear stress) for 30 s to remove non-adhered leukocytes with endothelial complete media. Leukocyte-endothelial interactions were recorded (Additional file 1: Video S1) for 5.5 min and firm leukocyte adhesion was quantified. Firm adhesion was defined by leukocytes that remained adhered on human brain endothelium in the field of view (FOV 640 × 480 µm) throughout the accumulation time and after increasing the flow to 1.5 dyn/cm$^2$ and manually counted using Image J software in five different FOVs. Image acquisition was performed using a X10 objective of an inverted fluorescence microscope (Olympus IX70, Tokyo, Japan) controlled by the Image Pro Plus software (Media Cybernetics Inc. Bethesda, USA) using a Q-IMAGING QICAM FAST 1394 on a 12-bit camera (40 images/min). For more details refer to Additional file 2: Fig. S1, Table S1 and Table S2.

### ELISA for adhesion molecules
Brain endothelial expression of VCAM1 and ICAM1 was measured by cell-surface ELISA performed as previously described [15] using 2 µg/ml mouse primary antibody against VCAM1 or ICAM1 (R&D SYSTEMS, Abingdon, UK) and the corresponding secondary antibodies conjugated to horseradish peroxidase. The optical density (OD) was then measured using a FLUOstar Optima

spectrometer (BMG LABTECH, Aylesbury, UK) at a wavelength of 450 nm.

## Statistics

All data are presented as mean ± SEM from a number of independent experiments (n) with replicates specified in each legend. $P$ values were calculated using paired Student's $t$ tests. Statistically significant differences are presented as probability levels of $P < 0.05$ (*), $P < 0.01$ (**). Calculations and figures were performed using the statistical software GraphPad Prism 5 (GraphPad Software).

## Results

### MiR-155 modulates Jurkat and THP-1 firm adhesion to hCMEC/D3 cells

We first investigated whether increased levels of miR-155 in unstimulated brain endothelial cells affected firm leukocyte adhesion under shear stress. In human brain endothelium, miR-155 overexpression simulates, to a certain extent, the effect of proinflammatory cytokines [13], which are known to increase T cell firm adhesion [10]. We observed strong increase in adhesion of both T cell (Jurkat ~twofold increase) and monocyte (THP-1 ~threefold

increase) to unstimulated hCMEC/D3 cells transfected with miR-155 precursor (pre-miR-155) compared with control (scrambled pre-miR) (Fig. 1a, b; Additional file 3: Video S2, Additional file 4: Video S3, Additional file 5: Video S4, Additional file 6: Video S5). Inhibition of endogenous miR-155 in hCMEC/D3 cells by transfection with anti-miR-155 reduced Jurkat and THP-1 firm adhesion to unstimulated brain endothelium compared to its control (scrambled anti-miR) (Fig. 1a and c; Additional file 7: Video S6, Additional file 8: Video S7, Additional file 9: Video S8, Additional file 10: Video S9). To better understand the contribution of endothelial miR-155 in leukocyte adhesion, in the context of inflammation, we then explored the effect of miR-155 modulation on monocytic and T cell adhesion on brain endothelial cells stimulated with pro-inflammatory cytokines (TNFα and IFNγ at 1 ng/ml for 24 h), a treatment that increases brain endothelial miR-155 expression, hence monocytic and T cell adhesion (Fig. 1d, e; controls). Over-expression of miR-155 slightly increased shear resistant leukocyte adhesion to cytokine-treated brain endothelium compared to control (cytokine-treated scrambled pre-miR) (Fig. 1 a, d; Additional file 11: Video S10, Additional

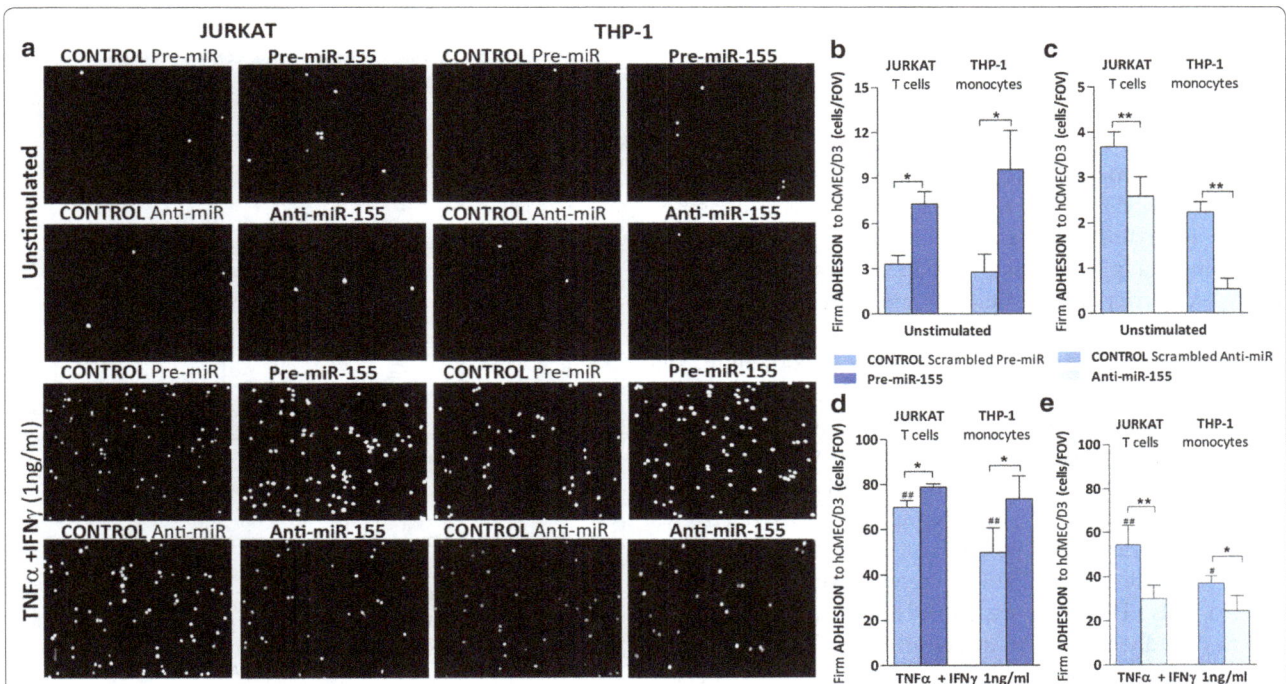

**Fig. 1** miR-155 modulates Jurkat and THP-1 firm adhesion to brain endothelial hCMEC/D3 cells. hCMEC/D3 cell monolayers were transfected with control scrambled Pre-miR and Pre-miR-155 (**a, c, d**) or control scrambled Anti-miR and Anti-miR-155 (**a, c, e**) followed by treatment with a combination of cytokines (TNFα + IFNγ) at 1 ng/ml for 24 h (**a, d, e**) or left unstimulated (**a, b, c**). **a** Representative images of shear-resistant firmly adhered Jurkat and THP-1 cells to hCMEC/D3 monolayer (field of view (FOV): 640 × 480 μm) used for quantification and **b-e** analysis of shear-resistant firmly adhered Jurkat and THP-1 cells to hCMEC/D3 expressed in number of cells/FOV. Experiments were carried out three to six times with five FOVs each. Data are mean ± SEM. Statistical analysis was performed using paired Student's $t$ test (*,#$P < 0.05$, **,##$P < 0.01$, #compared to unstimulated)

file 12: Video S11, Additional file 13: Video S12, Additional file 14: Video S13). Reduction of endogenous miR-155 reduced monocytic and T cell adhesion by ~50 and ~35 %, respectively, to cytokine-stimulated endothelial cells when compared to control (cytokine-treated scrambled anti-miR) (Fig. 1a and e; Additional file 15: Video S14, Additional file 16: Video S15, Additional file 17: Video S16, Additional file 18: Video S17).

## MiR-155 modulates expression of cell adhesion molecules in hCMEC/D3 cells

To further elucidate the role of miR-155 in leukocyte adhesion, we explored whether miR-155-induced changes in monocyte and T cell adhesion to endothelium were associated with modulation of cell adhesion molecules VCAM1 and ICAM1 on the endothelial surface, master mediators of leukocyte trafficking to the BBB [16]. ICAM1 plays a critical role in T cell adhesion as previously demonstrated [17], but VCAM1 is a main player in leukocyte adhesion and mediated both monocyte and T cells adhesion to brain endothelium (Fig. 2a, b). Overexpression of miR-155 enhanced VCAM1 and ICAM1 levels on unstimulated hCMEC/D3 cells (Fig. 2c) whereas decreasing the levels of miR-155 caused a small reduction in VCAM1 and ICAM1 expression (Fig. 2d). No changes in VCAM1 or ICAM1 expression by miR-155 were observed in cytokine-stimulated endothelium (Fig. 2e, f).

## Discussion

MiR-155 is strongly upregulated in cytokine-stimulated hCMEC/D3 cells and in EAE spinal cord vessels at acute stages of the disease, when the BBB is compromised [13]. The same study found that miR-155 acts as a novel regulator of barrier permeability by affecting expression of genes involved in modulation of tight junctions and cell to matrix interactions in human brain endothelium. In this study, we show that modulation of brain endothelial miR-155 levels led to significant changes on firm T cell and monocytic cell line adhesion to hCMEC/D3 cells. However, miR-155 induction of ICAM1 and VCAM1 endothelial expression, while significant, was relatively small in unstimulated conditions, and, no changes in CAM expression by miR-155 were observed in cytokine-treated cells. Therefore we consider that modulation of leukocyte adhesion to brain endothelium by endothelial miR-155 can only be partly accounted for by its effects in the expression of these adhesion molecules, in particular in the early stages of inflammation as miR-155 is one of the earliest microRNAs to be rapidly induced

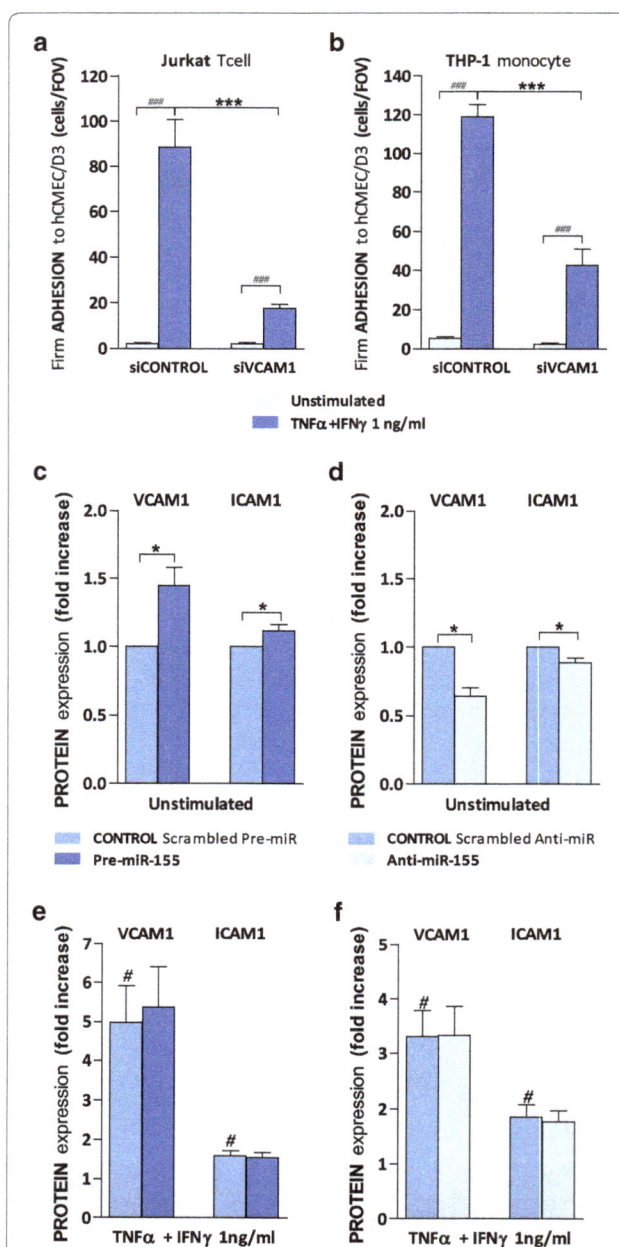

**Fig. 2** miR-155 modulates VCAM1 and ICAM1 expression on brain endothelial hCMEC/D3 cells. hCMEC/D3 cell monolayers were transfected with control siRNA (**a**, **b**) or scrambled Pre-miR and Pre-miR-155 (**c**, **e**) or Anti-miR and Anti-miR-155 (**d**, **f**) followed by treatment with a combination of cytokines (TNFα + IFNγ) at 1 ng/ml for 24 h or left unstimulated. **a**, **b** Number of shear-resistant firmly adhered Jurkat and THP-1 cells to siVCAM1-hCMEC/D3 monolayer per FOV (640 × 480 μm). **c–f** VCAM1 and ICAM1 expression levels were quantified by ELISA. Experiments were carried out three and four times with three replicates each. Data are mean ± SEM. Statistical analysis was performed using paired Student's $t$ test ($^{*,#}P < 0.05$, $^{***,###}P < 0.001$, $^#$compared to unstimulated)

following inflammatory stimuli [13]. Indeed, increased levels of miR-155 enhanced by two fold the expression of two other adhesion-related genes, CCL5 and TNFSF10 in hCMEC/D3 cells (Geo accession GSE44694, platform GPL6883).

Indirect mechanisms other than directly regulating expression of cell adhesion molecules could account for the effect of endothelial miR-155 on leukocyte firm-adhesion. MiRs act by suppressing the expression of genes that contain the miR-target sequence in their mRNA and hence they directly reduce protein expression. Therefore, in order to modulate leukocyte adhesion, miR-155 may regulate the expression of genes which control adhesion indirectly. In this context, it is possible that miR-155 could target NFκB pathway in brain endothelium as it does in HUVEC [18]. This pathway is activated by TNFα leading to the phosphorylation and breakdown of IκB which releases NFκB, allowing it to enter the nucleus and activate several genes involved in neuroinflammation, including VCAM1 and ICAM1. IκB, the inhibitor of NFκB does not contain target sites for miR-155, but 'Inhibitor of nuclear factor kappa-B kinase-interacting protein' (IKBIP) is a potential target for miR-155 (Diana Tools, miRTarbase), previously validated by proteomics [19]. It is therefore conceivable that a reduction in IKBIP expression due to cytokine-induced miR-155 would promote IκB kinase (IKK) to mediate phosphorylation and degradation of IκB, thereby leading to increased nuclear translocation of NFκB, with wide-ranging down-stream effects including the one resulting in increased leukocyte adhesion. This goes hand in hand with our previous observation where inhibition of RelA, NFκB associated protein crucial for NFκB nuclear translocation and activation, decreased T cell adhesion by 60 % to hCMEC/D3 cells [10].

Another possible mechanism by which endothelial miR-155 may modulate leukocyte adhesion involves the small GTPase RhoA, a validated target of miR-155 [20]. Indeed, RhoA controls Rho-associated kinase (ROCK) which in turn modulates ICAM1 expression, cell adhesion, the NFκB pathway [21]. In addition, RhoA is thought to affect leukocyte adhesion and migration by its actions in controlling the organisation of the brain endothelial cytoskeleton [22]. In hCMEC/D3, reduced levels of RhoA induced decreased VCAM1 expression and T cell adhesion [10]. It is certainly possible that miR-155 targets more than one gene controlling either leukocyte adhesion or endothelial activation, and the two genes discussed here both have several important down-stream effects in controlling molecules involved in neuroinflammation and leukocyte adhesion.

## Conclusions

Taken together, our findings support the notion that in neuroinflammatory conditions, miR-155 is itself up-regulated and can promote many pro-inflammatory processes including leukocyte adhesion to brain endothelium. Because of their multiple effects on cellular processes, targeting an individual miR such as miR-155 for therapeutic purposes may lead to modulation of different activation pathways that promote inflammation. Together, these results reinforce the role of endothelial miR-155 in the pathophysiology of the BBB, with a wide range of pro-inflammatory effects.

## Additional files

**Additional file 1: Video S1.** Representative video of flow-based leukocyte adhesion assay using live cell imaging. Brightfield (Left Panel) and FITC (Right Panel) are displayed in parallel to show that the flow-based leukocyte adhesion assay used allows to perform live cell imaging recording both the endothelial monolayer by light microscopy and the fluorescent labelled leukocytes by fluorescent microscopy. The number of arrested JURKAT cells constantly increased along the channel of Ibidi® Slide VI, the yellow arrows (Right Panel) indicate arrested Jurkat cells. Objective 10x, phase-contrast illumination and FITC channel (1 phase-contrast and 1 FITC), field of view 640 μm × 480 μm.

**Additional file 2:** Fig. S1, Table S1, Table S2.

**Additional file 3: Video S2.** Shear-resistant firm adhesion of JURKAT cells to CONTROL Scrambled-Pre-miR transfected and unstimulated hCMECD3 cells. JURKAT cells were pulled through the channel over hCMEC/D3 monolayers under low shear (0.5 dyn/cm²). After 5 min, flow shear stress was increased (1.5 dyn/cm²) to challenge non-firmly adherent JURKAT. The number of arrested JURKAT constantly increased during the accumulation phase and only the one that remained stationary on the endothelial monolayer were manually counted in 5 different FOV along the channel of Ibidi m-Slide VI. FITC channel was used to count fluorescently firmly adhered Jurkat cells. Objective 10x, at 40 images per min (1 phase-contrast and 1 FITC), field of view 640 μm × 480 μm, recording time 5.5 min.

**Additional file 4: Video S3.** Shear-resistant firm adhesion of JURKAT cells to Pre-miR-155 transfected and unstimulated hCMECD3 cells. JURKAT cells were pulled through the channel over hCMEC/D3 monolayers under low shear (0.5 dyn/cm²). After 5 min, flow shear stress was increased (1.5 dyn/cm²) to challenge non-firmly adherent JURKAT. The number of arrested JURKAT constantly increased during the accumulation phase and only the one that remained stationary on the endothelial monolayer were manually counted in 5 different FOV along the channel of Ibidi m-Slide VI. FITC channel was used to count fluorescently firmly adhered Jurkat cells. Objective 10x, at 40 images per min (1 phase-contrast and 1 FITC), field of view 640 μm × 480 μm, recording time 5.5 min.

**Additional file 5: Video S4.** Shear-resistant firm adhesion of THP1 cells to CONTROL Scrambled-Pre-miR transfected and unstimulated hCMECD3 cells. THP1 cells were pulled through the channel over hCMEC/D3 monolayers under low shear (0.5 dyn/cm²). After 5 min, flow shear stress was increased (1.5 dyn/cm²) to challenge non-firmly adherent THP1. The number of arrested THP1 constantly increased during the accumulation phase and only the one that remained stationary on the endothelial monolayer were manually counted in 5 different FOV along the channel of Ibidi m-Slide VI. FITC channel was used to count fluorescently firmly adhered THP1 cells. Objective 10x, at 40 images per min (1 phase-contrast and 1 FITC), field of view 640 μm × 480 μm, recording time 5.5 min.

**Additional file 6: Video S5.** Shear-resistant firm adhesion of THP1 cells to Pre-miR-155 transfected and unstimulated hCMECD3 cells. THP1 cells were pulled through the channel over hCMEC/D3 monolayers under low shear (0.5 dyn/cm²). After 5 min, flow shear stress was increased (1.5 dyn/cm²) to challenge non-firmly adherent THP1. The number of arrested THP1 constantly increased during the accumulation phase and only the one that remained stationary on the endothelial monolayer were manually counted in 5 different FOV along the channel of Ibidi m-Slide VI. FITC channel was used to count fluorescently firmly adhered THP1 cells. Objective 10x, at 40 images per min (1 phase-contrast and 1 FITC), field of view 640 μm × 480 μm, recording time 5.5 min.

**Additional file 7: Video S6.** Shear-resistant firm adhesion of JURKAT cells to CONTROL Scrambled-Anti-miR transfected and unstimulated hCMECD3 cells. JURKAT cells were pulled through the channel over hCMEC/D3 monolayers under low shear (0.5 dyn/cm²). After 5 min, flow shear stress was increased (1.5 dyn/cm²) to challenge non-firmly adherent JURKAT. The number of arrested JURKAT constantly increased during the accumulation phase and only the one that remained stationary on the endothelial monolayer were manually counted in 5 different FOV along the channel of Ibidi m-Slide VI. FITC channel was used to count fluorescently firmly adhered Jurkat cells. Objective 10x, at 40 images per min (1 phase-contrast and 1 FITC), field of view 640 μm × 480 μm, recording time 5.5 min.

**Additional file 8: Video S7.** Shear-resistant firm adhesion of JURKAT cells to Anti-miR-155 transfected and unstimulated hCMECD3 cells. JURKAT cells were pulled through the channel over hCMEC/D3 monolayers under low shear (0.5 dyn/cm²). After 5 min, flow shear stress was increased (1.5 dyn/cm²) to challenge non-firmly adherent JURKAT. The number of arrested JURKAT constantly increased during the accumulation phase and only the one that remained stationary on the endothelial monolayer were manually counted in 5 different FOV along the channel of Ibidi m-Slide VI. FITC channel was used to count fluorescently firmly adhered Jurkat cells. Objective 10x, at 40 images per min (1 phase-contrast and 1 FITC), field of view 640 μm × 480 μm, recording time 5.5 min.

**Additional file 9: Video S8.** Shear-resistant firm adhesion of THP1 cells to CONTROL Scrambled-Anti-miR transfected and unstimulated hCMECD3 cells. THP1 cells were pulled through the channel over hCMEC/D3 monolayers under low shear (0.5 dyn/cm²). After 5 min, flow shear stress was increased (1.5 dyn/cm²) to challenge non-firmly adherent THP1. The number of arrested THP1 constantly increased during the accumulation phase and only the one that remained stationary on the endothelial monolayer were manually counted in 5 different FOV along the channel of Ibidi m-Slide VI. FITC channel was used to count fluorescently firmly adhered THP1 cells. Objective 10x, at 40 images per min (1 phase-contrast and 1 FITC), field of view 640 μm × 480 μm, recording time 5.5 min.

**Additional file 10: Video S9.** Shear-resistant firm adhesion of THP1 cells to Anti-miR-155 unstimulated transfected and unstimulated hCMECD3 cells. THP1 cells were pulled through the channel over hCMEC/D3 monolayers under low shear (0.5 dyn/cm²). After 5 min, flow shear stress was increased (1.5 dyn/cm²) to challenge non-firmly adherent THP1. The number of arrested THP1 constantly increased during the accumulation phase and only the one that remained stationary on the endothelial monolayer were manually counted in 5 different FOV along the channel of Ibidi m-Slide VI. FITC channel was used to count fluorescently firmly adhered THP1cells. Objective 10x, at 40 images per min (1 phase-contrast and 1 FITC), field of view 640 μm × 480 μm, recording time 5.5 min.

**Additional file 11: Video S10.** Shear-resistant firm adhesion of JURKAT cells to CONTROL Scrambled-Pre-miR transfected and stimulated with TNFα and IFNγ hCMECD3 cells. JURKAT cells were pulled through the channel over hCMEC/D3 monolayers under low shear (0.5 dyn/cm²). After 5 min, flow shear stress was increased (1.5 dyn/cm²) to challenge non-firmly adherent JURKAT. The number of arrested JURKAT constantly increased during the accumulation phase and only the one that remained stationary on the endothelial monolayer were manually counted in 5 different FOV along the channel of Ibidi m-Slide VI. FITC channel was used to count fluorescently firmly adhered Jurkat cells. Objective 10x, at 40 images per min (1 phase-contrast and 1 FITC), field of view 640 μm × 480 μm, recording time 5.5 min.

**Additional file 12: Video S11.** Shear-resistant firm adhesion of THP1 cells to CONTROL Scrambled-Pre-miR transfected and stimulated with TNFα and IFNγ hCMECD3 cells. THP1 cells were pulled through the channel over hCMEC/D3 monolayers under low shear (0.5 dyn/cm²). After 5 min, flow shear stress was increased (1.5 dyn/cm²) to challenge non-firmly adherent THP1. The number of arrested THP1 constantly increased during the accumulation phase and only the one that remained stationary on the endothelial monolayer were manually counted in 5 different FOV along the channel of Ibidi m-Slide VI. FITC channel was used to count fluorescently firmly adhered THP1 cells. Objective 10x, at 40 images per min (1 phase-contrast and 1 FITC), field of view 640 μm × 480 μm, recording time 5.5 min.

**Additional file 13: Video S12.** Shear-resistant firm adhesion of THP1 cells to Pre-miR-155 transfected and stimulated with TNFα and IFNγ hCMECD3 cells. THP1 cells were pulled through the channel over hCMEC/D3 monolayers under low shear (0.5 dyn/cm²). After 5 min, flow shear stress was increased (1.5 dyn/cm²) to challenge non-firmly adherent THP1. The number of arrested THP1 constantly increased during the accumulation phase and only the one that remained stationary on the endothelial monolayer were manually counted in 5 different FOV along the channel of Ibidi m-Slide VI. FITC channel was used to count fluorescently firmly adhered THP1 cells. Objective 10x, at 40 images per min (1 phase-contrast and 1 FITC), field of view 640 μm × 480 μm, recording time 5.5 min.

**Additional file 14: Video S13.** Shear-resistant firm adhesion of JURKAT cells to CONTROL Scrambled-Anti-miR transfected and stimulated with TNFα and IFNγ hCMECD3 cells. JURKAT cells were pulled through the channel over hCMEC/D3 monolayers under low shear (0.5 dyn/cm²). After 5 min, flow shear stress was increased (1.5 dyn/cm²) to challenge non-firmly adherent JURKAT. The number of arrested JURKAT constantly increased during the accumulation phase and only the one that remained stationary on the endothelial monolayer were manually counted in 5 different FOV along the channel of Ibidi m-Slide VI. FITC channel was used to count fluorescently firmly adhered Jurkat cells. Objective 10x, at 40 images per min (1 phase-contrast and 1 FITC), field of view 640 μm × 480 μm, recording time 5.5 min.

**Additional file 15: Video S14.** Shear-resistant firm adhesion of JURKAT cells to CONTROL Scrambled-Anti-miR transfected and stimulated with TNFα and IFNγ hCMECD3 cells. JURKAT cells were pulled through the channel over hCMEC/D3 monolayers under low shear (0.5 dyn/cm²). After 5 min, flow shear stress was increased (1.5 dyn/cm²) to challenge non-firmly adherent JURKAT. The number of arrested JURKAT constantly increased during the accumulation phase and only the one that remained stationary on the endothelial monolayer were manually counted in 5 different FOV along the channel of Ibidi m-Slide VI. FITC channel was used to count fluorescently firmly adhered Jurkat cells. Objective 10x, at 40 images per min (1 phase-contrast and 1 FITC), field of view 640 μm × 480 μm, recording time 5.5 min.

**Additional file 16: Video S15.** Shear-resistant firm adhesion of THP1 cells to CONTROL Scrambled-Anti-miR transfected and stimulated with TNFα and IFNγ hCMECD3 cells. THP1 cells were pulled through the channel over hCMEC/D3 monolayers under low shear (0.5 dyn/cm²). After 5 min, flow shear stress was increased (1.5 dyn/cm²) to challenge non-firmly adherent THP1. The number of arrested THP1 constantly increased during the accumulation phase and only the one that remained stationary on the endothelial monolayer were manually counted in 5 different FOV along the channel of Ibidi m-Slide VI. FITC channel was used to count fluorescently firmly adhered THP1 cells. Objective 10x, at 40 images per min (1 phase-contrast and 1 FITC), field of view 640 μm × 480 μm, recording time 5.5 min.

**Additional file 17: Video S16.** Shear-resistant firm adhesion of THP1 cells to Anti-miR-155 transfected and stimulated with TNFα and IFNγ hCMECD3 cells. THP1 cells were pulled through the channel over hCMEC/D3 monolayers under low shear (0.5 dyn/cm²). After 5 min, flow shear stress was increased (1.5 dyn/cm²) to challenge non-firmly adherent THP1. The number of arrested THP1 constantly increased during the accumulation phase and only the one that remained stationary on the endothelial monolayer were manually counted in 5 different FOV along the channel of Ibidi m-Slide VI. FITC channel was used to count fluorescently firmly adhered THP1 cells. Objective 10x, at 40 images per min (1 phase-contrast and 1 FITC), field of view 640 μm × 480 μm, recording time 5.5 min.

**Additional file 18: Video S17.** Shear-resistant firm adhesion of THP1 cells to Anti-miR-155 transfected and stimulated with TNFα and IFNγ hCMECD3 cells. THP1 cells were pulled through the channel over hCMEC/D3 monolayers under low shear (0.5 dyn/cm²). After 5 min, flow shear stress was increased (1.5 dyn/cm²) to challenge non-firmly adherent THP1. The number of arrested THP1 constantly increased during the accumulation phase and only the one that remained stationary on the endothelial monolayer were manually counted in 5 different FOV along the channel of Ibidi m-Slide VI. FITC channel was used to count fluorescently firmly adhered THP1 cells. Objective 10x, at 40 images per min (1 phase-contrast and 1 FITC), field of view 640 μm × 480 μm, recording time 5.5 min.

## Abbreviations
BBB: blood–brain barrier; CNS: central nervous system; EAE: experimental autoimmune encephalomyelitis; ICAM1: intercellular adhesion molecule 1; IFNγ: interferon gamma; IKBIP: inhibitor of nuclear factor kappa-B kinase-interacting protein; IKK: IkB kinase; LFA-1: lymphocyte function-associated antigen 1; miRs: microRNAs; MS: multiple sclerosis; NFκB: nuclear factor kappa-light-chain-enhancer of activated B cells; ROCK: rho-associated kinase; VCAM1: vascular cell adhesion molecule 1; VLA-4: very late antigen-4; TNFα: tumor necrosis factor alpha.

## Authors' contributions
CC performed research, analysed and interpreted the data; PSM contributed to flow based adhesion assay and analysis; DW contributed to siVCAM1 study; IAR, DKM, BS, HdV and MALR, provided support with analysis of data and interpretation of results; CC, DKM and IAR designed the study and wrote the manuscript. All authors read and approved the final manuscript.

## Author details
[1] Department of Life, Health and Chemical Sciences, Biomedical Research Network, Open University, Walton Hall, Milton Keynes MK7 6AA, UK. [2] Department of Neuroscience, Sheffield University, 385a Glossop Road, Sheffield S10 2HQ, UK. [3] Randall Division of Cell and Molecular Biophysics, King's College London, New Hunt's House, Guy's Campus, London SE1 1UL, UK. [4] School of Engineering and Materials Science, Queen Mary University of London, Mile End Road, London E1 4NS, UK. [5] Department of Medicine, University of California, San Diego, La Jolla, CA 92093, USA. [6] Department of Molecular Cell Biology and Immunology, MS Centre Amsterdam, VU University Medical Centre, Amsterdam, The Netherlands.

## Acknowledgements
The authors are grateful to Julia Barkans for general laboratory infrastructure assistance and Radka Gromnicova for helpful discussions. This work was founded by the Multiple Sclerosis Society of Great Britain and Northern Ireland and BBSRC.

## Competing interests
The authors declare that they have no competing interests.

## References
1. Nourshargh S, Hordijk PL, Sixt M. Breaching multiple barriers: leukocyte motility through venular walls and the interstitium. Nat Rev Mol Cell Biol. 2010;11(5):366–78.
2. Ortiz GG, Pacheco-Moises FP, Macias-Islas MA, Flores-Alvarado LJ, Mireles-Ramirez MA, Gonzalez-Renovato ED, et al. Role of the blood–brain barrier in multiple sclerosis. Arch Med Res. 2014;45(8):687–97. doi:10.1016/j.arcmed.2014.11.013.
3. Aird WC. Phenotypic heterogeneity of the endothelium: I. Structure, function, and mechanisms. Circ Res. 2007;100(2):158–73. doi:10.1161/01.RES.0000255691.76142.4a.
4. Engelhardt B, Ransohoff RM. Capture, crawl, cross: the T cell code to breach the blood–brain barriers. Trends Immunol. 2012;33(12):579–89. doi:10.1016/j.it.2012.07.004.
5. Lucchinetti C, Brück W, Parisi J, Scheithauer B, Rodriguez M, Lassmann H. Heterogeneity of multiple sclerosis lesions: implications for the pathogenesis of demyelination. Annals of Neurology. 2000;47(6):707–17.
6. Bartel DP. MicroRNAs: target recognition and regulatory functions. Cell. 2009;136(2):215–33.
7. Thamilarasan M, Koczan D, Hecker M, Paap B, Zettl UK. MicroRNAs in multiple sclerosis and experimental autoimmune encephalomyelitis. Autoimmun Rev. 2012;11(3):174–9. doi:10.1016/j.autrev.2011.05.009.
8. Ksiazek-Winiarek DJ, Kacperska MJ, Glabinski A. MicroRNAs as novel regulators of neuroinflammation. Mediators Inflamm. 2013;2013:11.
9. Rom S, Dykstra H, Zuluaga-Ramirez V, Reichenbach NL, Persidsky Y. miR-98 and let-7 g* protect the blood–brain barrier under neuroinflammatory conditions. J Cereb Blood Flow Metab. 2015;35(12):1957–65.
10. Wu D, Cerutti C, Lopez-Ramirez MA, Pryce G, King-Robson J, Simpson JE, et al. Brain endothelial miR-146a negatively modulates T-cell adhesion through repressing multiple targets to inhibit NF-kappaB activation. J Cereb Blood Flow Metab. 2015;35(3):412–23. doi:10.1038/jcbfm.2014.207.
11. Faraoni I, Antonetti FR, Cardone J, Bonmassar E. miR-155 gene: a typical multifunctional microRNA. Biochim Biophys Acta. 2009;1792(6):497–505.
12. Vigorito E, Kohlhaas S, Lu D, Leyland R. miR-155: an ancient regulator of the immune system. Immunol Rev. 2013;253(1):146–57. doi:10.1111/imr.12057.
13. Lopez-Ramirez MA, Wu D, Pryce G, Simpson JE, Reijerkerk A, King-Robson J, et al. MicroRNA-155 negatively affects blood–brain barrier function during neuroinflammation. FASEB J. 2014;28(6):2551–65. doi:10.1096/fj.13-248880.
14. Weksler BB, Subileau EA, Perriere N, Charneau P, Holloway K, Leveque M, et al. Blood-brain barrier-specific properties of a human adult brain endothelial cell line. FASEB J. 2005:04-3458fje. doi:10.1096/fj.04-3458fje.
15. Male DK, Pryce G, Hughes CC. Antigen presentation in brain: MHC induction on brain endothelium and astrocytes compared. Immunology. 1987;60(3):453–9.
16. Greenwood J, Heasman SJ, Alvarez JI, Prat A, Lyck R, Engelhardt B. Review: leucocyte–endothelial cell crosstalk at the blood–brain barrier: a prerequisite for successful immune cell entry to the brain. Neuropathol Appl Neurobiol. 2011;37(1):24–39. doi:10.1111/j.1365-2990.2010.01140.x.
17. Steiner O, Coisne C, Cecchelli R, Boscacci R, Deutsch U, Engelhardt B, et al. Differential roles for endothelial ICAM-1, ICAM-2, and VCAM-1 in shear-resistant T cell arrest, polarization, and directed crawling on blood–brain barrier endothelium. J Immunol. 2010;185(8):4846–55. doi:10.4049/jimmunol.0903732.
18. Wu XY, Fan WD, Fang R, Wu GF. Regulation of microRNA-155 in endothelial inflammation by targeting nuclear factor (NF)-kappaB P65. J Cell Biochem. 2014;115(11):1928–36.
19. Selbach M, Schwanhausser B, Thierfelder N, Fang Z, Khanin R, Rajewsky N. Widespread changes in protein synthesis induced by microRNAs. Nature. 2008;455(7209):58–63. doi:10.1038/nature07228.
20. Kong W, Yang H, He L, Zhao JJ, Coppola D, Dalton WS, et al. MicroRNA-155 is regulated by the transforming growth factor beta/Smad pathway and contributes to epithelial cell plasticity by targeting RhoA. Mol Cell Biol. 2008;28(22):6773–84. doi:10.1128/MCB.00941-08.
21. Anwar KN, Fazal F, Malik AB, Rahman A. RhoA/Rho-associated kinase pathway selectively regulates thrombin-induced intercellular adhesion molecule-1 expression in endothelial cells via activation of I kappa B kinase beta and phosphorylation of RelA/p65. J Immunol. 2004;173(11):6965–72.
22. O'Connell RM, Rao DS, Baltimore D. microRNA regulation of inflammatory responses. Annu Rev Immunol. 2012;30:295–312. doi:10.1146/annurev-immunol-020711-075013.

# 2

# Correlation of CSF flow using phase-contrast MRI with ventriculomegaly and CSF opening pressure in mucopolysaccharidoses

Amauri Dalla Corte[1,2]* , Carolina F. M. de Souza[2], Maurício Anés[3], Fabio K. Maeda[4], Armelle Lokossou[5], Leonardo M. Vedolin[6], Maria Gabriela Longo[7], Monica M. Ferreira[8], Solanger G. P. Perrone[2], Olivier Balédent[5] and Roberto Giugliani[1,2]

## Abstract

**Background:** Very little is known about the incidence and prevalence of hydrocephalus in patients with mucopolysaccharidoses (MPS). The biggest challenge is to distinguish communicating hydrocephalus from ventricular dilatation secondary to brain atrophy, because both conditions share common clinical and neuroradiological features. The main purpose of this study is to assess the relationship between ventriculomegaly, brain and cerebrospinal fluid (CSF) volumes, aqueductal and cervical CSF flows, and CSF opening pressure in MPS patients, and to provide potential biomarkers for abnormal CSF circulation.

**Methods:** Forty-three MPS patients (12 MPS I, 15 MPS II, 5 MPS III, 9 MPS IV A and 2 MPS VI) performed clinical and developmental tests, and T1, T2, FLAIR and phase-contrast magnetic resonance imaging (MRI) followed by a lumbar puncture with the CSF opening pressure assessment. For the analysis of MRI variables, we measured the brain and CSF volumes, white matter (WM) lesion load, Evans' index, third ventricle width, callosal angle, dilated perivascular spaces (PVS), craniocervical junction stenosis, aqueductal and cervical CSF stroke volumes, and CSF glycosaminoglycans concentration.

**Results:** All the scores used to assess the supratentorial ventricles enlargement and the ventricular CSF volume presented a moderate correlation with the aqueductal CSF stroke volume (ACSV). The CSF opening pressure did not correlate either with the three measures of ventriculomegaly, or the ventricular CSF volume, or with the ACSV. Dilated PVS showed a significant association with the ventriculomegaly, ventricular CSF volume and elevated ACSV.

**Conclusions:** In MPS patients ventriculomegaly is associated with a severe phenotype, increased cognitive decline, WM lesion severity and enlarged PVS. The authors have shown that there are associations between CSF flow measurements and measurements related to CSF volumetrics. There was also an association of volumetric measurements with the degree of dilated PVS.

**Keywords:** Mucopolysaccharidoses, Brain MRI, Ventricular enlargement, Hydrocephalus, Cerebrospinal fluid

*Correspondence: dalacorte@gmail.com
[2] Medical Genetics Service, Hospital de Clínicas de Porto Alegre, Rua Ramiro Barcelos 2350, Porto Alegre, RS 90035-903, Brazil
Full list of author information is available at the end of the article

## Background

The mucopolysaccharidoses (MPS) are a group of rare genetic disorders of glycosaminoglycan (GAG) catabolism. Each MPS disorder is caused by a deficiency in the activity of a single, specific lysosomal enzyme required for GAG degradation. Lysosomal accumulation of GAGs results in chronic and progressive cellular damage, which can affect multiple organ systems. The neurologic expression of the disease varies among the different MPS types and sometimes also within the same type [1]. Ventricular enlargement is known to occur in patients with MPS and may be due to the combination of cortical atrophy secondary to central nervous system degeneration, a defect in cerebrospinal fluid (CSF) reabsorption due to thickening of the meninges and dysfunction of the Pacchionian granulations in the arachnoid villi, and venous hypertension secondary to reduced venous outflow through bone dysostosis of the skull base [2, 3]. The communicating hydrocephalus that occurs in MPS is usually slowly progressive and difficult to distinguish from the primary neurologic disease. Acute symptoms such as vomiting and papilledema are uncommon. The ventricular enlargement in severe forms of MPS I (Hurler syndrome) and MPS II (Hunter syndrome) may be associated with increased intracranial pressure (ICP), which can be used as indication for a shunting procedure. The degree to which hydrocephalus contributes to the neurologic deterioration in MPS is unknown [1].

Because brain atrophy and communicating hydrocephalus share common clinical and neuroradiological features in MPS patients, and in addition, they can potentially coexist, these two conditions were previously considered as one [4]. Ventriculomegaly is a cardinal feature of hydrocephalus and the severity can be defined by an Evans' index greater than 0.3 [5]. Several authors used magnetic resonance imaging (MRI) scoring systems to grade the ventricular enlargement and help differentiate between hydrocephalus and ex vacuo ventriculomegaly in MPS patients, taking into account mainly the width of the third ventricle and temporal horn dilatation [2, 6–9]. Measuring the callosal angle has been suggested as a convenient method for discriminating idiopathic normal pressure hydrocephalus (INPH) from neurodegenerative disease with large ventricles due to atrophy [10]. Excess build-up of CSF leads to an increase in ICP, which can be equated to CSF opening pressure. The relationship between size of cerebral ventricles and ICP has previously been investigated in adults and children with hydrocephalus, and conventional knowledge says that, with exception of some acute cases, brain imaging is rarely helpful in guessing value of ICP quantitatively [11–14]. We recently published an algorithm to aid in the diagnosis and management of hydrocephalus in MPS patients, considering neurologic deterioration, Evans' index, width of the third ventricle, callosal angle, CSF opening pressure and the presence of craniocervical stenosis [15].

At present, neuroimaging has only been only used to verify the extent of ventriculomegaly and exclude cases of gross cerebral atrophy and other pathological conditions that might explain the neurological deterioration in MPS patients. Phase-contrast (PC) MRI provides valuable additional information to conventional MRI and could help to distinguish hydrocephalus from brain atrophy in MPS patients by measuring the volume of CSF pulsating back and forth through the aqueduct with each cardiac cycle, the aqueductal CSF stroke volume (ACSV). According to Bradley, hyperdynamic CSF flow through the aqueduct is seen when there is ventricular enlargement without cerebral atrophy [16]. However, while some studies have supported the use of aqueductal flow rate for the diagnosis of INPH [17, 18] and related flow rate to a possible shunt response [19, 20], other studies have not been able to demonstrate any association between a clinical improvement after shunting and increased ACSV [21–23] or flow rate [24].

Currently, there is a lack of consensus as to which diagnostic test most reliably predicts which MPS patients will benefit from CSF diversion. Moreover, it has proved to be very difficult, using any objective measure, to demonstrate a neurological improvement after CSF drainage that could indicate an eventual positive response to ventriculoperitoneal shunting (VPS) [25]. There is also great difficulty in investigating these patients due to: rare disease, behavioral disturbances, high anesthetic risk, technical difficulties for lumbar puncture and low CSF drainage, for which invasive tests such as intermittent high volume spinal tap, prolonged lumbar drainage and continuous ICP monitoring are not feasible [15]. In this context, a noninvasive tool for selecting MPS patients with hydrocephalus for surgery would certainly be preferable, if the evidence for its utility was convincing.

The purpose of this study was to provide images of both structural and quantitative changes in the brain allowing access to and a better understanding of the brain disease and the consequences of hydrocephalus in patients with MPS. In that sense, we aimed to be able to identify noninvasive potential biomarkers for abnormal CSF circulation. Besides that, we analyzed the relationship between ventricular and cervical CSF flows and ventricular size, brain and CSF volumes, CSF opening pressure, CSF GAGs levels, dilated perivascular spaces (PVS), white matter (WM) lesion load, and craniocervical junction stenosis.

## Methods

### Subjects

This was a cross-sectional study. From July 2013 to June 2016, we examined all patients with MPS followed at the Medical Genetics Service of Hospital de Clínicas de Porto Alegre. Of these, 47 patients with confirmed biochemical diagnosis of MPS underwent evaluation for ventriculomegaly. We excluded three subjects who had VPS and one who was unable to undergo the MRI due to respiratory compromise and clinical instability. The remaining 43 patients formed the study group (12 patients with MPS I, 15 with MPS II, 5 with MPS III, 9 with MPS IV A, and 2 with MPS VI). Of the MPS I patients, 5 had Hurler syndrome, 2 had Hurler-Scheie syndrome and 5 had Scheie syndrome. Of the MPS II patients, 8 had the severe form and 7 had the attenuated form. Of the MPS III patients, 1 had type A, 3 had type B and 1 had type C. Twenty-five patients were male and 18 were female. Each patient presented with typical clinical manifestations of the disorder and had biochemical confirmation of a deficient enzymatic activity (α-L-iduronidase for MPS I, iduronate sulfatase for MPS II, heparan $N$-sulfatase for MPS III A, α-$N$-acetyl-glucosaminidase for MPS III B, acetyl-CoA: α-glucosaminide acetyltransferase for MPS III C, galactose 6-sulfatase for MPS IVA, and $N$-acetylgalactosamine 4-sulfatase for MPS VI). Multiple sulfatase deficiency was excluded by the observation of a normal activity of at least one other sulfatase. Twenty patients were receiving enzyme replacement therapy (7 with MPS I, 10 with MPS II, 1 with MPS IV A and 2 with MPS VI). Each patient had brain MR imaging immediately followed by lumbar puncture, and neurodevelopmental assessment performed within the same week, except one patient who died before intellectual test could be applied.

### Neurodevelopmental assessment

All patients received age-appropriate standardized neurodevelopmental assessments: Bayley Scales of Infant and Toddler Development Third Edition (Bayley-III) for children younger than 42 months, Wechsler Preschool and Primary Scale of Intelligence—Revised (WPPSI-R) for children between 42 months and 6 years, Wechsler Intelligence Scale for Children Third Edition (WISC-III) for patients between 6 and 16 years, and Wechsler Adult Intelligence Scale Third Edition (WAIS-III) for patients who were 16 years or older. All tests were performed according to their guidelines and to the developmental level of each patient by a psychologist (S.G.P.P.) who was experienced in development neurology. According to the study protocol, full-scale IQ scores were rated and patients presented as having cognitive impairment (CI) or not. CI was considered present when developmental tests (composite score) or intelligence quotient (IQ)

<70. Severely affected patients who could not respond to development tests were classified within the CI group.

### CSF sampling

Each patient underwent a lumbar puncture in a flexed lateral decubitus position whereby 7–10 cc of CSF was removed. The CSF opening pressure was measured with a standard spinal manometer calibrated in mm $H_2O$ (Hako, Germany) connected to a 20-G spinal needle. In five patients, it was not possible to obtain the opening pressure or the CSF sample due to technical difficulties (3 patients) or refusal to undergo the procedure after performing MRI (2 patients).

### Data acquisition

MRI studies were obtained on 1.5T Achieva (Philips Medical Systems, Best, The Netherlands) software version 2.6.3. For the acquisition of the cerebral images and the cervical region we used a 16-channel neurovascular coil manufactured by Invivo Devices. The research protocol for brain images included *fast spin echo* transversal plane FLAIR (TR 11000 ms; TE 140 ms; IT 2800 ms; flip 90°; NSA 3; slice thickness 5 mm; gap 1 mm; matrix 169 × 225; in plane resolution 1.3 × 1.03 mm; echo train length 55); *fast spin echo* transversal plane T2 (5054 ms; 100 ms; 90°; 2; 5 mm; 1 mm; 219 × 292; 0.75 × 0.59; 15); MPRAGE sagittal plane T1 (8.69 ms; 4 ms; 8°; 1 mm; 232 × 256; 1 × 1 mm; 232); cervical spine included *fast spin echo* T2 sagittal plane (4735 ms; 100 ms; 90°; 4; 3 mm; 0.5 mm; 247 × 198; 1 × 0.9 mm; 24); *fast spin echo* T2 axial plane (3800 ms; 120 ms; 90°; 4; 3 mm; 0.4 mm; 247 × 198; 1.11 × 0.85 mm; 44); *fast spin echo* T1 sagittal plane (958 ms; 7.8 ms; 90°; 3; 3 mm; 0.5 mm; 247 × 198; 1.25 × 0.9 mm; 4); throughout plane flow was measured with PC gradient echo for CSF at aqueduct and cervical subarachnoid space at C2–C3 spine level with velocity encoding (Venc) equal to 12 cm/s (TR 21 ms; TE 12 ms; flip 10°; NSA 2; slice thickness 5 mm; no gap; matrix 182 × 182; in plane resolution 0.55 × 0.55 mm) and 10 cm/s (21 ms; 12 ms; 10°; 2; 5 mm; 220 × 182; 0.55 × 0.5 mm), respectively. For those patients whose CSF flow was very distinct, the Venc was adjusted accordingly to reduce flow void artifacts and achieve higher image contrast.

### Imaging processing

Neuroimage post-processing was performed at a workstation by three researchers in agreement (A.D.C., M.A. and F.K.M.). They were blinded to the age, type, and clinical status of the patients.

### *Lesion load, CSF and brain volumes*

Cerebral segmentation and WM lesion load were measured with FLAIR brain images and CSF with T2-weighted images. The segmentation process and volume quantification were performed as described in detail elsewhere [26] to obtain brain volume, total CSF volume, ventricular CSF volume, subarachnoid CSF volume and lesion load. The skull size was used as denominator to correct brain and CSF volumes for variations in head size.

### Size of the supratentorial ventricles

Evans' index was calculated as the ratio of the greatest width of the frontal horns of the lateral ventricles to the maximal internal diameter of the skull [5]. The third ventricle enlargement was graded as follows: 1 = width of the third ventricle <5 mm; 2 = width of the third ventricle between 5 and 10 mm; 3 = width of the third ventricle >10 mm [9]. The callosal angle was measured on the coronal plane, which was perpendicular to the anteroposterior commissure plane on the posterior commissure of each subject [10]. The Evans' index, the width of third ventricle and the corpus callosal angle were calculated on the individual MPRAGE sagittal T1 reoriented to the parallel plane from the anteroposterior commissure plane consisting of 1.0-mm isotropic voxels. Ventriculomegaly was defined as Evans' index >0.3, width of the third ventricle >10 mm, or callosal angle <90°.

### Enlargement of the perivascular spaces

The PVS enlargement on T1-weighted images located in periventricular and subcortical WM, corpus callosum, basal ganglia, thalami and brainstem, were graded as follows: 0 = none; 1 = PVS number <10 and PVS size <3 mm; 2 = PVS number ≥10 and PVS size <3 mm; 3 = PVS number ≥10 and PVS size ≥3 mm [9].

### Craniocervical junction stenosis

For MRI evaluation of the craniocervical junction, sagittal and axial T1- and T2-weighted images were created. The T2-weighted images were also examined for increased signal intensity, suggesting myelomalacia. The presence or absence of a compression of the spinal cord was graded as follows: 0 = no spinal cord compression; 1 = spinal cord compression (absence of CSF in any direction); 2 = signs of myelomalacia [27].

### Aqueductal and cervical CSF stroke volume

Stroke volumes were defined as the average of craniocaudal and caudocranial volumes displaced through the region of interest (ROI) during the cardiac cycle (CC) [28]. They were measured for CSF in the aqueduct and cervical level and were expressed in milliliters per CC. Data were analyzed using validated image processing software [29] with an optimized CSF flow segmentation algorithm, which automatically extracts the ROI at each level, and calculates its flow curves over the 32 segments of the CC. Then, the CSF flow curve was generated within one CC (Figs. 1, 2). High CSF stroke volume was defined as aqueductal >0.05 ml/CC and C2–C3 >0.5 ml/CC [30].

### CSF GAGs analysis

Total CSF GAGs concentration was determined using a thrombin activity assay. The CSF samples were preincubated with human heparin cofactor II (HC II) and then incubated with a fixed amount of thrombin and with 0.5 mmol/l chromogenic substrate S-2238 in assay buffer. The quantification of the GAG concentrations was performed as described elsewhere [31].

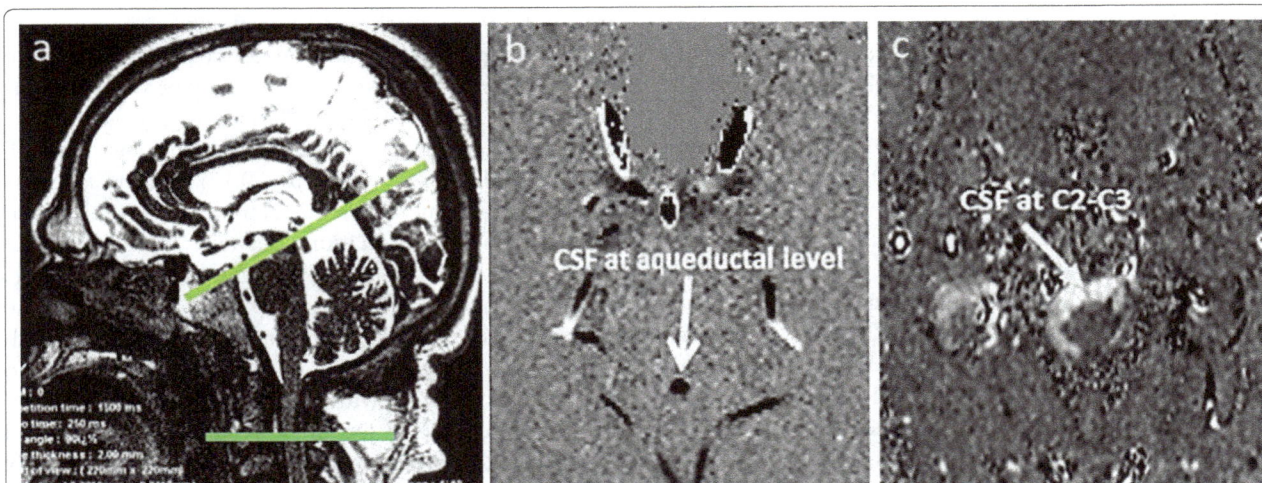

**Fig. 1** Data acquisition of a 34-year-old male patient with MPS II. Sagittal 3D scout view sequences were used as localizer to select the anatomical levels for flow quantification (**a**). The acquisition planes were selected perpendicular to the presumed direction of the flows. Sections through the cerebral aqueduct (**b**) and C2–C3 subarachnoid space level (**c**) were used for CSF flow measurement

**a** aqueductal CSF flow
mm3/s

**b** mm3/s cervical CSF flow

Number of images/cardiac cycle

Number of images/cardiac cycle

**Fig. 2** CSF oscillations were reconstructed during the cardiac cycle at aqueductal level (**a**) and cervical level (**b**). Aqueductal CSF stroke volume and cervical CSF stroke volume represent the mean volume of CSF under the curve of CSF flow during the cardiac cycle

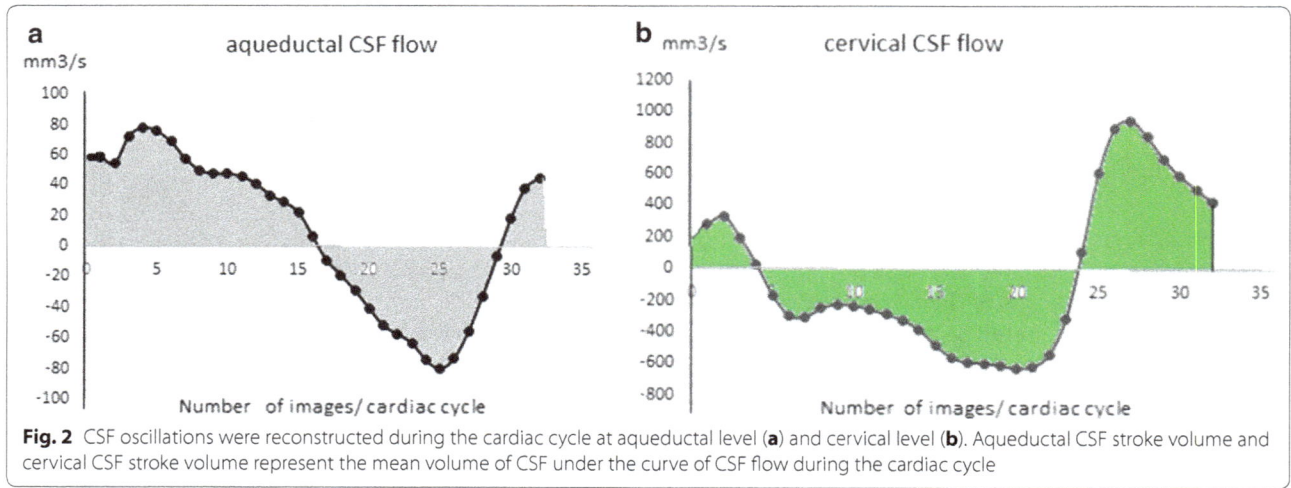

## Statistical analysis

Continuous variables were described using median and range, due to asymmetric distributions. Categorical data were presented as counts and percentages. Comparison of groups was conducted using Mann–Whitney U test or Fisher exact test, accordingly. To evaluate correlations between continuous and ordinal variables we used Spearman's rank correlation coefficient ($r_s$). Due to multiple comparisons, all p values in Table 1 were adjusted using Finner's adjustment procedure. Additionally, odds ratios were computed to estimate magnitude of association between categorical data. In situations where the odds ratio was undefined using traditional methods we approximated using Peto odds ratio.

Selected continuous measurements with no prior defined cut-off points were dichotomised using median values which are presented in Table 2. Therefore, adopted cut-off values were: CSF protein level >32 mg/dl, CSF GAGs >250 ng/ml, PVS ≥10; WM lesion load >0.4 cm³; ACSV >0.05 ml/CC; C2–C3 CSF stroke volume >0.5 ml/CC.

The significance level was set at p < 0.05. Data were analysed using IBM-SPSS version 22.0.

## Results

Forty-three MPS patients performed clinical and developmental tests, CSF and neuroimaging studies over 3 years. The mean age of the patients was 13.7 years (age range 0.9–36 years). Severe forms of the disease (Hurler syndrome and severe form of MPS II) were observed in thirteen patients (30.2%). Macrocephaly (+2SD or 98%) was present in 32.6% of the patients. Based on IQ and development testing, 41.9% of the patients had cognitive impairment.

All the scores (Evans' index, third ventricle width and callosal angle) used to assess the supratentorial ventricular enlargement in MPS patients presented a moderate correlation with the CSF aqueductal flow. Also, the ventricular CSF volume correlated with the CSF aqueductal flow, which did not occur with the total CSF volume and the subarachnoid CSF volume (Table 1). The third ventricle width showed a high inverse correlation with the brain volume ($r_s = -0.61$; p < 0.001) and Evans' index showed the highest correlation with the ventricular CSF volume ($r_s = 0.87$; p < 0.001). In addition, Evans and third ventricle width scores had large correlations ($r_s = 0.64$ and $r_s = 0.65$, p < 0.001, respectively) with the total CSF volume. The other factor tested that correlated with the total CSF volume was the dilated PVS. The craniocervical junction stenosis significantly correlated with the cervical CSF flow ($r_s = 0.46$; p < 0.002) and was inversely correlated with the subarachnoid CSF volume.

The CSF opening pressure did not correlate either with the three measures of ventriculomegaly or with the ventricular CSF volume (Table 1). Also, no correlation was found between the CSF opening pressure and the CSF aqueductal flow ($r_s = -0.23$, p = 0.177), or the score for craniocervical stenosis ($r_s = 0.19$, p = 0.258). Table 1 also shows significant correlations between the dilated PVS and the WM lesion load with the ventricular CSF volume.

Table 2 shows the relationship between the clinical, CSF and neuroimaging features of MPS patients with ventriculomegaly and CSF flow. CSF GAG levels had no significant association with ventricle enlargement or CSF flow. The presence of ten or more dilated PVS showed significant association with ventriculomegaly, especially to the third ventricle width (Peto odds ratio 8.56, 95% CI 2.23–32.88), and also with elevated CSF stroke volume at

**Table 1** Correlation between ventricular and CSF volume measurements, and CSF opening pressure, CSF flow and neuroimaging findings

| | CSF OP | | | ACSV | | | C2–C3 CSF SV | | | Dilated PVS | | | WML load | | | CCJ stenosis | | |
|---|---|---|---|---|---|---|---|---|---|---|---|---|---|---|---|---|---|---|
| | $r_s$ | p | p' | $r_s$ | p | p' | $r_s$ | p | p' | $r_s$ | p | p' | $r_s$ | p | p' | $r_s$ | p | p' |
| Evans' index | −0.08 | 0.646 | 0.702 | 0.35 | 0.023 | 0.040 | −0.05 | 0.762 | 0.813 | 0.39 | 0.011 | 0.019 | 0.51 | 0.001 | 0.004 | −0.01 | 0.933 | 0.933 |
| TVW | −0.29 | 0.073 | 0.412 | 0.46 | 0.002 | 0.014 | −0.12 | 0.469 | 0.773 | 0.54 | <0.001 | 0.003 | 0.34 | 0.030 | 0.052 | −0.08 | 0.619 | 0.730 |
| Callosal angle | 0.06 | 0.721 | 0.721 | −0.46 | 0.002 | 0.014 | −0.20 | 0.204 | 0.773 | −0.35 | 0.020 | 0.028 | −0.54 | <0.001 | 0.003 | 0.18 | 0.262 | 0.508 |
| Brain volume | 0.27 | 0.113 | 0.412 | −0.13 | 0.418 | 0.468 | 0.21 | 0.191 | 0.773 | −0.33 | 0.033 | 0.038 | −0.01 | 0.975 | 0.975 | 0.13 | 0.426 | 0.622 |
| TCSF volume | −0.18 | 0.300 | 0.460 | 0.29 | 0.071 | 0.098 | 0.09 | 0.596 | 0.773 | 0.49 | 0.001 | 0.004 | 0.26 | 0.097 | 0.133 | −0.30 | 0.054 | 0.177 |
| VCSF volume | −0.10 | 0.577 | 0.700 | 0.46 | 0.002 | 0.014 | 0.01 | 0.941 | 0.941 | 0.55 | <0.001 | 0.003 | 0.51 | 0.001 | 0.004 | −0.08 | 0.607 | 0.730 |
| SACSF volume | −0.26 | 0.124 | 0.412 | 0.06 | 0.694 | 0.694 | 0.16 | 0.325 | 0.773 | 0.29 | 0.071 | 0.071 | 0.03 | 0.871 | 0.908 | −0.37 | 0.016 | 0.107 |

Data are presented as Spearman's rank correlation coefficient ($r_s$), p value and adjusted p (p') using Finner's adjustment procedure

Italic values indicate significance of p value (p < 0.05)

CSF cerebrospinal fluid, CSF OP cerebrospinal fluid opening pressure, ACSV aqueductal cerebrospinal fluid stroke volume, C2–C3 CSF SV C2–C3 cerebrospinal fluid stroke volume, PVS perivascular spaces, WML white matter lesion, CCJ craniocervical junction, TVW third ventricle width, TCSF total cerebrospinal fluid, VCSF ventricular cerebrospinal fluid, SACSF subarachnoid cerebrospinal fluid

**Table 2** Association between ventriculomegaly and cerebrospinal fluid flow with clinical, cerebrospinal fluid and neuroimaging characteristics

| Characteristics | Ventriculomegaly | | | | | | | | | CSF stroke volume | | | | | |
| --- | --- | --- | --- | --- | --- | --- | --- | --- | --- | --- | --- | --- | --- | --- | --- |
| | Evans' index | | | Third ventricle width (mm) | | | Callosal angle (°) | | | Aqueductal (ml/CC) | | | C2–C3 (ml/CC) | | |
| | >0.3 n = 15 | ≤0.3 n = 28 | p | >10 n = 14 | ≤10 n = 29 | p | <90 n = 8 | ≥90 n = 35 | p | >0.05 n = 11 | ≤0.05 n = 31 | p | >0.5 n = 7 | ≤0.5 n = 35 | p |
| Age (years) | 9 (2–30) | 12 (1–36) | 0.483 | 10 (2–30) | 12 (1–36) | 0.577 | 9 (2–26) | 12 (1–36) | 0.502 | 6 (1–31) | 12 (1–36) | 0.229 | 12 (1–31) | 10 (1–36) | 0.774 |
| Male sex | 11 (73.3) | 14 (50.0) | 0.199 | 12 (85.7) | 13 (44.8) | 0.019 | 6 (75.0) | 19 (54.3) | 0.434 | 8 (72.7) | 16 (51.6) | 0.299 | 5 (71.4) | 19 (54.3) | 0.679 |
| Type | | | 0.709 | | | 0.373 | | | 0.333 | | | 0.183 | | | >0.99 |
| I | 4 (26.7) | 8 (28.6) | | 3 (21.4) | 9 (31.0) | | 2 (25.0) | 10 (28.6) | | 3 (27.3) | 8 (25.8) | | 2 (28.6) | 9 (25.7) | |
| II | 7 (46.7) | 8 (28.6) | | 7 (50.0) | 8 (27.6) | | 5 (62.5) | 10 (28.6) | | 6 (54.5) | 9 (29.0) | | 4 (57.1) | 11 (31.4) | |
| III | 1 (6.7) | 4 (14.3) | | 2 (14.3) | 3 (10.3) | | 1 (12.5) | 4 (11.4) | | 2 (18.2) | 3 (9.7) | | 1 (14.3) | 4 (11.4) | |
| IV | 2 (13.3) | 7 (25.0) | | 1 (7.1) | 8 (27.6) | | 0 (0.0) | 9 (25.7) | | 0 (0.0) | 9 (29.0) | | 0 (0.0) | 9 (25.7) | |
| VI | 1 (6.7) | 1 (3.6) | | 1 (7.1) | 1 (3.4) | | 0 (0.0) | 2 (5.7) | | 0 (0.0) | 2 (6.5) | | 0 (0.0) | 2 (5.7) | |
| Severe form | 9 (60.0) | 4 (14.3) | 0.004 | 8 (57.1) | 5 (17.2) | 0.013 | 6 (75.0) | 7 (20.0) | 0.006 | 6 (54.5) | 7 (22.6) | 0.066 | 2 (28.6) | 11 (31.4) | >0.99 |
| Macrocephaly | 9 (60.0) | 5 (17.9) | 0.008 | 8 (57.1) | 6 (20.7) | 0.035 | 5 (62.5) | 9 (25.7) | 0.089 | 6 (54.5) | 7 (22.6) | 0.066 | 2 (28.6) | 11 (31.4) | >0.99 |
| CI | 10 (66.7) | 8/27 (29.6) | 0.027 | 10 (71.4) | 8/28 (28.6) | 0.019 | 6 (75.0) | 12/34 (35.3) | 0.056 | 6 (54.5) | 11/30 (36.7) | 0.476 | 4 (57.1) | 13/34 (38.2) | 0.421 |
| eCSF protein | 6/12 (50.0) | 12/25 (48.0) | >0.99 | 5/12 (41.7) | 13/25 (52.0) | 0.728 | 3/7 (42.9) | 15/30 (50.0) | >0.99 | 2 (18.2) | 15/25 (60.0) | 0.031 | 2/6 (33.3) | 15/30 (50.0) | 0.662 |
| eCSF GAGs | 8/12 (66.7) | 13/25 (52.0) | 0.491 | 9/12 (75.0) | 12/25 (48.0) | 0.166 | 5/7 (71.4) | 16/30 (53.3) | 0.674 | 8 (72.7) | 13/25 (52.0) | 0.295 | 4/6 (66.7) | 17/30 (56.7) | >0.99 |
| dPVS | 14 (93.3) | 15 (53.6) | 0.015 | 14 (100.0) | 15 (51.7) | 0.001 | 7 (87.5) | 22 (62.9) | 0.240 | 11 (100.0) | 17 (54.8) | 0.007 | 7 (100.0) | 21 (60.0) | 0.075 |
| eWML load | 12/14 (85.7) | 9 (32.1) | 0.003 | 11/13 (84.6) | 10 (34.5) | 0.006 | 8 (100.0) | 13/34 (38.2) | 0.003 | 7 (63.6) | 14 (45.2) | 0.484 | 2 (28.6) | 19 (54.3) | 0.410 |
| SCC | 10 (66.7) | 20 (71.4) | 0.742 | 9 (64.3) | 21 (72.4) | 0.726 | 4 (50.0) | 26 (74.3) | 0.217 | 6 (54.5) | 23 (74.2) | 0.270 | 3 (42.9) | 26 (74.3) | 0.176 |

Data are presented as median (minimum–maximum) or counts (percentages)

Italic values indicate significance of p value (p < 0.05)

*p* statistical significance, *CSF* cerebrospinal fluid, *Severe form* Severe form Hurler syndrome (MPS I) and severe form of MPS II, *Macrocephaly* +2SD or 98%, *CI* cognitive impairment (score < 70), *eCSF protein* elevated cerebrospinal fluid protein (>32 mg/dl), *eCSF GAGs* elevated CSF glycosaminoglycans (>250 ng/ml), *dPVS* dilated perivascular spaces (number ≥ 10), *eWML load* elevated white matter lesion load (>0.4 cm³), *SCC* spinal cord compression (absence of CSF in any direction and/or myelomalacia) the level of the cerebral aqueduct (Peto odds ratio 7.27, 95% CI 1.72–30.74). The WM lesion severity was significantly higher in patients with ventriculomegaly. The presence of craniocervical stenosis showed no significant association with decreased cervical CSF stroke volume. Representative cases are described in Figs. 3 and 4.

## Discussion

One of the biggest challenges with MPS patients is to distinguish communicating hydrocephalus from ventricular dilatation secondary to brain atrophy. Although conventional MRI sequences reveal morphological findings, when there is concern that developing hydrocephalus may require surgical management dedicated neuroimaging studies, including CSF flow measurement, may be indicated [15]. Ventricular dilation may be related to ventricular wall modifications induced by an increase in the pressure gradient between ventricular CSF and extraventricular CSF [32]. PC-MRI has the ability to measure ACSV, the elevation of which is associated with hydrocephalus. This is the first time that this technique has been described in MPS patients.

Evans' index presented the highest correlation with ventricular CSF volumetrics and higher brain volume. Despite advances in brain imaging and volumetric analysis, this simple linear measurement continues to be fast, reliable and feasible for neurosurgical practice. The increased third ventricle width, which is a marker of brain atrophy in patients with multiple sclerosis [33, 34], might also be a surrogate marker of brain atrophy in MPS patients. The third ventricle divides the thalamic

hemispheres, and thalamic atrophy may give rise to ex vacuo enlargement of the third ventricle. The measurement of the callosal angle, another supportive marker for the diagnosis of hydrocephalus and predictor of a positive outcome after shunting [35], presented good correlation with the other scores and proved to be useful. For this reason, we recommend the assessment of ventricular size by these three indices, which may enhance the diagnostic accuracy of hydrocephalus in MPS patients [36].

Aqueductal CSF stroke volume was significantly correlated with ventricular measurements and CSF ventricular volume. Chiang et al. demonstrated that the magnitude of ACSV is linked to the ventricular morphology [37], which is consistent with the finding by Poncelet et al. that the lateral compressive motion of the thalami on the third ventricle during the cardiac cycle modulates the CSF flow in the aqueduct [38]. Cerebrospinal fluid oscillations through the aqueduct appear to depend directly on CSF venting from the cranial cavity, resulting from both arterial inflow and the compliance of the craniospinal cavity [29]. In patients with communicating hydrocephalus, ventricular pulsations play a major role in cerebral pressure damping during vascular brain expansion, and ventricular dilation seems to be an adaptive response to changes in subarachnoid intracranial CSF pulsations [32]. With regard to patients with MPS, we believe that the obstruction of CSF reabsorption associated with cortical venous system hypertension due to impaired venous drainage caused by deformation of the skull base involve a reduction in the compliance of the subarachnoid space and limit total arterial pulsation toward the ventricles, increasing the ACSV.

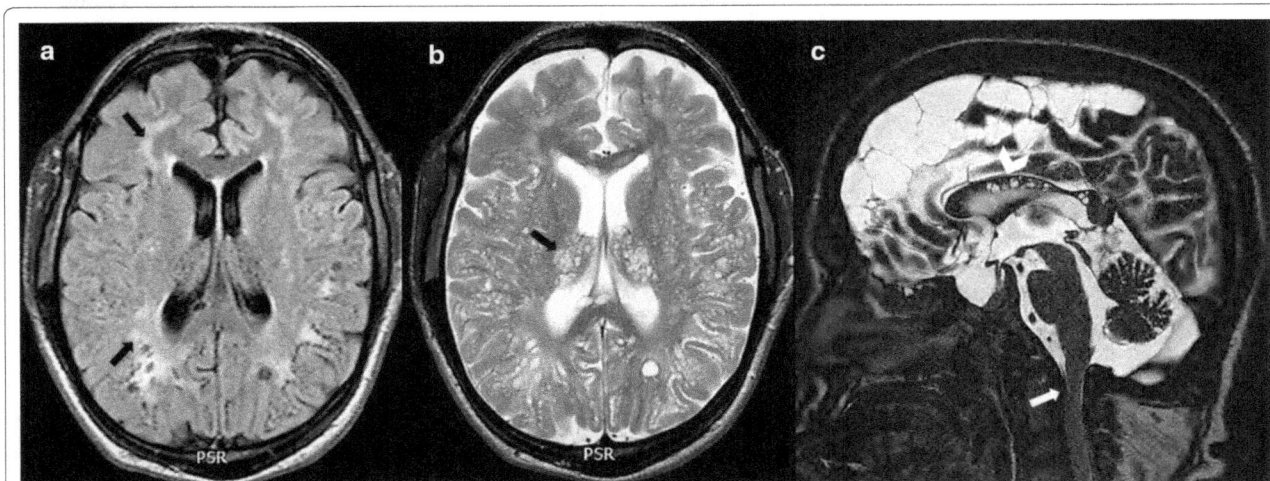

**Fig. 3** Brain MRI scans of a 20-year-old male patient affected by MPS II (attenuated form). Axial FLAIR image **a** shows periventricular and subcortical (arrows) white matter lesions (lesion load = 1.8%). Axial T2-weighted image **b** shows dilated perivascular spaces (score 3) prominently seen in the thalami and basal ganglia (arrow) and enlargement of subarachnoid spaces. Midsagittal T2-weighted image **c** shows dilated perivascular spaces within the corpus callosum (arrowhead), and effacement of CSF (arrow) and spinal stenosis at C1–C2 (score 1)

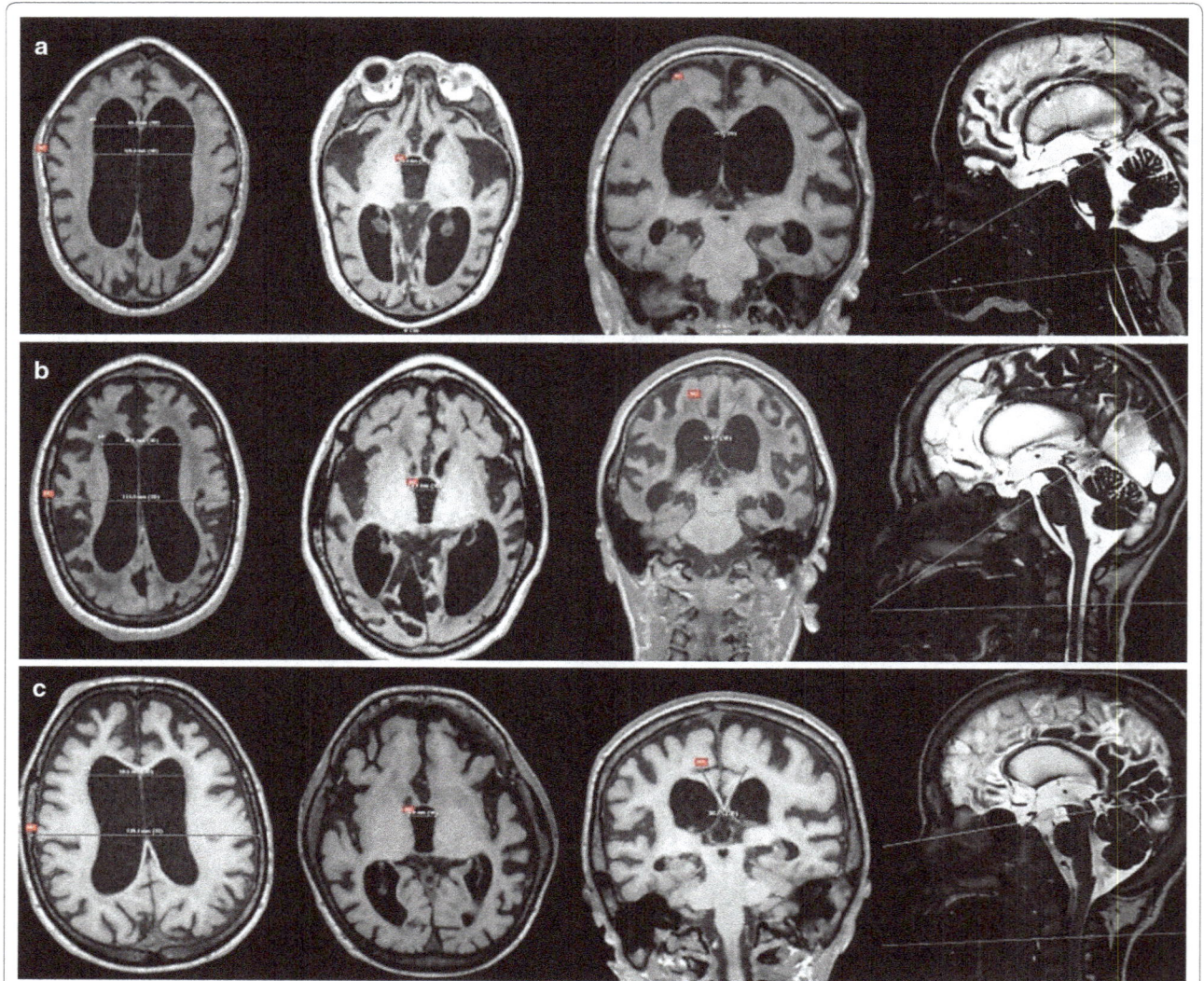

**Fig. 4** The three indices used for the assessment of ventricular size and the sagittal scout view sequences used for CSF flow quantifications at aqueductal level and C2–C3 level. **a** a 9-year-old girl with MPS I (Hurler syndrome): Evans' index (EI) = 0.51. Width of III ventricle (WTV) = 19.4 mm. Callosal angle (CA) = 77.9°. CSF opening pressure (CSF OP) = 17.5 cm $H_2O$. Aqueductal CSF stroke volume (ACSV) = 0.04 ml/CC. Cervical CSF stroke volume (CCSV) = 0 ml/CC; **b** a 10-year-old boy with MPS II (severe form): EI = 0.42. WTV = 14.9 mm. CA = 52.8°. CSF OP = 40 cm $H_2O$. ACSV = 0.03 ml/CC. CCSV = 0.13 ml/CC; **c** a 8-year-old boy with MPS III A. EI = 0.43. WTV = 16.8 mm. Callosal angle = 50.7°. CSF opening pressure = 17.5 cm $H_2O$. ACSV = 0.13 ml/CC. CCSV = 0.49 ml/CC

The relationship between ventricle enlargement and decreased brain volume, and also the increased total CSF volume, which includes the CSF of subarachnoid spaces, might lead straight to the conclusion that ventriculomegaly is mainly due to cerebral atrophy. However, using the acquired knowledge from the patients with INPH who have also been found to have larger intracranial CSF volumes [39], it is more likely that, with decreased uptake of CSF by the arachnoidal granulations due to the deposition of storage material in the meninges, MPS patients might have developed a parallel pathway for CSF reabsorption, which could be the extracellular space of the brain. In accordance with this theory, we found a correlation between an increased number of dilated PVS with high CSF flow through the aqueduct, but also with larger total CSF volumes.

Cerebrospinal fluid opening pressure did not correlate with ventriculomegaly, CSF volume or CSF flow. In accordance with our results, the relationship between ICP, also considered as CSF opening pressure, and cerebral ventricle indices was shown as unreliable in pediatric and adult patients with communicating hydrocephalus and INPH [12–14]. Also, the assessment of changes in ventricular size gave no reliable prediction of changes in ICP [13]. The possible explanations are: (1) the development of ventriculomegaly may require a longer time period as the arachnoid granulations fail to maintain their baseline removal of CSF, secondary to deposition of GAGs in subarachnoid spaces [40], which may initially result in elevation of the mean ICP, but as time elapses, assuming the PVS to serve as lymphatics of the brain, the CSF reabsorption may improve; (2) the compensatory enlargement of cerebral ventricles and subarachnoid spaces in response to loss of brain tissue (hydrocephalus ex vacuo) in severe forms of MPS, may contribute to a reduction in ICP. In daily clinical practice changes in ventricular size assessed by neuroimaging often are used as predictors of changes in ICP. In this context, short-term and long-term changes should be taken into account.

In MPS patients, the WM lesion severity is associated with ventriculomegaly. The loss of myelin, axons and oligodendoglial cells causes the environment to become more hydrophilic [41]. However minimal it might be, this is certain to increase the resistance to movement of free water through the extracellular space of the brain. Thus, there will be a tendency for CSF to back up in the ventricles, adding another mechanism to the impaired pathways of CSF egress from the ventricles to the subarachnoid space [39]. Based on our results, ventriculomegaly is associated with a severe phenotype, increased cognitive decline and brain structural changes. Moreover, ventriculomegaly can be hypertensive or not. Thus, it is possible that atrophy, visualized as dilated cortical sulci and ventriculomegaly, may represent parenchymal involvement of the disease and also may be a partial sequela of a form of communicating hydrocephalus [2].

This study provides new information for a better understanding of ventriculomegaly in MPS patients, including its relationship with the elevated aqueductal CSF flow. It also reinforces the importance of considering the amount of dilated PVS as a biomarker for the balance between production and CSF reabsorption. Moreover, our study describes a possible temporal correlation of the clinical and neuroimaging findings with some of the histopathological events in the brain of MPS patients. Lee et al. proposed the natural course of cerebral involvement in MPS based on the MRI findings, and also postulated that cribriform changes occurred first, followed by WM changes and, last, atrophy [6]. Our study provides new data about the association of these changes with reabsorption failure of CSF in MPS patients. Besides that, we believe that the accumulation of CSF within the intracranial tissue is a major determinant of the clinical signs of hydrocephalus, more so than ventriculomegaly or elevated aqueductal CSF flow.

However, a weakness of the present study is the lack of correlation between ventriculomegaly and intra- and extracranial venous mean flow to test the hypothesis that venous hypertension due to reduced venous blood outflow may also play a role in the genesis of ventricular dilatation. Therefore, further studies are necessary to correlate cerebral venous blood flow with obstruction in cerebral veins, venous drainage anomalies, skull base abnormalities and communicating hydrocephalus in MPS patients. The T2 through-plane used for CSF volumetrics has low resolution. This is a technical limitation of our study instead of using T1-MPRAGE sequence which could increase the sensitivity of volumetric measurements comparison. Moreover, because ventricular size has limited specificity with regard to pathophysiology of hydrocephalus, it is very likely that a stand-alone measurement of ACSV has poor specificity for differential diagnosis, as previously noted in INPH and in predicting the response to shunt surgery [23]. In addition, as ACSV is highly machine- and technique-dependent, it is recommended to first perform CSF flow studies on a number of healthy patients without dilated ventricles to determine what is normal on that scanner. Then, when a MPS patient with suspected hydrocephalus is evaluated, a stroke volume at least twice that value would be required before recommending shunting [16]. Taking all of these factors together, it is our opinion that a combination of positive supplemental tests coupled with neurological deterioration can increase predictive accuracy in the diagnosis of hydrocephalus in MPS patients.

## Conclusions

Brain ventricular size and ventricular CSF volume had significant association with ACSV in MPS patients. CSF opening pressure (ICP) had no association with any of the above measurements. It is possible that MPS patients are more heavily reliant on reabsorption via the extracellular space of the brain. Perivascular spaces may represent the initial phase of abnormal CSF circulation, and ventriculomegaly may represent the later stages.

Although we have a better understanding of biomarkers associated with ventriculomegaly in MPS patients, these still do not provide a certain diagnosis for hydrocephalus or improve the accuracy of patient selection for surgical treatment. Concomitant analysis of venous and CSF flows using PC-MRI is necessary to search for impaired venous outflow and reduced intracranial compliance due to jugular foramina narrowing and retrograde venous hypertension.

## Abbreviations

MPS: mucopolysaccharidoses; GAGs: glycosaminoglycans; CSF: cerebrospinal fluid; PC: phase-contrast; MRI: magnetic resonance imaging; INPH: idiopathic normal pressure hydrocephalus; ICP: intracranial pressure; ACSV: aqueductal CSF stroke volume; VPS: ventriculoperitoneal shunting; PVS: perivascular spaces; WM: white matter.

## Authors' contributions

ADC, LMV, CFMS and RG conceived the study and directed the research. ADC and CFMS collected the data. MA, FKM, AL, MGL and OB contributed to the data acquisition and analysis. ADC collected all the CSF samples. MMF performed the anesthesia for the procedures. SGPP performed all the neuropsychological testings. ADC, MA and FKM performed the calculations. ADC, CFMS and RG interpreted the results. OB participated in discussion of the data. ADC, MA and AL created the figures. ADC and RG drafted the paper. All authors read and approved the final manuscript.

## Author details

[1] Post-Graduate Program in Medical Sciences, Universidade Federal do Rio Grande do Sul, Porto Alegre, Brazil. [2] Medical Genetics Service, Hospital de Clínicas de Porto Alegre, Rua Ramiro Barcelos 2350, Porto Alegre, RS 90035-903, Brazil. [3] Medical Physics and Radioprotection Service, Hospital de Clínicas de Porto Alegre, Porto Alegre, Brazil. [4] Clinical Engineering, Santa Casa de Misericórdia de Porto Alegre, Porto Alegre, Brazil. [5] Image Processing Unit, Amiens University Hospital, Amiens, France. [6] Department of Neuroradiology, DASA Group, São Paulo, Brazil. [7] Department of Radiology, Massachusetts General Hospital, Boston, USA. [8] Anesthesiology Service, Hospital de Clínicas de Porto Alegre, Porto Alegre, Brazil.

## Acknowledgements

The authors thank the unrestricted grant received from Shire Pharmaceuticals, which enabled the MRI scans and CSF GAGs analyses.

## Competing interests

The authors declare that they have no competing interests.

## Funding

The study was supported by Shire Pharmaceuticals Grant IIR-BRA-000210. The funding body did not influence the design of the study and collection, analysis, and interpretation of data.

## References

1. Neufeld EF, Muenzer J. The mucopolysaccharidoses. In: Valle D, Beaudet AL, Vogelstein B, Kinzler KW, Antonarakis SE, Ballabio A, Gibson KM, Mitchell G, editors. The online metabolic and molecular bases of inherited disease, chapter 136. New York: McGraw-Hill; 2014. doi:10.1036/ommbid.165.
2. Matheus MG, Castillo M, Smith JK, Armao D, Towle D, Muenzer J. Brain MRI findings in patients with mucopolysaccharidosis types I and II and mild clinical presentation. Neuroradiology. 2004;46(8):666–72.
3. Vedolin LM, Schwartz IVD, Komlos M, Schuch A, Puga AC, Pinto LLC, et al. Correlation of MR imaging and MR spectroscopy findings with cognitive impairment in mucopolysaccharidosis II. AJNR Am J Neuroradiol. 2007;28(6):1029–33.
4. Manara R, Priante E, Grimaldi M, Santoro L, Astarita L, Barone R, et al. Brain and spine MRI features of Hunter disease: frequency, natural evolution and response to therapy. J Inherit Metab Dis. 2011;34(3):763–80.
5. Evans WA Jr. An encepahlographic ratio for estimating ventricular enlargement and cerebral atrophy. Arch Neurol Psychiatry. 1942;47:931–7.
6. Lee C, Dineen TE, Brack M, Kirsch JE, Runge VM. The mucopolysaccharidoses: characterization by cranial MR imaging. AJNR Am J Neuroradiol. 1993;14(6):1285–92.
7. Parsons VJ, Hughes DG, Wraith JE. Magnetic resonance imaging of the brain, neck and cervical spine in mild Hunter's syndrome (mucopolysaccharidoses type II). Clin Radiol. 1996;51(10):719–23.
8. Seto T, Kono K, Morimoto K, Inoue Y, Shintaku H, Hattori H, et al. Brain magnetic resonance imaging in 23 patients with mucopolysaccharidoses and the effect of bone marrow transplantation. Ann Neurol. 2001;50(1):79–92.
9. Lachman R, Martin KW, Castro S, Basto MA, Adams A, Teles EL. Radiologic and neuroradiologic findings in the mucopolysaccharidoses. J Pediatr Rehabil Med. 2010;3(2):109–18.
10. Ishii K, Kanda T, Harada A, Miyamoto N, Kawaguchi T, Shimada K, et al. Clinical impact of the callosal angle in the diagnosis of idiopathic normal pressure hydrocephalus. Eur Radiol. 2008;18(11):2678–83.
11. Kosteljanetz M, Ingstrup HM. Normal pressure hydrocephalus: correlation between CT and measurements of cerebrospinal fluid dynamics. Acta Neurochir (Wien). 1985;77(1–2):8–13.
12. Børgesen SE, Gjerris F. Relationships between intracranial pressure, ventricular size, and resistance to CSF outflow. J Neurosurg. 1987;67:535–9.
13. Eide PK. The relationship between intracranial pressure and size of cerebral ventricles assessed by computed tomography. Acta Neurochir (Wien). 2003;145(3):171–9.
14. Kim E, Lim YJ, Park HS, Kim SK, Jeon YT, Hwang JW, et al. The lack of relationship between intracranial pressure and cerebral ventricle indices based on brain computed tomography in patients undergoing ventriculoperitoneal shunt. Acta Neurochir. 2015;157(2):257–63.
15. Dalla Corte A, de Souza CFM, Anés M, Giugliani R. Hydrocephalus and mucopolysaccharidoses: what do we know and what do we not know? Childs Nerv Syst. 2017;33:1073–80.
16. Bradley WG Jr. CSF flow in the brain in the context of normal pressure hydrocephalus. AJNR Am J Neuroradiol. 2015;36(5):831–8.
17. Al-Zain FT, Rademacher G, Meier U, Mutze S, Lemcke J. The role of cerebrospinal fluid flow study using phase contrast MR imaging in diagnosing idiopathic normal pressure hydrocephalus. Acta Neurochir. 2008;Suppl 102:119–23.
18. Luetmer PH, Huston J, Friedman JA, Dixon GR, Petersen RC, Jack CR, et al. Measurement of cerebrospinal fluid flow at the cerebral aqueduct by use of phase-contrast magnetic resonance imaging: technique validation and utility in diagnosing idiopathic normal pressure hydrocephalus. Neurosurgery. 2002;50(3):534–43.
19. Sharma A, Gaikwad S, Gupta V, Garg A, Mishra N. Measurement of peak CSF flow velocity at cerebral aqueduct, before and after lumbar CSF drainage, by use of phase-contrast MRI: utility in the management of idiopathic normal pressure hydrocephalus. Clin Neurol Neurosurg. 2008;110:363–8.
20. El Sankari S, Fichten A, Gondry-Jouet C, Czosnyka M, Legars D, Deramond H, et al. Correlation between tap test and CSF aqueductal stroke volume in idiopathic normal pressure hydrocephalus. Acta Neurochir. 2012;Suppl 113:43–6.
21. Algin O, Hakyemez B, Parlak M. The efficiency of PC-MRI in diagnosis of normal pressure hydrocephalus and prediction of shunt response. Acad Radiol. 2010;17(2):181–7.
22. Kahlon B, Annertz M, Ståhlberg F, Rehncrona S. Is aqueductal stroke volume, measured with cine phase-contrast magnetic resonance imaging scans useful in redicting outcome of shunt surgery in suspected normal pressure hydrocephalus? Neurosurgery. 2007;60(1):124–9.
23. Bateman GA, Loiselle AM. Can MR measurement of intracranial hydrodynamics and compliance differentiate which patient with idiopathic

normal pressure hydrocephalus will improve following shunt insertion? Acta Neurochir (Wien). 2007;149(5):455–62.

24. Dixon GR, Friedman JA, Luetmer PH, Quast LM, McClelland RL, Petersen RC, et al. Use of cerebrospinal fluid flow rates measured by phase-contrast MR to predict outcome of ventriculoperitoneal shunting for idiopathic normal-pressure hydrocephalus. Mayo Clin Proc. 2002;77(6):509–14.

25. Aliabadi H, Reynolds R, Powers CJ, Grant G, Fuchs H, Kurtzberg J. Clinical outcome of cerebrospinal fluid shunting for communicating hydrocephalus in mucopolysaccharidoses I, II, and III: a retrospective analysis of 13 patients. Neurosurgery. 2010;67(6):1476–81.

26. Vedolin L, Schwartz IVD, Komlos M, Schuch A, Azevedo AC, Vieira T, et al. Brain MRI in mucopolysaccharidosis: effect of aging and correlation with biochemical findings. Neurology. 2007;69(9):917–24.

27. Lampe C, Lampe C, Schwarz M, Müller-forell W, Harmatz P, Mengel E. Craniocervical decompression in patients with mucopolysaccharidosis VI: development of a scoring system to determine indication and outcome of surgery. J Inherit Metab Dis. 2013;36(6):1005–13.

28. Enzmann DR, Pelc NJ. Cerebrospinal fluid flow measured by phase-contrast cine MR. AJNR Am J Neuroradiol. 1993;14(6):1301–10.

29. Balédent O, Henry-Feugeas MC, Idy-Peretti I. Cerebrospinal fluid dynamics and relation with blood flow: a magnetic resonance study with semiautomated cerebrospinal fluid segmentation. Invest Radiol. 2001;36(7):368–77.

30. Stoquart-ElSankari S, Balédent O, Gondry-Jouet C, Makki M, Godefroy O, Meyer M-E. Aging effects on cerebral blood and cerebrospinal fluid flows. J Cereb Blood Flow Metab. 2007;27(9):1563–72.

31. Hendriksz CJ, Muenzer J, Burton BK, Pan L, Wang N, Naimy H, et al. A cerebrospinal fluid collection study in pediatric and adult patients With Hunter syndrome. J Inborn Errors Metab Screen. 2015;3(3):1–5.

32. Balédent O, Gondry-Jouet C, Meyer ME, De Marco G, Le Gars D, Henry-Feugeas MC, et al. Relationship between cerebrospinal fluid and blood dynamics in healthy volunteers and patients with communicating hydrocephalus. Invest Radiol. 2004;39(1):45–55.

33. Benedict RHB, Bruce JM, Dwyer MG, Abdelrahman N, Hussein S, Weinstock-Guttman B, et al. Neocortical atrophy, third ventricular width, and cognitive dysfunction in multiple sclerosis. Arch Neurol. 2006;63(9):1301–6.

34. Müller M, Esser R, Kötter K, Voss J, Müller A, Stellmes P. Third ventricular enlargement in early stages of multiple sclerosis is a predictor of motor and neuropsychological deficits: a cross-sectional study. BMJ Open. 2013;3(9):e003582.

35. Virhammar J, Laurell K, Cesarini KG, Larsson E-M. Preoperative prognostic value of MRI findings in 108 patients with idiopathic normal pressure hydrocephalus. AJNR Am J Neuroradiol. 2014;58:1–8.

36. Dalla-Corte A, Souza CFM, Vairo F, Vedolin LM, Longo MG, Anés M, et al. An algorithm to assess the need for CSF shunting in mucopolysaccharidosis patients. Mol Genet Metab. 2017;120(1):S39.

37. Chiang WW, Takoudis CG, Lee SH, Weis-McNulty A, Glick R, Alperin N. Relationship between ventricular morphology and aqueductal cerebrospinal fluid flow in healthy and communicating hydrocephalus. Invest Radiol. 2009;44(4):192–9.

38. Poncelet BP, Wedeen VJ, Weisskoff RM, Cohen MS. Brain parenchyma motion: measurement with cine eco-planar MR imaging. Radiology. 1992;185(3):645–51.

39. Bradley WG, Safar FG, Hurtado C, Ord J, Alksne JF. Increased intracranial volume: a clue to the etiology of idiopathic normal-pressure hydrocephalus? AJNR Am J Neuroradiol. 2004;25(9):1479–84.

40. Fowler GW, Sukoff M, Hamilton A, Williams JP. Communicating hydrocephalus in children with genetic inborn errors of metabolism. Childs Brain. 1975;1(4):251–4.

41. Traboulsee A, Li D, Zhao G, Paty D. Conventional MRI Techniques in Multiple Sclerosis. In: Filippi M, De Stefano N, Dousset V, McGowan J, editors. MR imaging in white matter diseases of the brain and spinal cord. Berlin: Springer; 2005. p. 212.

# 3

# Improving the clinical management of traumatic brain injury through the pharmacokinetic modeling of peripheral  blood biomarkers

Aaron Dadas[1,2], Jolewis Washington[1,3], Nicola Marchi[4] and Damir Janigro[1,5*] [iD]

## Abstract

**Background:** Blood biomarkers of neurovascular damage are used clinically to diagnose the presence severity or absence of neurological diseases, but data interpretation is confounded by a limited understanding of their dependence on variables other than the disease condition itself. These include half-life in blood, molecular weight, and marker-specific biophysical properties, as well as the effects of glomerular filtration, age, gender, and ethnicity. To study these factors, and to provide a method for markers' analyses, we developed a kinetic model that allows the integrated interpretation of these properties.

**Methods:** The pharmacokinetic behaviors of S100B (monomer and homodimer), Glial Fibrillary Acidic Protein and Ubiquitin C-Terminal Hydrolase L1 were modeled using relevant chemical and physical properties; modeling results were validated by comparison with data obtained from healthy subjects or individuals affected by neurological diseases. Brain imaging data were used to model passage of biomarkers across the blood–brain barrier.

**Results:** Our results show the following: (1) changes in biomarker serum levels due to age or disease progression are accounted for by differences in kidney filtration; (2) a significant change in the brain-to-blood volumetric ratio, which is characteristic of infant and adult development, contributes to variation in blood concentration of biomarkers; (3) the effects of extracranial contribution at steady-state are predicted in our model to be less important than suspected, while the contribution of blood–brain barrier disruption is confirmed as a significant factor in controlling markers' appearance in blood, where the biomarkers are typically detected; (4) the contribution of skin to the marker S100B blood levels depends on a direct correlation with pigmentation and not ethnicity; the contribution of extracranial sources for other markers requires further investigation.

**Conclusions:** We developed a multi-compartment, pharmacokinetic model that integrates the biophysical properties of a given brain molecule and predicts its time-dependent concentration in blood, for populations of varying physical and anatomical characteristics. This model emphasizes the importance of the blood–brain barrier as a gatekeeper for markers' blood appearance and, ultimately, for rational clinical use of peripherally-detected brain protein.

**Keywords:** Physiologically-based pharmacokinetic model, Precision medicine, Traumatic brain injury, Glomerular filtration, Serum markers

*Correspondence: djanigro@flocel.com
[1] Flocel Inc., Cleveland, OH 44103, USA
Full list of author information is available at the end of the article

# Background

Peripheral biomarkers have myriad potential uses for prognostication, treatment and pharmacovigilance in many diseases, including those of neurological nature. For example, levels of the brain-derived glial fibrillary acidic protein (GFAP), S100B, tau and Ubiquitin C-Terminal Hydrolase L1 (UCHL-1) in biological fluids have been shown to correlate with presence and severity of many neurological disorders. Steady-state blood levels of these biomarkers are measurable, albeit at low concentrations, and increase rapidly after head injury. The most common use for peripheral biomarkers has been in the field of traumatic brain injury (TBI). The possibility of using serum S100B as a diagnostic tool for patients with mild head injury (MHI) was first reported in 1995 [1]. It was first thought that S100B release was a biomarker of subtle brain damage after MHI, although data suggests that an equally relevant mechanism may involve the release of S100B through a disrupted blood–brain barrier (BBB), without necessarily involving actual cellular damage [2–5]. Comparable results were obtained with GFAP and UCHL-1 [6] which suggests that these markers also appear in blood when the BBB is compromised.

The brain parenchyma is protected by a vascular barrier, referred to as BBB. The system of capillaries forming the human BBB has approximately 20 $m^2$ of exchange surface with brain tissue, and is separated from neurons by only a few microns. The BBB maintains a strict compartmentalization of brain-and-blood-specific substances through the presence of a tight-junctioned endothelial cell layer. During blood–brain barrier disruption (BBBD), proteins normally present in high concentrations in the CNS are free to diffuse into the blood following their concentration gradients [7]. An ideal and clinically significant biomarker should be: (1) present at low or undetectable levels in serum of normal subjects under steady-state conditions; (2) present in brain and cerebrospinal fluid (CSF) at higher concentrations than in blood; (3) susceptible to extravasation in the event of BBBD; (4) further released by brain cells in response to brain damage (e.g., during reactive gliosis).

Among the several reasons that made the use of brain biomarkers a holy grail for neurology is the minimally-invasive nature of the process required to obtain blood samples. While a venipuncture is typically required, such a procedure is clearly less morbid than CSF sampling or the use of intravascular contrast agents (e.g., gadolinium or iodinated contrast agents). In addition, imaging modalities such as computed tomography (CT) scans expose the patient to radiation. Last, but perhaps not least, is the cost differential between state-of-the-art medical imaging and a simple blood test.

While the advantages of peripheral biomarkers are well understood, their widespread use has been confounded by several factors including inter-individual variability in "reference values", the effect of age on markers' presence or levels, ethnic differences, etc. Many groups have described this variability, and most of the data presented so far has focused on the astrocytic protein S100B [8]. This biomarker has been studied for several years, and investigated as a tool to diagnose non-CNS conditions, mainly malignant melanoma [9]. Other markers are being investigated, and it's very likely that a number of new markers will become available in the next decade. We hypothesize that one of the obstacles in the acceptance of peripheral biomarker detection as a diagnostic approach for neurological diseases is the lack of understanding on how serum biomarker levels are holistically controlled by other physiological functions and parameters. For example, it has been suggested that S100B levels directly depend on body mass index (BMI) [10], while others have suggested that the increased BBB permeability in diabetes or conditions associated with obesity are the underlying factors contributing to this variability [11]. We developed a computer model that mimics, for a range of biomarker proteins, the key physiological features (e.g., BBB permeability, extracranial contribution) and pharmacokinetic properties (e.g., biomarker size and distribution, renal elimination) that contribute to changes in serum biomarker levels irrespective of neurological triggers.

# Methods

### Literature review for initial assignments of the model

The following sources were used to obtain the quantitative values used as initial conditions for our model. Values for total blood volume (TBV) were calculated using Nadler's formula shown in Eq. 1:

$$TBV, male = (0.3669 * height) \\ + (0.03219 * weight) + 0.6041 \quad (1)$$

$$TBV, female = (0.3561 * height) \\ + (0.03308 * weight) + 0.1833$$

where height and weight must be in units of meter and kilogram but are considered in the formula as unit-less quantities. Values for kidney function were acquired from [12]. Initial biomarker levels in brain were obtained from sources identified in Table 1. The values for maximal leakage of S100B and its homodimer were derived from our previous work [4, 11, 13]. The quantitative assignment of S100B levels in the human tissue of peripheral organs was similarly based on previous data [11].

**Table 1  Initial parameter values used within model**

| Model feature | Parameter | Value | References |
|---|---|---|---|
| Brain biomarker concentration | S100b monomer (10.7 kD) | 10.0 ng/ml = 1.0 nM | [23, 25, 36, 37] |
| | S100b dimer (21.0 kD) | 10.0 ng/ml = 0.5 nM | |
| | GFAP (26.0 kD) | 1.0 ng/ml = 0.038 nM | |
| | UCHL-1 (26.0 kD) | 7.6 ng/ml = 0.292 nM | |
| Blood–brain barrier | Steady-state, newborn | 10% of maximal BBBD | [4, 11, 13] |
| | Steady-state, adult | 1–5% of maximal BBBD | |
| Central nervous system | Brain volume, newborn | 0.42 l | [38] |
| | Brain volume, adult | 1.42 l (male) 1.05 l (female) | [15, 16] |
| | Blood volume, newborn | 0.28 l | [39] |
| | Blood volume, adult | 6.0 l | [15, 16] |
| Skin | Skin volume, adult | 7.8 l | [15] |
| | S100b in light skin | 0.288 ng/ml | [11] |
| | S100b in dark skin | 2.0 ng/ml | |
| Kidneys | Glomerular filtration rate | GFR (ml/min) = ((A*((SrCr/B)) ^ 1.209) * (0.993 ^ Age) | [12] |
| | Coefficient A (Caucasian) | 141 (male) 144 (female) | |
| | Coefficient A (African American) | 163 (male) 166 (female) | |
| | Coefficient B | 0.9 (male) 0.7 (female) | |

Glomerular filtration rate (GFR) was calculated using the Cockcroft–Gault formula shown in Eq. 2:

$$\text{GFR} = \left(\text{GFR}_{\text{Function}} * \left(A * \left((\text{SrCr}/B)^{\exp}\right) * \left(0.993^{\text{age}}\right)\right)\right) * 60 \tag{2}$$

where the variables A, B, exp and serum creatinine (SrCr) are race-and-gender-dependent, and $\text{GFR}_{\text{Function}}$ ranges from 0 to 1 and is indicative of kidney health. Due to the nature of the Cockcroft–Gault formula, changing age does little to influence the outcome of the model; as such, the value of Age was standardized to 45 years.

### Physiologically-based biomarker kinetic model development

Our model was developed using the SimBiology extension of MatLab (MathWorks, Natick MA), and results were analyzed in the Origin Pro 9.0 (Northampton, MA) and JMP 11 (SAS) programs. Our methods were derived from a generic Physiologically-Based Pharmacokinetic (PBPK) model developed by others [14], which was further based on a previous multi-compartment system in which several organs were represented with realistic dimensions [15, 16]. In the aforementioned model, the organs were connected by arterial and venous circulation with appropriate hemodynamic values, also obtained from the literature. For the model described herein, we simplified this arterial-to-venous transfer of biomarkers by assuming a homogeneous distribution of the biomarker in the systemic circulation, and that the volume of this idealized vascular compartment was equal to the total volemia. An additional consideration was made for the cerebral circulation, where permeability across the BBB was incorporated as a governing factor to free diffusion of brain-specific biomarkers. This dynamic range theoretically extends from a biomarker diffusivity (cm²/s) of zero to a diffusivity that equals the concentration-driven diffusion of a given molecule in bodily fluids. This spectrum of values is biologically unrealistic, but was established for convenience (see also Eq. 3 and paragraphs below). The extent of "opening" for the BBB was based on clinical observations (see Fig. 2b), and the kinetic property of molecule extravasation was based on empirical results (see Fig. 2a) [4, 5, 17, 18]. While there is a large difference between measurements based on contrast-enhancement versus diffusion of a molecule from brain to blood, we suggest that this "Radiologic Index" is currently the best comparative approach to model the behavior of a diffusible marker against clinically acceptable means. Please note that markers' concentrations in the blood were set to 0 ng/ml at the beginning of the simulation so that a kinetic progression toward steady-state levels could be observed.

Biological markers, as the ones modeled in this manuscript, are present in different CNS compartments. For example, S100B and GFAP are expressed at high levels in astrocytes (but not neurons or other brain cell types) but can also be detected in CSF as well as in interstitial fluid (ISF). Since the kinetics governing intracellular-to-extracellular exchange for these biomarkers is poorly understood, we used clinically available data to assign each biomarker an initial brain concentration (Fig. 1). The initial assignments used reflect what can be measured in extracellular fluid in normal brain. In spite of this simplification, our approach and modeling allow to replicate the common features of many neurological diseases (i.e., gliosis) if the increase in marker's source concentration can be estimated or measured. Gliosis is a secondary sequela of many acute injuries such as TBI, stroke, etc. During the gliotic process, GFAP and S100B are increased in astrocytes as well as in ISF and CSF.

## Model background

We used available data from patients undergoing BBBD by osmotic means [5, 17, 18] to determine the rate of S100B increase in blood. The time-dependent data corresponding to sudden increases in S100B for these patients was fitted to Eq. 3:

$$[S100B]_{serum} = 0.29 - 0.20 * 0.79^{time} \quad (3)$$

where time is expressed in minutes after the osmotic shock. For details see [5] and Fig. 2a.

Cross-validation of "goodness of BBB opening" measured by peripheral S100B and CT enhancement was performed as described [17, 18]. Maximal osmotic and bi-hemispheric BBBD was set as 100% while no effect of BBBD was computed as 0%. S100B was measured at time of imaging by contrast CT and plotted in Fig. 2b as the difference between post- and pre-disruption S100B values in serum. In the model, we expressed the time-dependent change in BBB permeability according to Eq. 3 and the subsequent change in blood S100B according to Eq. 4. We assumed in the simulation a steady-state, physiological "leak" of S100B across a healthy BBB as 1–5% of maximal possible hemispheric disruption, as per Eq. 4:

$$[S100B]_{serum} = 0.0022 * [Radiologic Index] \quad (4)$$

The relationship between molecular weight (MW) of a biomarker and its propensity to be filtered by the kidneys, referred to herein as the filtration coefficient ($C_F$), was based on Eq. 5:

$$C_F = \left( -0.04094 + (1.19614)/\left(1 + 10^{((27096-MW)*-3.1E-5)}\right)\right) \quad (5)$$

where the value of $C_F$ falls between 0 (no filtration) and 1.0 (complete filtration). Empirical data used to create this fitted equation was obtained from [19]. A graphic description of the model is provided in Additional file 1: Figure S1.

## BBB disruption in patients

All patients signed an informed consent according to institutional review protocols of The Cleveland Clinic Foundation and the Declaration of Helsinki. Eight patients with the histologically-proven, non-acquired immunodeficiency syndrome Primary Central Nervous System lymphoma (PCNSL) consented to participate in an institutional, review board-approved protocol for the management of this disease at the Cleveland Clinic Foundation. This protocol involved the concurrent administration of intravenous chemotherapy and a treatment that included BBB disruption [20] followed by the instillation of intra-arterial chemotherapy (IAC). This subset of patients also agreed to additional blood draws for serum S100B sampling. The appropriate inclusion and exclusion of patients on this protocol was documented previously [21]. Specifically, these patients were treated with intra-arterial injection of mannitol causing a temporary disruption of the BBB, followed by a selective, intra-carotid chemotherapeutic injection. The procedure consisted of the following steps: (1) patient is taken to the operating room and general thiopental anesthesia is induced; (2) catheterization of a selected intracranial artery (either an internal carotid or vertebral artery) is performed via a percutaneous, trans-femoral puncture on a given treatment day; (3) mannitol (25%; osmolarity 1372) is administered intra-arterially via the catheter at a predetermined rate of 3–12 cc/s for 30 s; (4) after the BBB is "opened" with mannitol, intra-arterial methotrexate is infused. Immediately following delivery of chemotherapy, non-ionic contrast dye is given intravenously; (5) the patient is transported, still anesthetized, for a CT scan. This step is essential to determine and document the extent of BBB opening since better disruption portends better delivery

(See figure on next page.)
**Fig. 1** Initial assignments and assumptions for the pharmacokinetic model. The illustrations provide a region-specific grouping of all initial assignments and assumptions considered in our kinetic modeling of biomarker distribution. A detailed graphic and mathematical description of the model is in Additional file 2: Figure S2. Parameters incorporated into the CNS **a** included: (1) molecular weight and concentration of biomarkers; (2) neonatal brain volume and volemia; (3) adult male/female brain volume and volemia; and (4) homeostatic (pre-BBBD) permeability levels across the BBB (see "Methods" section). Extracranial contributions to serum biomarker levels **b** do not significantly differ from a model whose only contribution comes from the brain. Extracranial sources of S100B were quantified using data from [11], and each organ was set to a fixed (1–5%) rate of marker's transfer to blood. The corresponding *bar plot* shows organ-specific contribution to serum levels. The flowchart in the inset shows a simplified diagram of the skin-to-blood contribution of S100B in the pharmacokinetic model. Arterial and venous blood volumes were combined into a common, systemic blood compartment **c** and an assumption of homogeneity was employed for serum biomarker levels. The blood compartment was provided an initial biomarker concentration of 0 ng/ml. Passage of biomarker mass into the kidneys **d** was dependent on initial assignment of glomerular filtration rate (GFR), as calculated by the Cockroft-Gault formula for both African American (A–A) and Caucasian male and female adults. Neonatal kidney filtration was preset to 47 ml/min/1.73 m$^2$ (see Table 1)

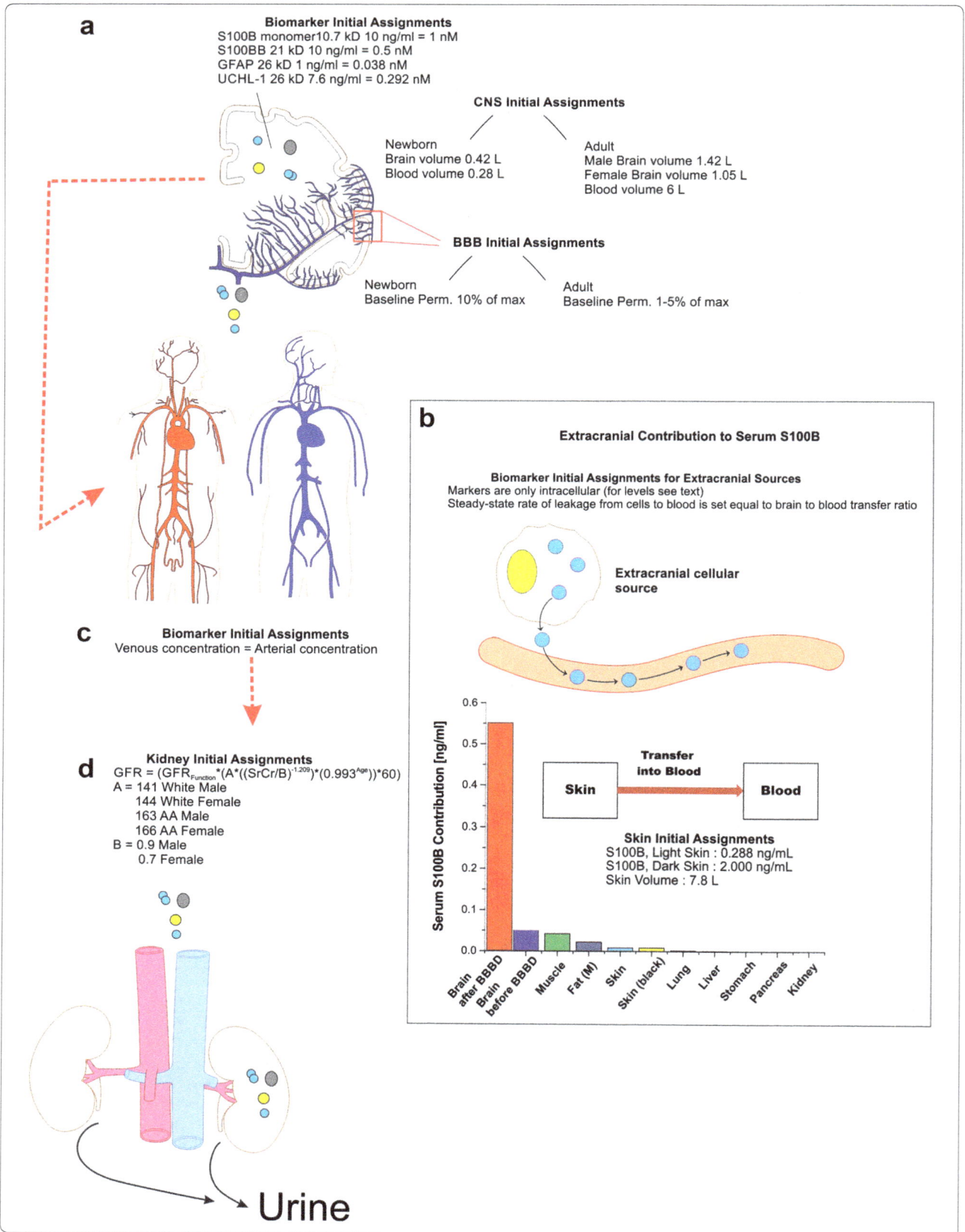

**a**

**Biomarker Initial Assignments**
S100B monomer 10.7 kD 10 ng/ml = 1 nM
S100BB 21 kD 10 ng/ml = 0.5 nM
GFAP 26 kD 1 ng/ml = 0.038 nM
UCHL-1 26 kD 7.6 ng/ml = 0.292 nM

**CNS Initial Assignments**

Newborn
Brain volume 0.42 L
Blood volume 0.28 L

Adult
Male Brain volume 1.42 L
Female Brain volume 1.05 L
Blood volume 6 L

**BBB Initial Assignments**

Newborn
Baseline Perm. 10% of max

Adult
Baseline Perm. 1-5% of max

**c**

**Biomarker Initial Assignments**
Venous concentration = Arterial concentration

**d**

**Kidney Initial Assignments**
$GFR = (GFR_{Function}*(A*((SrCr/B)^{-1.209}*(0.993^{Age})))*60)$
A = 141 White Male
     144 White Female
     163 AA Male
     166 AA Female
B = 0.9 Male
     0.7 Female

**Urine**

**b**

**Extracranial Contribution to Serum S100B**

**Biomarker Initial Assignments for Extracranial Sources**
Markers are only intracellular (for levels see text)
Steady-state rate of leakage from cells to blood is set equal to brain to blood transfer ratio

Extracranial cellular source

Transfer into Blood

**Skin** → **Blood**

**Skin Initial Assignments**
S100B, Light Skin : 0.288 ng/mL
S100B, Dark Skin : 2.000 ng/mL
Skin Volume : 7.8 L

Serum S100B Contribution [ng/ml]

Brain after BBBD, Brain before BBBD, Muscle, Fat (M), Skin, Skin (black), Lung, Liver, Stomach, Pancreas, Kidney

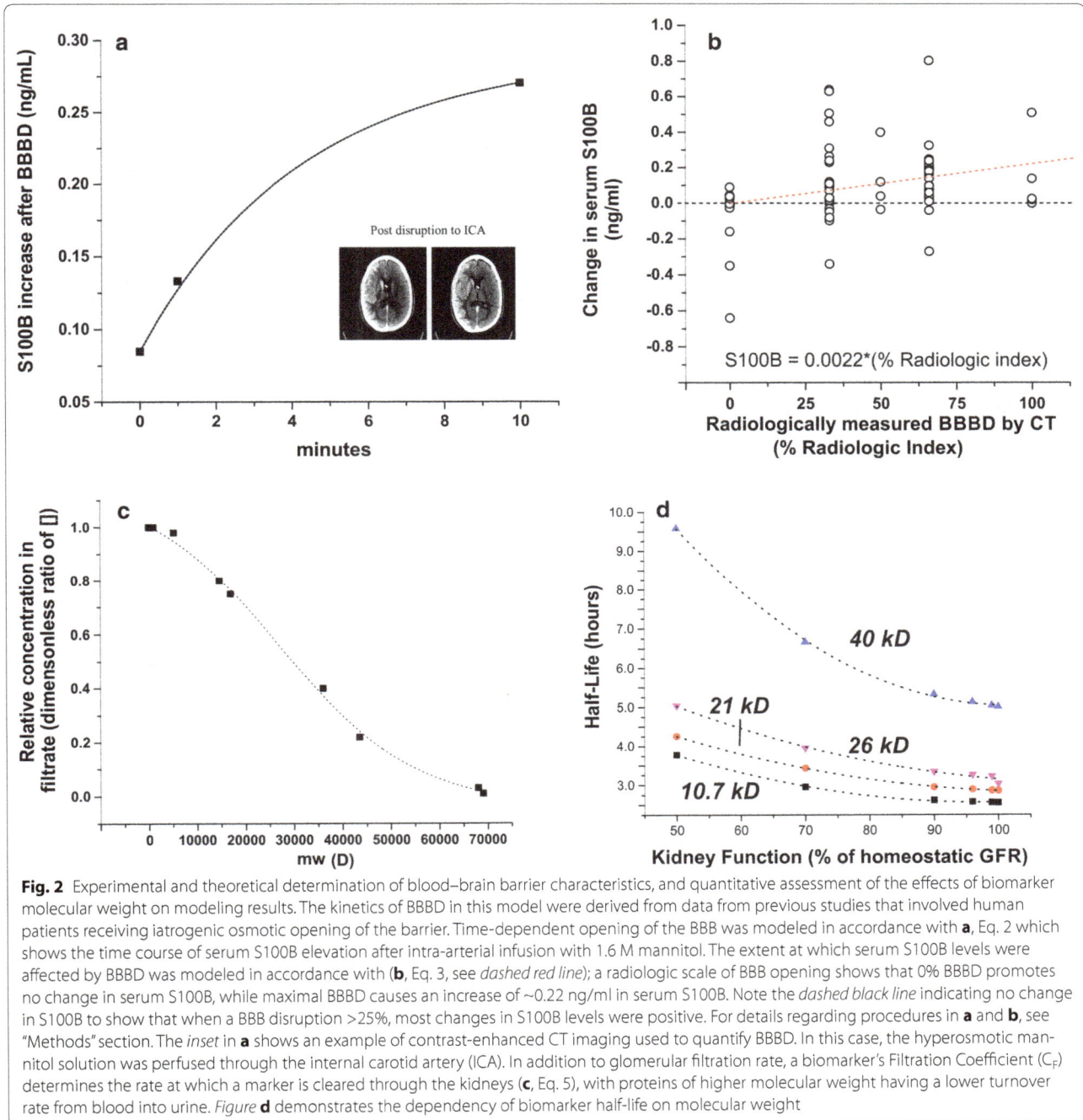

**Fig. 2** Experimental and theoretical determination of blood–brain barrier characteristics, and quantitative assessment of the effects of biomarker molecular weight on modeling results. The kinetics of BBBD in this model were derived from data from previous studies that involved human patients receiving iatrogenic osmotic opening of the barrier. Time-dependent opening of the BBB was modeled in accordance with **a**, Eq. 2 which shows the time course of serum S100B elevation after intra-arterial infusion with 1.6 M mannitol. The extent at which serum S100B levels were affected by BBBD was modeled in accordance with (**b**, Eq. 3, see *dashed red line*); a radiologic scale of BBB opening shows that 0% BBBD promotes no change in serum S100B, while maximal BBBD causes an increase of ~0.22 ng/ml in serum S100B. Note the *dashed black line* indicating no change in S100B to show that when a BBB disruption >25%, most changes in S100B levels were positive. For details regarding procedures in **a** and **b**, see "Methods" section. The *inset* in **a** shows an example of contrast-enhanced CT imaging used to quantify BBBD. In this case, the hyperosmotic mannitol solution was perfused through the internal carotid artery (ICA). In addition to glomerular filtration rate, a biomarker's Filtration Coefficient ($C_F$) determines the rate at which a marker is cleared through the kidneys (**c**, Eq. 5), with proteins of higher molecular weight having a lower turnover rate from blood into urine. *Figure* **d** demonstrates the dependency of biomarker half-life on molecular weight

of chemotherapeutic drugs across the barrier. Methods for grading the degree of BBBD and correlation of these grades with Hounsfield units were previously described [22]; degree of BBBD was graded by visual inspection as nil, fair, good, or excellent; (6) after the CT scan is completed the patient is awakened, extubated and monitored in the hospital overnight. Blood samples were drawn 10 min prior to mannitol injection and 2–5 min after mannitol injection. S100B was measured on all available blood samples by techniques described elsewhere [5, 13]. A total of 102 BBBD procedures in eight patients were studied. The results in Fig. 1 refer to 14 procedures consisting of intra-arterial chemotherapy not preceded by BBBD.

### Serum S100B measurements

Serum samples of S100B were obtained after induction of anesthesia, immediately prior to and immediately after intra-arterial mannitol infusion (Fig. 2a). At each time point, blood samples were collected and immediately centrifuged at $1200 \times g$ for 10 min, and the supernatant sera were stored at $-80$ °C. The S100B concentration was measured by the Sangtec 100 ELISA method (Diasorin, Stillwater, MN) using high and low level manufacturer-provided controls to ensure proper assay performance. A total of 267 apparently healthy subjects were prospectively enrolled in compliance with IRB regulations. Serum samples were collected in different seasons (summer and winter), from different regions of the USA (North, Central, and South), and of light and dark skin color. Dark skin color was defined according to FDA guidance ("dark skinned" is defined as Black or African–American, "light skinned" is defined as White, Hispanic, Asian, American Indian, Alaska Native, Native Hawaiian, and other Pacific Islander).

## Results

### Age-related differences in blood biomarkers dynamics

Since the model we developed encompasses several features of human physiology that are age-and-biomarker-dependent, we first analyzed the effects of age on serum values for biomarkers of varying molecular weight (MW). To our knowledge, data on UCHL-1 and GFAP levels in healthy newborns are not available, so we instead used S100B values which have been reported to decrease from an average of 0.9 to 0.3 ng/ml in the first postnatal months and further decrease to 0.11 ng/ml in adolescence [23]. For healthy adults, S100B levels in serum are below 0.1–0.12 ng/ml [3, 24, 25]. Of the physiological variables that may contribute to different biomarker concentrations between newborns and adults, we focused on three possible, non-mutually exclusive factors: (1) GFR is significantly lower in the neonatal stage of development, and does not reach fully mature levels until after infancy; (2) body size, and specifically the ratio of brain volume to volemia/body weight, is dramatically increased in babies; and (3) homeostatic BBB function may differ post-gestation compared to adulthood. The results of the modeling, and any discrepancy between experimental data and model results, are shown in Fig. 3a–c. The plot in Fig. 3a shows steady-state and BBBD-triggered changes in serum S100B for a newborn with a brain-to-blood volume ratio of 1.5 (0.42:0.28 l), compared to a ratio of 0.2 (1.4:6.0 l) for adults. This model also incorporated reference values for both neonatal and adult GFR which have been previously reported [12, 26–28]. For details regarding these parameters and other initial

assignments, see Fig. 1 and Table 1. The simulation was run as follows: we initially started with a level of 0 ng/ml for serum biomarker and observed an initial progression toward steady-state, which varies based on age-specific variables. After steady-state was established we simulated a maximal BBBD (see *vertical dashed line* in Fig. 3a), which gradually decreased to represent a time-dependent recovery of BBB integrity, and the return of leakage rates to steady-state levels. Serum biomarker levels decreased to steady-state at a rate dependent upon kidney function and therefore the MW of the biomarker. Note that newborn steady-state levels of S100B prior to BBBD were significantly elevated compared to that of a healthy adult. Similarly, the extent of the maximal BBBD-induced serum increase for S100B was exaggerated in the newborn. The *horizontal dashed lines* in Fig. 3a and c emphasize the strong correlation between experimental results and output of the model. Note the excellent agreement between predicted S100B values at pre-BBBD steady-state and the results of the model.

Since one of our goals was to expand this model to include other markers, we added a variable that takes into account protein excretion, at a given GFR, for different MWs. The results are shown in Fig. 3b and c while Eq. 5 shows the modeling relationship used to extrapolate kidney filtration for a marker's MW. In newborn (Fig. 3b), the steady-state and post-BBBD values for two brain markers with different MWs are shown alongside the kinetic curves of monomeric vs. homodimeric S100B [29]. Note that increased MW resulted in pronounced increases in clearance time, which translated into longer persistence of the signals. Similar results were obtained in adults (Fig. 3c). Please note that, although neonates and adults were modeled using physiological values for body size and kidney function, the initial concentration of brain markers in neonates was set equal to adults. These results emphasize how age-related differences in steady-state and post-BBBD serum levels of each marker may be explained by anatomic (e.g., brain volume) or physiological (e.g., steady-state BBB permeability) variations.

### Gender-related differences in blood biomarker levels

This model predicted minimal physiological changes in serum biomarker levels between an adult male and female. This is consistent with previously reported data showing no gender-specific variations in steady-state levels of S100B [30]. Although the Cockroft–Gault formula for estimating glomerular filtration rate provides a lower rate of elimination for females than males, extent of contribution by the brain is also decreased due to a smaller brain-to-blood volumetric ratio [31]. This deviation from the physiology of the adult male resulted in a

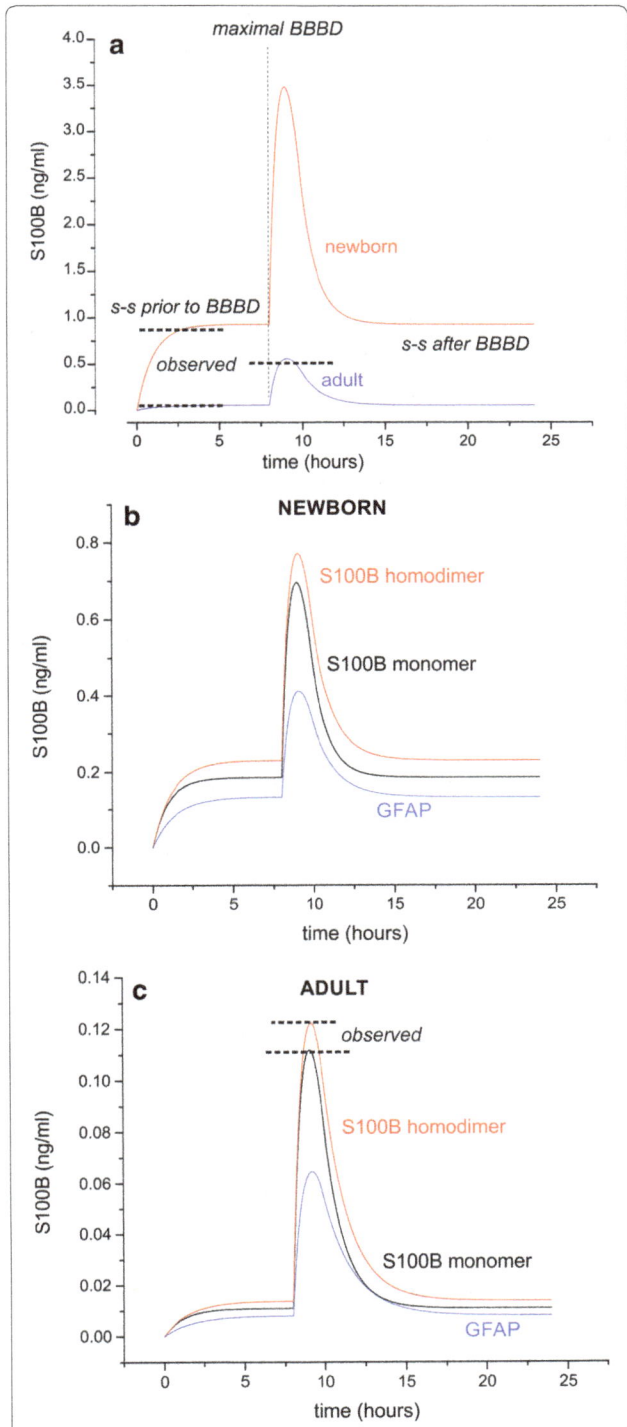

**Fig. 3** Predicted differences in biomarker kinetics between neonates and adults, based on GFR, body size, and steady-state BBB function. The plot shown in (**a**) demonstrates, for steady-state S100B levels in blood, a ~16-fold increase for newborns compared to adults (0.92 and 0.055 ng/ml, respectively). After maximal BBBD, newborns presented a more dramatic increase in serum S100B concentrations. The *horizontal dashed lines* in (**a**) show a consistency between the observed levels and results from prior literature, for steady-state as well as maximal BBBD in adults [3, 24, 40]. *Figure* **b** and **c** show the behavior for serum levels of the homodimeric form of S100B (21 kD), as well as GFAP (26 kD) and S100B monomer. The concentration profiles in a newborn **b** show a significantly increased steady-state and post-BBBD serum level for all biomarkers, compared to an adult (**c**). The differences among markers within a neonatal or adult population was entirely attributed in our model to GFR values. The *horizontal dashed lines* in **c** again show consistency between model predictions and results from previous studies [3, 24, 40]

### Ethnicity-related differences in blood biomarker levels

Recent literature has demonstrated a clinically relevant difference in serum S100B levels based on race and regional/seasonal variance, where individuals of a darker complexion have been reported to have higher steady-state S100B levels than those of lighter complexion (i.e., Caucasians during summer compared to winter in the Northern hemisphere [32], or individuals of African–American (A–A) compared to Caucasian descent [30, 33]). It was initially believed that ethnicity is the main driving force for elevated S100B in African–American subjects [30, 33]. If this were the case, based on available GFR data [12], our model would predict a *lower* biomarker level in this population due to increased clearance. Since this is obviously not the true reason for the observed elevations in steady-state levels, we added a skin compartment to the model to predict the following: (1) the contribution of dermal tissue to S100B levels for a given biomarker present in dermal tissue, at steady-state tissue-to-blood transfer rates (2% of maximal), and (2) sensitivity of this contribution value to changes in dermal biomarker tissue concentrations (Fig. 4). We also measured S100B in serum of 267 apparently healthy subjects in different seasons (summer and winter), regions of the USA (North, Central, and South), and in light or dark skinned individuals as described in "Methods" section. This was done to test the hypothesis that varied levels of sun exposure are sufficient to account for the differences originally attributed to ethnic factors. The initial assignment of skin S100B concentration in light-skinned subjects was derived from a previous study of organ-specific S100B levels, which indicated that brain tissue has a 34.7:1 concentration ratio with skin. This initial value was accompanied by a set secretion rate equaling 2% of free diffusion for a small molecule, a rate

slightly varied kinetic curve, due to reduced clearance of biomarkers from female subjects' serum. The difference predicted by the model is not clinically relevant as gender-driven differences have not been reported.

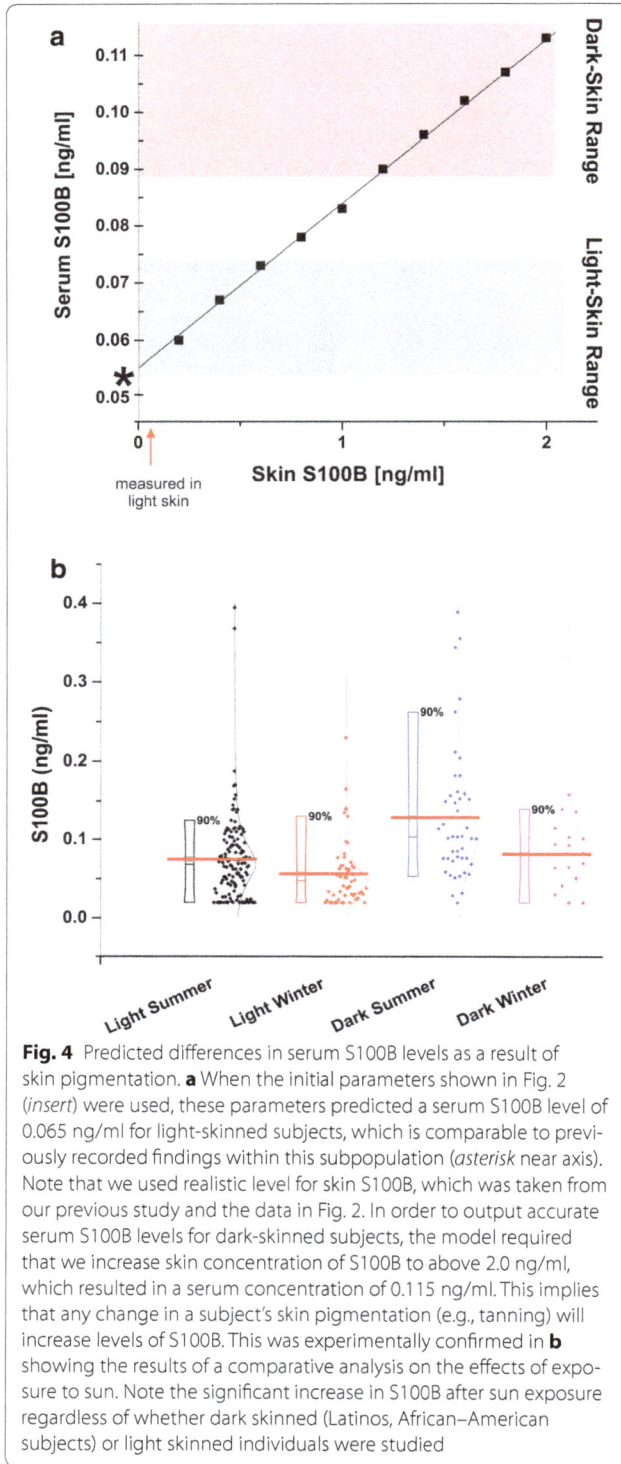

**Fig. 4** Predicted differences in serum S100B levels as a result of skin pigmentation. **a** When the initial parameters shown in Fig. 2 (*insert*) were used, these parameters predicted a serum S100B level of 0.065 ng/ml for light-skinned subjects, which is comparable to previously recorded findings within this subpopulation (*asterisk* near axis). Note that we used realistic level for skin S100B, which was taken from our previous study and the data in Fig. 2. In order to output accurate serum S100B levels for dark-skinned subjects, the model required that we increase skin concentration of S100B to above 2.0 ng/ml, which resulted in a serum concentration of 0.115 ng/ml. This implies that any change in a subject's skin pigmentation (e.g., tanning) will increase levels of S100B. This was experimentally confirmed in **b** showing the results of a comparative analysis on the effects of exposure to sun. Note the significant increase in S100B after sun exposure regardless of whether dark skinned (Latinos, African–American subjects) or light skinned individuals were studied

S100B or any other organ contributing to serum levels. We therefore measured levels of S100B by ELISA in freshly resected surgical samples from normal access tissue (Fig. 1) and these values were added to an appropriate volume of skin [14]. Only adult males were considered for this portion of the simulation. The results confirmed our hypothesis: when using the measured values of skin [S100B] and the appropriate volumetric ratios, the model accurately predicted increases in serum S100B based on sun exposure or skin pigmentation differences due to race. Note that sun exposure resulted in different levels of S100B even within a light (or dark) skinned population. Unlike in the modeling results presented in Fig. 3, changes in BBBD-induced S100B were minimally effected (*not shown*). This is to be expected, given that BBBD only effects cerebral vasculature permeability.

## Discussion

The main outcome of this study was the implementation of a MatLab-based pharmacokinetic model that allows to study or interpret the fate and excretion, levels and half-life of markers derived from the CNS but sampled in the blood compartment. A corollary set of hypotheses, which were largely confirmed by cross-validation of the model with existing data, implicated the variation of markers' levels due to: (1) physiological parameters (e.g., GFR); (2) somatic properties (volumetric size of different organs during development); and (3) environmental factors such as sun exposure.

### Strengths of the model

One of the key strengths of this model, and the results presented herein, is the extent to which these results can be validated by empirical data. These data were primarily obtained from our own work but we also used findings by others in the public domain. In addition, we used a realistic model of the human body, based on the success of PBPK analysis of drug AMDE [14]. In these models, and in the variation adopted by us, the body is represented as a network of intercommunicating compartments; each organ has an adjustable volume to accommodate anatomical variations, and the organs are interconnected by a realistic vascular tree with arteries and veins. However, the capillary compartment is not included.

The main strength and uniqueness of this approach resides in the clinical data we used to model permeability of the blood-brain barrier. Our results are based on uncommon inter-arterial procedures used to treat brain neoplasms. For details and rationale of this procedure, see [20]. Pertinent to this effort is the fact that "opening" of the BBB was clinically measured at time of

corresponding to that of the BBB under steady-state conditions.

An obvious limitation of this approach is that one needs to input an initial concentration for dermal blood testing by contrast-enhanced CT scans. Figure 2b shows the quantitative relationship between radiological measurements of BBBD and associated changes in blood S100B. Please note that because of the clinical nature of this trial and the large number of subjects enrolled, the data are not as clear-cut as one desires. Human studies were still utilized over available data from animal studies, however, due to increased translatability and clinical relevance.

Another significant feature of our modeling effort is the presence of excretive systems. This may come as a surprise given that the main focus of our research is in neurosciences. However, the modeling results demonstrate that one of the chief regulators of markers' presence in blood is the level of GFR. We were able to show that kidney function (both physiologic and pathologic; Fig. 2d) also affects markers' half-life in a size-dependent manner. In other words, with physiologic kidney function, half-life was linearly related to markers' molecular size. However, when approaching kidney failure, the effect was overwhelmingly shifted toward markers with higher (over 40 kD) molecular weight. This is important because markers of brain and BBB damage can be very small (S100B, 10 kD), of intermediate size (tau, 46 kD), or large (autoreactive IgG, 140 kD). We underscore that without adjusting for molecular weight and kidney function, one may misinterpret the true clinical meaning of a given marker. For example, if one wishes to determine the delayed sequelae of a given event (e.g., stroke, TBI) it is best to use a marker with a longer half-life (higher molecular weight).

An additional aspect that we wish to discuss is the use of accepted values for the markers' initial levels in the brain (Fig. 1a). We also modeled the relative changes in brain-to-blood volume due to changes in age and gender, as well as extracranial biomarker sources. In the case of S100B, it is widely reported that skin and fat contain substantial levels of S100B [10, 34]. In our model we used measured values for fat and skin S100B content (Fig. 1b). By doing so, we were able to show that skin levels directly affect steady-state serum S100B levels, and what is more important, they also reproduce changes in basal S100B levels due to ethnicity, exposure to sun and skin complexion. As in the other modeling efforts, we used real data to confirm or disprove the output of the model (Fig. 4). Fat tissue, when measured in a broad range of BMI, has been reported not to influence blood S100B [11]. This may be surprising since the measured levels of S100B in skin were in fact lower than levels in fat. This discrepancy can be explained by two mechanisms, namely the high cellular turnover and death rate of dermal cells [9] and the poor vascularization of adipose tissue compared to dermal tissue [35].

In every modeling effort, the source of modeling inputs is essential. Despite our efforts to use meaningful input values, some aspects of this approach require further studies to improve output accuracy. For example, MRI is the recognized quantitative tool to measure BBBD and yet we used CT. This was due to the fact that, at the time of our experiments, not only was intraoperative MRI not available, the velocity of acquisition in CT scanning made their use more amenable for fast-paced, intra-arterial procedures. Furthermore, the length of time required for MRI signal acquisition was inconsistent with the time resolution required by the model (minutes, see Fig. 2a).

Another limitation of this approach is the fact that the transfer of intracellular markers to the extracellular space is not fully understood, and certainly not known for the biomarkers discussed herein. We used as a surrogate for the movements of S100B across the plasma membrane data from melanoma cell lines expressing high levels of S100B (see Additional file 1: Figure S1 and Reference [9]). However, since none of the markers studied or modeled appear to have endocrine or exocrine functions, we believe it is safe to assume that their rate of intracellular-to-extracellular transfer is low in healthy tissue. By the same token, it is reasonable to predict that physical trauma will mobilize the marker from soft tissues such as skin and fat, and that under condition of traumatic events, the contribution of extracranial sources may well be different than at steady-state. In addition, while every effort was made to use available knowledge on brain and body development and aging, we lacked quantitative values for the brain concentration of various biomarkers in the newborn population.

## Conclusions

In conclusion, we developed a multi-compartment, pharmacokinetic model that integrates the biophysical properties of a given brain molecule and predicts its time-dependent concentration in blood, for populations of varying physical and anatomical characteristics.

**Abbreviations**
CNS: central nervous system; MHI: mild head injury; TBI: traumatic brain injury; BBB: blood–brain barrier; GFAP: brain-derived glial fibrillary acidic protein; UCHL-1: Ubiquitin C-Terminal Hydrolase L1; AMDE: absorption, distribution, metabolism, and excretion.

**Authors' contributions**
DJ and NM designed the study and analyzed results, as acknowledged in their published work. DJ, AD and JW developed the Matlab program that was used for the modeling of markers' dynamic behavior in the human body. All authors read and approved the final manuscript.

**Author details**
[1] Flocel Inc., Cleveland, OH 44103, USA. [2] The Ohio State University, Columbus, OH, USA. [3] John Carroll University, University Heights, OH, USA. [4] Laboratory of Cerebrovascular Mechanisms of Brain Disorders, Institut de Génomique Fonctionnelle, Université Montpellier, Montpellier, France. [5] Case Western Reserve University, Cleveland, OH, USA.

**Competing interests**
Dr. Damir Janigro holds a patent for the use of S100B in neurological diseases.

**Funding**
The work was supported by R01NS078307 (NM, DJ). UH4TR000491, awarded to DJ. R01NS43284, R41MH093302, R21NS077236, R42MH093302, and R21HD057256, awarded to DJ.

**References**
1.  Schiavi P, Laccarino C, Servadei F. The value of the calcium binding protein S100 in the management of patients with traumatic brain injury. Acta Biomed. 2012;83(1):5–20.
2.  Janigro D, Barnett G, Mayberg M, Inventors. Peripheral marker of blood brain barrier permeability. US Patent 20030170747 A1. 2003. http://www.google.ch/patents/US20030170747.
3.  Kanner AA, Marchi N, Fazio V, Mayberg MR, Koltz MT, Siomin V, et al. Serum S100beta: a noninvasive marker of blood-brain barrier function and brain lesions. Cancer. 2003;97(11):2806–13.
4.  Kapural M, Krizanac-Bengez L, Barnett G, Perl J, Masaryk T, Apollo D, et al. Serum S-100beta as a possible marker of blood-brain barrier disruption. Brain Res. 2002;940(1–2):102–4.
5.  Marchi N, Rasmussen PA, Kapural M, Fazio V, Cavaglia M, Janigro D. Peripheral markers of brain damage and blood-brain barrier dysfunction. Restorative Neurol Neurosci. 2003;21(3–4):109–21.
6.  Welch RD, Ayaz SI, Lewis LM, Unden J, Chen JY, Mika VH, et al. Ability of serum glial fibrillary acidic protein, ubiquitin C-terminal hydrolase-L1, and S100B to differentiate normal and abnormal head computed tomography findings in patients with suspected mild or moderate traumatic brain injury. J Neurotrauma. 2016;33(2):203–14.
7.  Reiber H. Dynamics of brain-derived proteins in cerebrospinal fluid. Clin Chim Acta. 2001;310(2):173–86.
8.  Heidari K, Vafaee A, Rastekenari AM, Taghizadeh M, Shad EG, Eley R, et al. S100B protein as a screening tool for computed tomography findings after mild traumatic brain injury: systematic review and meta-analysis. Brain Inj. 2015;11:1–12.
9.  Ghanem G, Loir B, Morandini R, Sales F, Lienard D, Eggermont A, et al. On the release and half-life of S100B protein in the peripheral blood of melanoma patients. Int J Cancer. 2001;94(4):586–90.
10. Steiner J, Schiltz K, Walter M, Wunderlich MT, Keilhoff G, Brisch R, et al. S100B serum levels are closely correlated with body mass index: an important caveat in neuropsychiatric research. Psychoneuroendocrinology. 2010;35(2):321–4.
11. Pham N, Fazio V, Cucullo L, Teng Q, Biberthaler P, Bazarian JJ, et al. Extracranial sources of S100B do not affect serum levels. PLoS ONE. 2010;5(9):e12691.
12. Stevens LA, Levey AS. Measured GFR as a confirmatory test for estimated GFR. J Am Soc Nephrol. 2009;20(11):2305–13.
13. Marchi N, Fazio V, Cucullo L, Kight K, Masaryk TJ, Barnett G, et al. Serum transthyretin as a possible marker of blood-to-CSF barrier disruption. J Neurosci. 2003;23(5):1949–55.
14. Peters SA. Evaluation of a generic physiologically based pharmacokinetic model for lineshape analysis. Clin Pharmacokinet. 2008;47(4):261–75.
15. Bernareggi A. Clinical pharmacokinetics of nimesulide. Clin Pharmacokinet. 1998;35(4):247–74.
16. Bernareggi A, Rowland M. Physiologic modeling of cyclosporin kinetics in rat and man. J Pharmacokinet Biopharm. 1991;19(1):21–50.
17. Marchi N, Angelov L, Masaryk T, Fazio V, Granata T, Hernandez N, et al. Seizure-promoting effect of blood-brain barrier disruption. Epilepsia. 2007;48(4):732–42.
18. Angelov L, Doolittle ND, Kraemer DF, Siegal T, Barnett GH, Peereboom DM, et al. Blood-brain barrier disruption and intra-arterial methotrexate-based therapy for newly diagnosed primary CNS lymphoma: a multi-institutional experience. J Clin Oncol. 2009;27(21):3503–9.
19. Boron WF, Boulpaep EL. Glomerular filtration and renal blood flow. In: Medical physiology. Philadelphia, PA: Elsevier; 2003. p. 757–73.
20. Kroll RA, Neuwelt EA. Outwitting the blood-brain barrier for therapeutic purposes: osmotic opening and other means. Neurosurgery. 1998;42(5):1083–99.
21. Neuwelt EA, Goldman DL, Dahlborg SA, Crossen J, Ramsey F, Roman Goldstein S, et al. Primary CNS lymphoma treated with osmotic blood-brain barrier disruption: prolonged survival and preservation of cognitive function. J Clin Oncol. 1991;9:1580–90.
22. Roman-Goldstein S, Clunie DA, Stevens J, Hogan R, Monard J, Ramsey F, et al. Osmotic blood-brain barrier disruption: CT and radionuclide imaging. AJNR Am J Neuroradiol. 1994;15(3):581–90.
23. Bouvier D, Duret T, Rouzaire P, Jabaudon M, Rouzaire M, Nourrisson C, et al. Preanalytical, analytical, gestational and pediatric aspects of the S100B immuno-assays. Clin Chem Lab Med. 2016;54(5):833–42.
24. Vogelbaum MA, Masaryk T, Mazzone P, Mekhail T, Fazio V, McCartney S, et al. S100beta as a predictor of brain metastases: brain versus cerebrovascular damage. Cancer. 2005;104(4):817–24.
25. Biberthaler P, Mussack T, Wiedemann E, Kanz KG, Mutschler W, Linsenmaier U, et al. Rapid identification of high-risk patients after minor head trauma (MHT) by assessment of S-100B: ascertainment of a cut-off level. Eur J Med Res. 2002;7(4):164–70.
26. Astor BC, Levey AS, Stevens LA, Van LF, Selvin E, Coresh J. Method of glomerular filtration rate estimation affects prediction of mortality risk. J Am Soc Nephrol. 2009;20(10):2214–22.
27. Hostetter TH, Levey AS, Stevens LA. Clinical impact of reporting estimated glomerular filtration rates. Clin Chem. 2010;56(9):1381–3.
28. Stevens LA, Claybon MA, Schmid CH, Chen J, Horio M, Imai E, et al. Evaluation of the chronic kidney disease epidemiology collaboration equation for estimating the glomerular filtration rate in multiple ethnicities. Kidney Int. 2011;79(5):555–62.
29. Nylen K, Ost M, Csajbok LZ, Nilsson I, Hall C, Blennow K, et al. Serum levels of S100B, S100A1B and S100BB are all related to outcome after severe traumatic brain injury. Acta Neurochir (Wien). 2008;150(3):221–7.
30. Ben AO, Vally J, Adem C, Foglietti MJ, Beaudeux JL. Reference values for serum S-100B protein depend on the race of individuals. Clin Chem. 2003;49(5):836–7.
31. Allen JS, Damasio H, Grabowski TJ. Normal neuroanatomical variation in the human brain: an MRI-volumetric study. Am J Phys Anthropol. 2002;118(4):341–58.
32. Morera-Fumero AL, Abreu-Gonzalez P, Henry-Benitez M, Yelmo-Cruz S, Diaz-Mesa E. Summer/winter changes in serum S100B protein concentration as a source of research variance. J Psychiatr Res. 2013;47(6):791–5.
33. Bazarian JJ, Pope C, McClung J, Cheng YT, Flesher W. Ethnic and racial disparities in emergency department care for mild traumatic brain injury. Acad Emerg Med. 2003;10(11):1209–17.
34. Bargerstock E, Puvenna V, Iffland P, Falcone T, Hossain M, Vetter S, et al. Is peripheral immunity regulated by blood-brain barrier permeability changes? PLoS ONE. 2014;9(7):e101477.
35. Weiss L, Haydock K, Pickren JW, Lane WW. Organ vascularity and metastatic frequency. Am J Pathol. 1980;101(1):101–14.
36. Mayer CA, Brunkhorst R, Niessner M, Pfeilschifter W, Steinmetz H, Foerch C. Blood levels of glial fibrillary acidic protein (GFAP) in patients with neurological diseases. PLoS ONE. 2013;8(4):e62101.
37. Mondello S, Kobeissy F, Vestri A, Hayes RL, Kochanek PM, Berger RP. Serum concentrations of ubiquitin C-terminal hydrolase-L1 and glial fibrillary acidic protein after pediatric traumatic brain injury. Sci Rep. 2016;6:28203.
38. Orasanu E, Melbourne A, Cardoso MJ, Modat M, Taylor AM, Thayyil S, et al. Brain volume estimation from post-mortem newborn and fetal MRI. Neuroimage Clin. 2014;6:438–44.

# 4

# Barrier dysfunction or drainage reduction: differentiating causes of CSF protein increase

Mahdi Asgari[1,2], Diane A. de Zélicourt[1] and Vartan Kurtcuoglu[1,2,3*] ⓘ

## Abstract

**Background:** Cerebrospinal fluid (CSF) protein analysis is an important element in the diagnostic chain for various central nervous system (CNS) pathologies. Among multiple existing approaches to interpreting measured protein levels, the Reiber diagram is particularly robust with respect to physiologic inter-individual variability, as it uses multiple subject-specific anchoring values. Beyond reliable identification of abnormal protein levels, the Reiber diagram has the potential to elucidate their pathophysiologic origin. In particular, both reduction of CSF drainage from the cranio-spinal space as well as blood–CNS barrier dysfunction have been suggested pas possible causes of increased concentration of blood-derived proteins. However, there is disagreement on which of the two is the true cause.

**Methods:** We designed two computational models to investigate the mechanisms governing protein distribution in the spinal CSF. With a one-dimensional model, we evaluated the distribution of albumin and immunoglobulin G (IgG), accounting for protein transport rates across blood–CNS barriers, CSF dynamics (including both dispersion induced by CSF pulsations and advection by mean CSF flow) and CSF drainage. Dispersion coefficients were determined a priori by computing the axisymmetric three-dimensional CSF dynamics and solute transport in a representative segment of the spinal canal.

**Results:** Our models reproduce the empirically determined hyperbolic relation between albumin and IgG quotients. They indicate that variation in CSF drainage would yield a linear rather than the expected hyperbolic profile. In contrast, modelled barrier dysfunction reproduces the experimentally observed relation.

**Conclusions:** High levels of albumin identified in the Reiber diagram are more likely to originate from a barrier dysfunction than from a reduction in CSF drainage. Our in silico experiments further support the hypothesis of decreasing spinal CSF drainage in rostro-caudal direction and emphasize the physiological importance of pulsation-driven dispersion for the transport of large molecules in the CSF.

## Background

Despite continued advances in non-invasive medical imaging, cerebrospinal fluid (CSF) analysis in general and CSF protein analysis in particular have remained important tools for the diagnosis of various disorders of the central nervous system (CNS) [1]. Yet while it is accepted that abnormal changes in CSF protein content are indicative of pathological conditions, the reasons leading to the measured protein concentrations are often a matter of debate [2].

While some proteins found in the CSF are synthesized within the CNS (choroid plexus, brain and spine) or the meninges, most of them originate in the blood serum under normal conditions [2–4]. They pass through blood-CNS barriers (either the blood–brain barrier, BBB, or blood-CSF barrier, BCSFB) into CNS fluids [5]. Equilibrium between the rate-limited influx of serum derived proteins through these barriers and their efflux with CSF drainage determines the protein content of the CSF [6]. Changes in the concentrations of these proteins may thus

*Correspondence: vartan.kurtcuoglu@uzh.ch
[1] The Interface Group, Institute of Physiology, University of Zurich, Winterthurerstrasse 190, 8057 Zurich, Switzerland
Full list of author information is available at the end of the article

reflect alterations in either (1) serum protein levels, (2) intrathecal protein synthesis [7], (3) barrier properties [8], or (4) CSF dynamics and drainage [2].

Since protein levels in the CSF show normal fluctuations as serum protein concentrations change, and since there are inter-individual variations, it is helpful to use relative values for diagnostic purposes. The Reiber diagram constitutes a standardized approach to assessing such values. Should, for example, the immunoglobulin G (IgG) concentration in a patient's CSF sample be analyzed, its relative value with respect to serum IgG concentration (IgG quotient) is compared to the corresponding relative concentration of albumin (albumin quotient). Since albumin is not synthesized in the mature CNS [2], a higher than expected IgG quotient for the given albumin quotient is seen as evidence for intrathecal synthesis of IgG and thus for an inflammatory process in the CNS. When there is no intrathecal immunoglobulin synthesis, Reiber noted a hyperbolic relationship between immunoglobulin and albumin quotients as shown in Fig. 1, and stated that the albumin quotient should remain below 0.01 for normal subjects [2]. He further defined upper and lower bounds for the relationship between the two quotients, both of which also follow a hyperbolic function, and noted that the relative spread of these bounds, as quantified by a population variation coefficient, remains constant over the entire range of investigated albumin levels (Fig. 1b).

Of the four possible causes for changes in CSF protein concentration listed above, the Reiber diagram corrects for variations in serum protein levels and identifies intrathecal protein synthesis (see Fig. 1a). However, it cannot distinguish between changes in CNS barrier properties and changes in CSF dynamics and drainage, both of which have been hypothesized as possible causes for abnormal albumin quotients [2, 8, 9]. In this study, we have employed a set of computational tools to test these two competing hypotheses.

To this end, we have analysed how changes in barrier function, CSF drainage rates and pulsatility translate to changes of albumin and IgG quotients in the Reiber diagram, where IgG was chosen from the family of immunoglobulins arbitrarily as a common biomarker for inflammatory neurological disorders [10]. Our models reproduce the empirical mathematical relationship between the two quotients given by Reiber, quantify the effect of CSF pulsation on protein distribution and show that barrier dysfunction rather than decreased cerebrospinal fluid drainage is the likely cause of abnormally high albumin values in the Reiber diagram. Our results further emphasize the pathophysiological importance of dispersion, CSF drainage and blood-CNS barrier

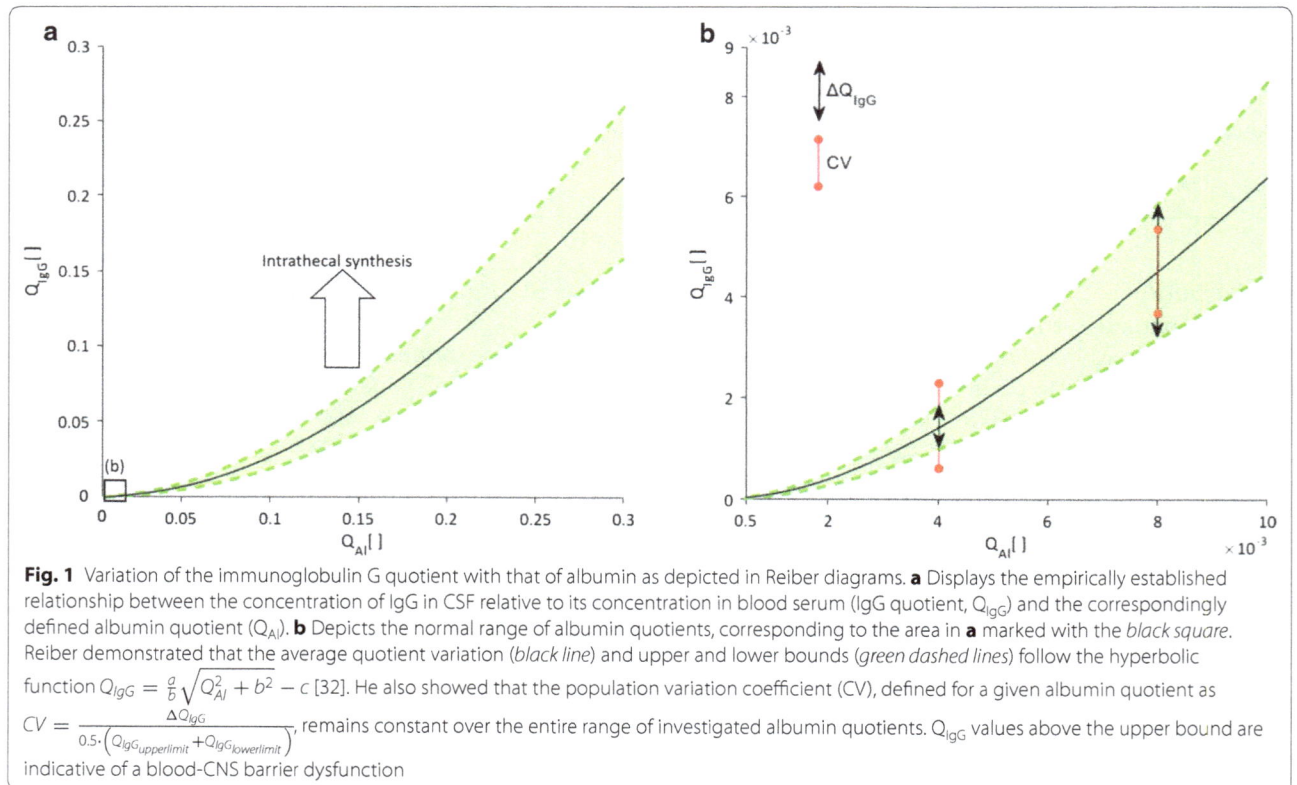

**Fig. 1** Variation of the immunoglobulin G quotient with that of albumin as depicted in Reiber diagrams. **a** Displays the empirically established relationship between the concentration of IgG in CSF relative to its concentration in blood serum (IgG quotient, $Q_{IgG}$) and the correspondingly defined albumin quotient ($Q_{Al}$). **b** Depicts the normal range of albumin quotients, corresponding to the area in **a** marked with the *black square*. Reiber demonstrated that the average quotient variation (*black line*) and upper and lower bounds (*green dashed lines*) follow the hyperbolic function $Q_{IgG} = \frac{a}{b}\sqrt{Q_{Al}^2 + b^2} - c$ [32]. He also showed that the population variation coefficient (CV), defined for a given albumin quotient as $CV = \frac{\Delta Q_{IgG}}{0.5 \cdot \left(Q_{IgG_{upperlimit}} + Q_{IgG_{lowerlimit}}\right)}$, remains constant over the entire range of investigated albumin quotients. $Q_{IgG}$ values above the upper bound are indicative of a blood-CNS barrier dysfunction

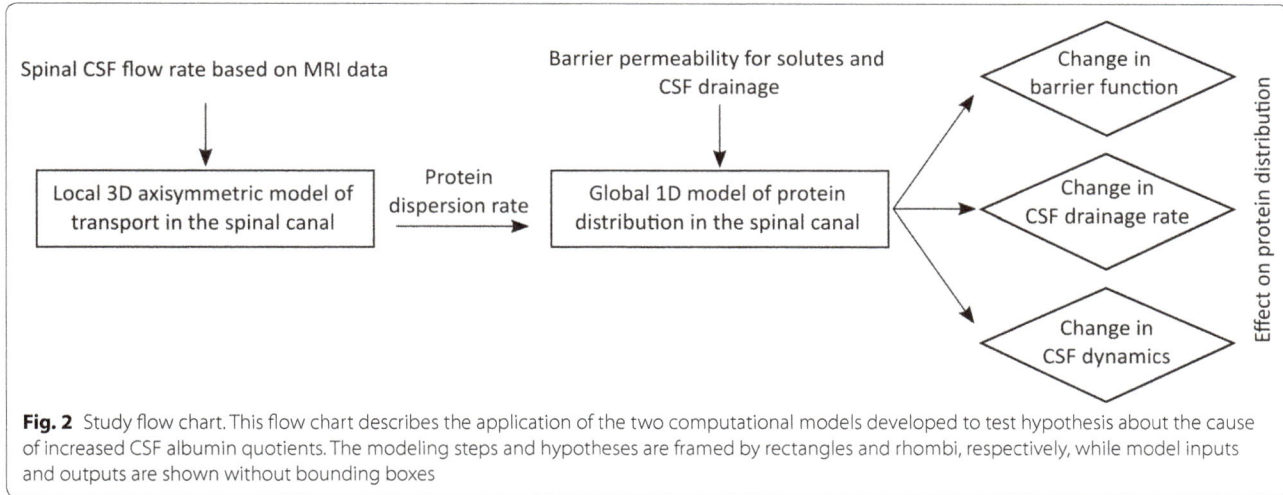

**Fig. 2** Study flow chart. This flow chart describes the application of the two computational models developed to test hypothesis about the cause of increased CSF albumin quotients. The modeling steps and hypotheses are framed by rectangles and rhombi, respectively, while model inputs and outputs are shown without bounding boxes

permeability for the transport of large molecules in the spinal subarachnoid space.

## Methods

We designed two computational models (Fig. 2) to investigate the mechanisms governing protein distribution in the spinal CSF and underlying reasons for pathological changes in protein levels. With a one-dimensional model (presented second), we evaluate the distribution of albumin and IgG in the spinal CSF, accounting for the protein transport rate across blood-CNS barriers, CSF dynamics (including both dispersion induced by CSF pulsations and advection by mean CSF flow) and CSF drainage from the cranio-spinal space. We also study the impact of pathological changes in barrier permeability, CSF dynamics and drainage on these distributions. The dispersion coefficients used in this one-dimensional model to account for CSF pulsations are determined a priori by computing the axisymmetric three-dimensional CSF dynamics and solute transport in a representative segment of the spinal canal.

### Three-dimensional model of protein dispersion induced by CSF pulsation

Dispersion as the combined effect of diffusion and advection by pulsatile fluid motion with zero net flow is the governing mechanism for the faster transport of solutes in the CSF compared to pure diffusion [11–14]. To determine dispersion coefficients of albumin and IgG along the spine, we first solve the axisymmetric three-dimensional Navier–Stokes equations and associated advection–diffusion equation for protein transport in a segment of the spinal canal.

### Model characteristics

The geometry of the spinal canal is idealized as an axisymmetric annular pipe (Fig. 3c) with dimensions

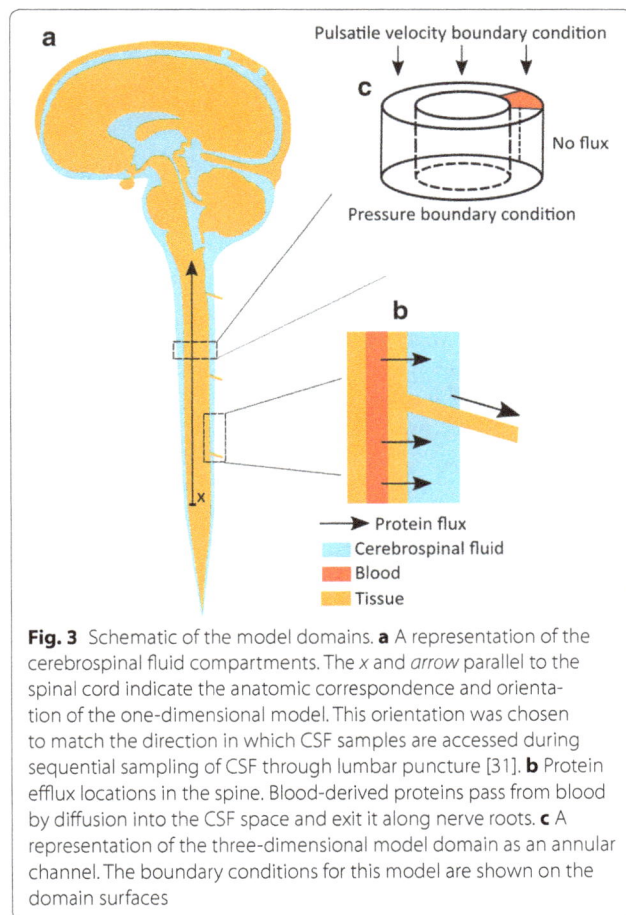

**Fig. 3** Schematic of the model domains. **a** A representation of the cerebrospinal fluid compartments. The x and *arrow* parallel to the spinal cord indicate the anatomic correspondence and orientation of the one-dimensional model. This orientation was chosen to match the direction in which CSF samples are accessed during sequential sampling of CSF through lumbar puncture [31]. **b** Protein efflux locations in the spine. Blood-derived proteins pass from blood by diffusion into the CSF space and exit it along nerve roots. **c** A representation of the three-dimensional model domain as an annular channel. The boundary conditions for this model are shown on the domain surfaces

based on statistical geometrical values reported in the literature [15, 16]. The thickness of the spinal subarachnoid space varies from cervical region to lumbar space within the range of 3.5–4.5 mm [17]. We have used the mean

**Table 1  Model parameters**

| Parameter | Value | References |
|---|---|---|
| **Barrier permeability for albumin $P_b$ [µg/min]** | | |
| In the cortical subarachnoid space | 29.4 | [27] |
| In the ventricular space | 7.6 | [27] |
| In the spinal space | 4.8 | [27] |
| **CSF compartments volume [ml]** | | |
| Ventricular space | 30 | |
| Cortical subarachnoid space | 90 | |
| Spinal subarachnoid space | 30 | |
| **Protein and pore size used in the membrane pore model for barrier permeability [nm]** | | |
| Pore radius, r | 19.4 | [6] |
| Albumin hydrodynamic radius, $a_{Al}$ | 3.58 | [6] |
| Immunoglobulin G hydrodynamic radius, $a_{IgG}$ | 5.34 | [6] |
| **CSF production and drainage rate** | | |
| CSF total production and drainage rate, F [ml/day] | 500 | [30] |
| CSF pulsation | | |
| CSF pulsation amplitude in the cervical region [mm/s] | 10 | [25] |
| CSF pulsation amplitude in the lumbar region [mm/s] | 0 | [24] |
| CSF pulsation time period [s] | 0.8 | [25] |
| **CSF physical properties** | | |
| Density, $\rho$ [kg/m$^3$] | 1000 | |
| Viscosity, $\mu$ [Pa s] | 0.001 | |
| **Spinal canal porosity and permeability** | | |
| Porosity, $\varepsilon$ | 0.99 | [21] |
| Permeability in the longitudinal direction, $K_{longitudinal}$ [m$^2$] | $1.45 \cdot 10^{-7}$ | [21] |
| Permeability in the radial direction, $K_{radial}$ [m$^2$] | $2.36 \cdot 10^{-8}$ | [21] |
| **CSF albumin concentrations** | | |
| Albumin concentration in the lumbar CSF [mg/ml] | 0.363 | [27] |
| Albumin CSF/blood quotient in the lumbar space | 0.002 | [31] |
| Albumin quotient ratio (lumbar to cisternal) | 2 | [27] |
| Albumin quotient ratio (cortical subarachnoid space to cisternal) | 3 | [27] |
| **Dimensions [mm]** | | |
| Spinal cord diameter | 10 | [16, 17] |
| Spinal subarachnoid space thickness, w | 4 | [16, 17] |
| Spinal segment length | 100 | |
| Spine length between cistern and lumbar space | 700 | |
| Protein properties [m$^2$/s] | | |
| Albumin diffusion coefficient, $D_{Al}$ | $6 \cdot 10^{-11}$ | |
| Immunoglobulin G diffusion coefficient, $D_{IgG}$ | $2.4 \cdot 10^{-11}$ | |

measured value for this thickness in the model, 4 mm [17]. The segment length is chosen to be long enough to avoid the influence of boundary conditions on protein transport rates. All geometrical parameters used are reported in Table 1.

The model domain is treated as porous, with permeability and porosity metrics according to literature values for the subarachnoid space [18]. A velocity (flow) boundary condition derived from MRI measurements of spinal CSF [19] is imposed at the inlet boundary (proximal site), while a constant pressure boundary condition is imposed at the outlet (distal site). Both the inner and outer boundaries of the spinal canal are treated as impermeable walls with zero slip and zero solute flux conditions. Constant solute concentration is imposed at the axial boundaries.

## Solution methodology

The time-dependent equations governing fluid motion and solute transport, namely modified Navier–Stokes with Darcy's law for the porous medium, continuity and advection–diffusion equations, are solved numerically using the open source finite volume code OpenFOAM [20]:

$$\frac{\partial u}{\partial t} + (u \cdot \nabla)u - \frac{\mu}{\rho}\nabla^2 u = -\frac{1}{\rho}\nabla P - \frac{\mu \varepsilon}{K\rho}u, \qquad (1)$$

$$\nabla \cdot u = 0, \qquad (2)$$

$$\frac{\partial C}{\partial t} = (u \cdot \nabla)C + D\nabla^2 C, \qquad (3)$$

where the unknowns u, P and C are, respectively, the fluid velocity, pressure, and protein concentration. The parameters $\mu$ and $\rho$ are the dynamic viscosity and density of the cerebrospinal fluid, respectively, $\varepsilon$ and K the porosity and permeability of the spinal canal, and D the diffusion coefficient of the respective protein. The permeability of the spinal subarachnoid space is derived using the solution presented by Gupta et al. [21]. The parameter values are reported in Table 1.

Equations (1) to (3) are discretized using an implicit Euler scheme for the temporal derivatives and central differencing for the first and second order spatial derivatives. All calculations are conducted with a time step size of $10^{-4}$ s and spatial resolution of 100 µm in both axial and radial directions. Grid and time-step independence were confirmed.

### Evaluation of the dispersion coefficient

The dispersion coefficient may be derived from the above three-dimensional model by fitting the simulated axial concentration with the analytical solution of the dispersion equation in a semi-infinite domain [11]:

$$\frac{C(x, t)}{C_0(x)} = \text{erfc}\left(\frac{x}{2\sqrt{D_L^* t}}\right), \qquad (4)$$

where x is the spatial coordinate in axial direction, t is time, $C_0$ is the initial concentration, and $D_L^*$ is the dispersion coefficient in a segment of length L. For a finite domain, this approximation is valid as long as the penetration Fourier number for the domain length remains small [22]. The value of $D_L^*$ is determined by fitting Eq. (4) to the results of the axisymmetric simulations at t = 8 s (10 cycles of pulsations). For further details on the dispersion coefficient evaluation, we refer the reader to [11].

## One dimensional model of protein distribution in the spinal CSF

Our one-dimensional domain represents protein transport in the spinal CSF between the lumbar and cervical regions. The model domain is illustrated in Fig. 3a. We solve the one-dimensional advection–diffusion equation modified to include sink and source terms representing protein drainage and influx, respectively, as schematically shown in Fig. 3b:

$$\frac{\partial C}{\partial t} = \frac{\partial^2 D^* C}{\partial x^2} + \frac{\partial u C}{\partial x} + S_i - S_o, \qquad (5)$$

where C(x,t) is the CSF protein concentration at time t and in axial location x, and u is the CSF bulk flow velocity. $D^*$ is the protein dispersion coefficient induced by CSF pulsation obtained from our three-dimensional model. The source term, $S_i$, represents the influx of serum proteins into the CSF, while the sink term, $S_o$, represents protein efflux due to CSF drainage [23]. The dimensions of the domain are reported in Table 1.

### Evaluation of the dispersion coefficient D*

The dispersion coefficient depends on both the solute considered and the amplitude of the CSF pulsations. The latter has been shown to increase from zero in the lumbar space [24] to a maximum of about 10 mm/s in the cervical region [25]. Accordingly, we applied our three-dimensional model to characterize the dispersion coefficients of albumin and IgG for CSF pulsation amplitudes ranging between 0 and 10 mm/s. The corresponding dispersion values are reported in results section. Expectedly, dispersion equals to diffusion for the pulsation amplitude of zero (i.e. in the lumbar space) and increases for the higher pulsation amplitudes, reaching a maximum for 10 mm/s velocity (i.e. in the cervical space). Since there is an almost linear relation between the imposed velocity and calculated dispersion coefficient, we consider a linear increase of the dispersion coefficient from $D_{\min}^*$ equal to the pure diffusion coefficient in the lumbar space to a value of $D_{\max}^*$ in the cervical region.

### Evaluation of the source term

In absence of active transporters in the blood vessel wall for albumin and immunoglobulins, the only transport mechanism for these larger proteins through the barrier is slow paracellular diffusion [26]. Therefore, the source term for the CSF concentration could be written as:

$$S_i = P_b \cdot (C_{blood} - C), \qquad (6)$$

where $P_b$ stands for the diffusive permeability of the blood-CNS barriers for the protein under consideration and $C_{blood}$ is the serum protein concentration. The permeability of the barrier to albumin molecules in different regions of the CSF compartments has been measured with radioactive studies [27]. However, it is not known how this permeability might change due to barrier opening. In order to model such permeability variations in pathological situations, we use the membrane pore model described in [6], which was demonstrated to accurately capture barrier permeability for different proteins. In this model, permeability depends on the ratio of protein size to pore size:

$$P_b \propto (1 - (a/r))^2 \cdot \left[1 - 2.1 \cdot (a/r) + 2.09 \cdot (a/r)^3 \right.$$
$$\left. -0.95 \cdot (a/r)^5 \right], \tag{7}$$

where $a$ and r are protein hydrodynamic radius and pore radius, respectively. These values are reported in Table 1. Barrier permeability to IgG molecules can be described in the same way.

### Evaluation of the sink term

Since protein efflux occurs by CSF drainage [23], the protein efflux pathways are the same as for CSF [28]. These include the arachnoid granulations mainly expressed in the cranial space but to a minor extent also in the spinal subarachnoid space, and outflow paths along nerves in both cranial and spinal spaces [29]. Thus, the drainage sink term can be written as

$$S_o = F \cdot C, \tag{8}$$

where $F$ is the CSF drainage rate. The total CSF turn-over rate has been estimated to 500 ml/day in humans [30]. However, the distribution of the corresponding drainage between cranial and spinal compartments is not fully known [30], let alone its distribution along the spinal axis. To address this issue, we leverage available data on the spatial distribution of albumin concentrations at steady state, namely the known relative concentrations of albumin in the cisterns, lumbar and cortical subarachnoid spaces, and reported albumin concentration gradients along the spinal subarachnoid space.

At steady state, the average concentration in a given compartment can be derived from Eq. 5 and is established by the balance of the source and sink terms. Equating the source and sink terms given in Eqs. 6 and 8, we obtain the following expression for the albumin quotient, $Q_{Al}$, in a given CSF compartment [6]:

$$Q_{Al} = \frac{P_{bc}}{P_{bc} + \overline{F_c}}, \tag{9}$$

where the subscript c represents the CSF compartment for which $Q_{Al}$ is known, namely the cisterns, cortical or

spinal subarachnoid spaces, $P_{bc}$ stands for the barrier permeability in that compartment and $\overline{F_c}$ for the mean CSF drainage rate to be determined. The corresponding results are reported in Table 3. The obtained mean drainage characteristics for the spinal compartment, $\overline{F_{spinal}}$, are then employed as baseline for other tested scenarios.

Having calculated the mean CSF drainage rate for the spinal compartment, we determine its local value by making use of reported albumin concentration gradients along the neuraxis. Due to the low CSF turnover rate, sequential sampling of CSF through a lumbar puncture allows one to sequentially access CSF portions from the lumbar, thoracic and finally cervical subarachnoid spaces. Using this method, a decrease of $Q_{Al}$ was observed from the first 0–3 ml of CSF to the last 27–30 ml of CSF obtained by lumbar puncture [31]. Having an opposite gradient in CSF drainage has been hypothesized as the most probable mechanism for these changing CSF protein concentrations [6]. Accordingly, we assume spinal CSF drainage to increase linearly from zero at x = 0 in the lumbar sac (end of lumbar region) to twice $\overline{F_{spinal}}$ in the cervical region, thereby ensuring that the average spinal drainage matches the above determined value, $\overline{F_{spinal}}$. Note that only at exactly x = 0 is CSF drainage zero, but that integrated over a segment, for example along the lumbar region, there is CSF drainage.

### Solution method

Equation (5) for solute transport is discretized using finite differences in Matlab with a forward Euler time stepping scheme and second order central differences for the spatial second derivatives. Neumann boundary conditions of zero flux for concentrations are imposed on the proximal end of the cervical region and the distal end of the lumbar space. These zero flux boundary conditions are reasonable due to the closed end of the lumbar and the steady-state equilibrium between protein influx and efflux in the lumped compartment of cranial space. The equation is solved with a time-step size of 6 s and a spatial resolution of 3.5 mm, with confirmed time-step and grid independence.

### The Reiber diagram

Reiber showed that a hyperbolic function can describe the relationship between albumin and immunoglobulin quotients seen in a population of patients without intrathecal production of immunoglobulins [32]:

$$Q_{IgG} = \frac{a}{b} \sqrt{Q_{Al}^2 + b^2} - c, \tag{10}$$

where a, b and c are parameters appropriately chosen to fit the measured patient values. We use this empirical relationship as a reference for the output of the protein distribution.

**Table 2 Calculated protein dispersion coefficients**

| Molecule | Diffusion coefficient (m²/s) | Maximum CSF velocity (mm/s) | Dispersion coefficient (m²/s) |
|---|---|---|---|
| Immunoglobulin G | $2.4 \cdot 10^{-11}$ | 10 | $4.0 \cdot 10^{-8}$ |
| Albumin | $6.0 \cdot 10^{-11}$ | 2.5 | $2.8 \cdot 10^{-9}$ |
| | | 5 | $2.2 \cdot 10^{-8}$ |
| | | 10 | $6.0 \cdot 10^{-8}$ |
| | | 20 | $1.3 \cdot 10^{-7}$ |
| | | 40 | $2.7 \cdot 10^{-7}$ |

**Table 3 CSF drainage distribution and albumin quotients in different CSF compartments**

| | |
|---|---|
| **CSF drainage distribution** | |
| Cortical region | 82% |
| Spinal region | 18% |
| **Albumin quotients in different CSF compartments** | |
| Lumbar region | 0.002 |
| Cortical subarachnoid space | 0.003 |
| Cistern | 0.001 |

Reiber further showed that the population variation coefficient, CV, stays constant as the albumin quotient changes. CV is defined as the ratio of the IgG variation to its mean value [32]:

$$CV = \frac{Q_{IgG_{upperlimit}} - Q_{IgG_{lowerlimit}}}{0.5 \cdot \left( Q_{IgG_{upperlimit}} + Q_{IgG_{lowerlimit}} \right)}, \quad (11)$$

## Results

### Transport of the molecules in the spinal canal

We interrogated the 3D axisymmetric model to evaluate protein transport resulting from pulsatile spinal CSF motion. The diffusion coefficients of albumin and IgG in CSF are $6 \cdot 10^{-11}$ and $2.4 \cdot 10^{-11}$ m²/s, respectively. A peak CSF velocity of 10 mm/s was considered as Ref. [25]. The resulting dispersion coefficients are summarized in Table 2. Since the CSF pulsation amplitude reduces along the spinal canal towards the lumbar space

[24], we also calculated the dispersion coefficient for lower velocities. Puy et al. showed that CSF pulsations can change in pathological situations [33], demonstrating an up to four fold increase in amplitude. To evaluate the impact of such pathological variations on protein distribution, we also calculated dispersion coefficients for accordingly increased velocities. We observed an almost linear increase in the dispersion coefficients with increasing velocity amplitude.

### Distribution of albumin and IgG in the spinal CSF: baseline condition

We first determined the distribution of CSF drainage between cortical and spinal spaces as outlined in the "Methods" section and then calculated albumin and IgG quotients using the one-dimensional model. Drainage distribution and albumin quotients in different regions of the CSF space are summarized in Table 3. The distribution of albumin and IgG quotients in the spinal canal between lumbar and cervical regions is shown in Fig. 4.

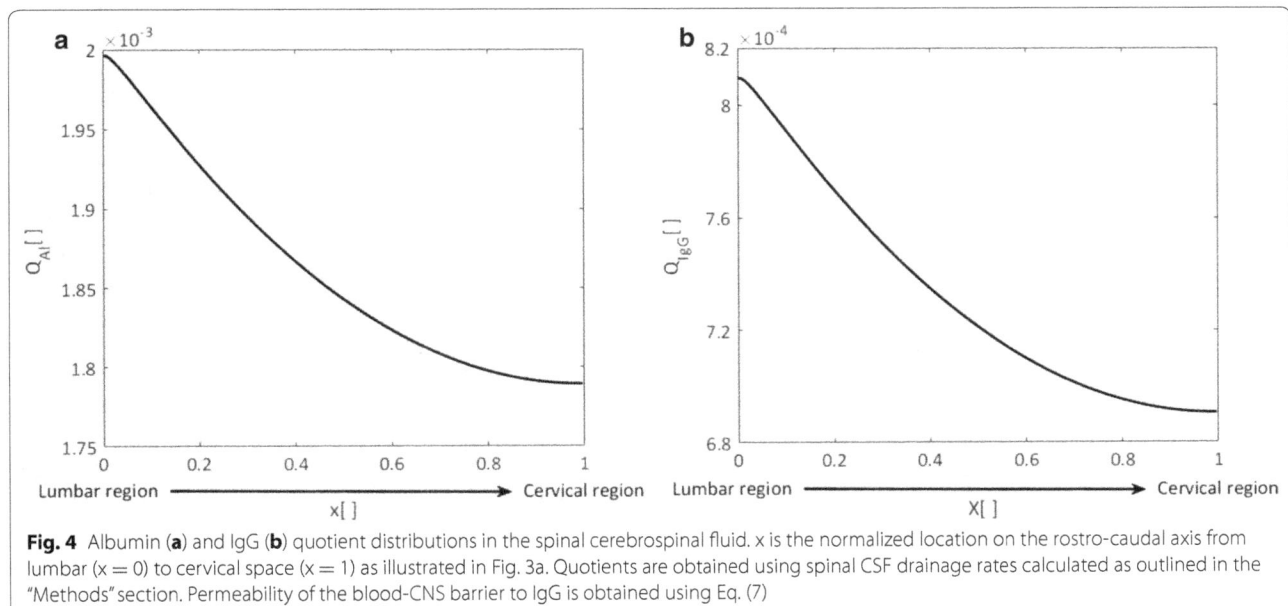

**Fig. 4** Albumin (**a**) and IgG (**b**) quotient distributions in the spinal cerebrospinal fluid. x is the normalized location on the rostro-caudal axis from lumbar (x = 0) to cervical space (x = 1) as illustrated in Fig. 3a. Quotients are obtained using spinal CSF drainage rates calculated as outlined in the "Methods" section. Permeability of the blood-CNS barrier to IgG is obtained using Eq. (7)

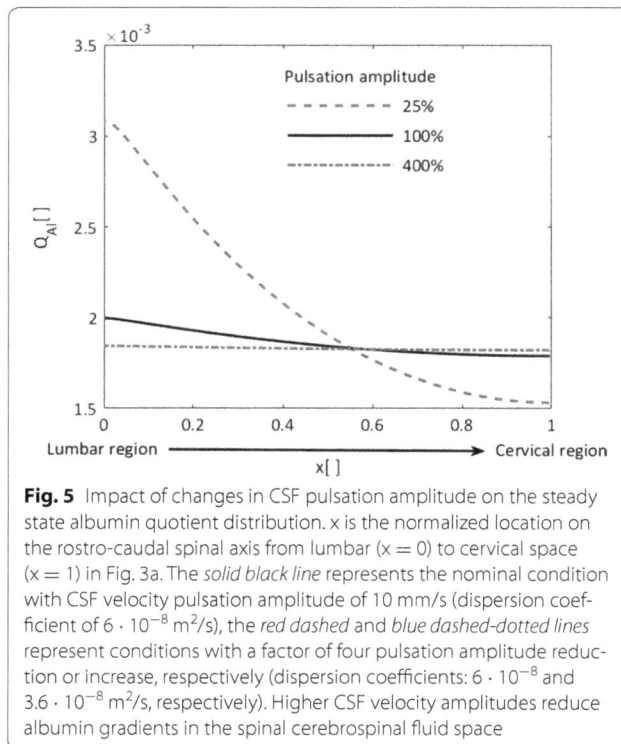

**Fig. 5** Impact of changes in CSF pulsation amplitude on the steady state albumin quotient distribution. x is the normalized location on the rostro-caudal spinal axis from lumbar (x = 0) to cervical space (x = 1) in Fig. 3a. The *solid black line* represents the nominal condition with CSF velocity pulsation amplitude of 10 mm/s (dispersion coefficient of $6 \cdot 10^{-8}$ m$^2$/s), the *red dashed* and *blue dashed-dotted lines* represent conditions with a factor of four pulsation amplitude reduction or increase, respectively (dispersion coefficients: $6 \cdot 10^{-8}$ and $3.6 \cdot 10^{-8}$ m$^2$/s, respectively). Higher CSF velocity amplitudes reduce albumin gradients in the spinal cerebrospinal fluid space

### Impact of CSF pulsation amplitude change on protein distribution

We employed the 1D model of albumin distribution in conjunction with the dispersion rates obtained using the 3D model of protein transport in the spinal space to assess the effect of changes in CSF pulsation amplitude. We investigated the effect of a fourfold increase in CSF pulsation amplitude observed in chronic hydrocephalus patients [33] and used the corresponding dispersion coefficient calculated in the previous section. Figure 5 shows the impact of CSF pulsation amplitude change on the steady state albumin distribution in the spinal CSF. An increase in CSF velocity amplitude results in a more even albumin distribution in the spinal canal, whereas a decrease intensifies the concentration gradient.

### Impact of barrier dysfunction and CSF drainage on protein quotients

We used the 1D model to investigate the effect of changes in blood-CNS barrier permeability and CSF drainage on albumin and IgG quotients in the lumbar cerebrospinal fluid. Figure 6a shows the relationship between IgG and albumin quotients in the cases of barrier permeability change (circles) and CSF drainage rate change (solid black line). An albumin quotient of 0.002 is taken as the nominal value. Decrease in CSF drainage and increase in barrier permeability lead to increased IgG and albumin

quotients, and vice versa. The empirical hyperbolic relation between albumin and IgG quotients derived by Reiber [2] from measurements in patients' CSF samples is shown to match well with our calculations for barrier permeability change (solid red line).

Figure 6b illustrates the effect of change in barrier permeability for three different constant CSF drainage rates. The center (dashed) curve corresponds to nominal drainage, while the upper and lower solid curves correspond to 30% increased and decreased drainage rates, respectively. All three curves are hyperbolic. We used the upper and lower curves to calculate representations of the population variation coefficient, obtaining values of 0.48, 0.44 and 0.4 for albumin quotients of 0.001, 0.002 and 0.003, respectively. Note that the population variation coefficient determined by Reiber based on patient data is constant over a range of albumin quotients.

Figure 6c illustrates the effect of change in barrier permeability for three different baseline IgG permeabilities, reflecting the variation of the barrier permeability to IgG to different extent than for albumin as shown by Seyfert et al. [34]. The center (dashed) curve corresponds to nominal baseline IgG permeability, while the upper and lower solid curves correspond to 30% increased and decreased baseline IgG permeability, respectively. The representation of the population variation coefficient is in this case 0.6 for all albumin quotients.

### Discussion

The biochemical analysis of the cerebrospinal fluid is an important diagnostic tool for pathologies of the CNS. For example, changes in CSF immunoglobulin content can be indicative of inflammatory reactions in the brain. To account for inter-individual and normal intra-individual variability, it is advantageous to assess relative rather than absolute values of protein concentration as done in the Reiber diagram. While the Reiber diagram can indicate intrathecal synthesis of proteins, it is debated whether higher than normal readings of relative albumin concentrations are indicative of CNS barrier dysfunction or reduction in CSF drainage. Here we have employed a set of computational models to assess which one of these two changes is the more likely cause of increased albumin concentration in CSF relative to that in the blood plasma.

The Reiber diagram features a hyperbolic relationship between albumin quotient and, for example, IgG quotient, where 'quotient' refers to the concentration of the respective protein in CSF relative to its concentration in blood plasma. Reiber derived this empirical relationship from measurements in a large set of patients in which intrathecal synthesis of the protein of interest could be

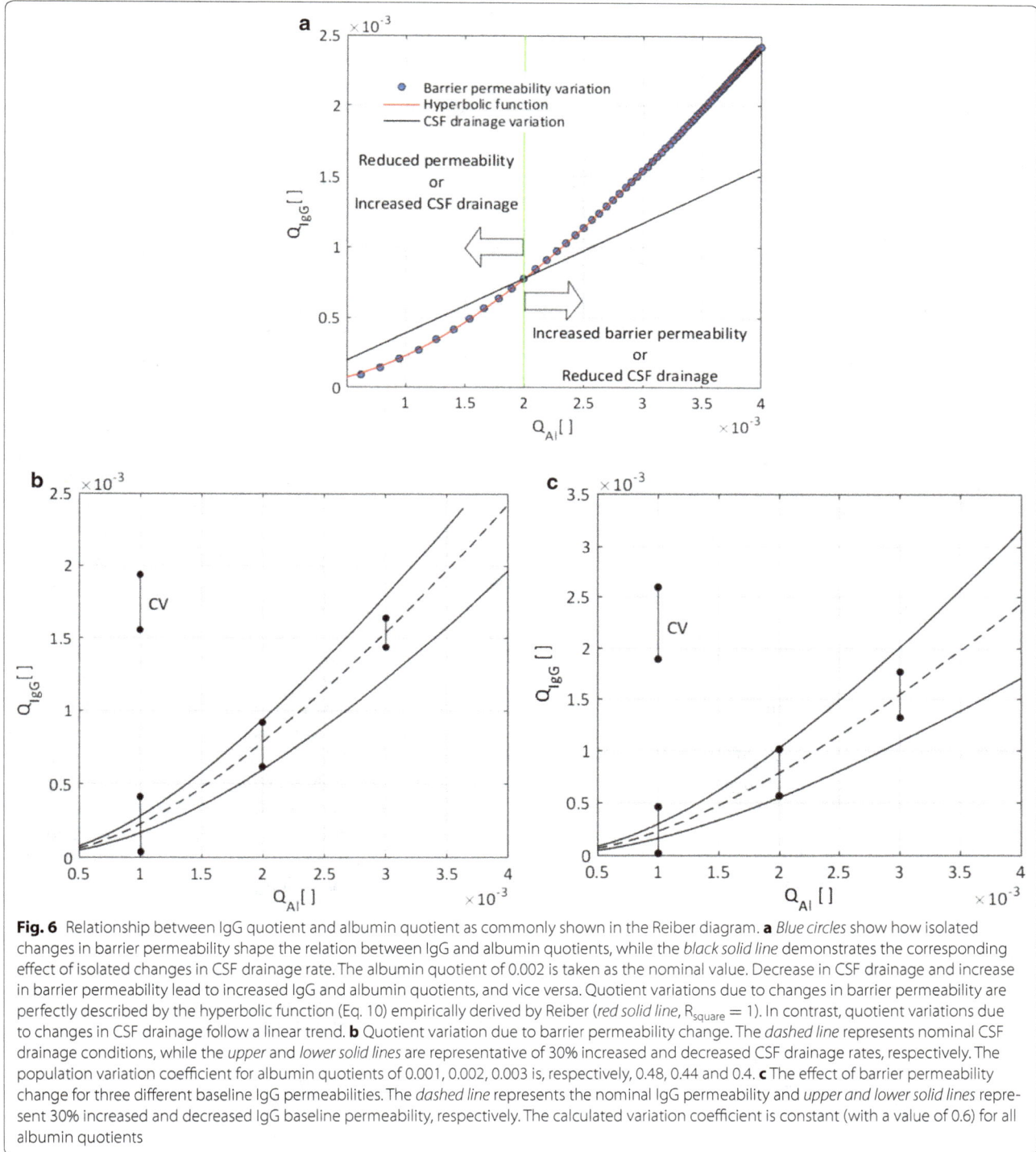

**Fig. 6** Relationship between IgG quotient and albumin quotient as commonly shown in the Reiber diagram. **a** *Blue circles* show how isolated changes in barrier permeability shape the relation between IgG and albumin quotients, while the *black solid line* demonstrates the corresponding effect of isolated changes in CSF drainage rate. The albumin quotient of 0.002 is taken as the nominal value. Decrease in CSF drainage and increase in barrier permeability lead to increased IgG and albumin quotients, and vice versa. Quotient variations due to changes in barrier permeability are perfectly described by the hyperbolic function (Eq. 10) empirically derived by Reiber (*red solid line*, $R_{square} = 1$). In contrast, quotient variations due to changes in CSF drainage follow a linear trend. **b** Quotient variation due to barrier permeability change. The *dashed line* represents nominal CSF drainage conditions, while the *upper* and *lower solid lines* are representative of 30% increased and decreased CSF drainage rates, respectively. The population variation coefficient for albumin quotients of 0.001, 0.002, 0.003 is, respectively, 0.48, 0.44 and 0.4. **c** The effect of barrier permeability change for three different baseline IgG permeabilities. The *dashed line* represents the nominal IgG permeability and *upper and lower solid lines* represent 30% increased and decreased IgG baseline permeability, respectively. The calculated variation coefficient is constant (with a value of 0.6) for all albumin quotients

excluded. He hypothesized that this non-linear relationship was caused by inter-patient variability in CSF drainage rates [32]. However, as shown in Fig. 6a, our models indicate that variations in the rate of CSF drainage would yield a linear relationship between the quotients rather than the experimentally determined hyperbolic one. Reiber also calculated the variation coefficient for his patient database and found it to be constant for a large range of albumin quotients. Our calculations show that the variation coefficient does not stay constant for different baseline CSF drainage values (Fig. 6b), indicating that inter-patient variability in CSF drainage alone may not result in the protein quotient relationship observed by Reiber. One should thus not, without further case-dependent evidence, attribute abnormally high albumin quotients identified in the Reiber diagram to reduced CSF drainage.

Others have attributed increased albumin quotients to blood-CNS barrier dysfunction. Indeed, as shown in Fig. 6a, variation in barrier permeability leads to the expected hyperbolic relationship between protein quotients. This is further confirmed by a constant population variation coefficient as illustrated in panel (c) for different baseline IgG permeabilities. Consequently, high albumin quotients identified in the Reiber diagram may be seen as indicative of a CNS barrier dysfunction.

Our calculations of the distribution of CSF efflux indicate 18% drainage in the spinal compartment and 82% drainage in the cranial compartment. This distribution matches well with the measurements of Marmarou et al. [35] in cats, where absorption in the spinal space accounted for 16% of the total CSF drainage and the cranial space contributed 84%. Similar results were obtained by Gehlen et al. using a lumped parameter model of coupled cardiovascular and CSF dynamics [36]. Albumin quotients calculated based on this drainage distribution are within the range of values obtained experimentally in healthy subjects [31].

Seyfert et al. measured albumin and immunoglobulin concentration gradients in the spinal CSF by sequential CSF sampling through lumbar puncture. They showed a decreasing protein concentration profile from lumbar to cervical space [31]. It was hypothesized that this concentration gradient results from the variation of CSF drainage along the spine [6]. Our calculations show that the hypothesized drainage gradient along the spinal canal with minimum drainage rate in the lumbar space would, indeed, result in a longitudinal concentration gradient for albumin and IgG (Fig. 4). Therefore, our results support the existence of rostro-caudally decreasing spinal CSF drainage.

Puy et al. correlated the magnitude of CSF pulsation with protein distribution in different CSF compartments [33]. We calculated the dispersion rate of albumin in the spinal CSF for different pulsation amplitudes as reported in Table 2, and employed these values in our global protein distribution model. Increased CSF pulsation diminishes the longitudinal concentration gradient in the spinal canal, while reduced pulsation intensifies it (Fig. 5). These results are in line with the measurements of Puy et al. [33]. Therefore, changed CSF dynamics in pathologies such as hydrocephalus and Chiari malformation could have an impact on protein distribution in the spinal canal.

The two computational models developed in this study have the following main limitations: First and foremost, we have simplified the spinal canal anatomy substantially to a 3D axisymmetric annular conduit and a 1D representation, respectively, considering the spinal subarachnoid space as a porous medium. Both the macroscopic anatomy as well as the microanatomy of the CSF spaces as defined by, e.g. arachnoid trabeculae, could play an important role in fluid and solute dynamics. Neglecting the microanatomy can lead to discrepancies between computed and measured metrics of spinal CSF dynamics [19]. In our models, the effect of microstructures is approximated by the introduction of anisotropic permeability of the porous medium representing the spinal subarachnoid space.

The second main limitation pertains to the issue of parameter uncertainty. For instance, we have considered the overall CSF drainage rate to be equal to the estimated value of CSF production, which itself is only known approximately [30]. We have dealt with parameter uncertainty by performing sensitivity analyses, which show that our main conclusions are robust with respect to reasonable variations of the model parameters. Concretely, we have shown that the hyperbolic protein quotient function in the Reiber diagram that results from variation in barrier permeability does not depend on baseline CSF drainage (Fig. 6b) or IgG permeability values (Fig. 6c). We have also made sure that the population variation coefficient does not only stay constant for a 30% change in IgG baseline permeability (Fig. 6c), but also for much larger and smaller changes (up to 100% change). Finally, we checked that the derived dispersion coefficients do not depend on the computational domain length and hydraulic conductivity of the domain.

### Authors' contributions

MA implemented the computational model and performed the calculations. DAZ supervised model implementation and calculations. VK conceived the study and directed the research. All authors analyzed the data and wrote the manuscript. All authors read and approved the final manuscript.

### Author details

[1] The Interface Group, Institute of Physiology, University of Zurich, Winterthurerstrasse 190, 8057 Zurich, Switzerland. [2] Neuroscience Center Zurich, University of Zurich, Zurich, Switzerland. [3] Zurich Center for Integrative Human Physiology, University of Zurich, Zurich, Switzerland.

### Acknowledgements

We gratefully acknowledge the financial support provided by the Swiss National Science Foundation through Grant 200021_147193 CINDY, Marie Heim-Vögtlin fellowship PMPDP2_151255 and NCCR Kindey.CH.

### Competing interests

The authors declare that they have no competing interests.

## Funding

The presented study was financially supported by the Swiss National Science Foundation through Grant 200021_147193 CINDY, Marie Heim-Vögtlin fellowship PMPDP2_151255 and NCCR Kindey.CH.

## References

1. Frankfort SV, Tulner LR, van Campen JP, Verbeek MM, Jansen RW, et al. Amyloid beta protein and tau in cerebrospinal fluid and plasma as biomarkers for dementia: a review of recent literature. Curr Clin Pharmacol. 2008;3(2):123–31.
2. Reiber H. Proteins in cerebrospinal fluid and blood: barriers, CSF flow rate and source-related dynamics. Restor Neurol Neurosci. 2003;21(3–4):79–96.
3. Reiber H, Padilla-Docal B, Jensenius JC, Dorta-Contreras AJ. Mannan-binding lectin in cerebrospinal fluid: a leptomeningeal protein. Fluids Barriers CNS. 2012;9(1):17.
4. Rosen H, Sunnerhagen KS, Herlitz J, Blomstrand C, Rosengren L. Serum levels of the brain-derived proteins S-100 and NSE predict long-term outcome after cardiac arrest. Resuscitation. 2001;49(2):183–91.
5. Engelhardt B, Sorokin L. The blood-brain and the blood-cerebrospinal fluid barriers: function and dysfunction. Semin Immunopathol. 2009;31(4):497–511.
6. Rapoport SI. Passage of proteins from blood to cerebrospinal fluid. Neurobiology of cerebrospinal fluid 2. New York: Springer; 1983. p. 233–45.
7. Winfield JB, Shaw M, Silverman LM, Eisenberg RA, Wilson HA 3rd, et al. Intrathecal IgG synthesis and blood-brain barrier impairment in patients with systemic lupus erythematosus and central nervous system dysfunction. Am J Med. 1983;74(5):837–44.
8. Sharief MK, Ciardi M, Thompson EJ. Blood-brain barrier damage in patients with bacterial meningitis: association with tumor necrosis factor-alpha but not interleukin-1 beta. J Infect Dis. 1992;166(2):350–8.
9. Zetterberg H, Jakobsson J, Redsater M, Andreasson U, Palsson E, et al. Blood-cerebrospinal fluid barrier dysfunction in patients with bipolar disorder in relation to antipsychotic treatment. Psychiatry Res. 2014;217(3):143–6.
10. Akaishi T, Narikawa K, Suzuki Y, Mitsuzawa S, Tsukita K, et al. Importance of the quotient of albumin, quotient of immunoglobulin G and Reibergram in inflammatory neurological disorders with disease-specific patterns of blood–brain barrier permeability. Neurol Clin Neurosci. 2015;3(3):94–100.
11. Asgari M, de Zélicourt D, Kurtcuoglu V. Glymphatic solute transport does not require bulk flow. Sci Rep. 2016;6:38635.
12. Kurtcuoglu V, Soellinger M, Summers P, Poulikakos D, Boesiger P. Mixing and modes of mass transfer in the third cerebral ventricle: a computational analysis. J Biomech. 2007;129(5):695–702.
13. Hettiarachchi HD, Hsu Y, Harris TJ Jr, Penn R, Linninger AA. The effect of pulsatile flow on intrathecal drug delivery in the spinal canal. Ann Biomed Eng. 2011;39(10):2592–602.
14. Siyahhan B, Knobloch V, de Zelicourt D, Asgari M, Schmid Daners M, et al. Flow induced by ependymal cilia dominates near-wall cerebrospinal fluid dynamics in the lateral ventricles. J R Soc Interface. 2014;11(94):20131189.
15. Panjabi MM, Oxland T, Takata K, Goel V, Duranceau J, et al. Articular facets of the human spine. Quantitative three-dimensional anatomy. Spine (Phila Pa 1976). 1993;18(10):1298–310.
16. Panjabi MM, Takata K, Goel V, Federico D, Oxland T, et al. Thoracic human vertebrae. Quantitative three-dimensional anatomy. Spine (Phila Pa 1976). 1991;16(8):888–901.
17. Zaaroor M, Kosa G, Peri-Eran A, Maharil I, Shoham M, et al. Morphological study of the spinal canal content for subarachnoid endoscopy. Minim Invasive Neurosurg. 2006;49(4):220–6.
18. Gupta S, Soellinger M, Grzybowski DM, Boesiger P, Biddiscombe J, et al. Cerebrospinal fluid dynamics in the human cranial subarachnoid space: an overlooked mediator of cerebral disease. I. Computational model. J R Soc Interface. 2010;7(49):1195–204.
19. Yiallourou TI, Kroger JR, Stergiopulos N, Maintz D, Martin BA, et al. Comparison of 4D phase-contrast MRI flow measurements to computational fluid dynamics simulations of cerebrospinal fluid motion in the cervical spine. PLoS ONE. 2012;7(12):e52284.
20. Jasak H. OpenFOAM: open source CFD in research and industry. Int J Nav Arch Ocean. 2009;1(2):89–94.
21. Gupta S, Soellinger M, Boesiger P, Poulikakos D, Kurtcuoglu V. Three-dimensional computational modeling of subject-specific cerebrospinal fluid flow in the subarachnoid space. J Biomech Eng. 2009;131(2):021010.
22. Pineda SM, Diaz G, Coimbra CFM. Approximation of transient 1D conduction in a finite domain using parametric fractional derivatives. J Heat Trans-T Asme. 2011;133(7):071301.
23. Abbott NJ. Evidence for bulk flow of brain interstitial fluid: significance for physiology and pathology. Neurochem Int. 2004;45(4):545–52.
24. Schellinger D, LeBihan D, Rajan SS, Cammarata CA, Patronas NJ, et al. MR of slow CSF flow in the spine. AJNR Am J Neuroradiol. 1992;13(5):1393–403.
25. Pahlavian SH, Bunck AC, Loth F, Tubbs RS, Yiallourou T, et al. Characterization of the discrepancies between four-dimensional phase-contrast magnetic resonance imaging and in silico simulations of cerebrospinal fluid dynamics. J Biomech Eng. 2015;137(5):051002.
26. Poduslo JF, Curran GL, Wengenack TM, Malester B, Duff K. Permeability of proteins at the blood–brain barrier in the normal adult mouse and double transgenic mouse model of Alzheimer's disease. Neurobiol Dis. 2001;8(4):555–67.
27. Cutler RW, Murray JE, Cornick LR. Variations in protein permeability in different regions of the cerebrospinal fluid. Exp Neurol. 1970;28(2):257–65.
28. Bechter K, Schmitz B. Cerebrospinal fluid outflow along lumbar nerves and possible relevance for pain research: case report and review. Croat Med J. 2014;55(4):399–404.
29. Bechter K, Benveniste H. Quinckes' pioneering 19th centuries CSF studies may inform 21th centuries research. Neurol Psychiatry Brain Re. 2015;21(2):79.
30. Brinker T, Stopa E, Morrison J, Klinge P. A new look at cerebrospinal fluid circulation. Fluids Barriers CNS. 2014;11:10.
31. Seyfert S, Faulstich A. Is the blood-CSF barrier altered in disease? Acta Neurol Scand. 2003;108(4):252–6.
32. Reiber H. Flow rate of cerebrospinal fluid (CSF)—a concept common to normal blood-CSF barrier function and to dysfunction in neurological diseases. J Neurol Sci. 1994;122(2):189–203.
33. Puy V, Zmudka-Attier J, Capel C, Bouzerar R, Serot J-M, et al. Interactions between flow oscillations and biochemical parameters in the cerebrospinal fluid. Front Aging Neurosci. 2016;8:154. doi:10.3389/fnagi.2016.00154.
34. Seyfert S, Quill S, Faulstich A. Variation of barrier permeability for albumin and immunoglobulin G influx into cerebrospinal fluid. Clin Chem Lab Med. 2009;47(8):955–8.
35. Marmarou A, Shulman K, LaMorgese J. Compartmental analysis of compliance and outflow resistance of the cerebrospinal fluid system. J Neurosurg. 1975;43(5):523–34.
36. Gehlen M, Kurtcuoglu V, Daners MS. Patient specific hardware-in-the-loop testing of cerebrospinal fluid shunt systems. IEEE Trans Biomed Eng. 2016;63(2):348–58.

# 5

# Human jugular vein collapse in the upright posture: implications for postural intracranial pressure regulation

Petter Holmlund[1]*[iD], Elias Johansson[2], Sara Qvarlander[1], Anders Wåhlin[1,3], Khalid Ambarki[1], Lars-Owe D. Koskinen[2], Jan Malm[2] and Anders Eklund[1]

## Abstract

**Background:** Intracranial pressure (ICP) is directly related to cranial dural venous pressure ($P_{dural}$). In the upright posture, $P_{dural}$ is affected by the collapse of the internal jugular veins (IJVs) but this regulation of the venous pressure has not been fully understood. A potential biomechanical description of this regulation involves a transmission of surrounding atmospheric pressure to the internal venous pressure of the collapsed IJVs. This can be accomplished if hydrostatic effects are cancelled by the viscous losses in these collapsed veins, resulting in specific IJV cross-sectional areas that can be predicted from flow velocity and vessel inclination.

**Methods:** We evaluated this potential mechanism in vivo by comparing predicted area to measured IJV area in healthy subjects. Seventeen healthy volunteers (age $45 \pm 9$ years) were examined using ultrasound to assess IJV area and flow velocity. Ultrasound measurements were performed in supine and sitting positions.

**Results:** IJV area was 94.5 mm$^2$ in supine and decreased to $6.5 \pm 5.1$ mm$^2$ in sitting position, which agreed with the predicted IJV area of $8.7 \pm 5.2$ mm$^2$ (equivalence limit $\pm 5$ mm$^2$, one-sided t tests, p = 0.03, 33 IJVs).

**Conclusions:** The agreement between predicted and measured IJV area in sitting supports the occurrence of a hydrostatic-viscous pressure balance in the IJVs, which would result in a constant pressure segment in these collapsed veins, corresponding to a zero transmural pressure. This balance could thus serve as the mechanism by which collapse of the IJVs regulates $P_{dural}$ and consequently ICP in the upright posture.

**Keywords:** Jugular vein, Collapse, Intracranial pressure, Posture, Physiology

## Background

Cerebral venous pressure and intracranial pressure (ICP) varies with body posture [1–5]. Since ICP has mostly been studied in the supine position, little is known about the underlying mechanisms controlling these variations. Increased knowledge of the mechanisms that regulate how ICP changes with posture may aid in understanding the pathophysiology and improving the treatment of diseases such as cerebral venous thrombosis [6], traumatic brain injury [7], idiopathic intracranial hypertension

(IIH) [8] and hydrocephalus [9]. Furthermore it has the potential to contribute to the design of new cerebrospinal fluid (CSF) shunts that better prevent over drainage when patients are upright [10].

In a recent study [5], we proposed a model where ICP in the upright posture is explained by a hydrostatic pressure reference point for the venous system at the level of the neck, and we suggested that this pressure reference point is related to the collapse of the internal jugular veins (IJVs). Furthermore, a recent theoretical analysis of CSF compliance has also indicated that IJV collapse likely plays an important role in the CSF dynamics in the upright human [11]. However, neither of these studies investigated how the suggested neck-level pressure reference point is formed and upheld by the well-known

*Correspondence: petter.holmlund@umu.se
[1] Department of Radiation Sciences, Umeå University, 901 87 Umeå, Sweden
Full list of author information is available at the end of the article

jugular venous collapse. This motivates further studies of IJV collapse and how it translates to an effect on ICP.

The link between equilibrium ICP and venous pressure is described by Davson's equation [12–14] for CSF absorption:

$$ICP = R_{out}\, I_{form} + P_{dural} \qquad (1)$$

where $R_{out}$ is the CSF outflow resistance, $I_{form}$ the formation rate of CSF and $P_{dural}$ the pressure in the dural veins. Equation 1 postulates that a change in venous pressure (and thus $P_{dural}$) should be followed by a corresponding change in ICP. It is known that venous pressure in the upper body decreases due to hydrostatic effects in the upright posture [15], with a venous hydrostatic indifference point slightly below the level of the heart [16], but due to collapse of the IJVs the cranial venous pressure is not as negative in the upright posture as these hydrostatic effects would suggest [17]. While the IJVs collapse in upright, in general they do not totally occlude in this position [18–20], which means that the fluid communication between the heart and brain is not disrupted; rather the collapse likely affects the IJV pressure more like a Starling resistor.

In this study, we evaluated a biomechanical description of the collapsing IJVs that could explain previous observations of upright ICP [3, 5] through a segment of zero transmural pressure in the neck. The description is based on the idea that the highly flexible IJVs adjust their shape to allow for transmission of the surrounding atmospheric pressure to the internal venous pressure of these collapsed vessels. This behaviour has been observed in experimental bench studies of collapsible rubber tubes inclined to some angle [21–24] and should be applicable in vivo if the IJVs are sufficiently flexible, i.e. wall forces are negligible, when in the collapsed state. Such a physiological mechanism should result in specific cross-sectional areas that are uniquely predicted by the IJV flow rate and body posture. For validation, we measured the IJV cross-sectional area and flow velocity in healthy volunteers using ultrasound. An agreement between measured and predicted IJV area in the upright posture would support the hypothesized description of IJV collapse and how venous collapse can allow for a venous pressure reference point at neck level in the upright human.

## Methods

In summary, a theoretical expression for the collapsed IJV cross-sectional area was derived based on the assumption of zero transmural pressure along the collapsed venous segment. This theoretical description was then evaluated by comparing the predicted IJV area with IJV area measurements in healthy volunteers.

## Theoretical expression for the cross-sectional area

For zero transmural pressure to hold along the collapsed IJVs at neck-level, assuming a constant surrounding pressure, the pressure at any two points along the collapsed segment must be the same and there will be no *pressure difference* between these two points (these principles are illustrated in Fig. 1). The pressure difference between two points in an inclined vessel is due to two major pressure contributions: the hydrostatic pressure of the blood column and the viscous losses due to flow resistance [22]. The hydrostatic pressure difference between two points of interest in a fluid column is described by:

$$\Delta P_{hydro} = \rho\, g\, h = \rho\, g\, L \sin\alpha \qquad (2)$$

where $h$ is the height of the fluid column, $L$ the total distance between the points of interest, $\alpha$ the tilt angle, $g$ the gravitational acceleration and $\rho$ the fluid density (Fig. 1). The viscous losses in a vein can be estimated by the modified Hagen–Poiseuille equation for elliptical tubes [21]:

$$\Delta P_{visc} = RQ = k\frac{8\,\pi\,\mu\,L}{A^2}Q \qquad (3)$$

where $R$ is the flow resistance, $Q$ the flow rate, $L$ the total distance between the points of interest, $\mu$ the viscosity and $A$ the cross-sectional area of the vein. The constant

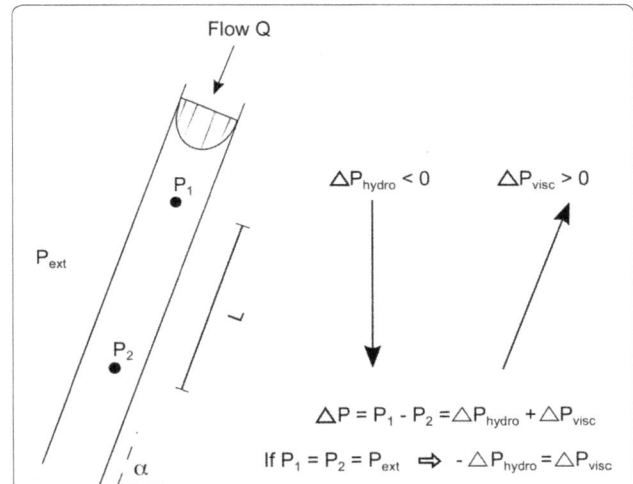

**Fig. 1** Description of pressure in a collapsed vessel. The description is based on the assumption of zero transmural pressure in the collapsed jugular vein. Thus, to achieve zero transmural pressure in the collapsed section of the vessel the *internal* pressures at any two levels 1 and 2 must be equal to the external pressure, i.e. $P_1 = P_2 = P_{ext}$. This means that internal pressure cannot change along the vein from level 1 to level 2 and the pressure (hydrostatic and viscous) components must cancel each other in this segment. The *arrows* indicate the direction of increasing pressure for the two pressure components inside the vessel. $L$ is the distance between the two points in question and $a$ is the tilt angle of the vessel. Since near-zero (i.e. near atmospheric) pressures are expected around the IJVs [24, 28, 29], the internal pressure should also be near-zero after collapse

$k = (a^2 + b^2)/2ab$ describes the shape of the vessel and is here called the ellipse factor; $a$ and $b$ are the semi-major and semi-minor axes of the ellipse [21]. For a circular tube, $k = 1$ and Eq. 3 then corresponds to the standard Hagen–Poiseuille equation. The rationale for the inclusion of the ellipse factor is to account for how the non-circular/semi elliptical shape of the collapsing IJVs (see Additional file 1: Figure S1) affects the flow resistance.

Then, equating Eqs. 2 and 3, gives us an expression for the IJV cross-sectional area ($A_c$) (Fig. 1) as a function of tilt angle $\alpha$ and maximum flow velocity $U_{max}$:

$$A_c = \frac{4\,\pi\,\mu\,k\,U_{max}}{\rho\,g\,\sin\alpha} \qquad (4)$$

where we made use of $Q = AU_{max}/2$, assuming a parabolic flow profile (applicable for both circular and elliptic cross-sections [25]). Equation 4 is the key relationship for the suggested IJV collapse mechanism and the relationship evaluated in this study. It is important to emphasize that the relationship is only meant to describe the collapsed state of a vessel. For positive transmural pressures, Eq. 4 should cease to be valid and IJV area should instead exceed $A_c$, e.g. in supine and at low upper body tilt angles where the hydrostatic column from the heart is small and the IJVs are inflated by the positive central venous pressure.

## Subjects

The study included 17 healthy volunteers (10 women) of age $45 \pm 9$ years (mean $\pm$ SD). Volunteers were recruited via an advertisement in a local newspaper and were considered eligible if they were without any past or present neurological, cardiovascular or psychiatric diseases. In addition, they had to have normal blood pressure (<140/90) and be within the age range 30–60 years. Subjects using any medication affecting the cardiovascular system or central nervous system were excluded.

## Ultrasound measurement protocol

To study the validity of Eq. 4, we measured jugular cross-sectional area, ellipse factor $k$ and maximum velocity $U_{max}$ with ultrasound. The jugular veins were examined using a GE Vivid E9 ultrasound system with a 9L linear probe (4–8 MHz) (General Electric Healthcare, Chicago, IL, USA). Brightness-mode was used for investigating the cross-sectional area of the IJVs at three different neck levels, on both sides (located $23 \pm 2$, $27 \pm 3$ and $29 \pm 3$ cm from the bottom of the sternum, respectively). The rationale for using three levels was to identify the segment with the smallest area in sitting posture, in order to ensure that the cross-sectional area was investigated in the collapsed region of the vein. This segment was then used in the analysis of agreement between measured and predicted IJV area.

The subjects were placed on their backs on a bed with an adjustable backrest and the ultrasound measurements were performed with the upper body/backrest at tilt angles of 0° (supine), 16° (half-sitting) and 71° (sitting). The half-sitting position was included to test Eq. 4 as a potential tool for determining the occurrence of collapse, as this angle is close to where our previous study suggested that venous collapse may start to influence ICP [5]. The angles were measured using a digital inclinometer (mini digital protractor) placed on the backrest of the bed. The leg rest was kept horizontal at all times. Each level was maintained for at least 8 min, during which the measurements took place. To avoid any local increase in the external pressure, the ultrasound probe was held so that only the ultrasound gel was in contact with the skin, i.e. the probe and the skin were only held together by the surface tension of the gel, as indicated by a lack of signal at the edges of the ultrasound images. An ultrasound sequence was saved for each measurement, consisting of 89–90 frames and a time span of roughly 3 s.

## Measuring the IJV cross-sectional area

In the ultrasound images, a region of interest (ROI) was manually drawn along the circumference of the jugular vein, and the cross-sectional area was calculated as the area within the ROI (see Additional file 1: Figure S1). We assessed the absolute minimum and maximum for each sequence and the average of the two was used as an estimate of the mean area for each sequence ($A_{meas}$). In addition to the cross-sectional area, the major and minor axes of the IJVs were also measured (in the same frames as the minimum and maximum area), in order to get an estimate of the ellipse factor (Additional file 1: Figure S1). As was the case with the cross-sectional area, the mean ellipse factor for each sequence was estimated as the average of the two ellipse factors. MATLAB (version R2012b, The Mathworks, Natick, MA) was utilized for all calculations.

## Ultrasound blood flow velocity measurements

The blood flow velocity was measured directly after the three measurements of cross-sectional area, at the same three neck level locations. The velocity was estimated using angle-corrected pulsed-wave ultrasound. The time average velocity was calculated for each ultrasound sequence by manual analysis of the Doppler data. Velocity was measured at the centre of the vessel, with the assumption that we thus measured the maximum velocity in the vessel ($U_{max}$). The velocity analysis was performed using MATLAB. One vessel with no detectable blood flow (i.e. fully occluded somewhere) was excluded from the analysis, since the assumptions for the hydrostatic-viscous pressure balance (Fig. 1) would not be valid if flow was zero. This resulted in a total of 33 IJVs for the analysis.

### Predicting IJV collapse area

The main analysis consisted of comparing the predicted IJV collapse area $A_c$ (according to Eq. 4) with the measured mean IJV area $A_{meas}$. Constants were set to $\rho_{blood} = 1060$ kg/m$^3$, $\mu_{blood} = 3.8 \times 10^{-3}$ Pa s and $g = 9.81$ m/s$^2$. The IJV level used for the analysis was the one with the smallest area in sitting position: level 1 for 21 IJVs and level 2 for 12 IJVs. To calculate $A_c$ individual ellipse factors $k$, individual flow velocities and tilt angles of the backrest were inserted in Eq. 4.

### Statistics

A test of equivalence [26] was used for comparing the predicted and measured IJV area in sitting position. The equivalence limits for the difference were set to ±5 mm$^2$, and two one-sided t tests (TOST) were performed, one for each limit, with the alternative hypothesis representing equivalence. The equivalence limit was based on error estimations assuming a measurement inaccuracy and physiological variability (e.g. respiratory and autoregulatory effects) of 25% in $U_{max}$, $k$ and $A_{meas}$, and an IJV area in upright of around 10 mm$^2$ [20, 27]. The significance level was set to p < 0.05. All statistical calculations were performed using built-in MATLAB functions. Measurement results are presented as mean ± SD unless otherwise specified.

### Results

In sitting, the IJV cross-sectional area predicted by the pressure balance (Eq. 4) was found to be equivalent to the measured cross-sectional area ($A_{meas} = 6.5 \pm 5.1$ mm$^2$ and $A_c = 8.7 \pm 5.2$ mm$^2$, equivalence test: limits ±5 mm$^2$, p = 0.03). This was further supported by a paired t test, which showed no significant difference between $A_{meas}$ and $A_c$ (p = 0.14). A boxplot of the difference between $A_{meas}$ and $A_c$ is shown in Fig. 2. The analysis of the half-sitting position showed that 27% of the 33 IJVs had an $A_{meas}$ within the equivalence limits of $A_c \pm 5$ mm$^2$ or below $A_c$ (using individual values of $A_c$) indicating that in these cases collapse had occurred already at this tilt angle.

$A_{meas}$ was $94.5 \pm 53.3$, $40.1 \pm 33.8$ and $6.5 \pm 5.1$ mm$^2$ in supine, half-sitting and sitting position, respectively. The change in area going from supine to sitting was thus $88.0 \pm 53.1$ mm$^2$ (one-sided paired t test, p < 0.01). The area while sitting was 11 ± 14% of the supine value. The average maximum and minimum $A_{meas}$ observed in sitting position were 8.1 and 5.0 mm$^2$, respectively. The ellipse factor $k$ was $1.2 \pm 0.3$, $1.6 \pm 0.7$ and $2.1 \pm 1.0$, illustrating a change in IJV shape from close to circular

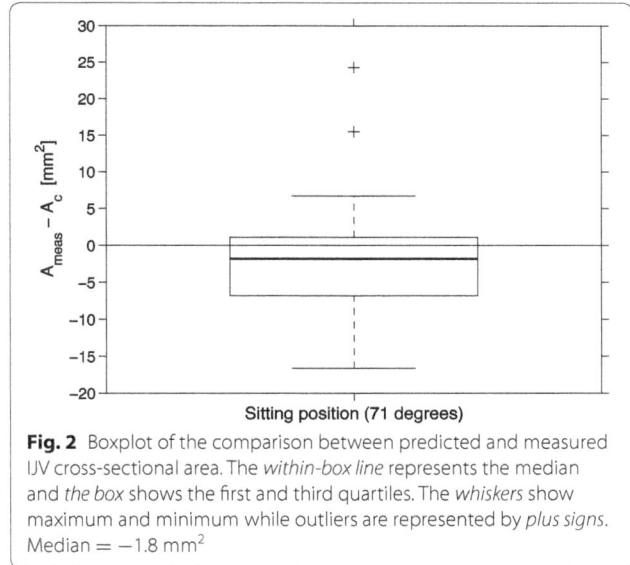

**Fig. 2** Boxplot of the comparison between predicted and measured IJV cross-sectional area. The *within-box line* represents the median and *the box* shows the first and third quartiles. The *whiskers* show maximum and minimum while outliers are represented by *plus signs*. Median = −1.8 mm$^2$

in supine to more elliptical in sitting position. The maximum velocity $U_{max}$ increased from 18 ± 19 cm/s in supine to 38 ± 34 cm/s in half-sitting and 89 ± 39 cm/s in sitting position. In one IJV, an extremely high value for $U_{max}$ was observed in supine position. Without this value, the supine $U_{max}$ would have been 16 ± 10 cm/s.

### Discussion

This study investigated the collapse of the IJVs in healthy subjects when going from supine to sitting. The results showed that measured IJV area and the area predicted by hydrostatic-viscous pressure balance agreed well in upright/sitting position, which supports zero transmural pressure in the collapsed IJVs in the upright human. The pressure balance could thus serve as the mechanism by which collapse of the IJVs regulate ICP in the upright posture to the levels reported in ICP studies.

Our aim in this study was to investigate how the IJV collapse could explain the previously observed changes in ICP [3, 5] when going from supine to sitting position. A hydrostatic-viscous pressure balance in the collapsed IJVs would introduce a segment where pressure remains constant, and the top of this segment would then serve as a new pressure reference point for cranial venous pressure. Since the driving force behind the pressure balance is a zero transmural pressure, the surrounding tissue pressure should determine the actual internal venous pressure and thus the pressure at this reference point. Previous studies of pressure around the IJVs in the neck have indicated that the surrounding pressure may range from slightly negative [28] to slightly positive [24, 29], but still close to zero (i.e. atmospheric pressure). This would be in agreement with studies of internal IJV pressure, where the pressure has ranged from zero to slightly positive in the collapsed IJVs [15, 30]. Such magnitudes of the surrounding pressure would also explain the ICP changes observed previously [5].

$P_{dural}$, and subsequently ICP, will depend on the position of the top of the collapse. Inter-individual differences in collapse length can thus yield inter-individual variations in $P_{dural}$ and ICP. A collapse at neck level would result in a negative $P_{dural}$ corresponding to a hydrostatic column of around 10 cm and an ICP that is close to zero or slightly negative, which is in agreement with previous ICP observations [3, 5].

The results of this study further support the idea of IJV collapse as an active part in the regulation of cranial venous pressure and thus also ICP. Since humans spend most of their day in an upright position, alterations in the IJV collapse function might be of importance in diseases with a suspected disturbance of the ICP dynamics, e.g. hydrocephalus, IIH and postural headache. Furthermore, since both area and flow estimations can quickly be performed using ultrasound, determination of the angle where collapse occurs could contribute to treatment of traumatic brain injury, where slight head-of-bed tilt is used to lower ICP [31, 32] and the optimal degree of head elevation is a matter of debate [33, 34]. Understanding how gravity regulates ICP is also of utmost importance for understanding changes in ICP when gravity is removed, i.e. in microgravity. One case of particular interest is the visual impairment syndrome seen in astronauts on long-duration space missions [35, 36] where an ICP disturbance is believed to be the main cause [37].

With a confirmed zero transmural pressure in collapsed IJVs, the simple expression for $A_c$ (Eq. 4) could be used to identify a collapsed IJV. This approach could then easily be applied in a clinical setting when investigating cranial venous pressure and ICP, since the IJVs are superficial veins that are easy to assess with ultrasound. Our measurement results in this study indicated that about one-fourth of the IJVs (27%) had already collapsed in the half-sitting position, verifying an inter-individual variation in the angle where collapse first occurs. The reason for the differences in collapse angle should mainly be inter-individual variations in central venous pressure and height.

In this study we utilize the jugular venous pathway to understand the cranial venous pressure. Previous studies have successfully modelled the cranial venous drainage, including the IJVs, as a parallel system analogous to an electrical circuit in order to predict blood flow distributions [38, 39]. In such a system, all possible venous pathways from the brain to the heart affect the distribution of blood flow. However, when interested specifically in the

pressure dynamics, any single pathway can be analysed, since all of them must yield the same central venous pressure and cranial venous pressure regardless of the pathway chosen (Fig. 3). This supports our use of the single pathway through the IJVs, as this provides sufficient information as long as the IJVs are not totally occluded (in that case, fluid communication would be broken in the IJVs and cranial venous pressure would be regulated by other, non-occluded pathways, such as the vertebral veins [19, 38, 40]).

While equivalence of measured and predicted area was strongly supported by the results, the observed difference of 2.2 mm$^2$ still opens the possibility that $A_{meas}$ is slightly smaller than $A_c$, meaning that the viscous losses could be larger than the hydrostatic component, leading to a pressure increase along the collapsed jugulars (from the proximal to the distal end). For example, if the equivalence limit were decreased to 3 mm$^2$, the two areas would not be considered equivalent (p = 0.29). However, since the difference is well within reasonable limits for

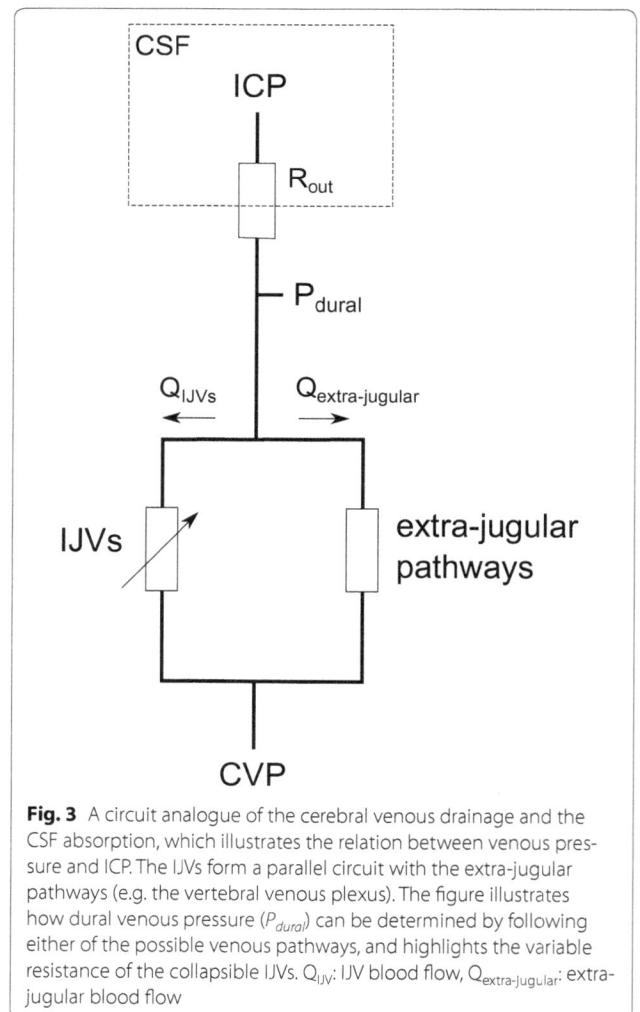

**Fig. 3** A circuit analogue of the cerebral venous drainage and the CSF absorption, which illustrates the relation between venous pressure and ICP. The IJVs form a parallel circuit with the extra-jugular pathways (e.g. the vertebral venous plexus). The figure illustrates how dural venous pressure ($P_{dural}$) can be determined by following either of the possible venous pathways, and highlights the variable resistance of the collapsible IJVs. Q$_{IJV}$: IJV blood flow, Q$_{extra-jugular}$: extra-jugular blood flow

measurement accuracy, this result could simply be due to systematic errors in the measurements.

The results in Fig. 2 reveal deviations from the predicted area in some specific cases. For the IJVs corresponding to the two extreme cases, it was the measured area that was unexpectedly large in the upright posture ($A_{meas}$ was 25.1 and 19.7 mm$^2$, respectively). Therefore, we believe it is possible that our three measurement sites did not successfully capture the collapse of these two IJVs during the ultrasound examination. The IJVs corresponding to the largest overestimation of the predicted area could possibly be explained by overestimation of the ellipse factor, as these IJVs had comparatively high ellipse factors (i.e. a very flattened shape) and since these measurements were sometimes difficult to perform for the smallest IJVs. However, it is also possible that the use of the correction by the ellipse factor was insufficient for these cases, i.e. that this assumption had reached its limit, and that the viscous losses were no longer well described by the modified Hagen–Poiseuille equation (Eq. 3). For example, if the IJVs with an ellipse factor $k > 2.5$ were excluded, the mean difference between $A_{meas}$ and $A_c$ was only 0.5 mm$^2$ (number of IJVs = 27). Thus, suggesting that highly flattened IJVs require a modified expression for the factor $k$, which is implicated by experimental studies of highly collapsed tubes [41].

In addition to the measurement uncertainties in ultrasound area and velocity measurements, the variability between predicted and measured IJV area (Fig. 2) could be due to variation in tissue pressure or in vessel rigidity along the IJVs. This would result in an IJV area that is expected to vary along the vessel, with a magnitude fluctuating around the predicted area. Furthermore, while we believe that the inertial effects, e.g. from variations in flow [42, 43], are relatively small in the upright IJVs, inertial effects are present [44] and can be a factor contributing to the observed differences, thus this is an area of improvement where further analysis would be interesting. In spite of these limitations, since the predicted area in the upright posture was in good agreement with the measured area on group level, the results support the hypothesized physiological mechanism, although we acknowledge that the limitations of the above assumptions need to be addressed before individual area predictions can be fully implemented.

## Conclusions

In conclusion, the agreement between predicted and measured IJV cross-sectional area in sitting indicates that hydrostatic effects are indeed cancelled by the viscous losses in the collapsed IJVs, which supports the occurrence of a zero transmural pressure segment in the IJVs in the upright human. The hydrostatic-viscous pressure balance could thus serve as the mechanism by which collapse of the IJVs regulates ICP in the upright posture.

### Abbreviations
CSF: cerebrospinal fluid; CVP: central venous pressure; ICP: intracranial pressure; IIH: idiopathic intracranial hypertension; IJV: internal jugular vein; ROI: region of interest; $P_{dural}$: dural venous pressure; $U_{max}$: maximum flow velocity; $A_{meas}$: measured jugular vein cross-sectional area; $A_c$: predicted jugular vein cross-sectional area; $k$: estimated ellipse factor.

### Authors' contributions
Concept and design by AE, JM, PH and LOK. PH, SQ, EJ, KA, AW and AE contributed to the data acquisition and analysis. PH, SQ, JM and AE interpreted the results, drafted the paper and created the figures. All authors critically edited and revised the manuscript. All authors read and approved the final manuscript.

### Author details
[1] Department of Radiation Sciences, Umeå University, 901 87 Umeå, Sweden. [2] Department of Pharmacology and Clinical Neuroscience, Umeå University, 901 87 Umeå, Sweden. [3] Umeå Centre for Functional Brain Imaging, Umeå University, 901 87 Umeå, Sweden.

### Acknowledgements
We thank research nurse Kristin Nyman for skilful assistance.

### Competing interests
The authors declare that they have no competing interests.

### Funding
The study was supported by the following grants: Swedish National Space Board and the Swedish Research Council Grant 2015-05616.

### References
1. Iwabuchi T, Sobata E, Suzuki M, Suzuki S, Yamashita M. Dural sinus pressure as related to neurosurgical positions. Neurosurgery. 1983;12:203–7.
2. Eklund A, Johannesson G, Johansson E, Holmlund P, Qvarlander S, Ambarki K, et al. The pressure difference between eye and brain changes with posture. Ann Neurol. 2016;80:269–76.
3. Petersen LG, Petersen JCG, Andresen M, Secher NH, Juhler M. Postural influence on intracranial and cerebral perfusion pressure in ambulatory neurosurgical patients. Am J Physiol Regul Integr Comp Physiol. 2016;310:R100–4.
4. Chapman PH, Cosman ER, Arnold MA. The relationship between ventricular fluid pressure and body position in normal subjects and subjects with shunts: a telemetric study. Neurosurgery. 1990;26:181–9.
5. Qvarlander S, Sundström N, Malm J, Eklund A. Postural effects on intracranial pressure: modeling and clinical evaluation. J Appl Physiol. 2013;115:1474–80.
6. Stam J. Thrombosis of the cerebral veins and sinuses. N Engl J Med. 2005;352:1791–8.
7. Grande P-O. The, "Lund Concept" for the treatment of severe head trauma—physiological principles and clinical application. Intensive Care Med. 2006;32:1475–84.
8. Malm J, Kristensen B, Markgren P, Ekstedt J. CSF hydrodynamics in idiopathic intracranial hypertension: a long-term study. Neurology. 1992;42:851–8.

9. Czosnyka M, Czosnyka Z, Momjian S, Pickard JD. Cerebrospinal fluid dynamics. Physiol Meas. 2004;25:R51–76.

10. Farahmand D, Qvarlander S, Malm J, Wikkelso C, Eklund A, Tisell M. Intracranial pressure in hydrocephalus: impact of shunt adjustments and body positions. J Neurol Neurosurg Psychiatry. 2015;86:222–8.

11. Gehlen M, Kurtcuoglu V, Schmid Daners M. Is posture-related craniospinal compliance shift caused by jugular vein collapse? A theoretical analysis. Fluids Barriers CNS. 2017;14:5.

12. Davson H. Formation and drainage of the cerebrospinal fluid. Sci Basis Med Annu Rev. 1966:238–59.

13. Davson H, Hollingsworth G, Segal MB. The mechanism of drainage of the cerebrospinal fluid. Brain. 1970;93:665–78.

14. Davson H, Domer FR, Hollingsworth JR. The mechanism of drainage of the cerebrospinal fluid. Brain. 1973;96:329–36.

15. Avasthey P. Venous pressure changes during orthostasis. Cardiovasc Res. 1972;6:657–63.

16. Gauer O, Thron H. Postural changes in the circulation. In: Hamilton WF, Dow P, editors. Handbook of physiology circulation. Washington, DC: American Physiological Society; 1965. p. 2409–40.

17. Guyton AC. The veins and their functions. In: Wonsiewicz MJ, editor. Textbook medical physiology. 8th ed. Philadelphia: W. B. Saunders Company; 1991. p. 164–8.

18. Chambers B, Chambers J, Churilov L, Cameron H, Macdonell R. Internal jugular and vertebral vein volume flow in patients with clinically isolated syndrome or mild multiple sclerosis and healthy controls: results from a prospective sonographer-blinded study. Phlebology. 2014;29:528–35.

19. Alperin N, Lee SH, Sivaramakrishnan A, Hushek SG. Quantifying the effect of posture on intracranial physiology in humans by MRI flow studies. J Magn Reson Imaging. 2005;22:591–6.

20. Ciuti G, Righi D, Forzoni L, Fabbri A, Pignone AM. Differences between internal jugular vein and vertebral vein flow examined in real time with the use of multigate ultrasound color Doppler. Am J Neuroradiol. 2013;34:2000–4.

21. Holt JP. Flow of liquids through "collapsible" tubes. Circ Res. 1959;7:342–53.

22. Hicks JW, Badeer HS. Siphon mechanism in collapsible tubes: application to circulation of the giraffe head. Am J Physiol. 1989;256:R567–71.

23. Seymour RS, Hargens AR, Pedley TJ. The heart works against gravity. Am J Physiol United States. 1993;265:R715–20.

24. Pedley TJ, Brook BS, Seymour RS. Blood pressure and flow rate in the giraffe jugular vein. Philos Trans R Soc Lond B Biol Sci. 1996;351:855–66.

25. Lekner J. Viscous flow through pipes of various cross-sections. Eur J Phys. 2007;28:521–7.

26. Walker E, Nowacki AS. Understanding equivalence and noninferiority testing. J Gen Intern Med United States. 2011;26:192–6.

27. Cirovic S, Walsh C, Fraser WD, Gulino A. The effect of posture and positive pressure breathing on the hemodynamics of the internal jugular vein. Aviat Sp Environ Med. 2003;74:125–31.

28. Parazynski SE, Hargens AR, Tucker B, Aratow M, Styf J, Crenshaw A. Transcapillary fluid shifts in tissues of the head and neck during and after simulated microgravity. J Appl Physiol United States. 1991;71:2469–75.

29. Guyton AC, Barber BJ, Moffatt DS. Theory of interstitial pressures. In: Hargens AR, editor. Tissue fluid pressure composition. London: Williams & Wilkins; 1981. p. 11–9.

30. Dawson EA, Secher NH, Dalsgaard MK, Ogoh S, Yoshiga CC, Gonza J, et al. Standing up to the challenge of standing : a siphon does not support cerebral blood flow in humans. Am J Physiol Regul Integr Comp Physiol. 2004;287:911–4.

31. Durward QJ, Amacher AL, Del Maestro RF, Sibbald WJ. Cerebral and cardiovascular responses to changes in head elevation in patients with intracranial hypertension. J Neurosurg. 1983;59:938–44.

32. Fan J-Y. Effect of backrest position on intracranial pressure and cerebral perfusion pressure in individuals with brain injury: a systematic review. J Neurosci Nurs. 2004;36:278–88.

33. A Brain Trauma Foundation; American Association of Neurological Surgeons; Congress of Neurological Surgeons. Guidelines for the management of severe traumatic brain injury (3rd Edition). J Neurotrauma. 2007;24:S1-106.

34. Koskinen L-OD, Olivecrona M, Grande PO. Severe traumatic brain injury management and clinical outcome using the Lund concept. Neuroscience. 2014;283:245–55.

35. Mader TH, Gibson CR, Pass AF, Kramer LA, Lee AG, Fogarty J, et al. Optic disc edema, globe flattening, choroidal folds, and hyperopic shifts observed in astronauts after long-duration space flight. Ophthalmology. 2011;118:2058–69.

36. Kramer LA, Sargsyan AE, Hasan KM, Polk JD, Hamilton DR. Orbital and intracranial effects of microgravity: findings at 3-T MR imaging. Radiology. 2012;263:819–27.

37. Berdahl JP, Yu DY, Morgan WH. The translaminar pressure gradient in sustained zero gravity, idiopathic intracranial hypertension, and glaucoma. Med Hypotheses. 2012;79:719–24.

38. Gisolf J, van Lieshout JJ, van Heusden K, Pott F, Stok WJ, Karemaker JM. Human cerebral venous outflow pathway depends on posture and central venous pressure. J Physiol. 2004;560:317–27.

39. Gadda G, Taibi A, Sisini F, Gambaccini M, Sethi SK, Utriainen DT, et al. Validation of a hemodynamic model for the study of the cerebral venous outflow system using mr imaging and echo-color Doppler data. Am J Neuroradiol. 2016;37:2100–9.

40. Valdueza JM, von Munster T, Hoffman O, Schreiber S, Einhaupl KM. Postural dependency of the cerebral venous outflow. Lancet. 2000;355:200–1.

41. Katz AI, Chen Y, Moreno AH. Flow through a collapsible tube: experimental analysis and mathematical model. Biophys J. 1969;9:1261–79.

42. Bertram CD, Pedley TJ. A mathematical model of unsteady collapsible tube behaviour. J Biomech. 1982;15:39–50.

43. Marchandise E, Flaud P. Accurate modelling of unsteady flows in collapsible tubes. Comput Methods Biomech Biomed Eng. 2010;13:279–90.

44. Kamm RD, Pedley TJ. Flow in collapsible tubes: a brief review. J Biomech Eng. 1989;111:177–9.

# 6

# Increased CSF aquaporin-4, and interleukin-6 levels in dogs with idiopathic communicating internal hydrocephalus and a decrease after ventriculo-peritoneal shunting

Martin J. Schmidt[1]*, Christoph Rummel[2], Jessica Hauer[1], Malgorzata Kolecka[1], Nele Ondreka[1], Vanessa McClure[3] and Joachim Roth[2]

## Abstract

**Background:** Studies in animal models, in which internal hydrocephalus has been induced by obstructing the cerebrospinal fluid pathways, have documented an up-regulation of the concentrations of aquaporin-4 (AQP4) in the brain. In this study, the concentrations of aquaporin-1 (AQP1), AQP1, AQP4 and interleukin-6 (IL-6) were determined in the CSF of dogs with idiopathic communicating hydrocephalus before and after the reduction of intraventricular volume following ventriculo-peritoneal shunt (VP-shunt) treatment.

**Results:** The concentrations of AQP4 and IL-6 were increased in the cerebrospinal fluid of dogs with hydrocephalus compared to controls. Both parameters significantly decreased after surgical treatment, accompanied by decrease of ventricular size and the clinical recovery of the dogs. AQP1 was not detectable in CSF.

**Conclusions:** Brain AQP4 up-regulation might be a compensatory response in dogs with hydrocephalus. Future determination of AQP4 at the mRNA and protein level in brain tissue is warranted to substantiate this hypothesis.

**Keywords:** Aquaporin, Communicating hydrocephalus, Dogs, Interleukin-6

## Background

Definitive treatment options for internal hydrocephalus in dogs and humans rely mostly on surgical implantation of CSF-draining shunt systems [1–4]. Medical treatment methods aiming at reducing CSF production have been reported to provide temporary relief of clinical signs, but are mostly ineffective [2, 5–7]. Therefore, improved medical treatment options, especially for immature hydrocephalic patients, are desirable. Aquaporins (AQPs) are a family of water channel proteins, which are found in cell membranes in a number of tissues, including the central nervous system (CNS) [8, 9]. In the brain, the predominant water channel is AQP4, which provides the molecular basis for bidirectional water transport across the cell membranes of the blood–brain- and blood-CSF boundaries. The driving force behind water movement can be both osmotic and hydraulic in nature, the latter allowing the bulk flow of water across cell membranes [9–11]. AQP4 is mainly located in the astrocyte foot processes that surround capillaries in the CNS. At this boundary, brain AQP4 regulates water removal from the pericapillary space into brain vessels suggesting it has a crucial role in fluid volume homeostasis [8–11].

Under certain pathological conditions changes in AQP4 expression have been found [12–14]. Studies in animal models, in which internal hydrocephalus has been induced by injection of kaolin into the subarachnoid space, documented an up-regulation of AQP4 in the periventricular white matter [15, 16] and cerebral cortex [17]. Increased levels of soluble AQP4 were also found in the CSF of children with naturally occurring internal hydrocephalus [18].

*Correspondence: Martin.J.Schmidt@vetmed.uni-giessen.de
[1] Department of Veterinary Clinical Sciences, Small Animal Clinic, Justus-Liebig-University, Frankfurter Strasse 108, 35392 Giessen, Germany
Full list of author information is available at the end of the article

It has been suggested that increased integration of AQP4 into the astrocyte membranes might have a compensatory effect in countering excess CSF [15, 19, 20] by increased astroglial clearance of excess brain water by transcellular routes and/or through the glia limitans [16].

A second water channel in the CNS, namely AQP1, is reported to be limited to choroid plexus epithelia within the CNS. Experimental depletion of the AQP1 gene in mice leads to a decrease in CSF production by the choroid plexus, demonstrating a role for AQP1 in CSF production [21]. The proposed adaptive and protective roles of AQP1 and-4 as regulators of CSF production and absorption in the pathophysiology of hydrocephalus, establishes these AQPs as interesting candidates for possible treatment options. Interleukin 6 (IL-6) is a pro-inflammatory cytokine. Increased levels of IL-6 have been associated with periventricular white matter damage [22]. Neurons, astrocytes, microglia and endothelial cells are the main sources of IL-6 in the CNS [23]. Internal hydrocephalus is primarily a white matter disease and IL-6 levels may be used as a surrogate marker for white matter injury. Thus, a correlation between IL-6 and AQP4 levels could be useful to indicate the extent of white matter damage.

The aim of the present study was to determine the concentration of AQP1 and AQP4 in the CSF of dogs with idiopathic communicating hydrocephalus, and possible changes in these levels after reduction of intra-ventricular pressure following ventriculo-peritoneal shunting. Given the previously-reported relationship between IL-6 and white matter damage in neonatal children and the presence of white matter damage in internal hydrocephalus, we also investigated the relationship between IL-6 and the aquaporins. We hypothesised that increased ventricular volume is positively correlated to CSF levels of AQP4 and IL-6, and negatively correlated to AQP1 in dogs with idiopathic communicating hydrocephalus.

## Methods
### Animals
Fourteen dogs with internal hydrocephalus, whose owners decided on surgical implantation of a ventriculo-peritoneal shunt (VP-shunt) system for permanent CSF drainage were prospectively selected between 2010 and 2014. The dogs had to meet the following criteria to be included in the study. (1) The hydrocephalus had to be diagnosed as idiopathic communicating, based on magnetic resonance imaging (MRI) of the brain without signs of parenchymal contrast enhancement or visual obstruction of CSF pathways. (2) Clinical re-evaluation, with CSF samples taken and immediately stored at −80 °C and both pre- and post-operative MRIs performed in our clinic to allow direct comparisons. (3) Medical pre-treatment using drugs to reduce CSF production (glucocorticoids,

omeprazole, acetazolamide, furosemide) excluded dogs from the study. (4) In the follow up MRI, a decrease in ventricular volume had to be demonstrated as an indication for effective shunt treatment.

CSF collection and MRI examination was also performed on a control group of 10 dogs that were donated to the clinic after euthanasia due to non-neurological diseases. CSF was taken within 2 min of death of the animals. Ventriculomegaly was an exclusion criterion for the dogs in this group.

### Clinical evaluation
Collected data included the breed, age, gender, bodyweight, type and duration of neurological deficits before and after surgery. Clinical data regarding the presenting signs and clinical improvement of the animals after shunting procedures were determined by a board certified neurologist. A standardised neurologic examination was performed prior to, and every day after surgery until discharge, and again 3 months after surgery.

### Magnetic resonance imaging
Diagnosis of idiopathic communicating hydrocephalus was made by MRI using a 1.0 Tesla scanner (Gyroscan Intera, Phillips, Hamburg, Germany) and a solenoid surface coil (C3). For the MRI examination dogs were premedicated with diazepam (0.5 mg/kg IV) and l-methadone (0.5 mg/kg IV). Anesthesia was induced with propofol (4 mg/kg IV) and maintained after endotracheal intubation with isoflurane in oxygen. Sagittal, dorsal, and transverse T2-weighted, transverse FLAIR sequences, T1-weighted before and after intravenous administration of 0.2 mL/kg gadodiamide (Omniscan®) were acquired in all animals pre-operatively. The administration of a contrast agent was of course not feasible in the post-mortem scans in the control dogs but was useful to exclude other neurological diseases in the study group. T2-weighted transverse images of the head were chosen from the whole MR-dataset for image segmentation, using T2-Turbospin echo sequences (TE: 120 ms, TR: 2900 ms). Slice thickness varied from 2–3 mm. The field of view measured $180 \times 180$ mm in small dogs and $210 \times 210$ mm in large dogs. The matrix was $288 \times 288$ in small dogs and $384 \times 384$ in large dogs leading to an in-plane pixel size between $0.625 \times 0.625$ and $0.54 \times 0.54$ mm.

Accumulation of CSF in the lateral cerebral ventricles, an absent septum pellucidum, dorsal bulging of the corpus callosum and dilation of the third ventricle all indicated active ventricular distension and were consistent with hydrocephalus [24]. Patency of the mesencephalic aqueduct was assessed in all image planes. A clearly visible hyperintense signal (CSF) within the aqueduct and a non-distended 4th ventricle determined the presence of communicating hydrocephalus [25]. The absence of any other visible lesion and lack of contrast enhancement within the brain parenchyma finally resulted in the diagnosis of idiopathic communicating hydrocephalus. MRI in the control group was without special findings. To assess the ventricular dimensions and restoration of the brain parenchyma, MRI was repeated 3 months after surgery in the study group (Fig. 1).

## Morphometric procedures

The volume of the cerebral ventricles and the brain tissue was determined based on the T2-weighted images. Image processing for volume rendering was achieved using specialised graphical software as described elsewhere [26] (AMIRA®, Mercury Computer Systems, Berlin, Germany), which allowed manual image segmentation of the ventricular system and brain parenchyma on a slice-by-slice basis. The segmented partitions were calculated and graphically presented by the programme (Fig. 2).

## Shunting procedures

Ventriculo-peritoneal shunting was performed as described elsewhere [3] (Fig. 3 Lateral radiograph of dog with shunt in place). A gravitational ball valve was used in all dogs (paediGAV®, Miethke GmbH & Co KG, Potsdam, Germany).

## CSF sampling

On the day of the diagnostic MRI, a routine CSF examination was performed (cytology and biochemical analysis) to rule out inflammatory diseases of the brain. CSF was collected from the cisterna magna (1 mL per 5 kg body weight).

The first CSF specimen for AQP and IL-6 analysis was collected from the pumping chamber during VP-shunt placement. After insertion of the ventricular catheter and connection of the pumping chamber, CSF was allowed to exit the ventricles via the shunt until pulsatile flow was observed in the transparent chamber. Depending on the ventricular volume and the size of the dog, 1–2 mL CSF was collected and stored in plastic tubes (Eppendorf tubes) at −80 °C for further analyses. The ventricular catheter was routinely tested for patency: 3 h after emptying the chamber via transcutaneous puncture, the chamber was checked for refilling by repeat puncture. The second CSF specimen was collected 3 months after shunt insertion from the subcutaneous pumping chamber.

## Ethical approval

Approval by an ethics committee for the CSF collection was not required as all procedures are part of the therapeutic procedure or routine diagnostic workup of clinical patients [German Animal Experiment Act ["Tierschutzgesetz"], paragraph 9.2]. Verbal approval to examine the CSF for research purposes was obtained from the owners.

## CSF AQP1, AQP4, and IL-6 measurements

Frozen CSF specimens were evaluated 4–26 months after sampling. A dog-specific ELISA Kit was used for analyses of AQP1 and AQP4 in CSF, according to the instructions provided by the manufacturer (Canine AQP ELISA kit, assay ID AQP4: E08A0467; AQP1: E08A0863, BlueGene Biotech, Shanghai, China). The kit applied the competitive immunoassay technique using a monoclonal anti-AQP4-antibody and an AQP4 horseradish- peroxidase conjugate. Standards containing 0, 2.5, 5.0, 10, 25 and 50 ng/mL AQP4 were used to create a standard curve, which was used to calculate AQP4 concentrations

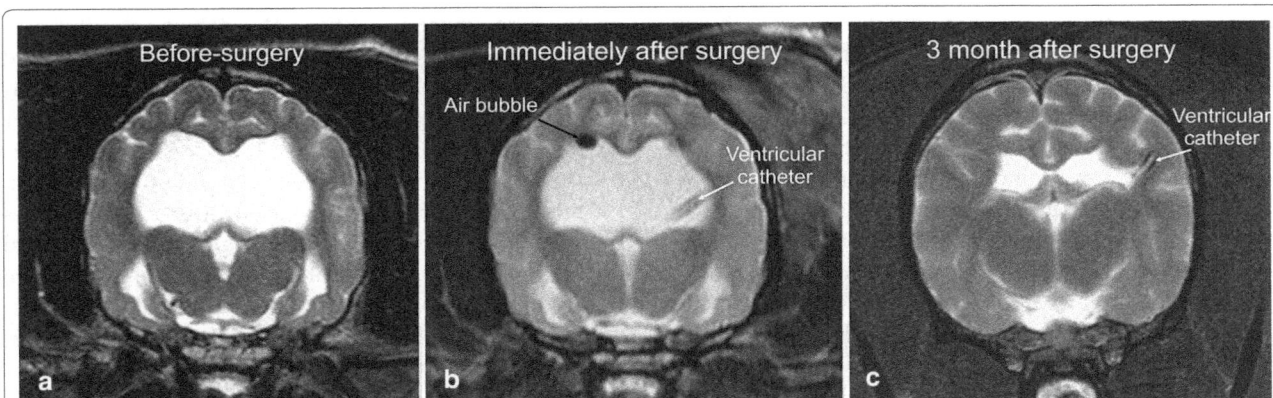

**Fig. 1** Transversal T2-weighted MR-image of the brain and ventricular system of a bullterrier with internal hydrocephalus at the time of diagnosis (**a**), directly post-operatively (**b**), and 3 months after surgery (**c**) showing the reduction of the ventricular volume and reconstitution of the cerebral parenchyma

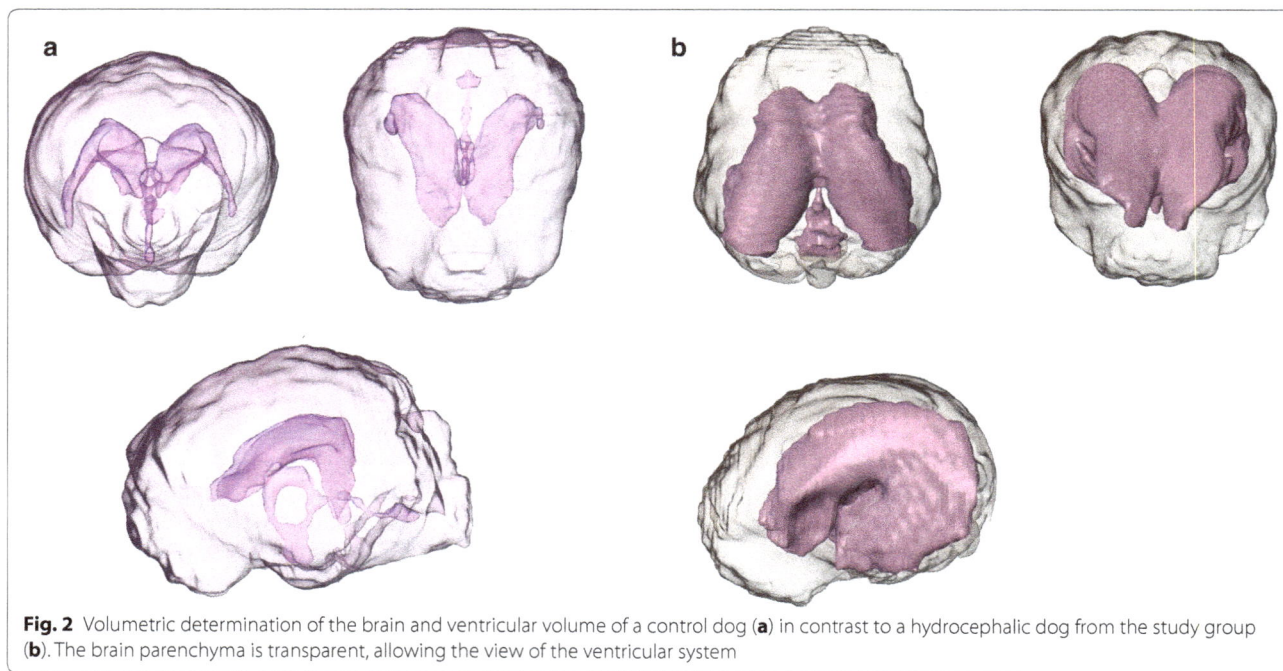

**Fig. 2** Volumetric determination of the brain and ventricular volume of a control dog (**a**) in contrast to a hydrocephalic dog from the study group (**b**). The brain parenchyma is transparent, allowing the view of the ventricular system

in the biological samples. According to the manufacturer's instructions no significant cross-reactivity or interference between AQP4 and its analogues was observed. The coefficient of variation within a given lot and between different lots was stated to be less than 10 %. Samples were determined in duplicate and the detection limit of the specific assay proved to be 0.1 ng/mL.

IL-6 concentrations were determined by a bioassay based on the dose-dependent growth stimulation of IL-6 on the B9 hybridoma cell line [27, 28]. This cell line requires IL-6 for survival and proliferation. The advantages of the B9 assay are its extreme sensitivity and its feature that only bioactive molecules are measured. The assay was performed in sterile, 96-well microtiter plates. In each well, 5000 B9 cells were incubated for 72 h with serial dilutions of biological samples (cerebrospinal fluid) or with different concentrations of a human IL-6 standard (code 89–548, National Institute for Biological Standards and Control, South Mimms, UK). Samples were prediluted so that serial dilutions of samples and standard dilution curves were made in parallel. The number of cells in each well was measured by the dimethylthiazol-diphenyl tetrazolium bromide (MTT) colorimetric assay [27]. The detection limit of the assay, after considering the dilution of samples, was set at 3 international units (IU)/mL.

### Statistical analysis

All data was analysed using a statistical software package (Graph Pad Prism 4.0, Graph Pad Software Inc.,

San Diego, California). AQP and IL-6 concentration before and after surgery were compared with controls. CSF volume before and after surgery may not only be dependent on ventricular distension, but also on the size of the dog (1.2–20 kg, see Table 1, Epidemiological data and clinical signs) as this also influences ventricular volume. Therefore, we considered that the concentrations of AQP4 and IL-6 could also be influenced by CSF volume. To take these morphological differences into account, the concentration of AQPs (ng/mL) and IL-6 (IU/mL) were additionally multiplied by the total ventricular volume (expressed as total AQP/-IL-6 quantity) to calculate the total amounts of AQPs and IL-6 in the ventricles.

After assessment of the normal distribution of this data using the Shapiro–Wilk test, one-way ANOVA was used to test for global differences between the mean concentration and total AQP4 quantity as well as the ventricular volume before and after surgery. If significant differences between the groups were present, post hoc Tukey's test for multiple comparisons was used to reveal differences between all pairs of groups. IL-6 concentration and total IL-6 quantity were not normally distributed. They were tested for global differences using a Kruskal–Wallis test followed by a post hoc Dunn's multiple comparison test.

Correlation between AQP4 and IL-6 concentration in the preoperative CSF specimen was tested using Spearman's correlation. Association of AQP4 and IL-6 with ventricular reduction was tested using the Chi

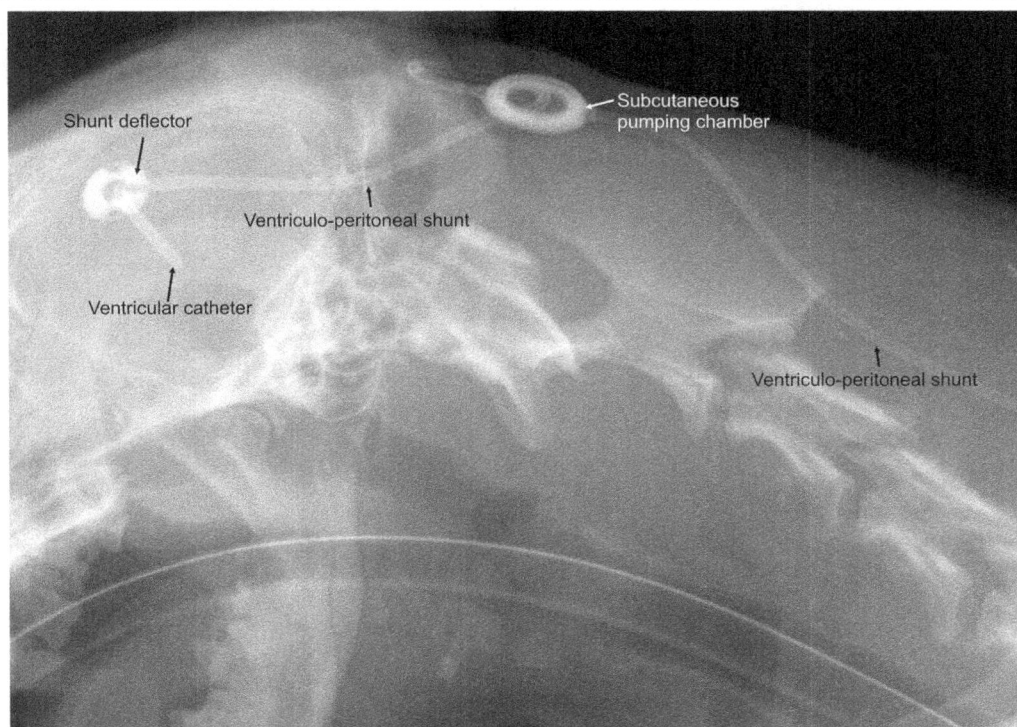

**Fig. 3** Laterolateral radiograph of the head and neck of a bullterrier after ventriculo-peritoneal shunting showing the proximal components and course of the shunt system

square test. *P* values less than 0.05 were considered to be statistically significant (95 % confidence interval).

## Results

### Animals and clinical examination

Breed, age, sex, clinical signs and duration of clinical signs are summarised in Table 1 (Study group dogs) and Table 3 (Control dogs). Two dogs were excluded from the study group because there was no postoperative reduction of ventricular volume.

### CSF analysis

Results of CSF analyses are presented in Table 2 (study group dogs) and Table 3 (control dogs).

### *AQP4*

Results of group comparisons are summarised in Fig. 4. The mean concentration of AQP4 was globally different between groups (*P* < 0.0127). Post hoc tests revealed a significant difference between the mean AQP4 concentrations before (11.32 ng/mL), and after surgery (9.3 ng/mL; *P* < 0.01), and before surgery compared to controls (9.5 ng/mL; *P* < 0.01). Postoperative AQP4 concentrations were not significantly different from controls (*P* > 0.05).

Total AQP4 quantities were globally different between groups (*P* < 0.0001). The mean total AQP4 quantity (325.8 ng) in dogs with internal hydrocephalus before surgery was significantly different from control dogs (32.12 ng, *P* < 0.0001). After shunting, mean total AQP4 quantity was significantly different from pre-operative values (60.49 ng, *P* < 0.0001), but not different from controls (*P* > 0.05). CSF volume was significantly reduced after surgery (*P* < 0.001). A reduction of ventricular volume was associated with AQP4 decrease (*P* < 0.001).

### *AQP1*

AQP1 levels remained below the detection limit in all CSF samples analysed. Using an AQP1 ELISA kit and the same procedure as for AQP4, OD values were around zero.

### *IL-6*

IL-6 concentrations (Fig. 4) were globally different between the groups (*P* < 0.0036). The median IL-6 concentrations before surgery (62 IU/mL) was significantly higher than postoperative values (34 IU/mL; *P* < 0.001) and higher when compared to controls (26 IU/mL; *P* < 0.001). Postoperative values were not different to

**Table 1** Epidemiological data and results of pre- and postoperative clinical examination of the study group

| Number | Breed | Gender, age, bodyweight | Clinical signs | Postoperative clinical signs |
|---|---|---|---|---|
| 1 | Boston terrier | Male, 3 months old, 2.5 kg | Obtundation, mild ataxia on all four limbs, circling, aimless barking | None |
| 2 | Mini Australian shepherd | Male-neutered, 26 months old, 12.5 kg | Visual deficits, reduced menace, circling | Visual deficits, reduced menace |
| 3 | Peruvian hairless dog | Male, 2 months old, 2.8 kg | Ataxia on all four limbs, ventro-lateral strabismus, obtundation | None |
| 4 | Austrian hound | Male, 54 months old, 20 kg | Obtundation, circling, head tremor, hypermetria in the front limbs | None |
| 5 | Cavalier King Charles spaniel | Male neutered, 60 months old, 9.9 kg | Obtundation | None |
| 6 | Pug | Male, 21 months old, 9.2 kg | Obtundation, ataxia on all four limbs | None |
| 7 | Papillon | Female, 7 months old 3.4 kg | Obtundation, ataxia, head tilt tremor | None |
| 8 | Chihuahua | Male neutered, 3 months old, 1.2 kg | Obtundation, mild ataxia, spasticity in all four limbs, reduced menace response | None |
| 9 | Australian shepherd | Male, 4 months old, 13.9 kg | Visual deficits. reduced menace, nystagmus, hypoactive | Visual deficits, reduced menace |
| 10 | Jack Russell terrier | Male, 4 months old, 4.7 kg | Obtundation, ataxia on all four limbs | None |
| 11 | Bullterrier | Female, 25 months old 12.5 kg | Intermittent obtundation, head pressing | None |
| 12 | Maltese mix | Male neutered, 6 months old, 6.1 kg | Circling, obtundation | None |

controls ($P > 0.05$). Total IL-6 quantities were significantly different between groups ($P < 0.0001$). Total IL-6 quantities were significantly higher in dogs with internal hydrocephalus than in control dogs before surgery (1083 vs. 86.3 IU; $P < 0.0001$) and significantly decreased after shunting (149.3 IU; $P < 0.0001$), but were still significantly higher than in the control group ($P < 0.01$).

Concentrations of AQP4 and IL-6 measured in the preoperative CSF specimens were not correlated ($P = 0.449$).

## Discussion

We found increased AQP4 and IL-6 concentrations in the CSF of dogs with idiopathic communicating hydrocephalus. AQP4 and IL-6 concentrations decreased significantly after reduction of lateral ventricular volume using an indwelling ventriculo-peritoneal shunt system. Upregulation of AQP4 channels has been documented in a variety of pathological processes in the brain that result in fluid overload, including internal hydrocephalus. In rats with inherited [19] and kaolin-induced hydrocephalus [15], an increase in AQP4 mRNA- and protein levels within the periventricular parenchyma was reported post-induction. It seems likely that the increase in AQP4 reflects the development of an alternative pathway for parenchymal CSF absorption [9, 15–17, 19, 20]. This notion is also supported by the observation that AQP4 null mice exhibit a more severe form of hydrocephalus with larger ventricular distension and pressure elevation after kaolin injection, than mice with unimpaired AQP4

expression [29]. Whereas AQP4 changes have been well described in experimentally-induced hydrocephalus, few publications have studied the association between AQPs and naturally-occurring hydrocephalus. This is important in that hydrocephalus is usually non-communicating in laboratory rodents, but communicating in the dogs reported in the present study. Hence, there are more similarities between human and canine communicating hydrocephalus, when compared to experimentally-induced hydrocephalus after intrathecal kaolin injection in rodents and the subsequent inflammatory reaction. It has been shown in dogs with induced hydrocephalus that after an initial rise, CSF pressure can return to normal levels as the ventricles enlarge [30].

In the classic model of CSF physiology in dogs the fluid is produced by the choroid plexus [31]. The primary sites of reabsorption are the arachnoid projections from the subarachnoid space into the sagittal dural venous sinus. There is evidence that extracellular fluid (ECF) from the brain parenchyma essentially contributes to CSF production and its bulk flow within the central nervous system [32]. Under normal conditions, arterial pulsation drives the ECF toward the veins and towards the ventricles in humans and dogs. It has been suggested that this physiological ECF flow is reduced in hydrocephalus, and the pericapillary space has been confirmed as playing a critical role in the reabsorption of ECF [9, 33]. The ependymal lining is frequently destroyed in hydrocephalus [34] and AQP4 can, therefore, leak more easily from the parenchyma to the CSF via the ECF [18].

**Table 2  Pre and post-operative concentrations for aquaporin 4 and interleukin 6 and CSF volumes for dogs with hydrocephalus**

| Dog number | Routine CSF examination | Pre-operative values AQP4 (ng/mL), total AQP4 (ng), IL-6 (IU/mL) total IL-6 (IU), CSF volume (mL) | Postoperative values AQP4 (ng/mL), total AQP4 (ng), IL-6 (IU/mL), total IL-6 (IU), CSF volume (mL) |
|---|---|---|---|
| 1 | *Protein* 252 mg/L<br>*RBC* 0/μL<br>*Cells* 3/μL | *AQP4* 12.78<br>*Total AQP4 quantity* 301.5<br>*IL-6* 63<br>*Total IL-6 quantity* 1486.8<br>*CSF volume* 23.6 | *AQP4* 10.81<br>*Total AQP4 quantity* 28.51<br>*IL-6* 30<br>*Total IL-6 quantity* 84<br>*CSF volume* 2.8 |
| 2 | *Protein* 276 mg/L<br>*RBC* 280/μL<br>*Cells* 1/μL | *AQP4* 10.77<br>*Total AQP4 quantity* 223.5<br>*IL-6* 87<br>*Total IL-6 quantity* 2260.8<br>*CSF volume* 26.4 | *AQP4* 10.2<br>*Total AQP4 quantity* 27.99<br>*IL6* 36<br>*Total IL-6 quantity* 96.62<br>*CSF volume* 2.6 |
| 3 | *Protein* 276 mg/L<br>*RBC* 291/μL<br>*Cells* 5/μL | *AQP4* 17.47<br>*Total AQP4 quantity* 391.33<br>*IL-6* 22<br>*Total IL-6 quantity* 492.8<br>*CSF volume* 22.4 | *AQP4* 14.23<br>*Total AQP4 quantity* 150<br>*IL-6* 15<br>*Total IL-6 quantity* 61.1<br>*CSF volume* 10.6 |
| 4 | *Protein* 240 mg/L<br>*RBC* 0/μL<br>*Cells* 1/μL | *AQP4* 15.29<br>*Total AQP4 quantity* 455.56<br>*IL-6* 28<br>*Total IL-6 quantity* 834.4<br>*CSF volume* 29.8 | *AQP* 49.71<br>*Total AQP4 quantity* 45.62<br>*IL-6* 13<br>*Total IL-6 quantity* 634.5<br>*CSF volume* 4.7 |
| 5 | *Protein* 240 mg/L<br>*RBC* 0/μL<br>*Cells* 5/μL | *AQP4* 13.51<br>*Total AQP4 quantity* 278.3<br>*IL-6* 39<br>*Total IL-6 quantity* 803.4<br>*CSF volume* 20.6 | *AQP4* 5.3<br>*Total AQP4 quantity* 34.45<br>*IL-6* 21<br>*Total IL-6 quantity* 136.5<br>*CSF volume* 6.5 |
| 6 | *Protein* 208 mg/L<br>*RBC* 0/μl<br>*Cells* 1/μl | *AQP4* 10.33<br>*Total AQP4 quantity* 133.3<br>*IL-6* 51<br>*Total IL-6 quantity* 658.41<br>*CSF volume* 12.91 | *AQP4* 9.9<br>*Total AQP4 quantity* 63.67<br>*IL-6* 32<br>*Total IL-6 quantity* 205.76<br>*CSF volume* 6.43 |
| 7 | Blood contamination | *AQP4* 17.96<br>*Total AQP4 quantity* 467.67<br>*IL-6* 87<br>*Total IL-6 quantity* 2265.48<br>*CSF volume* 26.04 | *AQP4* 8.93<br>*Total AQP4 quantity* 21.43<br>*IL-6* 37<br>*Total IL-6 quantity* 88.8<br>CSF volume 2.4 |
| 8 | *Protein* 246 mg/L<br>*RBC* 15/μL<br>*Cells* 5/μL | *AQP4* 8.46<br>*Total AQP4 quantity* 211.54<br>*IL-6* 62<br>*Total IL-6quantity* 1078.8<br>*CSF volume* 17.4 | *AQP4* 10.77<br>*Total AQP4 quantity* 3.95<br>*IL-6* 21<br>*Total IL-6 quantity* 13.4<br>*CSF volume* 1.64 |
| 9 | Blood contamination | *AQP4* 12.16<br>*Total AQP4 quantity* 472.45<br>*IL-6* 65<br>*Total IL-6 quantity* 1709.5<br>*CSF volume* 26.3 | *AQP4* 2.41<br>*Total AQP4 quantity* 58.03<br>*IL-6* 40<br>*Total IL-6 quantity* 260<br>*CSF volume* 6.5 |
| 10 | *Protein* 300.9 mg/L<br>*RBC* 18/μL<br>*Cells* 7/μL | *AQP4* 19.19<br>*Total AQP4 quantity* 675.31<br>*IL-6* 66<br>*Total IL-6 quantity* 2323.2<br>*CSF volume* 35.2 | *AQP4* 9.67<br>*Total AQP4 quantity* 190.95<br>*IL-6* 69<br>*Total IL-6 quantity* 1362.75<br>*CSF volume:*19.7 |
| 11 | *Protein* 374 mg/L<br>*RBC* 1/μL<br>*Cells* 1/μL | *AQP4* 14.63<br>*Total AQP4 quantity* 168.85<br>*IL-6* 54<br>*Total IL-6 quantity* 623.16<br>*CSF volume* 11.54 | *AQP4* 16.2<br>*Total AQP4 quantity* 58.31<br>*IL-6* 45<br>*Total IL-6 quantity* 162<br>*CSF volume* 3.6 |

**Table 2 continued**

| Dog number | Routine CSF examination | Pre-operative values AQP4 (ng/mL), total AQP4 (ng), IL-6 (IU/mL) total IL-6 (IU), CSF volume (mL) | Postoperative values AQP4 (ng/mL), total AQP4 (ng), IL-6 (IU/mL), total IL-6 (IU), CSF volume (mL) |
|---|---|---|---|
| 12 | Protein 204 mg/L<br>RBC 0/μL<br>Cells 4/μL | AQP4 7.1<br>Total AQP4 quantity 130.14<br>IL-6 89<br>Total IL-6 quantity 1631<br>CSF volume 18.33 | AQP4 4.5<br>Total AQP4 quantity 42.93<br>IL-6 46<br>Total IL-6 quantity 438.84<br>CSF volume 9.54 |

Pre-, and post-operative determination of the ventricular volume (CSF volume), aquaporin-4 (AQP4) and interleukin-6 (IL-6) of the study group of 12 dogs with hydrocephalus. AQP4 and IL-6 have been multiplied by the total CSF volume, to give the total quantity in the CSF. The underlined entries (dogs 8 and 11) are dogs in which no decrease of AQP4 and IL-6 concentration was found after surgery although the total quantities were decreased (CSF cerebrospinal fluid, RBC red blood cell count)

**Table 3 Epidemiological data and CSF analysis in the control group**

| Breed, age, gender, body weight | Routine CSF examination | CSF volume (mL) | AQP4 concentrations and total quantity | IL-6 concentrations and total quantity |
|---|---|---|---|---|
| Pug, 4 years male neutered, 4.6 kg | Protein 262 mg/L<br>RBC 0/μL<br>Cells 3/μL | 2.4 | AQP4: 11.25<br>Total AQP4 quantity 27 | IL-6: 25 IU<br>Total IL-6 quantity 60 |
| Dachshund, 9 years, male, 6 kg | Protein 256 mg/L<br>RBC 0/μL<br>Cells 1/μL | 3.2 | AQP4: 9.67<br>Total AQP4 quantity 30.94 | IL-6: 24 IU<br>Total IL-6 quantity 76.8 |
| Austrian hound, 3 years male, 26 kg | Protein 220 mg/L<br>RBC 0/μL<br>Cells 3/μL | 3.14 | AQP4: 9.0<br>Total AQP4 quantity 28.26 | IL-6: 27 IU<br>Total IL-6 quantity 85.87 |
| German Shepherd dog, male, 5 years, 22 kg | Protein 302 mg/L<br>RBC 0/μL<br>Cells 2/μL | 4.2 | AQP4: 12.33<br>Total AQP4 quantity 51.78 | IL-6: 19 IU<br>Total IL-6 quantity 79.8 |
| Beagle, male-neutered 2 years, 12 kg | Protein 286 mg/L<br>RBC 0/μL<br>Cells 1/μL | 2.45 | AQP4: 8.87<br>Total AQP4 quantity 21.74 | IL-6: 42 IU<br>Total IL-6 quantity 102.9 |
| Doberman, male, 4 years, 36 kg | Protein 120 mg/L<br>RBC 0/μL<br>Cells 1/μL | 3.04 | AQP4: 6.57<br>Total AQP4 quantity 19.97 | IL-6: 20 IU<br>Total IL-6 quantity 60.8 |
| French Bulldog female-neutered, 1,5 years, 8 kg | Protein 79 mg/L<br>RBC 0/μL<br>Cells 2/μL | 3.4 | AQP4: 9.1<br>Total AQP4 quantity 30.60 | IL-6: 27 IU<br>Total IL-6 quantity 91.8 |
| Bernese mountain dog, female, 6 years, 34 kg | Protein 265 mg/L<br>RBC 0/μL<br>Cells 3/μL | 4 | AQP4: 11.97<br>Total AQP4 quantity 47.86 | IL-6: 22 IU<br>Total IL-6 quantity 88 |
| Cavalier King Charles spaniel, female, 8 years, 6 kg | Protein 289 mg/L<br>RBC 0/μL<br>Cells 5/μL | 3.2 | AQP4: 11.52<br>Total AQP4 quantity 36.87 | IL-6: 34 IU<br>Total IL-6 quantity 108.8 |
| Doberman, female- neutered, 7 years, 29 kg | Protein 156 mg/L<br>RBC 0/μL<br>Cells 1/μL | 3.21 | AQP4: 8.03<br>Total AQP4 quantity 25.79 | IL-6: 55 IU<br>Total IL-6 quantity 176.55 |

CSF volume, aquaporin-4 (AQP4) and interleukin-6 (IL-6) concentrations in the control group. Both values have been multiplied with the total CSF volume, expressed as AQP4* and IL-6* to obtain the total quantity in CSF (CSF cerebrospinal fluid, RBC red blood cell count)

It remains unclear however, whether the increased AQP4 levels in the CSF of hydrocephalic dogs and humans is an unspecific finding related simply to the destruction of cell membranes. In this scenario, on the one hand, an increase of AQP4 would be a pure epiphenomenon reflecting damage to the structural integrity of the ependyma [35] and periventricular white matter. This might be the more likely cause of the increase in AQP4 in the CSF. On the other hand, it has also been suggested that higher AQP4 levels could also be a reflection of increased production and turnover of the protein and its release into the interstitial space and ventricular

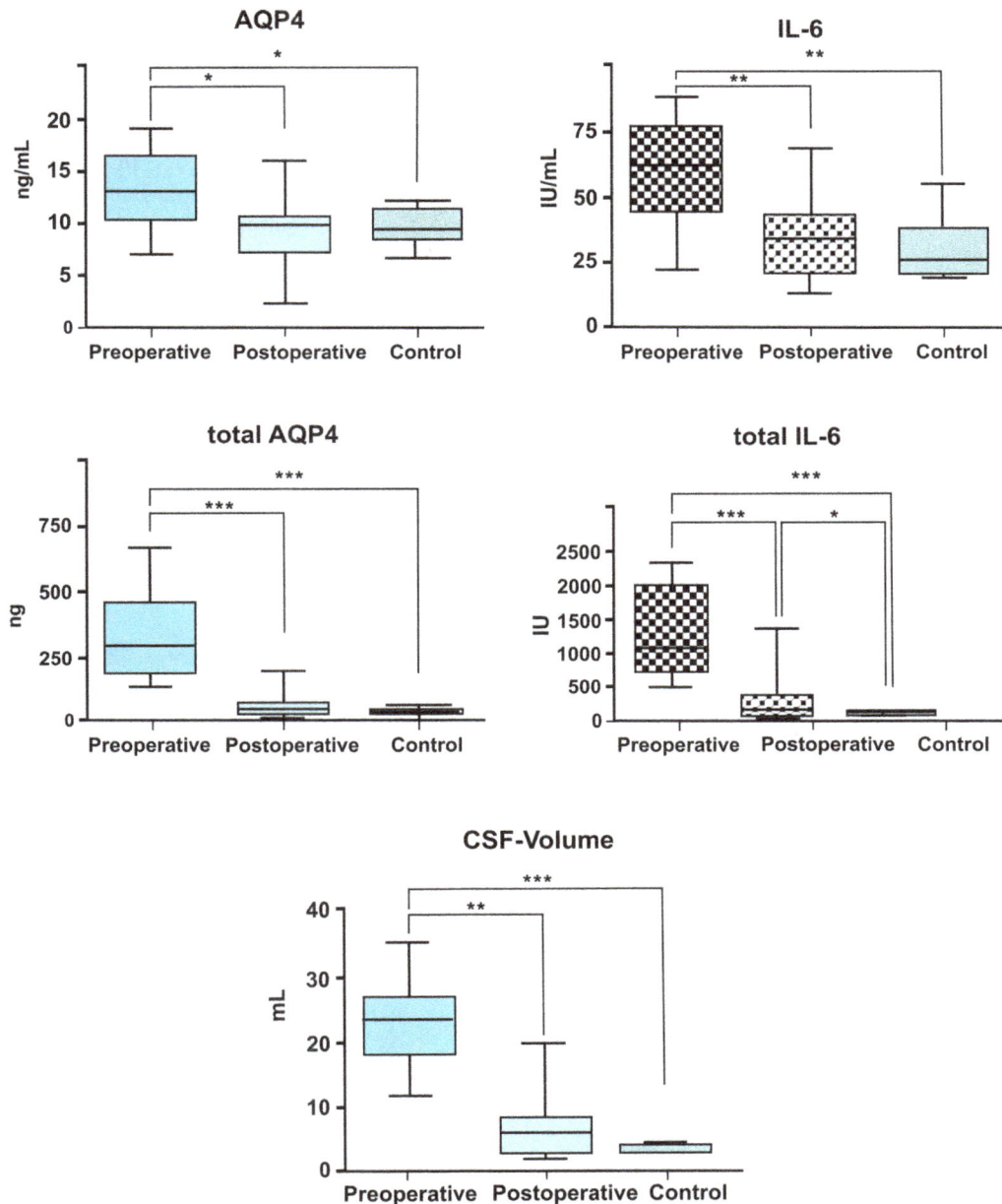

**Fig. 4** *Box* and *Whisker* diagrams demonstrating differences in the mean/median, 25/75 % percentile and minimum-maximum of the, aquaporin-4 (AQP4) and interleukin-6 (IL6) concentrations in the cerebrospinal fluid before and 3 months after surgery compared to controls (*top row*). The total quantity of both parameters AQP4 and IL6 (*middle row*) was calculated by multiplying by the ventricular volume (*bottom graph*). Significant differences are marked with *asterisks* (*$P < 0.01$; **$P < 0.001$; ***$P < 0.0001$, n = 14, 14, 10 for preoperative, postoperative and control groups, respectively

system. Such shedding of membrane proteins has been documented for renal AQPs. Wen et al. [36] showed that urinary excretion of AQP2 occurs under physiological conditions as part of its increased integration into the apical membrane of the collecting duct after vasopressin stimulation. During this process AQP2 is excreted into the urine in a proportion specific to the quantity of membrane-bound AQP [37–40].

It has been shown that distension of the ventricles and compression of periventricular white matter capillaries are accompanied by pro-inflammatory cytokine activation. Damage to the periventricular white matter is the main impact on brain integrity in hydrocephalus cases [34, 41]. IL-6 has been associated with periventricular white matter injury in newborn babies with peripartal hypoxia [22] and increases in IL-6 and IL-8 were more pronounced in the infants with a severe clinical course [42]. A correlation between IL-6 levels and white matter integrity has been documented in elderly humans [43, 44]. We therefore consider that changes in IL-6 concentrations in the CSF act as a surrogate marker for white matter injury in the present study. Here, it has become evident that AQP4 concentration was not correlated with IL-6 concentration in CSF taken preoperatively. This observation might favour the notion that CSF AQP4 level does not merely reflect white matter damage, however, the exact circumstances between pressure rise and AQP4 changes in the CSF remain to be further analysed in future studies.

Our study also showed that adjusting the concentrations of AQP4 and IL-6 to the total CSF volume was not necessary to detect significant differences in AQP4 and IL-6 concentrations. Following the rationale that CSF is constantly produced and the amount of the solute may depend on the amount of the total solvent (CSF), we considered it might be necessary to calculate AQP4 and IL-6 total quantities by multiplying by the ventricular volume. Although preoperative volumes in some dogs exceeded three times the volume of other hydrocephalic dogs, the differences in ventricular dimensions did not obscure differences in CSF AQP4 concentrations. In fact, the concentrations were comparable to those measured in children with hydrocephalus (13.3 in dogs vs. 11.32.ng/mL in children), as well as those in normal dogs to the values in unaffected children (9.5 in dogs vs. 8.61 ng/mL in children) [18].

The main limitation of this study is therefore the heterogeneity of the examined dogs. Different dog breeds were examined without knowledge of the underlying cause of the CSF accumulation or of intraventricular pressure, with different degrees of ventricular dilatation and different durations of clinical signs. Dogs with hydrocephalus were younger than control dogs. Furthermore, CSF from the control group was taken after euthanasia and also not from the intraventricular site, which might also have a potential influence on measured AQP4 and IL-6 levels.

While we were able to measure AQP4 in the CSF of normal and hydrocephalic dogs, AQP1 levels were below the detection limit in all samples. Interestingly, analysis of AQP1 expression after the induction of hydrocephalus in rodents has revealed conflicting results. In mice, it has been shown that AQP1 is down-regulated after induction of hydrocephalus, rather suggesting a compensatory response to hydrocephalus [41], however, another study showed unchanged AQP1 expression in a rat model of hydrocephalus [15]. Being confined to the choroid plexus, AQP1 expression is much lower than AQP4 expression in the rodent brain and CSF. This is also reflected in the fact that values remained below the detection limit in our current analyses for canine CSF AQP1.

## Conclusions

An increase in ventricular dimension is accompanied by increases in AQP4 and IL-6 concentrations in the CSF of dogs with idiopathic communicating hydrocephalus. All were greatly reduced or normalised after shunt treatment. Therefore AQP4 and IL-6 in CSF can be indicators of ventriculomegaly, of cellular damage, and of improvement after the treatment of hydrocephalus. Based on the results of this study, a brain tissue-based determination of AQP4 at the mRNA and protein level might be rewarding to analyse the potential role of AQP4 in the compensation of extracellular fluid overload in dogs with communicating hydrocephalus.

### Authors' contributions
MJS and NO authors helped to draft the manuscript and participated in its design. MK and JH collected the data for the study. JR analyzed the data. CR performed the statistical analysis of the data. All authors read and approved the final manuscript.

### Author details
[1] Department of Veterinary Clinical Sciences, Small Animal Clinic, Justus-Liebig-University, Frankfurter Strasse 108, 35392 Giessen, Germany. [2] Institute for Veterinary Physiology and Biochemistry, Justus-Liebig-University, Frankfurter Strasse 100, 35392 Giessen, Germany. [3] Department of Companion Animal Clinical Studies, Faculty of Veterinary Science, University of Pretoria, Private Bag X04, Onderstepoort, Pretoria 0110, Republic of South Africa.

### Competing interests
The authors declare that they have no competing interests.

### References
1. Shibab N, Davies E, Kenny PJ, Loderstedt S, Volk HA. Treatment of hydrocephalus with ventriculoperitoneal shunting in twelve dogs. Vet Surg. 2011;40:477–84.
2. Platt S, Garosi L. Hydrocephalus. In: Small Animal Neurological Emergencies. London: Manson Publishing Ltd/The Veterinary Press; 2012. p. 116–7.
3. Biel M, Kramer M, Forterre F, Jurina K, Failing K, Schmidt MJ. Outcome of ventriculoperitoneal shunt implantation for treatment of congenital internal hydrocephalus in dogs and cats: 36 cases (2001–2009). J Am Vet Med Assoc. 2013;242:948–58.
4. Cinalli G, Maixner WJ, Sainte-Rose CJ. Shunt hardware and surgical technique In: Pediatric Hydrocephalus. Springer: New York; 2004, p. 295–315.
5. Kolecka M, Ondreka N, Moritz A, Kramer M, Schmidt MJ. Effect of acetazolamide and subsequent ventriculo-peritoneal shunting on clinical signs and ventricular volumes in dogs with internal hydrocephalus. Acta Vet Scand. 2015;57:49.
6. Kennedy CR, Ayers S, Campbell MJ, Elbourne D, Hope P, Johnson A. Randomized controlled trial of acetazolamide and furosemide in posthemorrhagic ventricular dilation in infancy: follow-up at 1 year. Pediatrics. 2001;108:597–607.
7. Girod M, Allerton F, Gommeren K, Tutunaru AC, de Marchin J, Van Soens I, Ramery E, Peeters D. Evaluation of the effect of oral omeprazole on canine cerebrospinal fluid production: a pilot study. Vet J. 2016;209:119–24.
8. Yool A. Aquaporins: multiple roles in the central nervous system. Neuroscientist. 2007;13:470–85.
9. Neuroscience Nedergaard M. Garbage truck of the brain. Science. 2013;28:1529–30.
10. Abbott NJ. Evidence for bulk flow of brain interstitial fluid: significance for physiology and pathology. Neurochem Intern. 2004;45:545–52.

11. Papadopoulos MC, Verkman AS. Aquaporin water channels in the nervous system. Nat Rev Neurosci. 2013;14:265–77.

12. Vizuete ML, Venero JL, Vargas C, Ilundáin AA, Echevarría M, Machado A, Cano J. Differential upregulation of aquaporin-4 mRNA expression in reactive astrocytes after brain injury: potential role in brain edema. Neurobiol Dis. 1999;6:245–58.

13. Deng J, Zhao F, Yu X, Zhao Y, Li D, Shi H, Sun Y. Expression of aquaporin 4 and breakdown of the blood-brain barrier after hypoglycemia-induced brain edema in rats. PLoS ONE. 2014;9(9):e107022. doi:10.1371/journal.pone.0107022.

14. Vella J, Zammit C, Digiovanni G, Muscat R, Valentino M. The central role of aquaporins in the pathophysiology of ischemic stroke. Front Cell Neurosci. 2015;9:108.

15. Mao X, Enno TL, Del Bigio MR. Aquaporin 4 changes in rat brain with severe hydrocephalus. Eur J Neurosci. 2006;23:2929–36.

16. Skjolding AD, Rowland IJ, Søgaard LV, Praetorius J, Penkowa M, Juhler M. Hydrocephalus induces dynamic spatiotemporal regulation of aquaporin-4 expression in the rat brain. Cerebrospinal Fluid Res. 2010;7:20.

17. Skjolding AD, Holst AV, Broholm H, Laursen H, Juhler M. Differences in distribution and regulation of astrocytic aquaporin-4 in human and rat hydrocephalic brain. Neuropathol Appl Neurobiol. 2012;39:171–90.

18. Castañeyra-Ruiz L, González-Marrero I, González-Toledo JM, Castañeyra-Ruiz A, de Paz-Carmona H, Castañeyra-Perdomo A, et al. Aquaporin-4 expression in the cerebrospinal fluid in congenital human hydrocephalus. Fluid Barriers CNS. 2013;10:18.

19. Shen XQ, Miyajima M, Ogino I, Arai H. Expression of the water-channel protein aquaporin 4 in the H-Tx rat: possible compensatory role in spontaneously arrested hydrocephalus. J Neurosurg. 2006;105:459–64.

20. Tourdias T, Dragonu I, Fushimi Y, Deloire MSA, Boiziau C, Brochet B, et al. Aquaporin 4 correlates with apparent diffusion coefficient and hydrocephalus severity in the rat brain: a combined MRI-histological study. Neuroimage. 2009;47:659–66.

21. Kalani MY, Filippidis AS, Rekate H. Hydrocephalus and aquaporins: the role of aquaporin-1. Acta Neurochirurg. 2012;113:51–4.

22. Kaur C, Ling EA. Periventricular white matter damage in the hypoxic neonatal brain: role of microglial cells. Progr Neurobiol. 2009;87:264–80.

23. Erta M, Quintana A, Hidalgo J. Interleukin-6, a major cytokine in the central nervous system. Int J Biol Sci. 2012;8(9):1254–66.

24. Laubner S, Ondreka N, Failing K, Kramer M, Schmidt MJ. Magnetic resonance imaging signs of high intraventricular pressure—comparison of findings in dogs with clinically relevant internal hydrocephalus and asymptomatic dogs with ventriculomegaly. BMC Vet Sci. 2015;11:181.

25. Cinalli G, Maixner WJ, Sainte-Rose CJ. Classification and defnition of hydrocephalus. In: Pediatric Hydrocephalus. Springer: New York; 2004, p. 95–112.

26. Schmidt MJ, Oelschläger HA, Haddad D, Purea A, Haase A, Kramer M. Visualizing premature brain using 17.6 Tesla magnetic resonance imaging (magnetic resonance microscopy). Vet J. 2009;182:215–22.

27. Roth J, Martin D, Störr B. Zeisberger E Neutralization of pyrogen-induced tumour necrosis factor by its type 1 soluble receptor in guinea-pigs: effects on fever and interleukin-6 release. J Physiol. 1998;509(Pt 1):267–75.

28. Moeniralam HS, Bemelman WA, Endert E, Koopmans R, Sauerwein HP, Romijn JA. The decrease in nonsplenic interleukin-6 (IL-6) production after splenectomy indicates the existence of a positive feedback loop of IL-6 production during endotoxemia in dogs. Infect Immun. 1997;65(6):2299–305.

29. Bloch O, Auguste KI, Manley GT, Verkman AS. Accelerated progression of kaolin induced hydrocephalus in aquaporin-4-deficient mice. J Cer Blood Flow Metab. 2006;26:1527–37.

30. James AE, Burns B, Flor WF, Strecker EP, Merz T, Bush M, et al. Pathophysiology of chronic communicating hydrocephalus in dogs (Canis familiaris). Experimental studies. J Neurol Sci. 1975;24:151–78.

31. De Lahunta A, Glass EN. Cerebrospinal fluid and hydrocephalus. In: Veterinary neuroanatomy and clinical neurology. 3rd edn. Saunders: St. Louis; 2009. p.78–101.

32. Brinker T, Stopa E, Morrison J, Klinge P. A new look at cerebrospinal fluid circulation. Fluids Barriers CNS. 2014;11:10.

33. Page LK. Cerebrospinal fluid and extracellular fluid: their relationship to pressure and duration of canine hydrocephalus. Childs Nerv Syst. 1985;1:12–7.

34. Del Bigio MR. Neuropathological changes caused by hydrocephalus. Acta Neuropath. 1993;85:573–85.

35. Li X, Kong H, Wu W, Xiao M, Sun X, Hu G. AQP4 maintains ependymal integrity in adult mice. Neuroscience. 2009;162:67–77.

36. Wen H, Frokiaer J, Kwon TH, Nielsen S. Urinary excretion of aquaporin-2 in rat is mediated by a vasopressin-dependent apical pathway. J Am Soc Nephrol. 1999;10:1416–29.

37. Fushimi K, Uchida S, Hara Y, Hirata Y, Marumo F, Sasaki S. Cloning and expression of apical membrane water channel of rat kidney collecting tubule. Nature. 1993;361:549–52.

38. Kanno K, Sasaki S, Hirata Y, Ishikawa S, Fushimi K, Nakanishi S, et al. Urinary excretion of aquaporin-2 in patients with diabetes insipidus. New England J Med. 1995;332:1540–5.

39. Sasaki S, Fushimi K, Saito H. Cloning, characterization and chromosomal mapping of human aquaporin of collecting duct. J Clin Invest. 1994;93:1250–6.

40. Saito T, Ishikawa SE, Ando F, Okada N, Nakamura T, Kusaka I, et al. Exaggerated urinary excretion of aquaporin-2 in the pathological state of impaired water excretion dependent upon arginine vasopressin. J Clin Endocrinol Metab. 1998;83:4034–40.

41. Wang D, Nykanen M, Yang N, Winlaw D, North K, Verkman AS, Owler BK. Altered cellular localization of aquaporin-1 in experimental hydrocephalus in mice and reduced ventriculomegaly in aquaporin-1 deficiency. Mol Cell Neurosci. 2011;46:318–24.

42. Savman K, Blennow M, Gustafson K, Tarkowski E, Hagberg H. Cytokine response in cerebrospinal fluid after birth asphyxia. Pediatric Res. 1998;43:746–51.

43. Nagai K, Kozaki K, Sonohara K, Akishita M, Toba K. Relationship between interleukin-6 and cerebral deep white matter and periventricular hyperintensity in elderly women. Geriatr Geront Int. 2011;11:328–32.

44. Bettcher BM, Watson CL, Walsh CM, Lobach IV, Neuhaus J, Miller JW, et al. Interleukin-6, age, and corpus callosum integrity. PLoS ONE. 2004;4(9):e106521.

# 7

# Revisiting atenolol as a low passive permeability marker

Xiaomei Chen[1,2], Tim Slättengren[1], Elizabeth C. M. de Lange[3], David E. Smith[2] and Margareta Hammarlund-Udenaes[1]* (iD)

## Abstract

**Background:** Atenolol, a hydrophilic beta blocker, has been used as a model drug for studying passive permeability of biological membranes such as the blood–brain barrier (BBB) and the intestinal epithelium. However, the extent of S-atenolol (the active enantiomer) distribution in brain has never been evaluated, at equilibrium, to confirm that no transporters are involved in its transport at the BBB.

**Methods:** To assess whether S-atenolol, in fact, depicts the characteristics of a low passive permeable drug at the BBB, a microdialysis study was performed in rats to monitor the unbound concentrations of S-atenolol in brain extracellular fluid (ECF) and plasma during and after intravenous infusion. A pharmacokinetic model was developed, based on the microdialysis data, to estimate the permeability clearance of S-atenolol into and out of brain. In addition, the nonspecific binding of S-atenolol in brain homogenate was evaluated using equilibrium dialysis.

**Results:** The steady-state ratio of unbound S-atenolol concentrations in brain ECF to that in plasma (i.e., $K_{p,uu,brain}$) was 3.5% ± 0.4%, a value much less than unity. The unbound volume of distribution in brain ($V_{u, brain}$) of S-atenolol was also calculated as 0.69 ± 0.10 mL/g brain, indicating that S-atenolol is evenly distributed within brain parenchyma. Lastly, equilibrium dialysis showed limited nonspecific binding of S-atenolol in brain homogenate with an unbound fraction ($f_{u,brain}$) of 0.88 ± 0.07.

**Conclusions:** It is concluded, based on $K_{p,uu,brain}$ being much smaller than unity, that S-atenolol is actively effluxed at the BBB, indicating the need to re-consider S-atenolol as a model drug for passive permeability studies of BBB transport or intestinal absorption.

**Keywords:** Atenolol, Blood–brain barrier, Microdialysis, Unbound equilibrium partition coefficient ($K_{p,uu,brain}$), Unbound volume of distribution in brain ($V_{u,brain}$), Passive permeability, Transporters, Pharmacokinetics, Lipophilicity

## Background

Atenolol is a selective beta receptor blocker for the treatment of hypertension with the enantiomer S-atenolol responsible for the main active pharmacological effect [1–3]. For a long time, atenolol has been considered as a typical representative of a hydrophilic small molecule with low passive permeability and low paracellular diffusion across intestinal membrane and blood–brain barrier (BBB). Thus, it has been used as a model drug in developing and evaluating in vitro or in situ models for intestinal absorption and CNS penetration [4–6].

Like the intestinal epithelium, the BBB is characterized by tight junctions formed between adjacent cerebral capillary endothelial cells. These restrict paracellular transport, a pathway important for ions and other small hydrophilic molecules, which thus have lower permeability across the BBB and enterocytes. On the other hand, tight junctions have a limited effect on the BBB and intestinal permeability for lipophilic molecules that mainly use the transcellular pathway [7].

There have been several in vivo methods developed to assess the rate of drug transport across the BBB, including intravenous injection to measure the BBB

*Correspondence: mhu@farmbio.uu.se
[1] Department of Pharmaceutical Biosciences, Translational PKPD Research Group, Uppsala University, Box 591, SE-75124 Uppsala, Sweden
Full list of author information is available at the end of the article

permeability surface area product, intra-arterial injection to measure the brain uptake index, as well as in situ brain perfusion to assess BBB permeability using well-controlled perfusate [8–10]. From the above methods, if the samples are collected at very early time points, drug transport from brain back to blood is considered to be low and thus negligible, in which case the rate of initial brain uptake can be specifically studied. However, this includes possible influences of efflux transporters on the rate of brain uptake. Instead of assessing transport rate across the BBB, microdialysis can be used to evaluate the rate as well as extent of drug transport by measuring unbound drug concentrations in the extracellular fluid (ECF) of brain tissues over a longer duration. By modeling the microdialysis data with the information of unbound drug volume of distribution in brain ($V_{u,brain}$) the permeability in both directions, influx clearance into brain ($CL_{in}$) and efflux clearance from brain ($CL_{out}$), can also be estimated [11]. $CL_{in}$ and $CL_{out}$ values are determined by the contribution of both passive diffusion and active transport. Moreover, $CL_{out}$ may be affected by metabolism and ECF bulk flow [12]. The ratio of $CL_{in}$ over $CL_{out}$ values, is equal to the unbound equilibrium partition coefficient, $K_{p,uu,brain}$, which is defined as the ratio of unbound drug concentration in brain ECF to that in plasma at the steady state [13]. Even when steady state concentrations are not achieved, but with rate processes following first order kinetics (i.e. linear pharmacokinetics), $K_{p,uu,brain}$ can be estimated using the ratio of area under curve of unbound drug concentration–time profiles ($AUC_u$) in brain ECF to $AUC_u$ in plasma. It should be noted that the $K_{p,uu,brain}$ value reflects the *extent* of unbound drug concentration equilibration between brain and plasma, but not the rate with which a drug crosses the BBB [12]. Typically, BBB permeability is a measure of the *rate* of BBB transport of the drug. Compounds with lower lipophilicities tend to have lower BBB permeability, only if passive transport governs the exchange of drug molecules across the BBB.

For a drug with only passive transport across the BBB, it holds that $CL_{in} = CL_{out}$ with respect to unbound drug, making $K_{p,uu,brain}$ equal to unity. In other words, at steady state, the unbound drug concentration in brain ECF is equal to that in plasma. Drugs with a low BBB permeability just need more time to reach such equilibrium, but $K_{p,uu,brain}$ is independent of BBB permeability [12].

If atenolol were a typical drug of low passive BBB permeability, it would have equal $CL_{in}$ and $CL_{out}$, leading to the following characteristics: (1) without any carrier-mediated transport or being metabolized in brain, its $K_{p,uu,brain}$ value would be unity [12]; (2) as the net direction of mass transport for passive diffusion is only determined by unbound concentration gradient between the

two sides of BBB, its unbound brain concentration would keep increasing when higher unbound concentrations are present in blood than in brain (i.e. $C_{u,blood} > C_{u,brain}$) and $C_{u,brain}$ would start decreasing when $C_{u,blood} < C_{u,brain}$. However, a previous microdialysis study of atenolol in rats showed a ratio of $AUC_u$ in brain ECF to AUC in plasma of only $3.8 \pm 0.6\%$ after an intravenous 10 mg bolus dose. In addition, the peak of the $C_{u,brain}$ was at around 10 min, when the plasma concentration was much higher than $C_{u,brain}$. Moreover, both unbound brain and plasma concentration–time profiles had the same half-lives [14]. This is not consistent with the expected profile described above for compounds with only passive permeability. Instead, the reported $C_{u,brain}$-time profile of atenolol resembles that of compounds with active efflux, based on the simulations performed by Hammarlund-Udenaes et al. [15].

If indeed atenolol has a very low $K_{p,uu,brain}$ due to it being a substrate of an efflux transporter, it has important implications on the role of atenolol as a model drug for low passive permeability (i.e. low paracellular diffusion without any carrier-mediated transport), and thus the conclusions from the related research of biological membrane barriers may need reevaluation. Therefore, the aim of this study was to investigate in-depth the in vivo net flux of S-atenolol BBB transport. To that end, a detailed microdialysis study was carried out to evaluate the $K_{p,uu,brain}$ of S-atenolol, and investigate its intra-brain distribution by assessing the $V_{u,brain}$ and the unbound drug fraction in brain homogenate ($f_{u,brain}$). Modeling and simulation were used to describe the properties of atenolol from a rate and extent perspective.

## Methods
### Chemicals
S-(−)-atenolol and atenolol-D7 were purchased from Sigma-Aldrich (St. Louis, MO, USA). Isoflurane was obtained from Baxter Medical AB (Kista, Sweden). Ringer's solution was prepared to perfuse microdialysis probes and comprised 145 mM NaCl, 0.6 mM KCl, 1.0 mM $MgCl_2$, 1.2 mM $CaCl_2$, and 0.2 mM ascorbic acid in 2 mM phosphate buffer (pH 7.4). Normal saline was obtained from Braun Medical AB (Stockholm, Sweden), and water was purified using a Milli-Q system (Millipore, Bedford, MA, USA). Ammonium acetate and acetonitrile were purchased from Merck (Darmstadt, Germany). All other chemicals were of analytical grade.

### Animals
Male Sprague–Dawley rats (250–310 g) were obtained from Taconic (Lille Skensved, Denmark). The animals were acclimated for 1 week before the experiment and housed in groups with 12-hour day-night cycles at 22 °C.

The microdialysis study was approved by the Animal Ethics Committee of Uppsala University, Sweden (C328/10).

**Microdialysis study**

For the microdialysis study, vessel catheters and microdialysis probes were implanted in rats as previously described [13, 16]. Briefly, the rats were anesthetized using 2.5% isoflurane and their body temperature were maintained at 37 °C using CMA/150 temperature controller (CMA, Stockholm, Sweden) throughout the surgery. Firstly, a catheter made from PE-50 fused with silicon tubing was implanted into the femoral vein for S-atenolol infusion, followed by the insertion of a PE-50 catheter fused with PE-10 into the femoral artery for blood sampling. Secondly, an incision was made to insert a CMA/20 microdialysis probe (CMA, Stockholm, Sweden) with 10 mm flexible polyarylethersulphone (PAES) membrane into the right jugular vein for sampling unbound S-atenolol in plasma. Then, the head of the rat was fixed on a stereotaxic frame and a guide cannula was implanted into striatum with the coordinates 0.8 mm anterior, 2.7 mm lateral to the bregma, and 3.8 mm ventral to the surface of the skull. Dental cement was used to fix the guide cannula onto the skull with an anchor screw. The tubing of the vessel catheters and microdialysis probe were tunneled subcutaneously and fixed at the back of the neck. At the end of the surgery, the dummy inside the guide cannula was replaced by a CMA/12 microdialysis probe (CMA, Stockholm, Sweden) with a 3 mm PAES membrane (20 kDa cutoff) for sampling S-atenolol in brain ECF. The rats were allowed

to recover for 1 day before the microdialysis study and to move freely in a CMA 120 system with free access to food and water.

As shown in Fig. 1, the rats were divided into two groups with different dosing regimens. The infusion solution had a drug concentration of 5 mg/mL. Group 1 (n = 9) received S-atenolol starting with a fast infusion at 0.4 mg/min/kg for 15 min followed by a slow infusion of 0.182 mg/min/kg for 165 min using a Harvard 22 pump (Harvard Apparatus Inc., Holliston, MA, USA) in order to rapidly achieve steady state concentrations in plasma. Samples were collected for another 3 h after the end of drug infusion in four rats (Group 1a). The rats in Group 1b (n = 5) were decapitated at the end of the infusion to harvest the brains in order to measure the total S-atenolol amount in brain tissue. In Group 2 (n = 4), S-atenolol was given as a single constant infusion for 3 h at a rate of 0.167 mg/min/kg, and continuing sampling for 3 h thereafter. In all rats, the microdialysis perfusion was started at the beginning of the stabilization period, 90 min before S-atenolol dosing. Deuterated atenolol, atenolol-D7, was used to measure the relative recovery across the microdialysis probes throughout the study, using retrodialysis by the atenolol-D7 as a calibrator [17, 18]. Atenolol-D7 was added to the Ringer's solution at 50 ng/mL for brain probe and at 200 ng/mL for plasma probe, which were perfused through the microdialysis probes using a CMA 400 pump (CMA, Solna, Sweden) at a flow rate of 1 μL/min. The dialysates were collected every 15 min by a fraction collector (CMA 142, Solna, Sweden) until the end of experiment. For the animals with their drug elimination

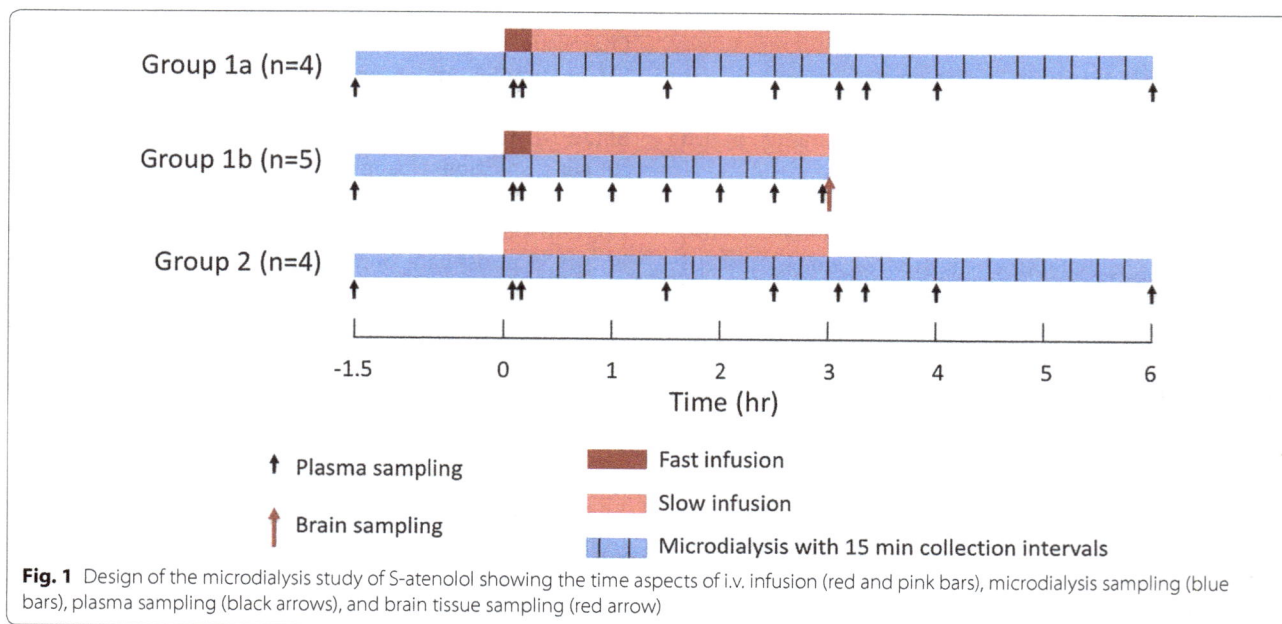

**Fig. 1** Design of the microdialysis study of S-atenolol showing the time aspects of i.v. infusion (red and pink bars), microdialysis sampling (blue bars), plasma sampling (black arrows), and brain tissue sampling (red arrow)

phase monitored, 100 µL of blood was drawn from the femoral artery pre-dose and at 5, 10, 90, 150, 185, 200, 240, and 360 min after the start of S-atenolol infusion. For the rats decapitated at the end of drug infusion, the blood was collected pre-dose and at 5, 10, 30, 60, 90, 120, 150, and 175 min. All blood samples were centrifuged at 7200g for 5 min to obtain plasma, which together with brain and microdialysis samples were frozen at − 20 °C until analysis.

### Equilibrium dialysis study

The $f_{u,brain}$ at three drug concentrations was measured in vitro using equilibrium dialysis of brain homogenate. Briefly, Sprague–Dawley rats were decapitated under isoflurane anesthesia and the brains were collected and homogenized in four volumes of 180 mM phosphate buffer. After being spiked with 132.5, 265, and 1325 ng/mL S-atenolol (corresponding to 0.5, 1, and 5 µM), 150 µL of the blank homogenate was dialyzed against PBS pH 7.4 for 6 h using a Pierce Rapid Equilibrium Dialysis Device (RED) (Thermo Scientific, Rockford, IL, USA) (n = 5 at each concentration) with a shaking speed of 200 rpm at 37 °C (MaxQ4450, Thermo Fisher Scientific, Nino Lab, Sweden). Samples were collected from both buffer and homogenate sides at the end of the incubation period of 6 h. The stability of S-atenolol in brain homogenate was evaluated by incubating homogenate containing the drug at the three concentrations and collecting samples before and after the incubation. In order to obtain the same matrix for all samples in the chemical assay, the same volume of buffer was added to brain homogenate samples and vice versa. All samples were stored at − 20 °C until assay. The unbound fraction of S-atenolol in diluted brain homogenate ($f_{u,hD}$) was calculated from the buffer/homogenate concentration ratio as:

$$f_{u,hD} = \frac{C_{buffer}}{C_{homogenate}} \quad (1)$$

The unbound fraction of S-atenolol in brain was calculated according to Eq. 2 after correction for the dilution factor D associated with the preparation of brain homogenate (D = 5 in this study):

$$f_{u,brain} = \frac{1}{1 + D\left(\frac{1}{f_{u,hD}} - 1\right)} \quad (2)$$

### Chemical analysis

Liquid chromatography coupled with tandem mass spectrometry (LC–MS/MS) was used to determine the concentrations of S-atenolol and atenolol-D7 in the microdialysis samples. Five microliters of the brain microdialysis samples were directly injected into the system. The plasma dialysate samples (15 µL) having

high drug concentrations were diluted by adding 150 µL Ringer's solution before analysis. After thawing to room temperature, the plasma samples were precipitated at a ratio of 1:3 with acetonitrile containing 500 ng/mL atenolol-D7 as internal standard. Following vortex mixing and centrifugation for 3 min at 7200g, 25 µL of the supernatant was further diluted by mixing it with 1 mL of 5 mM ammonium acetate solution and then injecting 10 µL of the mixture into the LC–MS/MS. The brain samples were homogenized with a tissue-saline ratio of 1:4 (w/v), prepared as described above. Then 150 µL of the homogenate was mixed with 150 µL of 50 ng/mL atenolol-D7 aqueous solution, and further precipitated with 150 µL acetonitrile. After 3 min centrifugation at 7200g, the supernatant was diluted tenfold with 5 mM ammonium acetate, injecting 50 µL. The homogenate samples from equilibrium dialysis were prepared with the same procedures as above. Standard curves were generated for all types of biological matrix (i.e., 0.5–500 ng/mL for dialysate; 50–10,000 ng/mL for plasma; 25–1000 ng/g brain for brain tissues from microdialysis study; 6.25–875 ng/mL for brain homogenate samples from equilibrium dialysis study) and quality control samples at low, medium and high concentrations were analyzed along with the samples for measurement validation. The coefficients of determination ($r^2$) were ≥ 0.994 for all standard curves.

The LC–MS/MS system consisted of two Shimadzu LC-10ADvp pumps (Shimadzu, Kyoto, Japan), a SIL-HTc autosampler (Shimadzu, Kyoto, Japan), and a Quattro Ultima mass spectrometer (Waters, Milford, MA, USA). A HyPurity C18 column (50 × 4.6 mm, 3 µm particle size), equipped with a HyPurity C18 guard column (10 × 4.0 mm, 3 µm particle size, Thermo Scientific Hypersil-Keystone, PA, USA), was used for chromatographic separation with a gradient elution involving mobile phase A (5 mM ammonium acetate in water) and mobile phase B (90:10 v/v acetonitrile:water). The flow rate was set to 0.8 mL/min, which was split to 0.3 mL/min before entering the mass spectrometer, where positive electrospray ionization (ESI +) was applied. The transition mode was $m/z$ 266.9 → 145 for S-atenolol and $m/z$ 273.8 → 145 for atenolol-D7. All chromatographs were acquired and analyzed using Masslynx 4.0 (Waters, Milford, MA, USA).

### Calculations and pharmacokinetic data analysis

The relative recovery of S-atenolol for each microdialysis probe was evaluated using retrodialysis with atenolol-D7 as a calibrator according to

$$Recovery = \frac{C_{in,ATD7} - C_{out,ATD7}}{C_{in,ATD7}} \quad (3)$$

where $C_{in,ATD7}$ and $C_{out,ATD7}$ are the concentrations of atenolol-D7 in perfusate and dialysate, respectively [18]. The relative recovery simultaneously determined by the retrodialysis of atenolol-D7 was $6.94 \pm 0.67\%$ for the microdialysis probes in brain and $50.1 \pm 1.9\%$ for the probes in blood without any time-dependence. The unbound concentration of S-atenolol in brain ECF and plasma was calculated by dividing the measured S-atenolol concentration in dialysate by the relative recovery.

The $K_{p,uu,brain}$ was calculated to characterize the extent of S-atenolol equilibration across the BBB as:

$$K_{p,uu,brain} = \frac{C_{u,ss,brainECF}}{C_{u,ss,plasma}} \qquad (4)$$

where $C_{u,ss,brainECF}$ and $C_{u,ss,plasma}$ are the unbound drug concentrations in brain ECF and plasma at the steady state, respectively.

The half-lives in brain ECF and plasma, $t_{1/2,brainECF}$ and $t_{1/2,plasma}$, were calculated based on the corresponding middle time points of microdialysis collection intervals of the elimination phase:

$$t_{1/2} = \frac{0.693}{\lambda_z} \qquad (5)$$

where $\lambda_z$ is the terminal rate constant obtained from the last seven observations. The half-lives of unbound S-atenolol in brain ECF and plasma were compared using paired t test.

A pharmacokinetic model was developed using nonlinear mixed effect modeling (NONMEM, version 7.3.0, ICON Development Solutions, Ellicott City, MD, US) to describe the rate of S-atenolol transport across the BBB via $CL_{in}$ and $CL_{out}$. The method of first-order conditional estimation with interaction (FOCEI) was used throughout the modeling procedure. The inter-individual variability was investigated for all pharmacokinetic parameters during the model development using an exponential model:

$$P_i = P_{pop}e^{\eta_i} \qquad (6)$$

where $P_i$ is the value of the parameter for the i-th individual, while $P_{pop}$ is the typical value of the parameter in the population. The inter-individual variability was described by $\eta$, which was assumed to follow a normal distribution with a mean at 0 and standard deviation $\omega$. In addition, different error models (proportional, additive, and slope-intercept error models) were explored to evaluate the residual variability, i.e. the difference between predicted and observed concentrations, for each type of observations.

The model selection was based on the objective function value (OFV), model parameter precision and graphical analysis. The likelihood ratio test was used to compare between nested models. Specifically, the difference in OFV between two nested models asymptotically follows $\chi2$ distribution, and a drop in OFV of $\geq 3.84$ indicates the superiority of the model for one-parameter difference with $p \leq 0.05$. The parameter precision was described by relative standard error, RSE %, which was calculated as the standard error (S.E.) divided by the parameter estimate. The graphical analyses were performed using PsN (version 4.4.0, Uppsala University, Uppsala, Sweden) and Xpose 4 (version 4.5.3, Uppsala University, Uppsala, Sweden) together with R (version 3.3.1, R Foundation for Statistical Computing, Vienna, Austria).

The previously developed integrated plasma-brain pharmacokinetic model for oxymorphone, oxycodone, and DAMGO was used in this study, with modification based on the data from the microdialysis study of S-atenolol [13, 19, 20]. All observed data of S-atenolol were included in the model comprising total plasma concentration in arterial sampling, unbound concentration in venous plasma from microdialysis sampling in jugular vein, and unbound concentration in brain ECF from microdialysis sampling in right striatum (Fig. 2). The model also took into account the relative recovery by including the concentrations of the calibrator atenolol-D7 in dialysate from both probes.

The model development started by building a plasma PK model, followed by adding the other compartments in steps. The parameters in the final model were estimated simultaneously based on all data. In the model, the central compartment was divided into two compartments, an arterial compartment for plasma concentration and a venous compartment for microdialysis sampling. The two compartments were assumed to have equal unbound volume of distribution, that is, $VA = VV$. The transport of S-atenolol across the BBB was parameterized by $CL_{in}$ and $K_{p,uu,brain}$, which were assessed according to:

$$CL_{in} = k_{in} \cdot VA \qquad (7)$$

$$K_{p,uu,brain} = \frac{CL_{in}}{CL_{out}} \qquad (8)$$

$$CL_{out} = k_{out} \cdot V_{u,brain} \qquad (9)$$

where $k_{in}$ and $k_{out}$ denote the rate constants between the arterial compartment and the brain compartment. $V_{u,brain}$ (mL/g brain) reflects the drug distribution within brain parenchyma since it describes the relationship between the total drug amount in brain and the unbound drug concentration in brain ECF:

$$V_{u,brain} = \frac{A_{brain} - C_p \times V_{bl} \times R_{bl-p}}{C_{u,ECF}} \qquad (10)$$

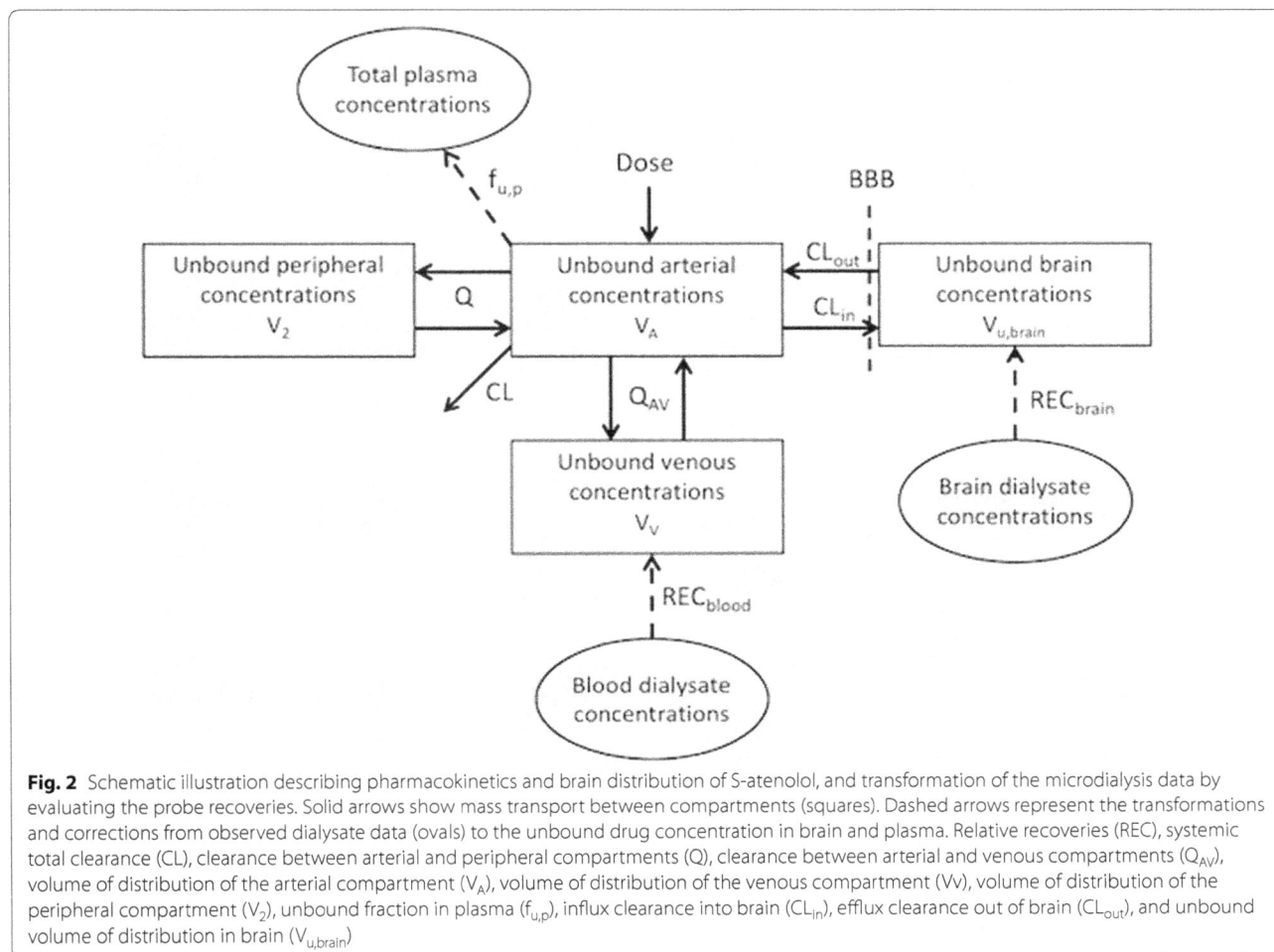

**Fig. 2** Schematic illustration describing pharmacokinetics and brain distribution of S-atenolol, and transformation of the microdialysis data by evaluating the probe recoveries. Solid arrows show mass transport between compartments (squares). Dashed arrows represent the transformations and corrections from observed dialysate data (ovals) to the unbound drug concentration in brain and plasma. Relative recoveries (REC), systemic total clearance (CL), clearance between arterial and peripheral compartments (Q), clearance between arterial and venous compartments ($Q_{AV}$), volume of distribution of the arterial compartment ($V_A$), volume of distribution of the venous compartment (Vv), volume of distribution of the peripheral compartment ($V_2$), unbound fraction in plasma ($f_{u,p}$), influx clearance into brain ($CL_{in}$), efflux clearance out of brain ($CL_{out}$), and unbound volume of distribution in brain ($V_{u,brain}$)

where $A_{brain}$ is the measured drug amount in brain and $C_p$ is the plasma concentration at the end of infusion. The volume of vascular space in rat brain ($V_{bl}$) is 0.014 mL/g brain [21], and the blood-to-plasma concentration ratio of atenolol ($R_{bl-p}$) is reported as 1.07 [22].

In order to illustrate the difference between efflux-transported drug and a drug with only passive diffusion across the BBB, simulations were performed for the cases: (1) $CL_{in} = CL_{out}$ and (2) $CL_{in} < CL_{out}$ with a constant i.v. infusion of 0.167 mg/min/kg (assuming a 280-g rat). The PK parameters were set as the typical values obtained from S-atenolol modeling.

All data are expressed as mean ± SEM in this report and GraphPad Prism v5.04 (GraphPad Software Inc., San Diego, CA) was used for statistical analysis and plots.

## Results

### Microdialysis study

In Group 1, the unbound S-atenolol concentration in plasma increased quickly during the 15-min fast infusion and was maintained at steady state ($C_{u,ss,plasma}$) during the following 165 min slow infusion (Fig. 3a). The concentrations in plasma were comparable to the unbound S-atenolol concentration in plasma, indicating little to no binding of drug in plasma ($f_{u,p}$ approaches 1). The steady state unbound concentration of S-atenolol in brain ECF was also quickly achieved and the concentration–time profile during elimination phase exhibited a similar shape to that in plasma. However, the brain ECF concentrations were much lower than in plasma throughout the whole experiment. The unbound S-atenolol steady-state concentration in plasma calculated from 90 to 180 min was 4429 ± 94 ng/mL, nearly 30-fold higher than in brain ECF (158 ± 20 ng/mL). The concentration–time profile of atenolol in Group 2 for the 3 h constant i.v. infusion followed a similar pattern (Fig. 3b). The unbound S-atenolol level gradually increased during the infusion in plasma and brain ECF to 4127 ± 103 ng/mL and 256 ± 41 ng/mL, respectively, at the last time point before the infusion ended.

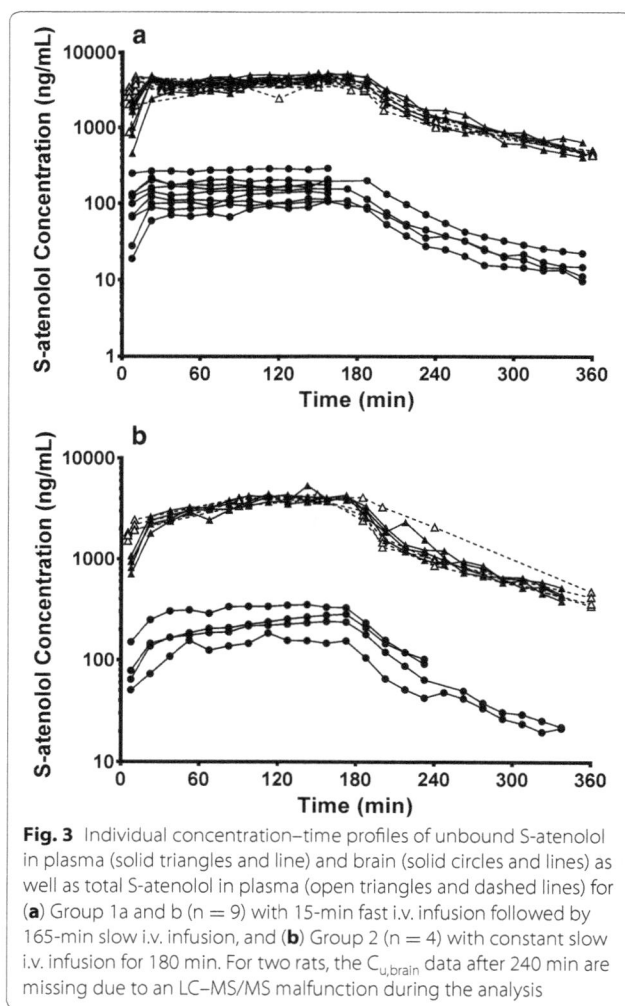

**Fig. 3** Individual concentration–time profiles of unbound S-atenolol in plasma (solid triangles and line) and brain (solid circles and lines) as well as total S-atenolol in plasma (open triangles and dashed lines) for (**a**) Group 1a and b (n = 9) with 15-min fast i.v. infusion followed by 165-min slow i.v. infusion, and (**b**) Group 2 (n = 4) with constant slow i.v. infusion for 180 min. For two rats, the $C_{u,brain}$ data after 240 min are missing due to an LC–MS/MS malfunction during the analysis

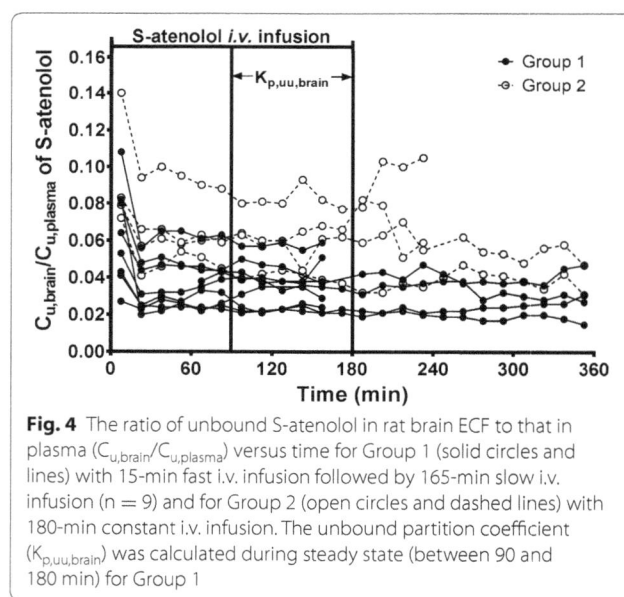

**Fig. 4** The ratio of unbound S-atenolol in rat brain ECF to that in plasma ($C_{u,brain}/C_{u,plasma}$) versus time for Group 1 (solid circles and lines) with 15-min fast i.v. infusion followed by 165-min slow i.v. infusion (n = 9) and for Group 2 (open circles and dashed lines) with 180-min constant i.v. infusion. The unbound partition coefficient ($K_{p,uu,brain}$) was calculated during steady state (between 90 and 180 min) for Group 1

There was a rapid exchange and equilibration of S-atenolol across the BBB in spite of its low passive permeability. For both groups during the elimination phase, brain ECF concentrations decreased at the same rate as in plasma, which was confirmed by similar terminal half-lives in brain ECF and plasma (82 ± 7 min vs 85 ± 10 min, p = 0.325, paired t-test). In addition, the unbound brain to plasma ratio with time was stable both during the infusion period and during the elimination phase (Fig. 4). The $K_{p,uu,brain}$ of S-atenolol was 3.55% ± 0.40% during 90–180 min.

The $V_{u,brain}$ of S-atenolol was 0.686 ± 0.104 mL/g brain calculated from Eq. 10, which was not significantly different from the brain total water volume (0.8 mL/g brain) (p = 0.137). This suggested an even distribution of atenolol in brain with nonsignificant binding to brain parenchymal tissue and similar drug concentration in brain ECF and intracellular fluid (ICF) [12].

## Equilibrium dialysis study

From the equilibrium dialysis of brain homogenates, it was found that the $f_{u,brain}$ of S-atenolol was 0.74 ± 0.04, 0.80 ± 0.04, and 1.09 ± 0.15 at the S-atenolol incubation concentrations of 0.5, 1.0, and 5.0 µM, respectively. There was no significant difference among the three S-atenolol levels with p = 0.0833 from one-way ANOVA analysis, suggesting that the nonspecific binding of S-atenolol in brain homogenate was independent of the incubation concentration. The average $f_{u,brain}$ from all the three concentration groups was 0.875 ± 0.067, comparable with a previously reported value of 0.90 ± 0.052 [23], indicating very limited binding in brain homogenate, in line with the $V_{u,brain}$ estimates presented above. S-atenolol was very stable in brain homogenate with zero degradation (100 ± 1% recovery) during the 6 h incubation at 37 °C.

## Pharmacokinetic modeling

To be able to calculate the BBB clearance values, and to better understand the kinetics of S-atenolol transport at the BBB, a pharmacokinetic model including a brain compartment was developed based on the microdialysis data. The individual plots in Fig. 5 show observations, individual predictions and population predictions of S-atenolol in plasma, blood dialysate, and brain dialysate. A noticeable discrepancy between population and individual profiles was observed for some individuals (e.g. ID11 in brain dialysate), which may explain the large inter-individual variation for some parameters (Table 1). Nevertheless, the model is appropriate for describing S-atenolol distribution in plasma and brain, given the close median lines of real data and model-based simulation data in the

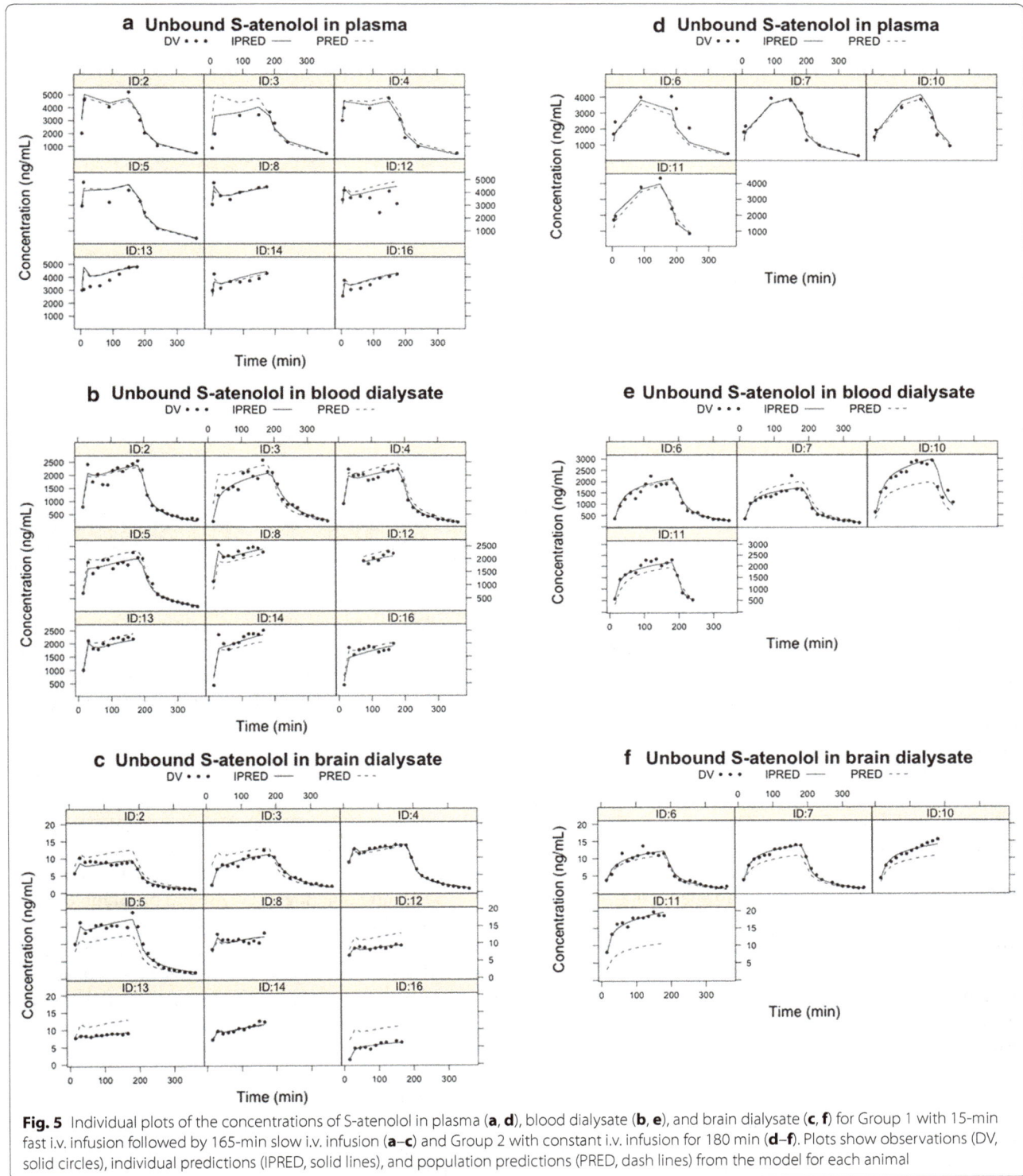

**Fig. 5** Individual plots of the concentrations of S-atenolol in plasma (**a**, **d**), blood dialysate (**b**, **e**), and brain dialysate (**c**, **f**) for Group 1 with 15-min fast i.v. infusion followed by 165-min slow i.v. infusion (**a–c**) and Group 2 with constant i.v. infusion for 180 min (**d–f**). Plots show observations (DV, solid circles), individual predictions (IPRED, solid lines), and population predictions (PRED, dash lines) from the model for each animal

visual predictive check based on 200 simulations (Fig. 6). The typical values of relative recoveries estimated from the model that included atenolol-D7 concentrations

in dialysates are comparable to the values calculated directly from Eq. 1, and the model-estimated $K_{p,uu,brain}$ of 4.00% is also comparable to the value of 3.55% from Eq. 4.

**Table 1** Parameter estimates of the S-atenolol pharmacokinetic model in rats

| Parameter | Unit | Estimate | RSE (%) | IIV (%) | RSE IIV (%) |
|---|---|---|---|---|---|
| $REC_{blood}$ | % | 49.9 | 3.5 | 12.2 | 24.8 |
| $REC_{brain}$ | % | 6.73 | 9.5 | 27.9 | 17.2 |
| CL | mL/min | 10.2 | 2.4 | 7.5 | 16.9 |
| $V_1$ | mL | 215 | 10.8 | 30.3 | 28.4 |
| Q | mL/min | 5.56 | 8.9 | | |
| $V_2$ | mL | 402 | 4.8 | | |
| $f_{u,p}$ | | 1.0 | Fixed | | |
| $Q_{AV}$ | mL/min | 15.4 | 9.2 | | |
| $CL_{in}$ | μL/min/gbrain | 17.0 | 48.8 | 134.2 | 27.5 |
| $K_{p,uu,brain}$ | | 0.040 | 11.3 | 35.5 | 18.0 |
| $V_{u,brain}$ | mL/g brain | 0.686 | Fixed | | |
| $\sigma_{proportional,RECbrain}$ | | 0.028 | 9.4 | | |
| $\sigma_{additive,RECblood}$ | ng/mL | 7.83 | 5.1 | | |
| $\sigma_{proportional,plasma}$ | | 0.184 | 20.3 | | |
| $\sigma_{proportional,blood}$ | | 0.112 | 8.8 | | |
| $\sigma_{proportional,brain}$ | | 0.0741 | 12.3 | | |
| $\sigma_{additive,brain}$ | ng/mL | 0.22 | 20.2 | | |

*RSE* relative standard error; *IIV* Inter-individual variation expressed as coefficient of variation; *REC* relative recoveries; *CL* systemic total clearance; $V_1$ volume of distribution of total arterial and venous compartments; *Q* clearance between arterial and peripheral compartments; $V_2$ volume of distribution of the peripheral compartment; $f_{u,p}$ unbound fraction in plasma; $Q_{AV}$ clearance between arterial and venous compartments; $Cl_{in}$ influx clearance into brain; $K_{p,uu,brain}$ unbound partition coefficient in brain; $V_{u,brain}$ unbound volume of distribution in brain; $\sigma$ variances of the proportional or additive residual errors

$CL_{in}$ is estimated as 17.0 μL/min/g brain, and the resultant $CL_{out}$ is 425 μL/min/g brain based on the definition of $K_{p,uu,brain}$, as the ratio of $CL_{in}$ to $CL_{out}$.

To illustrate the unbound concentration profile for a compound with only passive diffusion across the BBB, simulation was performed by assuming $CL_{out} = CL_{in}$ (17 μL/min/g brain) with a 12-h i.v. infusion (Fig. 7a). In this case, the unbound drug concentration is equal in plasma and brain at the steady state. Also, brain concentration decreased at a slower rate than the plasma concentration immediately after the infusion termination. On the other hand, a simulation was performed using the $CL_{in}$ and $CL_{out}$ values (17 and 425 μL/min/g brain, respectively) as estimated from the model of S-atenolol for the case of $CL_{in} < CL_{out}$ and as a result there is a considerable difference between $C_{u,brain}$ and $C_{u,plasma}$ (Fig. 7b) during and after the drug infusion. The simulation was also performed based on the permeability surface area product of sucrose across the BBB (0.3 μL/min/g brain) [24]. Sucrose is a well-known marker for low intrinsic permeability without any active transport (Fig. 7c). Due to the lack of pharmacokinetic information of sucrose as well as our focus on the impact of BBB transport ($CL_{in}$ and $CL_{out}$), the model structure and the other parameter estimates used for sucrose simulation were the same as those for S-atenolol. The bulk flow was not considered in the simulation as no study has been found to quantify its impact on drug elimination from brain ECF. Compared to the scenario of

$CL_{in} = CL_{out} = 17$ μL/min/g brain (Fig. 7a), the unbound brain concentration of sucrose in Fig. 7c takes much longer time to achieve 90% of steady state (3.7 days vs. 4 h) and has much longer half life during the elimination phase.

## Discussion

Beta blockers exhibit highly variable lipophilicity and accordingly diverse pharmacokinetic properties [25], catching the attention of scientists who study drug permeability across biological barriers. Therefore, the hydrophilic and lipophilic extremes in the beta blocker class, respectively, atenolol (logP of 0.23) and propranolol (logP of 3.65) have been used to study the relationship between lipophilicity and permeability in intestinal absorption and BBB penetration [25–27]. In addition, substantial efforts have been made to develop a variety of models to study and predict drug permeability, e.g. the in vitro Caco-2 cell model for intestinal absorption and in vitro brain capillary endothelial cell models for BBB transport. To evaluate and characterize these models, atenolol and propranolol are commonly used as model drugs for studying hydrophilic and lipophilic passive diffusion, respectively [5, 28, 29]. In addition to passive diffusion, carrier-mediated transport also plays a critical role in drug transport across biological barriers [30, 31]. Due to its importance, the function of transporters is usually evaluated by studying drug permeability across biological membranes in various in vivo, in situ, and in vitro

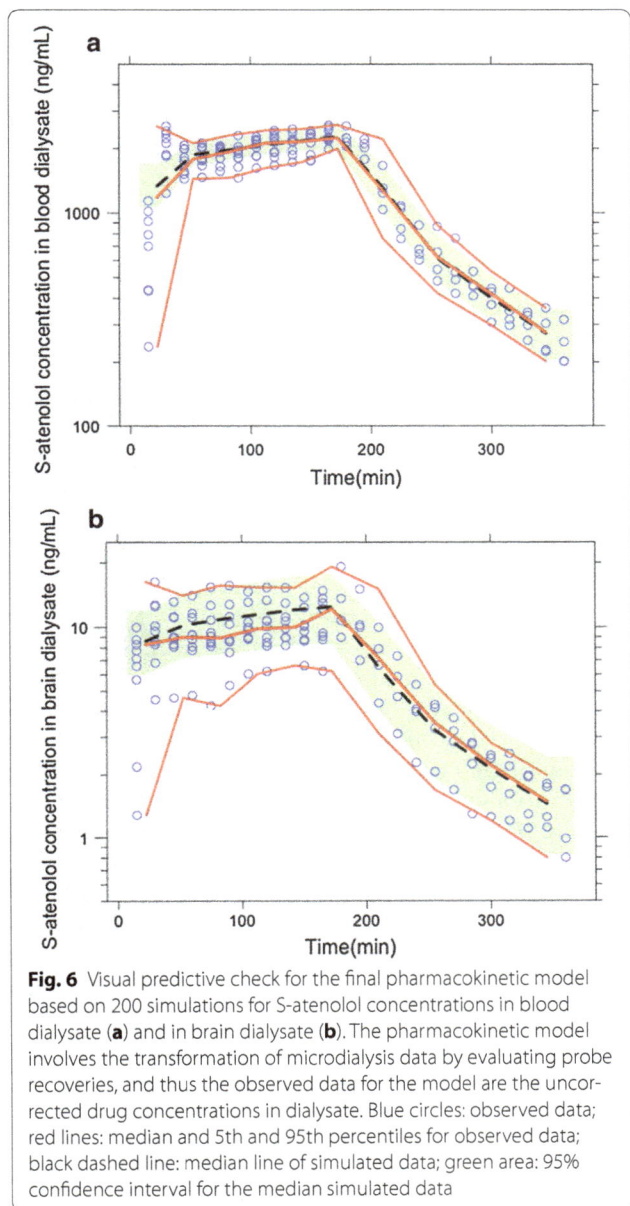

**Fig. 6** Visual predictive check for the final pharmacokinetic model based on 200 simulations for S-atenolol concentrations in blood dialysate (**a**) and in brain dialysate (**b**). The pharmacokinetic model involves the transformation of microdialysis data by evaluating probe recoveries, and thus the observed data for the model are the uncorrected drug concentrations in dialysate. Blue circles: observed data; red lines: median and 5th and 95th percentiles for observed data; black dashed line: median line of simulated data; green area: 95% confidence interval for the median simulated data

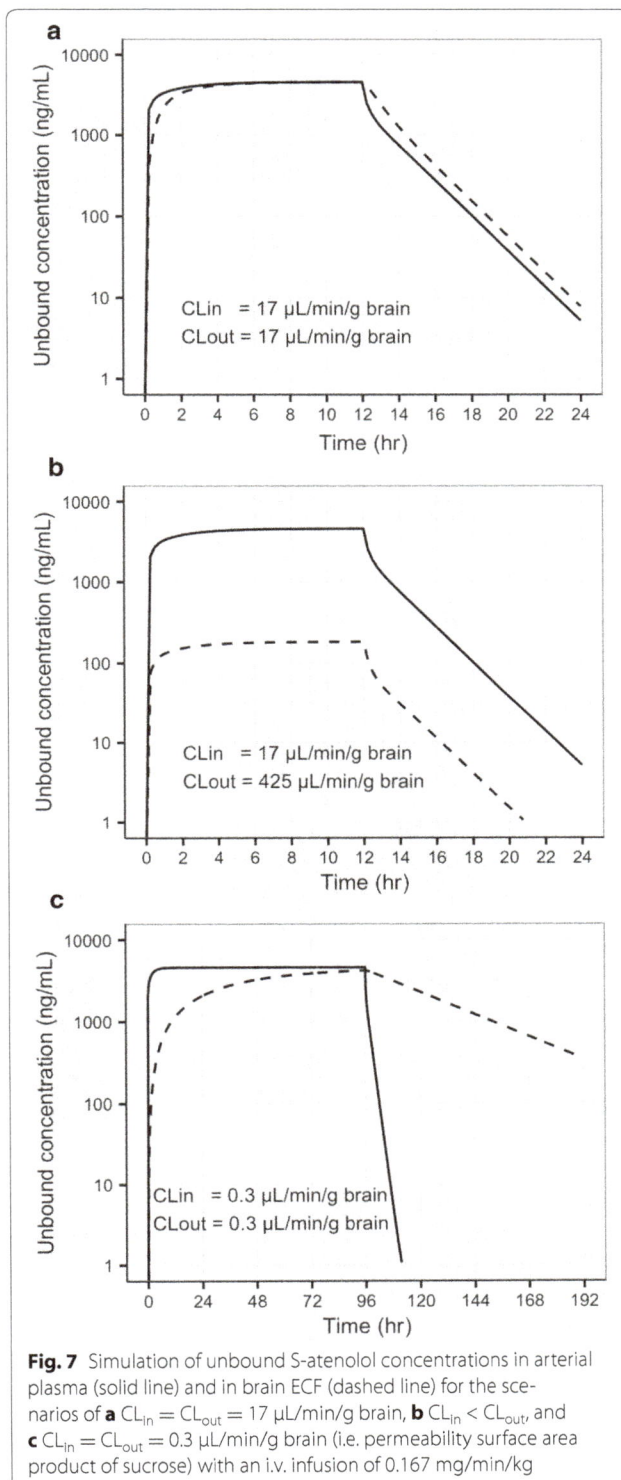

**Fig. 7** Simulation of unbound S-atenolol concentrations in arterial plasma (solid line) and in brain ECF (dashed line) for the scenarios of **a** $CL_{in} = CL_{out} = 17$ µL/min/g brain, **b** $CL_{in} < CL_{out}$, and **c** $CL_{in} = CL_{out} = 0.3$ µL/min/g brain (i.e. permeability surface area product of sucrose) with an i.v. infusion of 0.167 mg/min/kg

models. In this context, atenolol is still used as a model drug for low passive/paracellular diffusion in permeability-related studies without further systematic assessment of the possibility of it being a transporter substrate.

The current study monitored, for the first time, the unbound concentration of S-atenolol in brain ECF during steady state and estimated its $K_{p,uu,brain}$ to assess whether it is likely that any transporter is participating in the atenolol transport across the BBB. If atenolol is a hydrophilic drug without any involvement of transporters, it should have the profile of passive diffusion as in Fig. 7a with equal unbound concentration in plasma and brain at steady state. However, the present microdialysis study showed a profile with the S-atenolol $K_{p,uu,brain}$ much lower than unity ($3.55 \pm 0.40\%$), measured at steady state. The $C_{u,brain}/C_{u,plasma}$ was stable during both the steady state and the elimination phases (Fig. 4), and corresponds to the AUC ratio of brain ECF to plasma from a previous microdialysis study after an intravenous bolus dose (3.8 ± 0.6%) [14]. The lower-than-unity $K_{p,uu,brain}$ suggests that efflux transporters are involved in the atenolol transport at the BBB, leading to a higher $CL_{out}$ than $CL_{in}$. From the modeling approach, the $CL_{in}$ value of atenolol in rats was 17.0 μL/min/g brain (Table 1), much lower than the $CL_{out}$ of 425 μL/min/g brain (calculated according to Eq. 8). It should be noted that brain ECF bulk flow and metabolism may also contribute to discrepancies between $CL_{in}$ and $CL_{out}$ [12]. However, atenolol was found to be very stable in brain homogenate, thereby concluding that metabolism is not important. The relatively low bulk flow reported in rats of 0.1–0.3 μL/min/g brain [32, 33] is also of minor importance considering the estimation of $CL_{out}$ to be 425 μL/min/g brain. The inter-individual variation was high with 134%, which was probably due to its low permeability into brain and the resultant low precision. Avdeef et al. measured atenolol $K_{in}$ (unidirectional transfer constant into brain) under different pH values and concentrations, using the technique of in situ rat brain perfusion [34]. The $K_{in}$, which is similar to $CL_{in}$ for compounds with low permeability, was 1.8 μL/min/g brain for atenolol at 61.7 μM and pH 7.4, which is nearly 10% of the $CL_{in}$ estimated from the model in the current study based on in vivo data. However, their study also showed high inter-individual variation in $K_{in}$ with coefficient of variation (CV) ranging from 33.3% up to 1540% among the dosing groups. In another study published by Agon et al., positron emission tomography (PET) was used to monitor the brain uptake of atenolol in dogs after an i.v. bolus dose of 1.25 or 0.125 mg/kg [35]. By modeling the PET data, $K_{in}$ was estimated ranging from 0.7 to 1.5 μL/min/g brain and the rate constant out of brain ($k_{out}$) ranged from 0.0070 to 0.0151/min. Because of a lack of dog $V_{u,brain}$ information, $CL_{out}$ cannot be extracted from this PET study. However, it should be noted that instead of decreasing with blood concentration, the total drug concentration in dog brain remained at a stable level during the 90 min following the bolus dose. Given the low $f_{u,brain}$ of atenolol due to its hydrophilic property, the difference in the profile of atenolol brain concentration between rats and dogs suggests a species difference in the BBB transport of atenolol.

By correcting for the surface area of endothelial cells in brain (100 cm$^2$/g brain) [12], S-atenolol $CL_{in}$ and $Cl_{out}$ estimated from the model correspond to $2.83 \times 10^{-6}$ and $70.8 \times 10^{-6}$ cm/s of permeability coefficients into and out of rat brain, respectively. The permeability into brain was comparable to the $P_{app}$ value (apparent in vitro transcellular permeability coefficient) assessed from an in vitro BBB model using primary rat brain endothelial cells, pericytes, and astrocytes ($2.49 \times 10^{-6}$ cm/s) [5]. Compared to the above model, the $P_{app}$ values from in vitro BBB models composed of only brain microvessel endothelial cells were higher with $48.5 \times 10^{-6}$ cm/s for bovine (BBMEC) and $9.78 \times 10^{-6}$ cm/s for human (hBMEC) [36, 37]. The reported $P_{app}$ values from other in vitro cell models bearing tight junctions for both A–B and B–A directions were in the range of $0.18 \times 10^{-6} - 11 \times 10^{-6}$ cm/s for Caco-2 cells and $0.13 \times 10^{-6} - 0.8 \times 10^{-6}$ cm/s for MDCKII (Madin-Darby canine kidney II cells) [37–40]. Although showing large inter-laboratory variation, these values and ranges are lower than the out-of-brain permeability estimated in the current study ($70.8 \times 10^{-6}$ cm/s), also suggesting the involvement of transporters in removing atenolol from the brain. Compared to the penetration permeability into the brain, atenolol exhibited higher intestinal absorption permeability based on in situ intestinal perfusion ($5.5 \times 10^{-6}$ cm/s for rats and $15 \times 10^{-6}$ cm/s for human) [4, 41], which may be due to different characteristics of tight junctions and/or expression/function of related transporters.

Although being the most hydrophilic beta blocker, atenolol shows a much higher $CL_{in}$ than sucrose (17.0 vs. 0.3 μL/min/g brain) [24]. Thus, the unbound profile of sucrose brain concentration was simulated to illustrate the unbound brain concentration–time profile of low intrinsic permeability (i.e. due to physicochemical property). As shown in Fig. 7c with $CL_{in}$ and $CL_{out}$ being the same and as low as 0.3 μL/min/g brain, the unbound brain concentration increases very slowly taking approximately 3.7 days to achieve 90% steady state. The ratio of $C_{u,brain}$ to $C_{u,blood}$ is only 25% at 12 h, indicating the very long time that would be needed to reach equal concentrations for a compound with such low intrinsic BBB permeability, (which therefore, in practice, is never measured at true equilibrium time points) and also showing a slower decline in unbound brain concentrations relative to unbound blood concentrations. Unlike the results of sucrose with low intrinsic permeability, the simulation of atenolol in Fig. 7b showed lower unbound concentration in brain than in blood at steady state, indicating the involvement of efflux transporter(s) in decreasing atenolol's $K_{p,uu,brain}$ value. In summary, the atenolol delivery to the brain is limited by the extent but not the rate of BBB transport.

In addition to $K_{p,uu,brain}$ that is related to drug transport at the BBB, $f_{u,brain}$ and $V_{u,brain}$ are important measures to understand drug distribution within the brain, describing the intra-brain distribution [12]. Drug $f_{u,brain}$ describes nonspecific binding within brain tissue while $V_{u,brain}$ also describes intracellular distribution due to other reasons like transporters at some brain cell membranes. Similar to the nonspecific protein binding in plasma, hydrophilic drugs generally have low binding in brain homogenate [42]. From the equilibrium dialysis, atenolol had an $f_{u,brain}$

of 0.875 ± 0.067. In contrast, propranolol has extensive nonspecific binding in brain homogenate with an $f_{u,brain}$ of 0.029 [23]. If drug is evenly distributed within the brain parenchymal fluid, $V_{u,brain}$ is close to the water volume of brain (0.8 mL/g brain). If drug is mainly is distributed inside brain cells or bound to brain tissues, $V_{u,brain}$ tends to be larger than 0.8 mL/g brain [12]. The $V_{u,brain}$ of S-atenolol estimated from microdialysis and whole brain measurements was 0.686 ± 0.104 mL/g brain, indicating no effects of transporters at the brain cells on the drug intra-brain distribution, or that there are transporters with counteractive functions transporting the drug in both the inward and outward directions at the same clearances across brain cell membrane. The latter is however much less likely.

It should be noted that it is the unbound, free drug rather than the bound drug that directly interacts with pharmacological targets. As a result, unbound drug concentration is more relevant to drug therapeutic effect instead of total drug in brain. In addition, the unbound drug concentration in brain ECF rather than total concentration of drug in brain tissue is more relevant in understanding drug transport across BBB because the total concentration of drug is confounded by ECF-ICF and/or nonspecific binding equilibration (as characterized by $V_{u,brain}$ and $f_{u,brain}$). The conclusion about BBB transport based on total drug concentrations in brain could therefore be misleading [43]. Thus, the $K_{p,uu,brain}$ based on unbound concentration in plasma and brain ECF at steady state is a more clinically relevant measure to quantify drug transport at the BBB than rate measurements.

Our results suggest that some transporters actively eliminate atenolol from the brain, however no reports have been found to relate any possible BBB transporters with atenolol efflux. However, it was reported that fruit juices reduced the intestinal absorption of atenolol. The $C_{max}$ and AUC were decreased by 49% and 40%, respectively, by orange juice, and 68% and 81%, respectively, by apple juice, based on pharmacokinetic studies in human subjects [44, 45]. There is some controversy in the literature about the transporters responsible for the interaction between atenolol and fruit juices. The organic anion transporting polypeptide 1A2 (OATP1A2) is suggested to be responsible of the atenolol uptake in the OATP1A2-expressed *X. laevis* oocytes [46]. However, another study by Mimura et al. suggested that organic cation transporter 1 (OCT1) rather than OATP probably contributes to the interaction between atenolol and flavonoids in fruit juices [47]. It was also reported that hOCT2 at the basolateral membrane of kidney tubules lead to renal active secretion of atenolol [48]. Furthermore, the study performed by Yin et al. suggested that atenolol is also a substrate of multidrug and toxin extrusion proteins (hMATE-1 and hMATE2-K) located at the apical membrane of renal

tubule, thus contributing to the elimination of atenolol from blood to urine together with OCT2 [49]. Among these possible transporters for atenolol, only OATP has been found expressed at the BBB with bidirectional transport [50, 51]. OCT2 was also found to be expressed at the apical membrane of the blood-choroid plexus interface (i.e., CSF-facing), which may be relevant for efflux transport of substrates from cerebrospinal fluid to blood [52].

In addition to the solute carrier family (SLC), several members belonging to the ATP-binding cassette (ABC) transporter family are well known efflux transporters at the BBB with a wide range of substances, including P-glycoprotein (Pgp), multidrug resistance protein (MRP), and breast cancer resistance protein (BCRP) [53]. Studies are limited in evaluating the potential of atenolol as a substrate of MRP and BCRP, while controversial results have been reported for the role of brain and intestinal Pgp on atenolol efflux. Kallem et al. reported that coadministration of elacridar, a Pgp inhibitor, did not significantly change the total brain to plasma concentration ratio ($K_{p,brain}$) or brain-to-plasma AUC ratio of atenolol in rats and mice [54]. An in situ intestinal perfusion study showed that verapamil, a Pgp inhibitor, did not change the absorption or intestinal permeability of atenolol [55, 56]. Similar conclusions that atenolol is not a Pgp substrate were drawn from in vitro studies using Caco-2 or Pgp transfected cell lines [40, 57]. On the other hand, Pgp inhibitors (cyclosporin and itraconazole) were reported to slightly increase the absorption rate and bioavailability of atenolol [58, 59]. However, these inhibitors are not specific and also act on other transporters. In addition, polarized transport of atenolol was found in a Pgp-transfected IPEC-J2 cell lines and Caco-2 cell with an efflux ratio of 3.5 and 2.3, respectively, which were decreased by addition of Pgp inhibitors (zosuquidar and verapamil) [60, 61]. In a collaborative study comparing Caco-2 cells from 10 laboratories, atenolol showed highly variable permeability and its efflux ratios ranged from 0.18 to 3.76, indicating the possibility of an involvement of transporter-mediated transport [38]. In summary, it is not clear which transporter(s) are responsible for the efflux of atenolol from brain, even though more solid evidence of transporter involvement have been found related to the intestinal absorption and renal secretion of atenolol.

## Conclusions

The present study systematically evaluated the extent of S-atenolol distribution into and within the brain using microdialysis, and strongly suggests an involvement of carrier-mediated efflux of S-atenolol at the BBB, in addition to passive diffusion. Although it is currently unclear which transporter (or transporters) is responsible for atenolol efflux transport at the BBB, it is likely not appropriate to use atenolol as a model drug for paracellular transport or passive diffusion. For any other candidate as a model drug of passive diffusion at the BBB, measurement of $K_{p,uu,brain}$ based on unbound concentrations at steady state is useful to detect potential involvement of transporters in the BBB transport. The likely transporters may have different expression levels and functions in other organs (e.g. intestine and kidney), thus the importance of carrier-mediated transport is likely different depending on the organ studied.

## Abbreviations

$AUC_u$: unbound drug concentration–time profiles; BBB: blood-brain barrier; BCRP: breast cancer resistance protein; $C_{in,ATD7}$: concentrations of atenolol-D7 in perfusate; $C_{out,ATD7}$: concentrations of atenolol-D7 in dialysate; $C_{u,brain}$: unbound drug concentration in brain ECF; $C_{u,blood}$: unbound drug concentrations in blood; $C_{u,ss,brainECF}$: unbound drug concentrations in brain ECF at steady state; $C_{u,ss,plasma}$: unbound drug concentrations in plasma at steady state; $CL_{in}$: influx clearance into brain; $CL_{out}$: efflux clearance from brain; CV: coefficient of variation; ECF: extracellular fluid; $f_{u,brain}$: unbound drug fraction in brain homogenate; $f_{u,hD}$: unbound drug fraction in diluted brain homogenate; $f_{u,p}$: unbound drug fraction in plasma; ICF: intracellular fluid; $K_{in}$: unidirectional transfer constant into brain; $K_{p,uu,brain}$: unbound equilibrium partition coefficient; LC–MS/MS: liquid chromatography coupled with tandem mass spectrometry; hMATE: multidrug and toxin extrusion proteins; MRP: multidrug resistance protein; OATP: organic anion transporting polypeptide; OCT: organic cation transporter; PAES: polyarylethersulphone; Pgp: P-glycoprotein; $r^2$: coefficients of determination; $R_{bl-p}$: blood-to-plasma concentration ratio; RSE: relative standard error; $t_{1/2,brain}$: half-lives; $V_{u,brain}$: unbound volume of distribution in brain; $V_{bl}$: volume of vascular space in brain.

## Authors' contributions

XC contributed to the design of the study, carried out experiments, performed data collection and analysis, and drafted the manuscript. TS participated in the microdialysis study. ECMdL and DES contributed to data interpretation and drafting of the manuscript; MHU contributed to the design of the study, data interpretation, and drafting of the manuscript. All authors have read and approved the final manuscript.

## Author details

[1] Department of Pharmaceutical Biosciences, Translational PKPD Research Group, Uppsala University, Box 591, SE-75124 Uppsala, Sweden. [2] Department of Pharmaceutical Sciences, College of Pharmacy, University of Michigan, Ann Arbor, MI 48109, USA. [3] Department of Pharmacology, Leiden Academic Centre for Drug Research, Leiden, The Netherlands.

## Acknowledgements

The authors greatly appreciated the excellent technical support provided by Jessica Dunhall in the animal experiments and by Britt Jansson in the chemical analyses.

## Competing interests

The authors declare that they have no competing interests.

## Funding

This work was supported by the National Institutes of Health National Institute of General Medical Sciences grant R01-GM115481 (to DES).

## References

1. Ong HT. Beta blockers in hypertension and cardiovascular disease. BMJ. 2007;334:946–9.
2. Pearson AA, Gaffney TE, Walle T, Privitera PJ. A stereoselective central hypotensive action of atenolol. J Pharmacol Exp Ther. 1989;250:759–63.
3. Mehvar R, Brocks DR. Stereospecific pharmacokinetics and pharmacodynamics of beta-adrenergic blockers in humans. J Pharm Pharm Sci. 2001;4:185–200.
4. Lennernas H. Human intestinal permeability. J Pharm Sci. 1998;87:403–10.
5. Nakagawa S, Deli MA, Kawaguchi H, Shimizudani T, Shimono T, Kittel A, Tanaka K, Niwa M. A new blood-brain barrier model using primary rat brain endothelial cells, pericytes and astrocytes. Neurochem Int. 2009;54:253–63.
6. Smith D, Artursson P, Avdeef A, Di L, Ecker GF, Faller B, Houston JB, Kansy M, Kerns EH, Kramer SD, Lennernas H, van de Waterbeemd H, Sugano K, Testa B. Passive lipoidal diffusion and carrier-mediated cell uptake are both important mechanisms of membrane permeation in drug disposition. Mol Pharm. 2014;11:1727–38.
7. Abbott NJ, Ronnback L, Hansson E. Astrocyte-endothelial interactions at the blood-brain barrier. Nat Rev Neurosci. 2006;7:41–53.
8. Bickel U. How to measure drug transport across the blood–brain barrier. NeuroRx. 2005;2:15–26.
9. Oldendorf WH. Measurement of brain uptake of radiolabeled substances using a tritiated water internal standard. Brain Res. 1970;24:372–6.
10. Takasato Y, Rapoport SI, Smith QR. An in situ brain perfusion technique to study cerebrovascular transport in the rat. Am J Physiol. 1984;247:H484–93.
11. Hammarlund-Udenaes M. In vivo approaches to assessing the blood–brain barrier. Top Med Chem Ser. 2014;10:21–48.
12. Hammarlund-Udenaes M, Friden M, Syvanen S, Gupta A. On the rate and extent of drug delivery to the brain. Pharm Res. 2008;25:1737–50.
13. Lindqvist A, Jonsson S, Hammarlund-Udenaes M. Exploring factors causing low brain penetration of the opioid peptide DAMGO through experimental methods and modeling. Mol Pharm. 2016;13:1258–66.
14. Delange ECM, Danhof M, Deboer AG, Breimer DD. Critical factors of intracerebral microdialysis as a technique to determined the pharmacokinetics of drugs in rat-brain. Brain Res. 1994;666:1–8.
15. Hammarlund-Udenaes M, Paalzow LK, de Lange EC. Drug equilibration across the blood–brain barrier–pharmacokinetic considerations based on the microdialysis method. Pharm Res. 1997;14:128–34.
16. Sadiq MW, Borgs A, Okura T, Shimomura K, Kato S, Deguchi Y, Jansson B, Bjorkman S, Terasaki T, Hammarlund-Udenaes M. Diphenhydramine active uptake at the blood–brain barrier and its interaction with oxycodone in vitro and in vivo. J Pharm Sci. 2011;100:3912–23.
17. Bouw MR, Hammarlund-Udenaes M. Methodological aspects of the use of a calibrator in in vivo microdialysis-further development of the retrodialysis method. Pharm Res. 1998;15:1673–9.
18. Bengtsson J, Bostrom E, Hammarlund-Udenaes M. The use of a deuterated calibrator for in vivo recovery estimations in microdialysis studies. J Pharm Sci. 2008;97:3433–41.
19. Bostrom E, Simonsson US, Hammarlund-Udenaes M. In vivo blood–brain barrier transport of oxycodone in the rat: indications for active influx and implications for pharmacokinetics/pharmacodynamics. Drug Metab Dispos. 2006;34:1624–31.
20. Sadiq MW, Bostrom E, Keizer R, Bjorkman S, Hammarlund-Udenaes M. Oxymorphone active uptake at the blood–brain barrier and population modeling of its pharmacokinetic-pharmacodynamic relationship. J Pharm Sci. 2013;102:3320–31.
21. Bickel U, Schumacher OP, Kang YS, Voigt K. Poor permeability of morphine 3-glucuronide and morphine 6-glucuronide through the blood–brain barrier in the rat. J Pharmacol Exp Ther. 1996;278:107–13.
22. Taylor EA, Turner P. The distribution of propranolol, pindolol and atenolol between human-erythrocytes and plasma. Brit J Clin Pharmaco. 1981;12:543–8.
23. Friden M, Bergstrom F, Wan H, Rehngren M, Ahlin G, Hammarlund-Udenaes M, Bredberg U. Measurement of unbound drug exposure in brain: modeling of pH partitioning explains diverging results between the brain slice and brain homogenate methods. Drug Metab Dispos. 2011;39:353–62.

24. Ennis SR, Betz AL. Sucrose permeability of the blood-retinal and blood-brain barriers. Effects of diabetes, hypertonicity, and iodate. Invest Ophthalmol Vis Sci. 1986;27:1095–102.

25. Neildwyer G, Bartlett J, Mcainsh J, Cruickshank JM. Beta-adreno-ceptor blockers and the blood–brain-barrier. Brit J Clin Pharmaco. 1981;11:549–53.

26. Sun D, Lennernas H, Welage LS, Barnett JL, Landowski CP, Foster D, Fleisher D, Lee KD, Amidon GL. Comparison of human duodenum and Caco-2 gene expression profiles for 12,000 gene sequences tags and correlation with permeability of 26 drugs. Pharm Res. 2002;19:1400–16.

27. Camenisch G, Alsenz J, van de Waterbeemd H, Folkers G. Estimation of permeability by passive diffusion through Caco-2 cell monolayers using the drugs' lipophilicity and molecular weight. Eur J Pharm Sci. 1998;6:313–9.

28. Artursson P. Epithelial transport of drugs in cell-culture. 1. A model for studying the passive diffusion of drugs over intestinal absorptive (Caco-2) cells. J Pharm Sci. 1990;79:476–82.

29. Cheng Z, Zhang J, Liu H, Li Y, Zhao Y, Yang E. Central nervous system penetration for small molecule therapeutic agents does not increase in multiple sclerosis- and Alzheimer's disease-related animal models despite reported blood–brain barrier disruption. Drug Metab Dispos. 2010;38:1355–61.

30. Scherrmann JM. Drug delivery to brain via the blood–brain barrier. Vascul Pharmacol. 2002;38:349–54.

31. International Transporter C, Giacomini KM, Huang SM, Tweedie DJ, Benet LZ, Brouwer KL, Chu X, Dahlin A, Evers R, Fischer V, Hillgren KM, Hoffmaster KA, Ishikawa T, Keppler D, Kim RB, Lee CA, Niemi M, Polli JW, Sugiyama Y, Swaan PW, Ware JA, Wright SH, Yee SW, Zamek-Gliszczynski MJ, Zhang L. Membrane transporters in drug development. Nat Rev Drug Discov. 2010;9:215–36.

32. Rosenberg GA, Kyner WT, Estrada E. Bulk flow of brain interstitial fluid under normal and hyperosmolar conditions. Am J Physiol. 1980;238:F42–9.

33. Cserr HF, Cooper DN, Milhorat TH. Flow of cerebral interstitial fluid as indicated by the removal of extracellular markers from rat caudate nucleus. Exp Eye Res. 1977;25(Suppl):461–73.

34. Avdeef A, Sun N. A new in situ brain perfusion flow correction method for lipophilic drugs based on the pH-dependent Crone-Renkin equation. Pharm Res. 2011;28:517–30.

35. Agon P, Goethals P, Van Haver D, Kaufman JM. Permeability of the blood–brain barrier for atenolol studied by positron emission tomography. J Pharm Pharmacol. 1991;43:597–600.

36. Eigenmann DE, Jahne EA, Smiesko M, Hamburger M, Oufir M. Validation of an immortalized human (hBMEC) in vitro blood–brain barrier model. Anal Bioanal Chem. 2016;408:2095–107.

37. Hakkarainen JJ, Jalkanen AJ, Kaariainen TM, Keski-Rahkonen P, Venalainen T, Hokkanen J, Monkkonen J, Suhonen M, Forsberg MM. Comparison of in vitro cell models in predicting in vivo brain entry of drugs. Int J Pharm. 2010;402:27–36.

38. Hayeshi R, Hilgendorf C, Artursson P, Augustijns P, Brodin B, Dehertogh P, Fisher K, Fossati L, Hovenkamp E, Korjamo T, Masungi C, Maubon N, Mols R, Mullertz A, Monkkonen J, O'Driscoll C, Oppers-Tiemissen HM, Ragnarsson EG, Rooseboom M, Ungell AL. Comparison of drug transporter gene expression and functionality in Caco-2 cells from 10 different laboratories. Eur J Pharm Sci. 2008;35:383–96.

39. Wang Q, Rager JD, Weinstein K, Kardos PS, Dobson GL, Li JB, Hidalgo IJ. Evaluation of the MDR-MDCK cell line as a permeability screen for the blood-brain barrier. Int J Pharm. 2005;288:349–59.

40. Gartzke D, Delzer J, Laplanche L, Uchida Y, Hoshi Y, Tachikawa M, Terasaki T, Sydor J, Fricker G. Genomic knockout of endogenous canine P-glycoprotein in wild-type, human P-glycoprotein and human BCRP transfected MDCKII cell lines by zinc finger nucleases. Pharm Res. 2015;32:2060–71.

41. Fagerholm U, Johansson M, Lennernas H. Comparison between permeability coefficients in rat and human jejunum. Pharm Res. 1996;13:1336–42.

42. Wan H, Rehngren M, Giordanetto F, Bergstrom F, Tunek A. High-throughput screening of drug-brain tissue binding and in silico prediction for assessment of central nervous system drug delivery. J Med Chem. 2007;50:4606–15.

43. Chen X, Keep RF, Liang Y, Zhu HJ, Hammarlund-Udenaes M, Hu Y, Smith DE. Influence of peptide transporter 2 (PEPT2) on the distribution of cefadroxil in mouse brain: a microdialysis study. Biochem Pharmacol. 2017;131:89–97.

44. Lilja JJ, Raaska K, Neuvonen PJ. Effects of orange juice on the pharmacokinetics of atenolol. Eur J Clin Pharmacol. 2005;61:337–40.

45. Jeon H, Jang IJ, Lee S, Ohashi K, Kotegawa T, Ieiri I, Cho JY, Yoon SH, Shin SG, Yu KS, Lim KS. Apple juice greatly reduces systemic exposure to atenolol. Br J Clin Pharmacol. 2013;75:172–9.

46. Kato Y, Miyazaki T, Kano T, Sugiura T, Kubo Y, Tsuji A. Involvement of influx and efflux transport systems in gastrointestinal absorption of celiprolol. J Pharm Sci. 2009;98:2529–39.

47. Mimura Y, Yasujima T, Ohta K, Inoue K, Yuasa H. Atenolol transport by organic cation transporter 1 and its interference by flavonoids. Drug Metab Rev. 2015;47:263.

48. Ciarimboli G, Schroter R, Neugebauer U, Vollenbroker B, Gabriels G, Brzica H, Sabolic I, Pietig G, Pavenstadt H, Schlatter E, Edemir B. Kidney transplantation down-regulates expression of organic cation transporters, which translocate beta-blockers and fluoroquinolones. Mol Pharm. 2013;10:2370–80.

49. Yin J, Duan HC, Shirasaka Y, Prasad B, Wang J. Atenolol renal secretion is mediated by human organic cation transporter 2 and multidrug and toxin extrusion proteins. Drug Metab Dispos. 2015;43:1872–81.

50. Ronaldson PT, Davis TP. Targeted drug delivery to treat pain and cerebral hypoxia. Pharmacol Rev. 2013;65:291–314.

51. Westholm DE, Rumbley JN, Salo DR, Rich TP, Anderson GW. Organic anion-transporting polypeptides in the blood-brain and blood-cerebrospinal fluid barriers. Curr Top Dev Biol. 2008;80:135–70.

52. Sweet DH, Miller DS, Pritchard JB. Ventricular choline transport: a role for organic cation transporter 2 expressed in choroid plexus. J Biol Chem. 2001;276:41611–9.

53. Loscher W, Potschka H. Role of drug efflux transporters in the brain for drug disposition and treatment of brain diseases. Prog Neurobiol. 2005;76:22–76.

54. Kallem R, Kulkarni CP, Patel D, Thakur M, Sinz M, Singh SP, Mahammad SS, Mandlekar S. A simplified protocol employing elacridar in rodents: a screening model in drug discovery to assess P-gp mediated efflux at the blood brain barrier. Drug Metab Lett. 2012;6:134–44.

55. Mols R, Brouwers J, Schinkel AH, Annaert P, Augustijns P. Intestinal perfusion with mesenteric blood sampling in wild-type and knockout mice: evaluation of a novel tool in biopharmaceutical drug profiling. Drug Metab Dispos. 2009;37:1334–7.

56. Brouwers J, Mols R, Annaert P, Augustijns P. Validation of a differential in situ perfusion method with mesenteric blood sampling in rats for intestinal drug interaction profiling. Biopharm Drug Dispos. 2010;31:278–85.

57. Doppenschmitt S, Spahn-Langguth H, Regardh CG, Langguth P. Role of P-glycoprotein-mediated secretion in absorptive drug permeability: an approach using passive membrane permeability and affinity to P-glycoprotein. J Pharm Sci. 1999;88:1067–72.

58. Terao T, Hisanaga E, Sai Y, Tamai I, Tsuji A. Active secretion of drugs from the small intestinal epithelium in rats by P-glycoprotein functioning as an absorption barrier. J Pharm Pharmacol. 1996;48:1083–9.

59. Lilja JJ, Backman JT, Neuvonen PJ. Effect of itraconazole on the pharmacokinetics of atenolol. Basic Clin Pharmacol Toxicol. 2005;97:395–8.

60. Saaby L, Helms HC, Brodin B. IPEC-J2 MDR1, a novel high-resistance cell line with functional expression of human P-glycoprotein (ABCB1) for drug screening studies. Mol Pharm. 2016;5(13):640–52.

61. Augustijns P, Mols R. HPLC with programmed wavelength fluorescence detection for the simultaneous determination of marker compounds of integrity and P-gp functionality in the Caco-2 intestinal absorption model. J Pharm Biomed Anal. 2004;34:971–8.

# 8

# Patterns of relapse in primary central nervous system lymphoma: inferences regarding the role of the neuro-vascular unit and monoclonal antibodies in treating occult CNS disease

Prakash Ambady[1,2], Rongwei Fu[3,4], Joao Prola Netto[1,5], Cymon Kersch[1], Jenny Firkins[1], Nancy D. Doolittle[1] and Edward A. Neuwelt[1,2,6]* (iD)

## Abstract

**Background and purpose:** The radiologic features and patterns of primary central nervous system lymphoma (PCNSL) at initial presentation are well described. High response rates can be achieved with first-line high-dose methotrexate (HD-MTX) based regimens, yet many relapse within 2 years of diagnosis. We describe the pattern of relapse and review the potential mechanisms involved in relapse.

**Methods:** We identified 78 consecutive patients who attained complete radiographic response (CR) during or after first-line treatment for newly diagnosed PCNSL (CD20+, diffuse large B cell type). Patients were treated with HD-MTX based regimen in conjunction with blood–brain barrier disruption (HD-MTX/BBBD); 44 subsequently relapsed. Images and medical records of these 44 consecutive patients were retrospectively reviewed. The anatomical location of enhancing lesions at initial diagnosis and at the time of relapse were identified and compared.

**Results:** 37/44 patients fulfilled inclusion criteria and had new measureable enhancing lesions at relapse; the pattern and location of relapse of these 37 patients were identified. At relapse, the new enhancement was at a spatially distinct site in 30 of 37 patients. Local relapse was found only in seven patients.

**Discussion:** Unlike gliomas, the majority of PCNSL had radiographic relapse at spatially distinct anatomical locations within the brain behind a previously intact neurovascular unit (NVU), and in few cases outside, the central nervous system (CNS). This may suggest either (1) reactivation of occult reservoirs behind an intact NVU in the CNS (or ocular) or (2) seeding from bone marrow or other extra CNS sites.

**Conclusion:** Recognizing patterns of relapse is key for early detection and may provide insight into potential mechanisms of relapse as well as help develop strategies to extend duration of complete response.

## Background

Primary central nervous system lymphoma (PCNSL) in immunocompetent patients (non-acquired immune deficiency syndrome and non-post-transplant lymphoproliferative disease) is a rare, aggressive extranodal non-Hodgkin's lymphoma. The most common morphology consists primarily of diffuse large CD20+ B-cell aggregates confined to the CNS or eyes at initial presentation. First line high dose methotrexate (HD-MTX)-based chemotherapy regimens are the current backbone therapy for newly diagnosed PCNSL with high rates of complete response (CR) [1]. CR is defined by the

*Correspondence: neuwelte@ohsu.edu
[1] Department of Neurology, Oregon Health & Science University, 3181 SW Sam Jackson Park Road, L603, Portland, OR 97239, USA
Full list of author information is available at the end of the article

complete disappearance of all enhancing abnormalities on gadolinium-enhanced MRI with no evidence of disease in the CSF and ocular compartments after discontinuation of all corticosteroids for at least 2 weeks [2]. Despite high initial CR rates with MTX-based regimens, over 50% of patients relapse within 2 years of diagnosis [3–5]. Unlike systemic diffuse large B-cell lymphoma (DLBCL), PCNSL lack a plateau in progression-free survival rates; even patients who remain disease free for over 5 years continue to be at risk of relapse [6]. Understanding the mechanisms of relapse is particularly important to further improve overall survival by guiding therapies aimed at extending disease control [7].

Primary central nervous system lymphoma in immunocompetent patients typically presents as a solitary homogeneously enhancing mass in the subcortical white matter, predominantly in the periventricular or white matter of the cerebral hemispheres [8–10]. Contrast-enhanced MRI is the preferred imaging technique for diagnosis, response assessment and follow up. Lesions are typically hypo- or isointense on T1-weighted MR images and iso-, hypo-, or hyperintense on T2-weighted MR images with evidence of restricted diffusion [11–13]. Although the characteristic feature of newly diagnosed PCNSL in immunocompetent patients is well described, the pattern and location of relapses is not. Relapses are generally believed to be derived from the same clone as the initial presentation and not entirely new disease [14, 15]. It has been postulated that relapse may be due to seeding from occult CNS sites, ocular disease or from distant subclinical extra-CNS sites [7]. Better understanding of the pattern and mechanism of relapse is key to early detection and understanding the true extent of disease, potentially helping guide therapies aimed at maintaining response as well as better manage relapses. We report the site of relapse in PCNSL patients after attaining CR with HD-MTX in conjunction with blood–brain barrier disruption (BBBD).

## Methods

### Patients

Our institutional review board approved this study. This retrospective review identified all newly-diagnosed immunocompetent PCNSL patients treated with HD-MTX/BBBD between 02/1982 and 09/2013 at our institution. Inclusion criteria included: (1) histologically confirmed CD20+ DLBCL confined to the brain, cerebrospinal fluid or eyes; (2) treatment with intra-arterial HD-MTX/BBBD regimens with or without rituximab (treatment regimens were previously described) [16, 17]; (3) first relapse after achieving CR with first line treatment. Patients with primary low grade CNS lymphoma

and primary CNS T-cell lymphoma, evidence of lymphoma outside the CNS at initial presentation, having only ocular lymphoma but subsequently developed CNS lesion before CR in the eyes, and patients with no measurable radiologic lesions (diagnosis only by CSF analysis) were excluded. Patients who received alternative therapies/regimens (other than HD-MTX/BBBD) as first line therapy, whole-brain radiotherapy (WBRT), or maintenance immunotherapy after completion of initial year of therapy, were also excluded from the analysis. Only patients with documented radiologic relapse were included, since pattern of relapses were the focus of this analysis.

### Radiologic assessment

Imaging and response assessment was done as previously described and in line with current international consensus-based guidelines [16, 18]. Anatomical location of Axial and Coronal T1 and T2, and contrast enhanced T-1 weighted MR images at initial diagnosis and at relapse were determined. Anatomical sites of disease were categorized as involving the CNS, ocular or extra-CNS. CNS lesions were further divided into the following sites: (a) right or left cerebral hemispheres with further classification into frontal, temporal or occipital lobes based on neuroanatomical land marks, (b) lesions involving the corpus callosum, (c) infra-tentorial posterior fossa lesions including the brainstem and cerebellum, (d) subependymal, (e) spinal cord or (f) leptomeningeal, based on the predominant location of the enhancing lesion. At relapse, enhancing lesions inside or within a 2 cm margin of the T2 hyperintensity at initial presentation was considered to be local relapse, while those outside this margin were considered distant relapse. Since PCNSL is a diffusely infiltrative disease with no clear margins, this 2 cm margin was chosen based on the margins used for radiation planning and pattern of relapse seen in glioblastoma [19]. Clinical history, including pretreatment Karnofsky Performance Score (KPS), cranial MRI with and without contrast, and computed tomography (CT) staging (chest and abdomen) scans were reviewed. Contrast-enhanced cranial CT was used in some early cases when MRI was not readily available. Results of bone marrow biopsy and ophthalmologic examination were reviewed when available.

### Results

A total of 129 consecutive newly diagnosed PCNSL patients received first line HD-MTX/BBBD during the study period; one patient treated with WBRT and six patients treated with maintenance immunotherapy were excluded. Of the remaining 122 patients, CR was achieved in 78 (64%) during or at the end of treatment, and 44 (56%) subsequently progressed. Due to the retrospective nature of this study, imaging was not available to confirm location of new enhancement at progression in three patients; additional four had no measurable lesion at progression (clinical progression or by CSF analysis). These seven were excluded from further analysis. We describe the location of first relapses, defined as new measurable enhancing lesion on contrast enhanced MRI in the remaining 37 patients.

Among the 37 patients, ocular involvement at initial diagnosis was noted in seven patients. Bone marrow biopsy was performed in 29/37 patients, one patient had evidence of low grade lymphoma, and another had atypical polyclonal lymphoid aggregates, the remaining did not have any clinical evidence of lymphoma in the marrow. Demographics are described in Table 1. Median time to progression was 17.8 months (95% CI 11.7–41.7). At relapse, new enhancement was noted in a spatially distinct site in 30 of 37 (81%) patients with 15 (50%) relapses in an entirely different lobe. Six patients (20%) had systemic relapse (outside the CNS) with no new measurable lesion in the CNS (Table 2). Only 7/37 (19%) of relapses were contiguous (inside or within a 2 cm margin of T2 hyperintensity of at initial diagnosis; Table 2). Local relapses were more common when the initial lesion involved the corpus callosum, posterior fossa, sub-ependymal disease or the leptomeninges. Due to the small sample size, no formal statistical evaluation was performed. Representative cases are described in Figs. 1, 2, 3 and 4.

### Table 1  Demographics of patients with relapsing primary central nervous system lymphoma

| Number: 37 | |
|---|---|
| **Variables** | |
| Median age in years at diagnosis (Min, Max) | 63.7 (27.6, 80.1) |
| Gender (N, % Female) | 21 (57%) |
| Median KPS at diagnosis (Min, Max) | 80 (20, 100) |
| Ocular involvement (%) | 7 (18.9%) |
| Treatment regiment | HD-MTX/BBBD without rituximab: 30 (81.1%) |
| | HD-MTX/BBBD with rituximab: 7 (18.9%) |
| Median age in years at relapse (Min, Max) | 65.1 (31.6, 80.8) |
| Median time to progression in months | 17.8 (95% CI 11.7–41.7) |

KPS Karnofsky Performance status [55], HD-MTX/BBBD High dose methotrexate with blood–brain barrier disruption

### Table 2  Site of relapse in primary central nervous system lymphoma

| Site of relapse after complete response (n = 37) | |
|---|---|
| Distant | 30 (81%) |
| Different lobe | 15 |
| Systemic/non CNS | 6 |
| Ocular | 2 |
| Same lobe but distinct site | 3 |
| Corpus callosum | 2 |
| Leptomeningeal | 2 |
| Local | 7 (19%) |
| Corpus callosum | 3 |
| Cerebellum/posterior fossa | 2 |
| Sub-ependymal | 1 |
| Leptomeningeal | 1 |

The location of enhancement at relapse after complete response with high dose methotrexate was at an anatomically distant site compared to the site of enhancement at location of enhancement at presentation in a majority of cases. Local relapses were more frequent when the initial lesion was in the corpus callosum, posterior fossa, subependymal or in leptomeningeal lesions

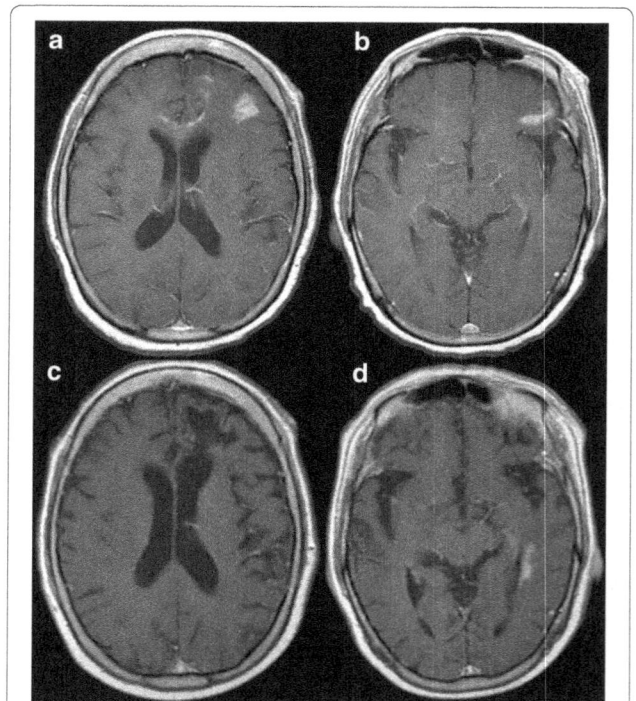

**Fig. 1** Case 1; Axial T1-weighted post contrast imaging at initial presentation (**a**, **b**), in complete response (**c**) after therapy and at relapse (**d**). At initial presentation, multiple scattered left frontal and callosal lesions are noted (**a**). Patient achieved complete response after 12 months of HD-MTX treatment (**c**). 1 year after finishing treatment, relapse was noted in the periventricular white matter of the left lateral ventricle (**d**)

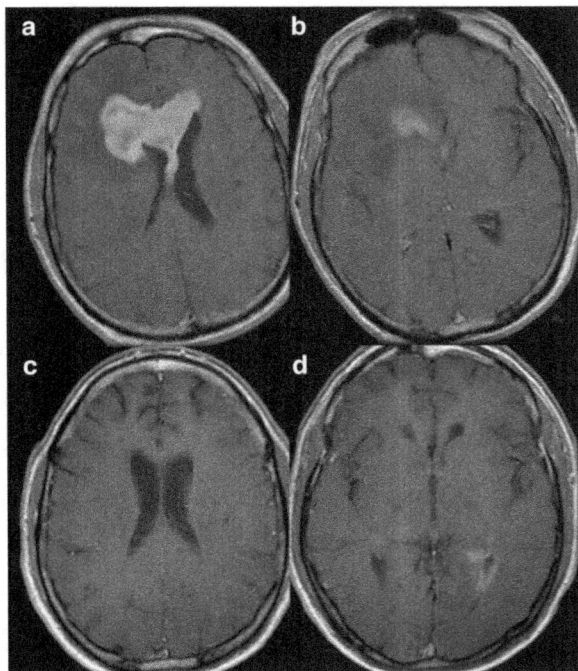

**Fig. 2** Case 2; Axial T1-weighted post contrast imaging at initial presentation (**a**, **b**) and relapse (**c**, **d**). Initial presentation shows a localized large enhancing lesion centered in the genus of the corpus callosum (CC) with extension mainly into the right frontal lobe (**a**, **b**). After 10 months of HD-MTX treatment there is relapse in the ependymal surface of the left lateral ventricle (**d**) with complete response in the CC lesion (**c**)

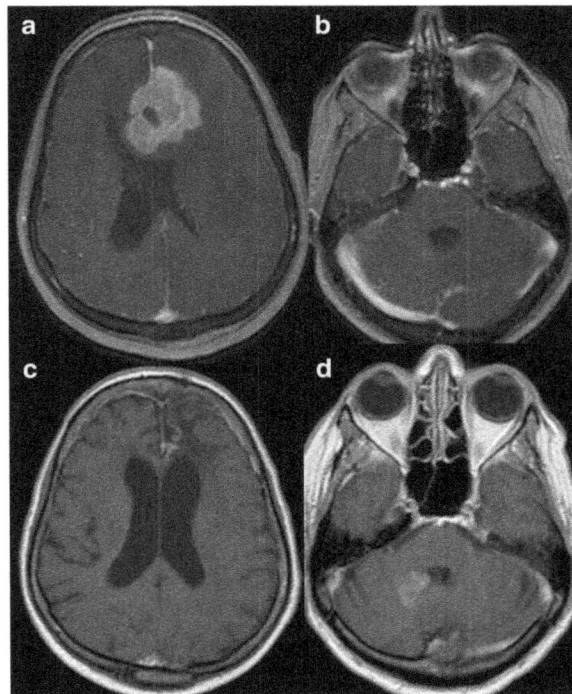

**Fig. 3** Case 3; Axial T1-weighted post contrast imaging at initial presentation (**a**, **b**), after completing therapy with HD-MTX (**c**) and relapse (**d**). Initial presentation shows a large enhancing lesion in the left frontal lobe (**a**) and normal cerebellum (**b**). Patient was in complete response after completing 1 year of HD-MTX treatment (**c**) with radiographic relapse in the right cerebellum, 6 years after the initial diagnosis (**d**)

## Discussion

Both glioma and lymphoma are well recognized to involve the whole brain even when imaging may deceivingly suggest anatomically localized disease sites. Our data suggests that unlike gliomas where local relapse is the norm, the majority of PCNSL relapses occur distal to the site of initial presentation. This difference in the pattern of relapse may allow an insight into the mechanism of relapse. Our data aligns with a smaller retrospective study (16 patients) that evaluated relapse pattern in 16 PCNSL patients where only four relapses were at the site of initial tumor [20]. This study provides a larger sample size and duration of follow-up for this rare disease.

HD-MTX based therapy is the backbone of most modern chemotherapy regimens for PCNSL. The majority of PCNSLs are CD20-expressing diffuse large B cell lymphomas; the addition of rituximab, a monoclonal antibody (mAb) targeted against CD-20, to HD-MTX-based regimens is intuitive. However, there is ongoing debate regarding the delivery of high molecular weight monoclonal antibodies across the blood–brain barrier (BBB) and neurovascular unit (NVU) [21]. Monoclonal antibodies to CD-20 have a long half-life, and in

pre-clinical studies have been shown to leak slowly and accumulate across diseased NVU around the enhancing tumor [22, 23]. Further, the addition of anti-CD20 mAb, rituximab to HD-MTX has substantially improved CR rates, progression free survival and OS in PCNSL [24, 25].

A similar pattern of distant relapses has also been reported in systemic DLBCL, where most relapses are believed to be derived from the same clones as the original tumor [14]. Similarly, small studies have suggested clonal relation of the primary and recurrent tumors in PCNSL [6, 15]. The possibility of late relapses and isolated CNS relapses of systemic lymphoma being new clones or the possibility of dual clonality has also been previously raised based on small studies [26, 27]. Although limited, there is emerging evidence suggesting that relapses after intravenous HD-MTX at sites distant from initial presentation within the CNS and in rare instances outside the CNS are not uncommon [20, 27–30]. The incidence and pattern of relapses distant from the site of initial tumor presentation with HD-MTX/BBBD (30/37, 81%) are comparable to those described with intravenous

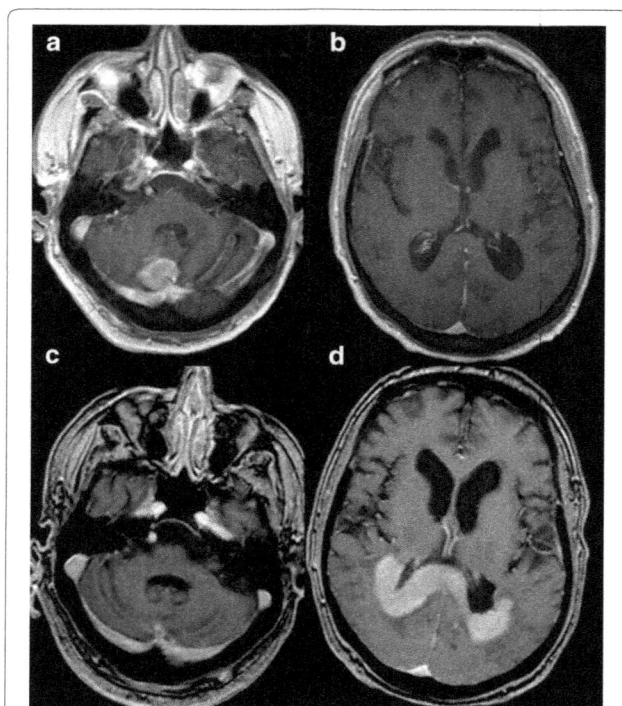

**Fig. 4** Case 4; Axial T1 WI post contrast imaging at initial presentation (**a**, **b**) and relapse (**c**, **d**). At initial presentation there is a solitary right cerebellar lesion (**a**) with normal supra-tentorial compartment (**b**). After 10 months of high-dose MTX treatment, relapse was noted in the splenium of the CC with extension to the periventricular white matter (**d**) with no evidence of residual disease in the cerebellum (**c**)

HD-MTX (12/16, 75%) [20]. These studies suggests that the pattern of distant relapse is unique to the natural history of PCNSL and unlikely related to BBBD.

The mechanism of relapse is unclear, but two mechanisms have been postulated (1) seeding from occult reservoir lesions within the CNS (including eye and CSF) or (2) seeding from the blood and bone marrow [7, 22, 31]. The first possibility is supported by preclinical studies that have demonstrated dormant microscopic PCNSL cells behind a minimally leaky NVU [22]. New contrast enhancement detected by MRI is generally considered to be a sensitive biomarker for disease progression. However, contrast enhancement is a sensitive marker for disrupted NVU which consists of the BBB (endothelial cells and their associated tight junctions) surrounded by neurons and non-neuronal cells such as pericyte and glial (astrocytes, microglia and oligodendroglia) foot processes [32–34]. Subclinical CNS tumor sites may remain undetected by conventional contrast enhanced MRI scanning behind an intact NVU or blood-cerebrospinal fluid barrier. At relapse, 10% (4/36) of our patients had radiographic evidence of leptomeningeal relapses; this raises the issue of

occult lymphoma cells in the CSF reservoirs that subsequently seed sites distant from the initial tumor [1]. We acknowledge that contrast enhanced MRI may be an inadequate tool to detect microscopic (occult) disease. The low sensitivity of CSF cytology and the retrospective nature of this study further limits extensive review of CSF as an occult reservoir. However, prior studies looking at this issue with CSF-flow cytometry and CSF-polymerase chain reaction (PCR) found similar low rates (11–16%) of CSF dissemination of PCNSL [35]. On the other hand, the detection of persistent monoclonal B cells in blood and bone marrow samples by PCR in patients with no other evidence of systemic involvement by routine staging procedures supports the notion of seeding from these sites [31]. Unusually high mutation frequency of *Ig* genes seen at relapse also suggests that these clones are derived from these occult sites with ongoing mutation [36, 37].

Although this study is limited by its retrospective nature and small sample size, our report is an independent confirmation of the pattern of relapses in a larger cohort of patients treated with first line HD-MTX/BBBD. At relapse, tumor biopsy and bone marrow biopsy samples are not routinely collected in PCNSL patients; these additional assays would further help in establishing the mechanism and source of relapse in this rare disease. There is emerging evidence and interest in evaluating the role of blood- and CSF-based biomarkers such as circulating tumor cells (CTC), as well as micro-RNA and DNA in the blood and CSF to improve the diagnostic sensitivity and specificity [38–41]. Although there is limited data in PCNSL, CTC have been detected in a variety of solid tumors, including systemic DLBCL, lung, breast and prostate cancer; they may help with effective surveillance and early detection of persistent clonal populations even after radiographic CR as well as potentially help modify therapy, based on response [40, 42, 43].

The role of the BBB and NVU need to be considered when developing strategies and approaches for new therapies and biomarkers for response assessment in PCNSL. Strategies aimed at delaying relapses including those that address seeding from occult reservoir lesions within the CNS (including the CSF and eye) and/or seeding from outside the CNS (blood and bone marrow), are currently being evaluated. WBRT after CR addresses the issue of occult CNS disease. However, WBRT is associated with significant concerns for neurocognitive toxicities [44, 45]. The efficacy and improved toxicity profile of reduced-dose radiotherapy after CR is an area of active investigation [46]. Intrathecal route of drug administration is an alternative approach to target the CSF reservoir [21, 47]. However, limited drug delivery into the brain parenchyma beyond the superficial (2–3 mm) around the subarachnoid space is expected due to the inherent interstitial fluid pressure in the brain. In spite of good cytological responses, the majority had disease progression within a year in a phase I trial evaluating intrathecal rituximab at relapse [23, 47, 48]. This approach needs further evaluation; however there is concern for increased neuro-toxicities, especially with intrathecal administration of drug combinations [49, 50]. On the other hand, myeloablative chemotherapy with autologous stem cell transplant, and systemic maintenance anti-CD20 immunotherapy, address the issue of seeding from extra CNS sites [7, 51–53]. Encouraging results were noted after autologous stem cell transplantation in patients who have attained CR, but this approach is associated with significant hematological and non-hematological grade-3 and 4 toxicities and up to 10% treatment related mortality [53, 54]. Maintenance immunotherapy with anti CD-20 antibody via systemic (iv) infusion is another approach that has been shown to be relatively safe and potentially beneficial in a preliminary retrospective review, most likely due to its action on subclinical disease sites outside the CNS and potentially on occult CNS sites [7, 51]. These antibodies can potentially address occult extra-CNS as well as CNS reservoir sites due to slow leak and accumulation across minimally disrupted BBB. This approach is being evaluated in a prospective multicenter randomized trial [7]. Currently available clinical imaging techniques and blood or CSF biomarkers cannot detect these occult disease sites behind an intact NVU or at other potential non-CNS sites, innovative strategies for early detection and targeting therapies to address these sites can further improve outcomes.

## Conclusion

Both gliomas and PCNSL are well recognized to be a whole brain disease, even if imaging may suggest anatomically localized lesions at presentation. It is important to recognize that contrast enhancement is a surrogate for BBBD and not for the true extent of tumor in the CNS. Our results suggest that unlike gliomas, majority of PCNSL recur at spatially distinct anatomical locations within, and in few cases, outside the CNS. This may either be due to seeding from occult lesions (areas of CNS with intact BBB or ocular) or other extra CNS sites such as the bone marrow. Recognizing patterns of relapse is key for early detection and may provide insight into potential mechanisms of relapse as well as help develop strategies to extend duration of complete response.

## Abbreviations

PCNSL: primary central nervous system lymphoma; CC: corpus callosum; CNS: central nervous system; CR: complete response; CTC: circulating tumor cells; DLBCL: diffuse large B-cell lymphoma; BBB: blood-brain barrier; BBBD: blood–brain barrier disruption; HD-MTX: high dose methotrexate; MRI: magnetic resonance imaging; NVU: neurovascular unit; WBRT: whole brain radiotherapy.

## Authors' contributions

JP and PA interpreted the imaging findings, JF and CK collected the data, PA, RF, JF, ND and ED interpreted analyzed and interpreted the patient data. PA, ND and ED were major contributors in writing the manuscript. All authors read and approved the final manuscript.

## Author details

[1] Department of Neurology, Oregon Health & Science University, 3181 SW Sam Jackson Park Road, L603, Portland, OR 97239, USA. [2] Portland Veterans Affairs Medical Center, Portland, OR, USA. [3] School of Public Health, Oregon Health & Science University, Portland, OR, USA. [4] Department of Emergency Medicine, Oregon Health & Science University, Portland, OR, USA. [5] Department of Radiology, Oregon Health & Science University, Portland, OR, USA. [6] Department of Neurosurgery, Oregon Health & Science University, Portland, OR, USA.

## Acknowledgements

We thank Emily Youngers for her editorial assistance with this manuscript.

## Competing interests

The authors declare that they have no competing interests.

## Funding

This work was supported by the National Institutes of Health National Cancer Institute Grant CA137488, a Veterans Administration Merit Review grant and the Walter S. and Lucienne Driskill Foundation, all to Edward A. Neuwelt.

## References

1. Hoang-Xuan K, Bessell E, Bromberg J, Hottinger AF, Preusser M, Ruda R, Schlegel U, Siegal T, Soussain C, Abacioglu U, et al. Diagnosis and treatment of primary CNS lymphoma in immunocompetent patients: guidelines from the European Association for Neuro-Oncology. Lancet Oncol. 2015;16:e322–32.
2. Abrey LE, Batchelor TT, Ferreri AJ, Gospodarowicz M, Pulczynski EJ, Zucca E, Smith JR, Korfel A, Soussain C, DeAngelis LM, et al. Report of an international workshop to standardize baseline evaluation and response criteria for primary CNS lymphoma. J Clin Oncol. 2005;23:5034–43.
3. Thiel E, Korfel A, Martus P, Kanz L, Griesinger F, Rauch M, Roth A, Hertenstein B, von Toll T, Hundsberger T, et al. High-dose methotrexate with or without whole brain radiotherapy for primary CNS lymphoma (G-PCNSL-SG-1): a phase 3, randomised, non-inferiority trial. Lancet Oncol. 2010;11:1036–47.
4. Jahnke K, Thiel E, Martus P, Herrlinger U, Weller M, Fischer L, Korfel A. Relapse of primary central nervous system lymphoma: clinical features, outcome and prognostic factors. J Neurooncol. 2006;80:159–65.
5. Herrlinger U, Kuker W, Uhl M, Blaicher HP, Karnath HO, Kanz L, Bamberg M, Weller M. NOA-03 trial of high-dose methotrexate in primary central nervous system lymphoma: final report. Ann Neurol. 2005;57:843–7.
6. Ambady P, Holdhoff M, Bonekamp D, Wong F, Grossman SA. Late relapses in primary CNS lymphoma after complete remissions with high-dose methotrexate monotherapy. CNS Oncol. 2015;4:393–8.
7. Neuwelt EA, Schiff D. Primary CNS lymphoma: a landmark trial and the next steps. Neurology. 2015;84:1194–5.
8. Haldorsen IS, Krakenes J, Krossnes BK, Mella O, Espeland A. CT and MR imaging features of primary central nervous system lymphoma in Norway, 1989–2003. Am J Neuroradiol. 2009;30:744–51.
9. Go JL, Lee SC, Kim PE. Imaging of primary central nervous system lymphoma. Neurosurg Focus. 2006;21:E4.
10. Erdag N, Bhorade RM, Alberico RA, Yousuf N, Patel MR. Primary lymphoma of the central nervous system: typical and atypical CT and MR imaging appearances. Am J Roentgenol. 2001;176:1319–26.
11. Haldorsen IS, Espeland A, Larsson EM. Central nervous system lymphoma: characteristic findings on traditional and advanced imaging. Am J Neuroradiol. 2011;32:984–92.
12. Slone HW, Blake JJ, Shah R, Guttikonda S, Bourekas EC. CT and MRI findings of intracranial lymphoma. Am J Roentgenol. 2005;184:1679–85.
13. Zacharia TT, Law M, Naidich TP, Leeds NE. Central nervous system lymphoma characterization by diffusion-weighted imaging and MR spectroscopy. J Neuroimaging. 2008;18:411–7.

14. de Jong D, Glas AM, Boerrigter L, Hermus MC, Dalesio O, Willemse E, Nederlof PM, Kersten MJ. Very late relapse in diffuse large B-cell lymphoma represents clonally related disease and is marked by germinal center cell features. Blood. 2003;102:324–7.

15. Nayak L, Hedvat C, Rosenblum MK, Abrey LE, DeAngelis LM. Late relapse in primary central nervous system lymphoma: clonal persistence. Neuro-oncology. 2011;13:525–9.

16. Angelov L, Doolittle ND, Kraemer DF, Siegal T, Barnett GH, Peereboom DM, Stevens G, McGregor J, Jahnke K, Lacy CA, et al. Blood-brain barrier disruption and intra-arterial methotrexate-based therapy for newly diagnosed primary CNS lymphoma: a multi-institutional experience. J Clin Oncol. 2009;27:3503–9.

17. Doolittle ND, Fu R, Muldoon LL, Tyson RM, Lacy CA, Neuwelt EA. Rituximab in combination with methotrexate-based chemotherapy with blood–brain barrier disruption in newly diagnosed primary CNS lymphoma. In: 12th international conference on malignant lymphoma. Lugano, Switzerland; 2013.

18. Abrey LE, Batchelor TT, Ferreri AJ, Gospodarowicz M, Pulczynski EJ, Zucca E, Smith JR, Korfel A, Soussain C, DeAngelis LM, et al. Report of an international workshop to standardize baseline evaluation and response criteria for primary CNS lymphoma. J Clin Oncol. 2005;23:5034–43.

19. Hochberg FH, Pruitt A. Assumptions in the radiotherapy of glioblastoma. Neurology. 1980;30:907–11.

20. Schulte-Altedorneburg G, Heuser L, Pels H. MRI patterns in recurrence of primary CNS lymphoma in immunocompetent patients. Eur J Radiol. 2012;81:2380–5.

21. Rubenstein JL, Combs D, Rosenberg J, Levy A, McDermott M, Damon L, Ignoffo R, Aldape K, Shen A, Lee D, et al. Rituximab therapy for CNS lymphomas: targeting the leptomeningeal compartment. Blood. 2003;101:466–8.

22. Muldoon LL, Lewin SJ, Dosa E, Kraemer DF, Pagel MA, Doolittle ND, Neuwelt EA. Imaging and therapy with rituximab anti-CD20 immunotherapy in an animal model of central nervous system lymphoma. Clin Cancer Res. 2011;17:2207–15.

23. Muldoon LL, Soussain C, Jahnke K, Johanson C, Siegal T, Smith QR, Hall WA, Hynynen K, Senter PD, Peereboom DM, Neuwelt EA. Chemotherapy delivery issues in central nervous system malignancy: a reality check. J Clin Oncol. 2007;25:2295–305.

24. Morris PG, Correa DD, Yahalom J, Raizer JJ, Schiff D, Grant B, Grimm S, Lai RK, Reiner AS, Panageas K, et al. Rituximab, methotrexate, procarbazine, and vincristine followed by consolidation reduced-dose whole-brain radiotherapy and cytarabine in newly diagnosed primary CNS lymphoma: final results and long-term outcome. J Clin Oncol. 2013;31:3971–9.

25. Holdhoff M, Ambady P, Abdelaziz A, Sarai G, Bonekamp D, Blakeley J, Grossman SA, Ye X. High-dose methotrexate with or without rituximab in newly diagnosed primary CNS lymphoma. Neurology. 2014;83:235–9.

26. Pels H, Montesinos-Rongen M, Schaller C, Van Roost D, Schlegel U, Wiestler OD, Deckert M. Clonal evolution as pathogenetic mechanism in relapse of primary CNS lymphoma. Neurology. 2004;63:167–9.

27. Igala M. Unusual relapse of primary central nervous system lymphoma. Springerplus. 2016;5:301.

28. Jahnke K, Thiel E, Martus P, Herrlinger U, Weller M, Fischer L, Korfel A, German Primary Central Nervous System Lymphoma Study G. Relapse of primary central nervous system lymphoma: clinical features, outcome and prognostic factors. J Neurooncol. 2006;80:159–65.

29. Mylam KJ, Michaelsen TY, Hutchings M, Jacobsen Pulczynski E, Pedersen LM, Braendstrup P, Gade IL, Eberlein TR, Gang AO, Bogsted M, et al. Little value of surveillance magnetic resonance imaging for primary CNS lymphomas in first remission: results from a Danish Multicentre Study. Br J Haematol. 2017;176(4):671–3.

30. Tabouret E, Houillier C, Marint-Duverneuil N, Blonski M, Soussain C, Ghesquieres H, Houot R, Delwail V, Soubeyran P, Gressin R, et al. Patterns of response and relapse of primary central nervous system lymphomas (PCNSL) following first line of high-dose methotrexate-based chemotherapy (hdMTX): analysis of a prospective ANOCEF randomized phase II trial. In: 2015 ASCO Annual Meeting. 2015.

31. Jahnke K, Hummel M, Korfel A, Burmeister T, Kiewe P, Klasen HA, Muller HH, Stein H, Thiel E. Detection of subclinical systemic disease in primary

CNS lymphoma by polymerase chain reaction of the rearranged immunoglobulin heavy-chain genes. J Clin Oncol. 2006;24:4754–7.

32. McConnell HL, Kersch CN, Woltjer RL, Neuwelt EA. The translational significance of the neurovascular unit. J Biol Chem. 2017;292:762–70.

33. Zlokovic BV. The blood-brain barrier in health and chronic neurodegenerative disorders. Neuron. 2008;57:178–201.

34. Zlokovic BV. Neurovascular mechanisms of Alzheimer's neurodegeneration. Trends Neurosci. 2005;28:202–8.

35. Fischer L, Martus P, Weller M, Klasen HA, Rohden B, Roth A, Storek B, Hummel M, Nagele T, Thiel E, Korfel A. Meningeal dissemination in primary CNS lymphoma: prospective evaluation of 282 patients. Neurology. 2008;71:1102–8.

36. Thompsett AR, Ellison DW, Stevenson FK, Zhu D. V(H) gene sequences from primary central nervous system lymphomas indicate derivation from highly mutated germinal center B cells with ongoing mutational activity. Blood. 1999;94:1738–46.

37. Montesinos-Rongen M, Kuppers R, Schluter D, Spieker T, Van Roost D, Schaller C, Reifenberger G, Wiestler OD, Deckert-Schluter M. Primary central nervous system lymphomas are derived from germinal-center B cells and show a preferential usage of the V4-34 gene segment. Am J Pathol. 1999;155:2077–86.

38. Baraniskin A, Kuhnhenn J, Schlegel U, Chan A, Deckert M, Gold R, Maghnouj A, Zollner H, Reinacher-Schick A, Schmiegel W, et al. Identification of microRNAs in the cerebrospinal fluid as marker for primary diffuse large B-cell lymphoma of the central nervous system. Blood. 2011;117:3140–6.

39. Wang Y, Springer S, Zhang M, McMahon KW, Kinde I, Dobbyn L, Ptak J, Brem H, Chaichana K, Gallia GL, et al. Detection of tumor-derived DNA in cerebrospinal fluid of patients with primary tumors of the brain and spinal cord. Proc Natl Acad Sci USA. 2015;112:9704–9.

40. Ambady P, Bettegowda C, Holdhoff M. Emerging methods for disease monitoring in malignant gliomas. CNS Oncol. 2013;2:511–22.

41. Holdhoff M, Schmidt K, Donehower R, Diaz LA Jr. Analysis of circulating tumor DNA to confirm somatic KRAS mutations. J Natl Cancer Inst. 2009;101:1284–5.

42. Roschewski M, Dunleavy K, Pittaluga S, Moorhead M, Pepin F, Kong K, Shovlin M, Jaffe ES, Staudt LM, Lai C, et al. Circulating tumour DNA and CT monitoring in patients with untreated diffuse large B-cell lymphoma: a correlative biomarker study. Lancet Oncol. 2015;16:541–9.

43. Kwok M, Wu SP, Mo C, Summers T, Roschewski M. Circulating tumor DNA to monitor therapy for aggressive B-cell lymphomas. Curr Treat Options Oncol. 2016;17:47.

44. DeAngelis LM. Whither whole brain radiotherapy for primary CNS lymphoma? Neuro Oncol. 2014;16:1032–4.

45. Doolittle ND, Dosa E, Fu R, Muldoon LL, Maron LM, Lubow MA, Tyson RM, Lacy CA, Kraemer DF, Butler RW, Neuwelt EA. Preservation of cognitive function in primary CNS lymphoma survivors a median of 12 years after enhanced chemotherapy delivery. J Clin Oncol. 2013;31:4026–7.

46. Correa DD, Rocco-Donovan M, DeAngelis LM, Dolgoff-Kaspar R, Iwamoto F, Yahalom J, Abrey LE. Prospective cognitive follow-up in primary CNS lymphoma patients treated with chemotherapy and reduced-dose radiotherapy. J Neurooncol. 2009;91:315–21.

47. Rubenstein JL, Fridlyand J, Abrey L, Shen A, Karch J, Wang E, Issa S, Damon L, Prados M, McDermott M, et al. Phase I study of intraventricular administration of rituximab in patients with recurrent CNS and intraocular lymphoma. J Clin Oncol. 2007;25:1350–6.

48. Blasberg RG, Patlak C, Fenstermacher JD. Intrathecal chemotherapy: brain tissue profiles after ventriculocisternal perfusion. J Pharmacol Exp Ther. 1975;195:73–83.

49. Jabbour E, O'Brien S, Kantarjian H, Garcia-Manero G, Ferrajoli A, Ravandi F, Cabanillas M, Thomas DA. Neurologic complications associated with intrathecal liposomal cytarabine given prophylactically in combination with high-dose methotrexate and cytarabine to patients with acute lymphocytic leukemia. Blood. 2007;109:3214–8.

50. Khan RB, Shi W, Thaler HT, DeAngelis LM, Abrey LE. Is intrathecal methotrexate necessary in the treatment of primary CNS lymphoma? J Neurooncol. 2002;58:175–8.

51. Ney DE, Abrey LE. Maintenance therapy for central nervous system lymphoma with rituximab. Leuk Lymphoma. 2009;50:1548–51.

52. Abrey LE, Moskowitz CH, Mason WP, Crump M, Stewart D, Forsyth P, Paleologos N, Correa DD, Anderson ND, Caron D, et al. Intensive methotrexate and cytarabine followed by high-dose chemotherapy with autologous

# 9

# The opioid epidemic: a central role for the blood brain barrier in opioid analgesia and abuse

Charles P. Schaefer, Margaret E. Tome* and Thomas P. Davis

## Abstract

Opioids are currently the primary treatment method used to manage both acute and chronic pain. In the past two to three decades, there has been a surge in the use, abuse and misuse of opioids. The mechanism by which opioids relieve pain and induce euphoria is dependent on the drug crossing the blood–brain barrier and accessing the central nervous system. This suggests the blood brain barrier plays a central role in both the benefits and risks of opioid use. The complex physiological responses to opioids that provide the benefits and drive the abuse also needs to be considered in the resolution of the opioid epidemic.

**Keywords:** Opioids, Morphine, Pain, Blood–brain barrier, P-Glycoprotein, Opioid tolerance

## Background

In the United States, the abuse of opioids is currently described as an epidemic. On average, 3900 individuals begin the non-medical use of prescription opioids, and 580 individuals begin heroin use every day [1]. Drug overdose deaths related to opioids, including both opioid pain relievers and heroin, increased 200% between 2000 and 2014 [2]. This trend is continuing unabated. Yet, opioids are the most effective therapy for reducing reported pain in most patients. For example, pain management is an important component of post-surgical recovery. Poor pain management can impair recovery, increase the probability of readmission, increase the cost of care and decrease patient satisfaction [3]. Intravenous opioid analgesics, such as morphine, are currently the standard of care for post-surgical pain. The yin and yang of the opioid response leads to the clinical challenge of how to treat short/moderate duration post-surgical pain without causing opioid dependence that could lead to abuse.

The purpose of this review is to first, trace the history of the use and abuse of opioids and put this into the context of our current understanding of the physiology

of pain. Next, we examine the role that the blood brain barrier (BBB) plays in opioid analgesia and euphoria. We have highlighted the central role of the BBB in opioid analgesia and abuse because it is a critical regulator of opioid access to the central nervous system (CNS).

### Physiology of pain

In his famous novel *1984*, George Orwell describes "Of pain you could wish only one thing: that it should stop. Nothing in the world was so bad as physical pain. In the face of pain there are no heroes".

Pain and the negative emotions associated with it serve as invaluable tools for survival. Acute pain acts as a signal of noxious stimuli and the negative emotional response associated with the pain reinforces behaviors that avoid these stimuli. Persistent pain acts as a clue of internal injuries such as muscular damage or broken bones. Changes can occur in pain pathways resulting in an altered, chronic state. When chronic pain is associated with an injury, this can alter behavior to protect the site of an injury allowing the injury to heal without further harm. In some cases, chronic pain will persist at the site of an injury well past the time protective pain is beneficial to healing.

The physical component of pain, nociception, is the process by which nociceptors, a group of nerve cells

*Correspondence: mtome@pathology.arizona.edu
Department of Pharmacology, University of Arizona, P.O. Box 245050, Tucson, AZ 85724, USA

found in the peripheral nervous system, recognize intense thermal, mechanical or chemical stimuli [4]. Nociceptors have a unique physiology; they have cell bodies in specific regions known as ganglia. In the periphery, the cell bodies of nociceptors are located in the dorsal root ganglion. Nociceptors have two axonal branches, a peripheral branch that innervates the target organ and a central axon that innervates the spinal cord [5]. A key feature of nociceptors is the ability to limit the initiation of a signal in response to noxious stimuli by requiring a relatively high activation signal. Nociceptors are divided into two groups of fibers. The Aδ-fibers and Aβ-fibers are thinly myelinated fibers responsible for transmitting "acute, well-localized, fast pain," specifying the location of the stimulus [4]. The second type of fiber is the unmyelinated C-fiber which is responsible for poorly-localized "slow" pain often described as an ache. Both of these fiber types can be organized into subtypes that are more or less sensitive to thermal or mechanical stimulation.

In the central nervous system, nociceptors project to differing laminae of the dorsal horn of the spinal cord depending on the type of nociceptive fiber. A variety of signaling molecules act at the synapses between the central terminal of the nociceptors and the laminae of the spinal cord [5]. Neurons within these laminae are responsible for transmitting the nociceptive signal through the spinal cord in a contralateral manner to the thalamus of the brain. From here, signals are sent to the somatosensory cortex and limbic system. While this process is short-lived for acute pain, persistent or chronic pain can arise when there is an anomaly in this system. The anomaly can be caused by either over sensitization or spontaneous firing of nociceptors. Pharmacological modification of this pathway is used as a strategy to reduce or eliminate pain.

### History of opioid use for pain treatment

Opioids are a key drug in our arsenal for the treatment of pain. However, the addictive and destructive properties of opioids and their derivatives present both a clinical challenge and a public health problem that we have yet to resolve. The exact origins of the use of opium for pain treatment are not known. The original use of opium was probably as a euphoriant in religious ceremonies as described in pictographs from ancient Sumerian sites. Knowledge of the process used to isolate opium was likely limited to priests [6]. Brownstein states that the earliest written records of medicinal use of the opium poppy date back to the dawn of human civilization [6]. The Sumerians were the first people to record the production and use of opium. Clay tablets dating around 3000 BC describe the process by which the opium poppy was cultivated. The tablets also describe how to extract

the juice from the cultivated flowers and the process by which this juice is processed into opium. Cultivation of this plant remained popular, spanning many centuries and empires and eventually led to the distribution of opium throughout Eurasia.

The complex issues surrounding opioid use are illustrated by the history of opium use in China. As documented in Schiff, Arabian traders brought opium and knowledge of the medicinal use of the drug to the country at some point between the 11th and 13th centuries AD [7]. This review goes on to say that following a ban on smoking tobacco by Tsung Chen in 1644, smoking opium became a popular replacement for many Chinese citizens. Opium sold in China originated from large growing operations in India distributed by the East India Company. Following the acquisition of the East India Company by the British government, large quantities of opium were sold to smaller companies that would smuggle the drug into China. These companies sold the opium through Canton. Following the replacement of the Viceroy of Canton in 1838, opium distribution was severely reduced. In 1839, millions of pounds of British and American opium were confiscated and destroyed by the Viceroy. This sparked the first opium war resulting in Britain being awarded control of the island of Hong Kong for over 150 years. By 1913, 25% of the Chinese population was addicted to opium. This epidemic prompted the British government to suspend the sale of opium, but this action came too late. Widespread use of opium would not stop in China until the years following World War II with the establishment of the People's Republic of China.

The search for opioid derivatives that retain efficacy and decrease addiction also has a long history. In 1806, morphine was isolated from the opium poppy by Sertüner [8]. Morphine could be produced in large quantities and became popular to use for minor surgical procedures and for the management of post-surgical and chronic pain. This discovery was not the solution for opiate addiction that many had hoped for and triggered the widespread search for a non-addictive replacement. In 1898, heroin was first synthesized with the claim of being more potent than morphine and being free from an addictive nature like other opioids [9]. Only one of these claims would prove to be true, and both heroin abuse and the search for a non-addictive opioid continue today [6]. The search for a non-addictive replacement resulted in the synthesis of methadone in 1946 which led to the first potential treatment for opioid addiction [10]. The symptoms of withdrawal syndrome associated with methadone use were markedly more manageable than those associated with traditional opioids. While these symptoms have a longer duration, the effects experienced are milder. This observation inspired a treatment plan in which patients would be switched from an opioid to methadone with the goal that administration would be tapered off entirely [6]. These programs rely on very careful monitoring of drug intake combined with the addition of supportive behavioral therapies and lead to lowered mortality rates than in those who do not use this therapy [11]. Those using this therapy are also able to maintain mostly normal lives, easing the transition out of addiction [6].

Use of opioids for pain management has waxed and waned through history in part because of changing attitudes toward the risk/benefit balance of such treatment. For example, chronic opioid therapy for non-cancer related chronic pain has been a standard use of these drugs throughout history. While this did fall out of favor though much of the 20th century due to the danger of addiction and other adverse effects, attitudes began to change in the 1980s [12]. A letter written to the New England Journal of Medicine made a significant impact on attitudes towards the addictive nature of opioids in chronic pain patients [13]. The letter explained that of the 11,882 examined patients who received at least one prescription of a narcotic, only four had well-documented addiction after leaving the hospital. The feeling of safety related to chronic opioid use was further reinforced by letters and scholarly reviews throughout the following decades. These studies often involved patients with a history of opioid use presenting little to no evidence of addiction [14–16]. Of these studies, an article published in *Pain* was particularly notable. This study followed 38 patients who had received opioids for an extended period reporting misuse in only two patients [15]. This gave the impression that if an opioid was prescribed for pain, there was little danger of addiction. The shift in attitudes towards opioids as a complete solution for all types of pain management seemed to answer the increasing demand for pain management in clinical settings [12]. The relaxed attitudes surrounding opioids began to be questioned again after a decade long trend, beginning in 2000, resulted in large changes of opioid use. Articles and reviews were published detailing the increase in opioid prescriptions across all types of clinical settings [17, 18]. Increasing trends in opioid use, as well as the increase in opioid prescriptions, are currently raising public safety concerns.

### Physiology of the opioid response: crossing the blood brain barrier

Opioids are a class of drugs with several useful effects including cough suppression, gastric slowing, and as they are most commonly prescribed, analgesia. Opioid analgesics can be administered through suppository or intrathecally, intravenously, or orally. More lipophilic opioids can also be administered transdermally. As described by Yaksh and Wallace in *Goodman and Gilman's: The Pharmacological Basis of Therapeutics*, oral opioids are subject to the first pass effect in the liver as well as poor absorption due to gastric ion trapping and have a bioavailability of about 25% [19]. Intravenous administration of opioids results in prompt action [19]. The speed of action is affected by the lipophilicity of the compound which contributes to differences in the speed at which the compound can cross the BBB and enter the CNS. Morphine does not persist in tissue and is found in trace quantities 24 h after the last administered dose. Metabolism of morphine relies on conjugation with glucuronic acid producing two metabolites, morphine-6-glucuronide (M6G) and morphine-3-glucuronide (M3G). M6G has an analgesic effect. It is twice as potent as morphine, and is thought to make up a significant portion of morphine's analgesic effect in patients treated with long-term opioid therapy [20]. The more prevalent metabolite, M3G, is known to have neuroexcitatory effects [21]. M3G is also the primary form excreted from the body [19]. While almost no unmodified morphine is excreted, morphine's metabolites are excreted through the kidneys.

The analgesic effect of opioids is due to pharmacological action in the brain, in the spinal cord, and potentially in the periphery. In the brain, opioids act at mu opioid receptors (MOR). Mutations in the MOR at position 118 are sufficient to modify post-cesarean pain perceptions and the amount of morphine used by patients through a patient-controlled analgesia system [22]. Experiments involving microinjections at the medulla, substantia nigra, nucleus accumbens, and periaqueductal gray (PAG) resulted in the reduction of pain behaviors in animal models [23]. The action in the PAG causes a disinhibition of the medulla at tonically active neurons [19]. This disinhibition leads to the release of norepinephrine and serotonin to the spinal dorsal horn, attenuating dorsal horn excitability [23]. This attenuation results in a reduction of nociceptive signaling through the spinal cord.

### The blood–brain barrier: opioid access to the CNS and the role of P-glycoprotein

The main analgesic response to opioids occurs at the level of the CNS. To exert this effect, the opioids must cross the BBB. The BBB serves as a selectively permeable physical and biochemical barrier that contributes to the maintenance of the ionic homeostatic environment required for proper neuronal function in the CNS. Evolutionary studies have shown that this type of barrier was essential for the development and function of increasing complex brains in vertebrates [24, 25]. The BBB also plays a major role in protecting the CNS from pathogens and toxins in the bloodstream. The ability of the BBB to exclude xenobiotics from the CNS serves as a challenge for delivery of pharmacological agents, including opioids, to the brain [26, 27].

Anatomically, the BBB is a barrier formed by endothelial cells surrounding the lumen of the brain microvasculature (Fig. 1). Adjacent endothelial cells attach themselves to each other via specific proteins forming tight junctions of high transendothelial electrical resistance. These tight junctions are made up of a complex of transmembrane proteins and prevent paracellular movement of substances from the blood into the brain [28]. Adherens junctions, which help establish cell polarity, also link endothelial cells to each other and contribute to barrier integrity. Pericytes surround the endothelial cells. Pericytes belong to the vascular smooth muscle cell family. They play an important role in the establishment of the BBB and provide structural support and maintenance signals for the mature BBB [29]. Astrocytes, which surround the endothelial cells and pericytes also contribute to BBB maintenance and regulation of barrier properties [30]. The interaction of these cell types, known as the neurovascular unit, is a critical regulator of

barrier properties in response to physiological changes and under pathological conditions.

The ability of the BBB to act as a selectively permeable barrier is heavily reliant on transport proteins in the endothelial cells that regulate transcellular movement of substances. Transport proteins are essential for the movement of nutrients into the brain while keeping pathogens and toxins out. Some of the transporters are highly specific. For example, glucose, essential for brain function, requires a transporter to cross the BBB. The GLUT1 transporter is responsible for glucose transport and allows glucose to travel into the brain along its concentration gradient [31]. Some transporters act to export compounds from the BBB, most notably the ATP-Binding Cassette (ABC) proteins [32]. Of these, P-glycoprotein (P-gp), also known as multiple drug resistant protein 1 (Mdr1), plays a major role in the mechanism by which toxins and xenobiotics are excluded [33, 34]. P-gp is of particular interest because it has a wide range of substrates, including opioids, and a poorly understood system of regulators. Numerous other transporters are

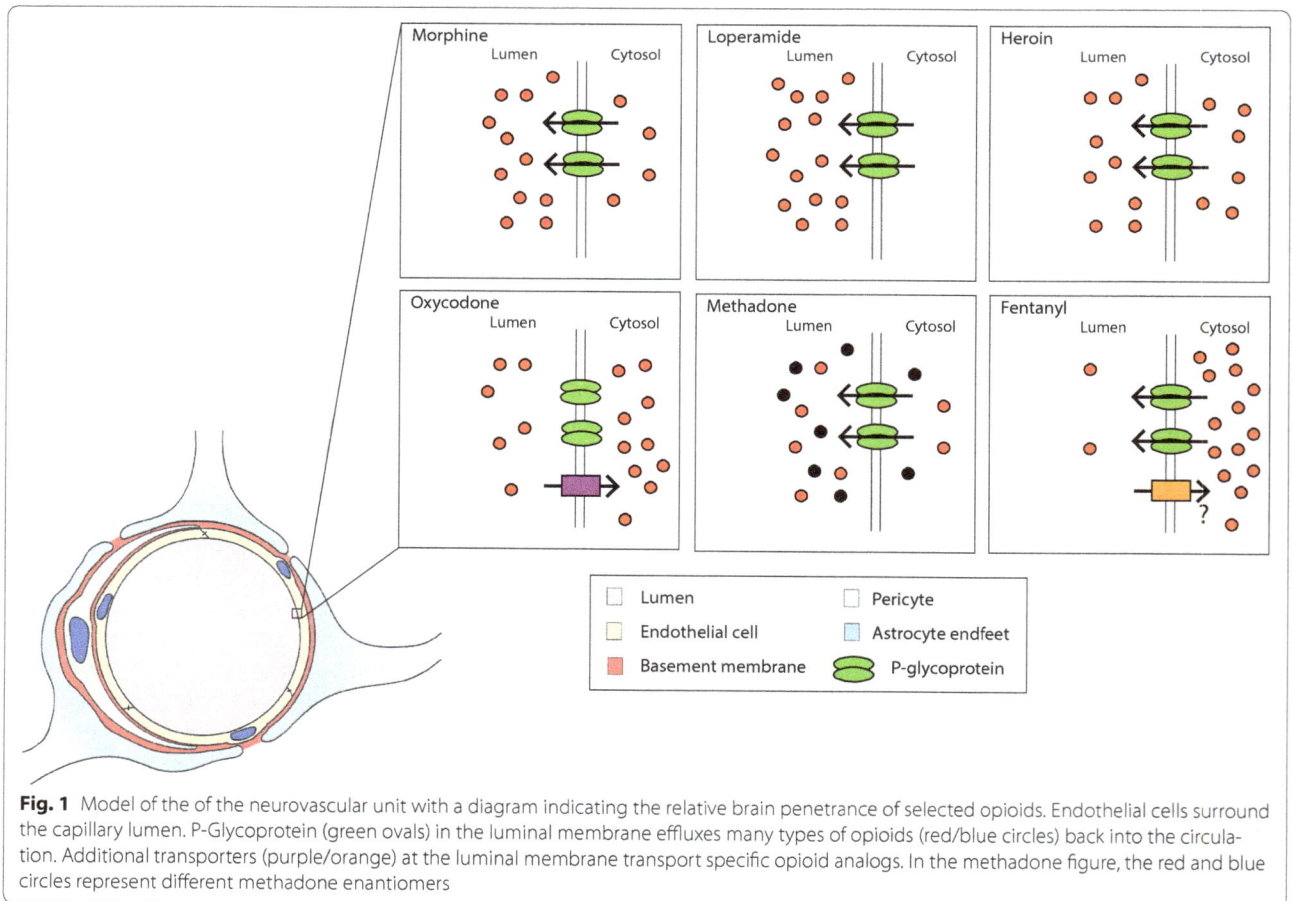

**Fig. 1** Model of the of the neurovascular unit with a diagram indicating the relative brain penetrance of selected opioids. Endothelial cells surround the capillary lumen. P-Glycoprotein (green ovals) in the luminal membrane effluxes many types of opioids (red/blue circles) back into the circulation. Additional transporters (purple/orange) at the luminal membrane transport specific opioid analogs. In the methadone figure, the red and blue circles represent different methadone enantiomers

expressed in the BBB endothelial cells and contribute to the selective barrier properties of the BBB [26].

## The blood brain barrier: delivery of opioids to the CNS

Analgesic efficacy of opioids depends on the relative ability to cross the BBB. Opioids currently in clinical use alleviate pain mostly by binding to MOR in the CNS; uptake into the brain, therefore, is critical for efficacy. P-gp is the major drug exporter at the BBB; it is very efficient at exporting opioids [35]. In the luminal membrane, P-gp binds to drug both as it is diffusing through the endothelial cell membrane and from inside the endothelial cells [36]. It effluxes drug back into the circulation via an ATP-dependent mechanism [36]. Inhibition of P-gp to improve CNS drug delivery has not proven clinically viable because of the risk of death due to infection and toxicity [37, 38]. Therefore, an analysis of the efficacy of opioids and their derivatives depends in part on the ability of P-gp to exclude them from the CNS. An appreciation for the central role of P-gp in opioid analgesia is illustrated by the relative effects of several structurally divergent opioids (Fig. 1).

Morphine is the international standard for opioid analgesic therapy. As previously discussed, morphine is metabolized into M3G and M6G via glucuronidation, leading to blood concentrations of these metabolites several times higher than that of the parent compound. Morphine can also be metabolized to M3G and M6G in the brain directly [39]. Morphine is a substrate for P-gp [39, 40]. The analgesic efficacy of morphine is roughly proportional to the concentration of morphine in the blood and the amount of active P-gp at the BBB [41]. M6G, the metabolite with higher analgesic potency than the parent compound, is not a P-gp substrate, but may be a substrate of other transporters at the BBB [42, 43]. Genetic polymorphisms in ABCB1, the gene which encodes P-gp, in cancer patients play a major role in intracellular concentrations of morphine and both metabolites [42]. Inhibition of P-gp at the time of administration of morphine increases the observed analgesic effect, confirming P-gp inhibits the analgesic effect of morphine [44]. Multidrug resistance protein 3 effects the transport of morphine metabolites; additional studies to determine whether morphine metabolites are substrates of other members of the MDR protein family are needed [45].

Loperamide is a synthetic MOR agonist that is a stronger P-gp substrate than morphine, leading to its clinical use as an anti-diarrheal [46]. Both in vitro and in vivo models indicate that P-gp efficiently effluxes loperamide [46, 47]. The brain penetrance is minimal in humans; loperamide is marketed as an anti-diarrheal because the major effect is opioid-mediated constipation in the GI track [48]. P-gp knockout mice accumulated loperamide in the CNS and displayed opioid-mediated effects [49]. These data indicate that P-gp, by regulating brain uptake of loperamide, determines the analgesic efficacy of loperamide.

Heroin has a potency twofold greater than morphine and crosses the BBB more readily than morphine [50]. Although heroin is similar in structure to morphine, this drug is acetylated and therefore more lipophilic than morphine leading to an increased potency. Heroin is metabolized into 6-monoacetylmorphine (6-MAM) and subsequently to morphine in the blood [51]. In a study by Seleman et al. in which the effect of a P-gp inhibitor co-administered with heroin, 6-MAM, and morphine, only morphine transport was increased [27]. This study showed the transport of heroin and 6-MAM were unaffected by P-gp inhibition, suggesting that this may also play a role in the higher potency of heroin over morphine. 6-MAM has been shown to have an even greater affinity for MOR than morphine and a greater analgesic effect [51]. 6-MAM has a short half-life in humans and is rapidly metabolized into morphine. Although heroin and 6-MAM can enter the BBB, P-gp still plays a role in the effect of heroin on the CNS because of the rapid metabolism to morphine [52].

Oxycodone is a potent opioid often prescribed to manage moderate to severe pain. When co-administered with the P-gp inhibitor valspodar, transport of oxycodone into the brain was not affected [53]. Oxycodone has a lower affinity for MOR than morphine, but in similar doses is as effective as morphine in the management of post-surgical pain [54]. This prompted experimentation examining the relative BBB transport of oxycodone into the brain compared with morphine. Oxycodone is transported into the mouse brain in concentrations six times higher than morphine [35]. The relationship between the BBB and oxycodone is unique because oxycodone can be found at concentrations three times higher in the brain than in the blood [55]. A cation/H+ antiporter in the BBB endothelial cells has been implicated in the uptake of oxycodone into the brain [27, 56].

Methadone is a synthetic opioid that is used in the treatment of, especially, chronic pain and for opioid dependence [11, 57]. Methadone has lesser side effects than many other opioids, so chronic administration is often considered more manageable than for other opioids [11]. Methadone is administered as a racemic mixture of both the R- and S-enantiomers of the drug [58]. Methadone is metabolized into the pharmacologically inactive compound 2-ethylidene-1,5-dimethyl-3,3-diphenylpyrrolidine (EDDP) [59]. A study by Wang et al. showed both the R- and S-enantiomers of methadone are substrates of P-gp, limiting the delivery of the clinically used racemic methadone across the BBB [58]. This study compared concentrations of methadone found in multiple tissues throughout the body in wild-type and ABCB1a (the gene encoding P-gp in mice) knockout animals. Significantly higher concentrations of both enantiomers of methadone occurred only in the brain. Although there is minimal stereoselectivity of P-gp for methadone enantiomers, resulting in similar brain penetrance of both enantiomers, the (R)-enantiomer (levomethadone) is responsible for the action of methadone as a MOR agonist [40, 58, 60–62].

Fentanyl is a synthetic opioid with a potency 100-fold greater than morphine [63]. Fentanyl has become important due to its contribution to the epidemic of opioid related deaths [1]. A study by Henthorn et al. in which the CNS uptake of radiolabeled fentanyl was quantified, demonstrated that the presence of a P-gp inhibitor increased transport across bovine brain endothelial cells (an in vitro model of the BBB) [64]. This study also demonstrated that there is likely a transporter that contributes to direct transport of fentanyl across these endothelial cells. A study by Wandel et al. demonstrated that cells with an increased expression of P-gp did not have significantly lower transport of fentanyl across endothelial cells in vitro [46]. This suggests that other components of the neurovascular unit may play a significant role in fentanyl transport at the BBB. Further investigation into this mechanism would provide a path to reducing the dangers and addictive nature of this drug.

Analgesic efficacy of the opioids is complicated by additional factors in the clinic. The comparison studies on the relative ability of P-gp to efflux opioids are based on the same genetic variant of P-gp. Genetic polymorphisms in P-gp will affect the amount of drug excluded from the CNS at a given dose in humans [65]. As mentioned above, the ability of opioids (or their active metabolites) to cross the BBB can also depend on other transport mechanisms, as suggested by the data on oxycodone [56]. Once in the brain, the relative binding to MOR, rate of metabolism of the native compound, and relative activity of the metabolites will all contribute to analgesic efficacy (e.g., [52, 54]). Genetic polymorphisms that alter proteins in these pathways increase the difficulty of predicting the analgesic efficacy for a given patient [65]. In this review, we have chosen to discuss a few opioids in detail to illustrate the central role of the BBB. Many additional opioid derivatives exist. The complexity illustrated by our examples, however, indicates the extent to which opioids need to be studied to determine their best clinical use; an analysis of their ability to cross the BBB is an important component.

## The blood brain barrier: opioid-induced euphoria
Opioid transport across the BBB into the CNS is essential for the euphoric effects of opioids [19]. A review by

Xi and Stein summarizes the reward associated with opioids as, disinhibition of GABAergic neurons in the nucleus accumbens by dopaminergic neurons from the ventral tegmental area (VTA) which increases activity in the ventral pallidum and causes an increase of dopamine release [66]. Animals with the ability to deliver morphine directly to the VTA will continue to do so [66]. This suggests a feeling of reward for the animal and the presence of opioids in the brain is therefore capable of eliciting this response. This response to the presence of morphine in the brain demonstrates that the reduction of opioids in the brain may reduce the reward associated with these compounds.

## Opioid tolerance and dependence
One of the most challenging aspects of prolonged treatment with opioids is the progressive loss of efficacy referred to as opioid tolerance. Opioid tolerance is defined by Yaksh and Wallace as the reduction of analgesic efficacy of a particular dose of an opioid as that dose is repeatedly given over time [19]. Opioid tolerance occurs in as little as 2 weeks [67]. Tolerance is observable at the level of reduced analgesic and sedative effects. At the level of the cell, adenyl cyclase activity is disinhibited [68]. Research regarding the effect of chronic morphine exposure on the BBB is sparse. Whole brain and larger cortical blood vessels show an increase in expression of genes in the Mdr family including P-gp [69, 70]. These changes are correlated with decreased CNS uptake of morphine in rodents [69, 70]. Two studies suggest that the NMDA receptor signaling through the cyclooxygenase 2 pathway is involved in P-gp upregulation by morphine [69, 71], however, additional work is needed to understand the mechanistic details. Different physiological responses to opioids develop tolerance at different rates [19]. The constriction of the pupil (pupillary miosis) is an example of a response with little development of tolerance. Analgesia, sedation, respiratory depression, and constipation are examples of responses to which tolerance will build at a slower, more moderate pace. Cross-tolerance between different opioids can occur, but this is not always the case, suggesting small but meaningful differences in the action of different types of opioid agonists. Tolerance is reversible and suspension of administration of the drug will, over time, return efficacy of a particular dose to the original, basal levels.

Chronic administration of opioids will also lead to the development of a state of dependence. Dependence presents as a state in which cessation of opioid use, or administration of an opioid receptor antagonist such as naloxone or naltrexone, will result in the precipitation of withdrawal syndrome symptoms. Because opioids are an inhibitory signal to the cell, cells will increase signaling to compensate and return to normal function. Removing the inhibitory signal will result in an overactivation of affected cellular pathways leading to a variety of symptoms caused by the overactivation of the somatomotor cortex and autonomic nervous system [19]. Work by Nakagawa et al. showed that a glutamate transport activator, MS-153, was sufficient to prevent opioid dependence and withdrawal, suggesting glutamate may play a role in the formation of opioid dependence and withdrawal [72]. A study by Chaves et al. described that in the case of naloxone precipitated opioid withdrawals following sub-chronic morphine exposure, there was little change on P-gp at the BBB [73]. The major physical symptoms of withdrawal syndrome include diarrhea, vomiting, agitation, hyperalgesia, hyperthermia and hypertension. Feelings of depression, dysphoria and anxiety are also associated with withdrawal. Due to the fact these symptoms are highly aversive, prevention of withdrawal can act as a major motivator to continue use of the drug. This incentive to continue use can lead to overuse of, abuse of and addiction to opioids [74].

Tolerance to the euphoric effects of opioids develops rapidly and at a rate higher than many other effects [19]. Diminishing euphoria means users seeking this feeling are prone to ingesting a dose which can elicit a dangerous effect from a different response with a slower rate of tolerance. Because of this and severe withdrawal symptoms, addiction and abuse are problems for many individuals including both those who began as therapeutic users and exclusively recreational users [75]. Opioid addiction, also known as opioid use disorder, is a psychological condition defined as "compulsive, prolonged self-administration of opioid substances that are used for no legitimate medical purpose or, if another medical condition is present that requires opioid treatment, that are used in doses greatly in excess of the amount needed for that medical condition," [76]. Both those using opioids recreationally for euphoric effects and those who begin using them for medical conditions are at risk of addiction. Tolerance, dependence and the risk of addiction should be considered when prescribing opioids for post-surgical pain management.

The presence of a mental health condition can increase the likelihood of substance abuse. As many as 50% of patients with dipolar disorder have been found to have a substance abuse problem at some time in their life [77]. A survey by Martins et al. showed that several psychopathologies, especially anxiety disorders and bipolar I disorder, are associated with an increased incidence of opioid use [78]. This was an increased risk for those with a pre-existing condition as well as in individuals with newly diagnosed disorders in which the patient had a history of non-medical opioid use. This study suggests

individuals with anxiety disorders and with bipolar I disorder will use opioids as a means of "self-medication". In a disease like bipolar disorder with many different presenting episodes, the use of heroin is consistent across all types of episodes [79]. The use of opioids as a "self-medication" is a major public health concern. The comorbidity of substance abuse disorders and other psychopathologies demonstrates that this population must be treated with increased care and attention.

**An epidemic**

Opioid abuse has reached epidemic proportions in the United States. This has raised the awareness of opioid abuse as a public health issue. Several states have increased funding for treatment of opioid dependence to combat the trends of increased abuse and overdose deaths [1, 80]. However, there is insufficient treatment capacity to address the opioid dependence problem [1]. Cost of treatment is a challenge that significantly impacts the ability to increase capacity; approximately 25 billion dollars was spent in 2007 on extra healthcare costs related to opioid abuse [81]. New affordable, effective treatments and government funding for these programs will be essential to changing these trends.

Multiple societal, physiological and psychological factors contribute to the increasing opioid abuse. A majority of modern recreational opioid users begin their experience with opioids as therapeutics [82]. A study of patients diagnosed with opioid abuse disorder showed that almost 80% of these patients had a prescription for opioids before the first diagnosis of opioid abuse [83]. This study was also able to show that of the 20% that did not have a previous prescription, over half of them had a close family member who had a prescription before the first diagnosis of opioid abuse. This suggests that the availability of opioids from a family member can be a risk factor for abuse. Misuse of prescription refills and "doctor shopping," a situation where an individual seeking opioids may go to several different doctors to receive multiple prescriptions for the drugs, are common problems associated with prescribed opioids [12, 84, 85]. Use of online pharmacies, some of which require little documentation, and the dark web system of encrypted websites which is designed to allow the user complete anonymity has opened the door for illicit sale of prescription opioids [86]. Early refills are a subset of prescription abuse that requires additional scrutiny [87]. Some chronic opioid users increase use because opioids lose analgesic effectiveness over time, and the patient may resort to taking more pills to manage pain [88]. However, in other cases the additional pills are given to others or sold.

Physicians prescribing opioids must be examined as a factor contributing to the opioid epidemic, but must also be part of the solution of the problem. Physicians prescribe opioids at different rates due to many factors including: patient satisfaction surveys online [89]; professional repercussions for using (or not using) prudent judgment [89]; and how concerned a physician is about opioids as a public health problem (physicians less concerned with opioids as a problem are more likely to have patients on long-term opioid therapy for chronic pain as well [90]). Since 2014, the changing opinions of physicians towards opioids caused a decrease in the number of opioid prescriptions dispensed in the United States relative to predicted rates [91]. While these rates have dropped, the overall opioid epidemic has not changed [92].

Several studies suggest that a switch from prescription opioids to heroin is fueling the opioid epidemic. Heroin use has increased in the United States over the last decade [93]. This is likely due to the increase in popularity of opioid pain pills. A review of surveys interviewing heroin users who used opioid pain pills before the first time the individual used heroin range from 40 to 86% but was enough to suggest a relationship [82]. From 2010 to 2013, individuals who had used an opioid in the past month began to use only prescription opioids less and used a combination of opioids and heroin more, according to a self-administered survey of diagnosed opioid abusers [94]. The availability of heroin in the United States is increasing [95]. This report also states heroin is less expensive than prescription opioids on the streets. The estimated cost of a 10 mg dose of oxycodone is approximately $10 while it is estimated 50 mg of 50% pure heroin is around the same price. Heroin use may also be favorable because of the increased potency of the drug compared to morphine; a larger amount of heroin is able to cross the BBB compared to morphine [27]. Addressing this epidemic requires: (1) the development of better options for treating pain that takes into account the necessity of crossing the BBB to elicit an effect; (2) the societal and political will to develop strategies to combat the problem; (3) increased capacity to treat opioid dependence; and (4) a change in attitude such that opioid addiction is viewed as a medical problem rather than a criminal offense.

## Conclusion

Opioids are a powerful tool for the treatment of pain. Effective and responsible clinical use of opioids and their derivatives is complicated by P-gp at the BBB, tolerance and dependence. For the treatment of short/moderate duration post-surgical pain the analgesic benefit must be balanced with the risk of dependence, addiction and abuse. Regulation of opioid access to the CNS by the blood brain barrier is central to the ability of currently

available opioids to alleviate pain, but also to induce euphoria. This BBB effect contributes to the addiction and abuse that is fueling the opioid epidemic.

Continued research to develop new strategies and agents to alleviate pain is required. Some strategies, such as the development of opioid derivatives that act locally show promise in pre-clinical models [96]. The basis of this strategy is using the inherent challenges associated with designing therapeutics that will cross the blood–brain barrier to design opioid-based treatment strategies so that the opioids do not cross the BBB. Peripherally acting opioid analgesics are generally free from the addictive nature of traditional centrally acting opioid analgesics [97]. This type of analgesic was traditionally thought to be less effective, but there is increasing evidence this may be a promising strategy for pain management under certain conditions [98]. A recent study by Spahn et al. demonstrated that computer modeling could be used to design a novel therapeutic effective at relieving pain without exhibiting addiction potential [96]. The opioid fentanyl was fluorinated resulting in selection for mu opioid receptors in environments with lower pH, such as those associated with inflamed tissue. The modified fentanyl demonstrated no addictive properties in a conditioned place preference test. Because of the power of computer based research in receptor affinities and the increasingly complex computer modeling systems, this approach may represent a way to modify already available opioid analgesics. Alternative routes of administration of already existing opioids are also showing promise. A study by Arti and Mehdinsab demonstrated that an intra-articular injection of opioid analgesics reduced pain following arthroscopic surgery compared to control [99]. This study demonstrated this effect using a variety of different opioid analgesics including: morphine, methadone, pethidine, and tramadol. By demonstrating analgesia can be achieved by multiple opioid analgesics in this way, this study demonstrated the potential the peripheral opioid system has in analgesia. An advantage to this approach is it can be performed with already available opioid analgesics. This route of administration is selective in nature and works only in inflamed tissue, similar to the previously described study [100]. An understanding of the BBB and how it can be used to keep opioids out of the CNS combined with further study into peripheral action of opioid analgesics, represents a potential new path into systemically administered opioids that only act in inflamed or painful areas without the unwanted side effects of dependence or addiction.

The opioid epidemic has sparked renewed interest in non-opioid-based pain treatment strategies. An extensive discussion of these approaches to pain treatment/management are beyond the scope of this review. However, some strategies with clinical promise include: identification of alternate pain pathways that can be targeted by therapeutics [101, 102]; use of non-opioid drugs [103, 104]; first line treatment of pain with physical therapy [105]; and development innovative alternatives such as the use of green light [106]. Dealing with the opioid epidemic, however, is more complex than just developing novel pain treatments. It will also require: responsible use of opioids where medically warranted; acceptance of these new treatment options by patients and insurance companies; and funding for opioid addiction treatment combined with social and political changes.

## Abbreviations
BBB: blood–brain barrier; P-gp: P-glycoprotein; OIH: opioid induced hyperalgesia; PAG: periaqueductal grey; M3G: morphine-3-glucuronide; M6G: morphine-6-glucuronide; 6-MAM: 6-monoacytylmorphine; EDDP: 2-ethylidene-1,5-dimethyl-3,3-diphenylpyrrolidine; CNS: central nervous system.

## Authors' contributions
Review concept and writing (CPS, MET); Review concept and edit for critical intellectual content and accuracy (TPD). All authors read and approved the final manuscript.

## Acknowledgements
We thank anonymous reviewers for helpful comments to improve this review.

## Competing interests
The authors declare that they have no competing interests.

## Funding
The author(s) disclose receipt of the following financial support from the NIH: 5 R01 DA011271 and 5 R01 NS042652 (to T.P.D.)

## References
1. United States Department of Health and Human Services. The opioid epidemic: by the numbers. 2016;60. http://www.hhs.gov/sites/default/files/Factsheet-opioids-061516.pdf. Accessed 6 June 2016.
2. Rudd RA, Aleshire N, Zibbell JE, Gladden RM. Increases in drug and opioid overdose deaths—United States, 2000–2014. MMWR Morb Mortal Wkly Rep. 2016;64:1378–82.
3. Joshi GP, Beck D, Emerson R, Halaszynki T, Jahr J, Lipman A, et al. Defining new directions for more effective management of surgical pain in the United States: highlights of the inaugural surgical pain congress ä. Highlights Inaug Surg Pain Congr. 2014;80:219–28.
4. Basbaum AI, Bautista DM, Scherrer G, Julius D. Cellular and molecular mechanisms of pain. Cell. 2009;139:267–84.
5. Woolf CJ, Ma Q. Nociceptors–noxious stimulus detectors. Neuron. 2007;55:353–64.
6. Brownstein MJ. A brief history of opiates, opioid peptides, and opioid receptors. Proc Natl Acad Sci USA. 1993;90:5391–3.
7. Schiff PL. Opium and its alkaloids. Am J Pharm Educ. 2002;66:186–94.
8. Sertuner F. Trommsdorff's J Pharm. 1806;47–93.
9. Wright CRA. On the action of organic acids and their anhydrides on the natural alkaloids. Part I. J Chem Soc. 1872;27:1031–43.
10. Bockmuhl VM, Ehrhart G. Uber eine neue Klasse von spasmolytisch und aiialgetisch wirkenden Verbindungen. I. Eur J Org Chem. 1947;561:52–85.
11. Fugelstad A, Stenbacka M, Leifman A, Nylander M, Thiblin I. Methadone maintenance treatment: the balance between life-saving treatment and fatal poisonings. Addiction. 2007;102:406–12.
12. Wilkerson RG, Kim HK, Windsor TA, Mareiniss DP. The opioid epidemic in the United States. Emerg Med Clin N Am. 2016;34:e1–23. https://doi.org/10.1016/j.emc.2015.11.002.
13. Porter J, Jick H. Addiction rare in patients treated with narcotics. N Engl J Med. 1980;302:123.
14. Zenz M, Strumpf M, Tryba M. Long-term oral opioid therapy in patients with chronic nonmalignant pain. J Pain Symptom Manage. 1992;7:69–77.
15. Portenoy RK, Foley KM. Chronic use of opioid analgesics in non-malignant pain [letter]. Pain. 1987;29:257–62.
16. Weingarten MA. Chrnoic opioid therapy in patients with a remote history of substance abuse. J Pain Symptom Manage. 1991;6:2–3.
17. Okie S. A Flood of Opioids, a Rising Tide of Deaths. New England journal. N Engl J Med. 2010;363:1981–5. https://doi.org/10.1056/NEJMp1002530.
18. Cantrill SV, Brown MD, Carlisle RJ, Delaney KA, Hays DP, Nelson LS, et al. Clinical policy: critical issues in the prescribing of opioids for adult patients in the emergency department. Ann Emerg Med. 2012;60:499–525. https://doi.org/10.1016/j.annemergmed.2012.06.013.
19. Yaksh TL, Wallace MS. Chapter 18 : opioids, analgesia, and pain management. In: Goodman and Gilman's: the pharmacological basis of therapeutics, 12th ed. New York: McGraw-Hill; 2011.
20. Osbourne R, Joel S, Trew D, Slevin M. analgesic activity of morphine-6-glucuronide. Lancet. 1988;1:828.
21. Smith MT. Neuroexcitatory effects of morphine and hydromorphone: evidence implicating the 3-glucuronide metabolites. Clin Exp Pharmacol Physiol. 2000;27:524–8.
22. Sia AT, Lim Y, Lim ECP, Goh RWC, Law HY, Landau R, et al. A118G single nucleotide polymorphism of human mu-opioid receptor gene influences pain perception and patient-controlled intravenous morphine consumption after intrathecal morphine for postcesarean analgesia. Anesthesiology. 2008;109:520–6.
23. Yaksh TL. Pharmacology and mechanisms of opioid analgesic activity. Acta Anaesthesiol Scand. 1997;41(1 Pt 2):94–111.
24. Bundgaard M, Abbott NJ. All vertebrates started out with a glial blood-brain barrier 4–500 million years ago. Glia. 2008;56:699–708.
25. Mayer F, Mayer N, Chinn L, Pinsonneault RL, Bainton RJ. Evolutionary conservation of vertebrate blood–brain barrier chemoprotective mechanisms in Drosophila. J Neurosci. 2011;29:3538–50.
26. Mahringer A, Ott M, Fricker G. The blood brain barrier (BBB). Heidelberg: Springer; 2014. p. 1–20.
27. Seleman M, Chapy H, Cisternino S, Courtin C, Smirnova M, Schlatter J, et al. Impact of P-glycoprotein at the blood–brain barrier on the uptake of heroin and its main metabolites: behavioral effects and consequences on the transcriptional responses and reinforcing properties. Psychopharmacology. 2014;231:3139–49.
28. Campbell AW. The blood–brain barrier. Altern Ther. 2016;22:6–7.
29. Nakagawa S, Deli MA, Kawaguchi H, Shimizudani T, Shimono T, Kittel Á, et al. A new blood–brain barrier model using primary rat brain endothelial cells, pericytes and astrocytes. Neurochem Int. 2009;54:253–63.
30. Abbott NJ, Patabendige AAK, Dolman DEM, Yusof SR, Begley DJ. Structure and function of the blood-brain barrier. Neurobiol Dis. 2010;37:13–25.

31. Dick AP, Harik SI, Klip A, Walker DM. Identification and characterization of the glucose transporter of the blood–brain barrier by cytochalasin B binding and immunological reactivity. Proc Natl Acad Sci USA. 1984;81:7233–7.

32. Jones PM, George AM. The ABC transporter structure and mechanism: perspectives on recent research. Cell Mol Life Sci. 2004;61:682–99.

33. Cordon-Cardo C, O'Brien JP, Casals D, Rittman-Grauer L, Biedler JL, Melamed MR, et al. Multidrug-resistance gene (P-glycoprotein) is expressed by endothelial cells at blood–brain barrier sites. Proc Natl Acad Sci USA. 1989;86:695–8.

34. Schinkel AH, Smit JJM, van Tellingen O, Beijnen JH, Wagenaar E, van Deemter L, et al. Disruption of the mouse mdr1a P-glycoprotein gene leads to a deficiency in the blood–brain barrier and to increased sensitivity to drugs. Cell. 1994;77:491–502.

35. Bostrom E, Hammarlund-Udenaes M, Simonsson US. Blood–brain barrier transport helps to explain discrepancies in in vivo potency between oxycodone and morphine. Anesthesiology. 2008;108:495–505. https://doi.org/10.1097/ALN.0b013e318164cf9e.

36. Ambudkar SV, Kim I, Sauna ZE. The power of the pump: mechanisms of action of P-glycoprotein (ABCB1). Eur J Pharm Sci. 2006;27:392–400.

37. Thomas H, Coley H. Overcoming multidrug resistance in cancer: an update on the clinical strategy of inhibiting p-glycoprotein. Cancer Control. 2003;10:159–65.

38. Liang X, Aszalos A. Multidrug transporters as drug targets. Curr Drug Targets. 2006;7:911–21.

39. Yamada H, Ishii K, Ishii Y, Ieiri I, Nishio S, Morioka T, et al. Formation of highly analgesic morphine-6-glucuronide following physiologic concentration of morphine in human brain. J Toxicol Sci. 2003;28:395–401.

40. Tournier N, Chevillard L, Megarbane B, Scherrmann J, Pirnay S, Decleves X. Interaction of drugs of abuse and maintenance treatments with human P-glycoprotein (ABCB1) and breast cancer resistance protein (ABCG2). Int J Neurophychopharmacology. 2010;13:905–15.

41. Fujita KI, Ando Y, Yamamoto W, Miya T, Endo H, Sunakawa Y, et al. Association of UGT2B7 and ABCB1 genotypes with morphine-induced adverse drug reactions in Japanese patients with cancer. Cancer Chemother Pharmacol. 2010;65:251–8.

42. De Gregori S, De Gregori M, Ranzani GN, Allegri M, Minella C, Regazzi M. Morphine metabolism, transport and brain disposition. Metab Brain Dis. 2012;27:1–5.

43. Bourasset F, Cisternino S, Temsamani J, Scherrmann J. Evidence for an active transport of morphine-6-β-D-glucuronide but not P-glycoprotein-mediated at the blood–brain barrier. J Neurochem. 2003;86:1564–7.

44. Balayssac D, Cayre A, Ling B, Maublant J, Penault-Llorca F, Eschalier A, et al. Increase in morphine antinociceptive activity by a P-glycoprotein inhibitor in cisplatin-induced neuropathy. Neurosci Lett. 2009;465:108–12.

45. Zelcer N, van de Wetering K, Hillebrand M, Sarton E, Kuil A, Wielinga PR, et al. Mice lacking multidrug resistance protein 3 show altered morphine pharmacokinetics and morphine-6-glucuronide antinociception. Proc Natl Acad Sci USA. 2005;102:7274–9. https://doi.org/10.1073/pnas.0502530102.

46. Wandel C, Kim R, Wood M, Ch MBB, Wood A, Ch MBB. Interaction of morphine, fentanyl, sufentanil, alfentanil, and loperamide with the efflux drug transporter P-glycoprotein. Anesthesiology. 2002;86:913–20.

47. Montesinos RN, Moulari B, Gromand J, Beduneau A, Lamprecht A. Coadministration of P-glycoprotein modulators on loperamide pharmacokinetics and brain distribution. Drug Metab Dispos. 2014;42:700–6.

48. Regnard C, Twycross R, Mihalyo M, Wilcock A. Loperamide. J Pain Symptom Manag. 2011;42:319–23.

49. Schinkel AH, Wagenaar E, Mol CAAM, Van Deemter L. P-Glycoprotein in the blood–brain barrier of mice influences the brain penetration and pharmacological activity of many drugs. J Clin Invest. 1996;97:2517–24.

50. Kaiko RF, Wallenstein SL, Rogers A. Relative analgesic potency of intramuscular heroin and morphine in cancer patients with postoperative pain and chronic pain due to cancer. NIDA Res Minigr Ser. 1981;34:213–9.

51. Selley DE, Cao CC, Sexton T, Schwegel JA, Martin TJ, Childers SR. μ opioid receptor-mediated G-protein activation by heroin metabolites: evidence for greater efficacy of 6-monoacetylmorphine compared with morphine. Biochem Pharmacol. 2001;62:447–55.

52. Boix F, Andersen JM, Mørland J. Pharmacokinetic modeling of subcutaneous heroin and its metabolites in blood and brain of mice. Addict Biol. 2013;18:1–7.

53. Boström E, Simonsson USH, Hammarlund-Udenaes M. Oxycodone pharmacokinetics and pharmacodynamics in the rat in the presence of the P-glycoprotein inhibitor PSC833. J Pharm Sci. 2005;94:1060–6.

54. Silvasti M, Rosenburg P, Seppala T, Svartling N, Pitkanen M. Comparison of analgesic efficacy of oxycodone and morphine in postoperative intravenous patient-controlled analgesia. Acta Anaesthesiol Scand. 1998;42:576–80.

55. Bostrom E, Simonsson USH, Hamarlund-Udenases M. In vivo blood–brain barrier transport of oxycodone in the rat: indications for active influx and implications for pharmacokinetics/pharmacodynamics. Drug Metab Dispos. 2006;34:1624–31.

56. Okura T, Hattori A, Takano Y, Sato T, Hammarlund-udenaes M, Terasaki T, et al. Involvement of the pyrilamine transporter, a putative organic cation transporter, in blood–brain barrier transport of oxycodone. Drug Metab Dispos. 2008;36:2005–13.

57. Hagen NA, Wasylenko E. Methadone: outpatient titration and monitoring strategies in cancer patients. J Pain Symptom Manage. 1999;18:369–75.

58. Wang JS, Ruan Y, Taylor RM, Donovan JL, Markowitz JS, DeVane CL. Brain penetration of methadone (R)- and (S)-enantiomers is greatly increased by P-glycoprotein deficiency in the blood–brain barrier of Abcb1a gene knockout mice. Psychopharmacology. 2004;173:132–8.

59. Sullivan HR, Due SL. Urinary metabolites of dl-methadone in maintenance subjects. J Med Chem. 1973;16:909–13.

60. Mccance-katz EF. (R)-methadone versus racemic methadone: what is best for patient care? Addiction. 2011;106:687–8.

61. Crettol S, Digon P, Powell Golay K, Brawand M, Eap CB. In vitro P-glycoprotein-mediated transport of (R)-, (S)-, (R,S)-methadone, LAAM and their main metabolites. Pharmacology. 2007;80:304–11.

62. Mercer SL, Coop A. Opioid analgesics and P-glycoprotein efflux transporters: a potential systems-level contribution to analgesic tolerance. Curr Top Med Chem. 2011;11:1157–64.

63. Volpe DA, Mcmahon GA, Mellon RD, Katki AG, Parker RJ, Colatsky T, et al. Uniform assessment and ranking of opioid Mu receptor binding constants for selected opioid drugs. Regul Toxicol Pharmacol. 2011;59:385–90. https://doi.org/10.1016/j.yrtph.2010.12.007.

64. Henthorn TK, Liu Y, Mahapatro M, Ng K. Active transport of fentanyl by the blood–brain barrier 1. J Pharmacol Exp Ther. 1999;289:1084–9.

65. Klepstad P, Dale O, Skorpen F, Borchgrevink PC, Kaasa S. Genetic variability and clinical efficacy of morphine. Acta Anaesthesiol Scand. 2005;49:902–8.

66. Xi Z, Stein EA. GABAergic mechanisms of opiate reinforcement. Alcohol Alcohol. 2002;37:485–94.

67. Doi K, Gibbons G. Improving postoperative pain management in orthopedic total joint surgical patients with opioid tolerance using the iowa model of evidence-based practice. ASPAN Natl Conf Abstr. 2014;29:e38.

68. Pasternak GW. Molecular biology of opioid analgesia. J Pain Symptom Manage. 2005;29:2–9.

69. Yousif S, Saubamea B, Cisternino S, Marie-Claire C, Dauchy S, Scherrmann J-M, et al. Effect of chronic exposure to morphine on the rat blood–brain barrier: focus on the P-glycoprotein. J Neurochem. 2008;107:647–57.

70. Aquilante CL, Letrent SP, Pollack GM, Brouwer KL. Increased brain P-glycoprotein in morphine tolerant rats. Life Sci. 2000;66:L47–51.

71. Li Y, Yue H, Xing Y, Sun H, Pan Z, Xie G. Oxymatrine inhibits development of morphine-induced tolerance associated with decreased expression of P-glycoprotein in rats. Integr Cancer Ther. 2010;9:213–8.

72. Nakagawa T, Ozawa T, Shige K, Yamamoto R, Minami M. Inhibition of morphine tolerance and dependence by MS-153, a glutamate transporter activator. Eur J Pharmacol. 2001;419:39–45.

73. Chaves C, Gomez-Zepeda D, Auvity S, Menet M-C, Crete D, Labat L, et al. Effect of subchronic intravenous morphine infusion and naloxone-precipitated morphine withdrawal on P-gp and Bcrp at the rat blood–brain barrier. J Pharm Sci. 2015;105:350–8.

74. Kahan M, Srivastava A, Wilson L, Gourlay D, Midmer D. Misuse of and dependence on opioids: study of chronic pain patients. Can Fam Physician. 2006;52(9):1081–7.

75. Gupta A, Christo PJ. Opioid abuse and dependence. J Nurse Pract. 2009;5:132–4.

76. Author. Substance-related and addictive disorders. In: Diagnostic and statistical manual of mental disorders. 5th ed. Washington, DC: American Psychiatric Association; 2013.

77. Sonne S, Brady K. Substance abuse and bipolar comorbidity. Psychiatr Clin N Am. 1999;22:609–27.

78. Martins SS, Keyes KM, Storr CL, Zhu H, Chilcoat HD. Pathways between nonmedical opioid use/dependence and psychiatric disorders: results from the National Epidemiologic Survey on Alcohol and Related Conditions. Drug Alcohol Depend. 2009;103:16–24.

79. Maremmani I, Giovanni A, Maremmani I, Rugani F, Rovai L, Pacini M, et al. Clinical presentations of substance abuse in bipolar heroin addicts at time of treatment entry. Ann Gen Psychiatry. 2012;11:1–7. https://doi.org/10.1186/1744-859X-11-23.

80. Executive Office of Health and Humand Serivices. Recovery Support. http://www.mass.gov. 2017. http://www.mass.gov/eohhs/gov/departments/dph/programs/substance-abuse/recovery-support.html. Accessed 1 Jan 2017.

81. Birnbaum HG, White AG, Schiller M, Waldman T, Cleveland JJM, Setnik B, et al. Societal costs of opioid abuse, dependence and misuse in the United States. Value Health. 2010;13:A111. https://doi.org/10.1016/S1098-3015(10)72532-8.

82. Kanouse AB, Compton P. The epidemic of prescription opioid abuse, the subsequent rising prevalence of heroin use, and the federal response. J Pain Palliat Care Pharmacother. 2015;29:102–14. https://doi.org/10.3109/15360288.2015.1037521.

83. Shei A, Rice JB, Kirson NY, Bodnar K, Birnbaum HG, Holly P, et al. Sources of prescription opioids among diagnosed opioid abusers. Curr Med Res Opin. 2015;31:779–84. https://doi.org/10.1185/03007995.2015.1016607.

84. McDonald DC, Carlson KE. Estimating the prevalence of opioid diversion by "doctor shoppers" in the United States. PLoS ONE. 2013;8:e69241.

85. Han H, Kass PH, Wilsey BL, Li C-S. Increasing trends in Schedule II opioid use and doctor shopping during 1999–2007 in California. Pharmacoepidemiol Drug Saf. 2014;23:26–35.

86. Aldridge J, Decary-Hetu D. Hidden wholesale: the drug diffusing capacity of online drug cryptomarkets. Int J Drug Policy. 2016;35:7–15.

87. Lange A, Lasser KE, Xuan Z, Khalid L, Beers D, Heymann OD, et al. Variability in opioid prescription monitoring and evidence of aberrant medication taking behaviors in urban safety-net clinics. Pain. 2015;156:335–40.

88. Katz N, Panas L, Kim M, Audet A, Bilansky A, Eadie J, et al. Usefulness of prescription monitoring programs for surveillance—analysis of Schedule II opioid prescription data in Massachusetts, 1996–2006. Pharmacoepidemiol Drug Saf. 2010;19:115–23.

89. Lembke A. Why doctors prescribe opioids to known opioid abusers. N Engl J Med. 2012;367:1580–1.

90. Wilson HD, Dansie EJ, Kim MS, Moskovitz BL, Chow W, Turk DC, et al. Clinicians' attitudes and beliefs about opioids survey (CAOS): instrument development and results of a national physician survey. J Pain. 2013;14:613–27. https://doi.org/10.1016/j.jpain.2013.01.769.

91. Jones CM, Lurie PG, Throckmorton DC. Effect of US drug enforcement administration's rescheduling of hydrocodone combination analgesic products on opioid analgesic prescribing. J Am Med Assoc Intern Med. 2017;176:399–402.

92. Kertesz S. Turning the tide or riptide? The changing opioid epidemic. Subst Abus. 2017;38:3–8.

93. Center for Behavioral Health Statistics and Quality. Behavioral health trends in the United States: results from the 2014 national survey on drug use and health. 2015. http://www.samhsa.gov/data/sites/default/files/NSDUH-FRR1-2014/NSDUH-FRR1-2014.pdf%5Cn, http://www.samhsa.gov/data/. Accessed 23 Dec 2016.

94. Cicero TJ, Ellis MS, Harney J. Shifting patterns of prescription opioid and heroin abuse in the United States. N Engl J Med. 2015;373:1789–90.

95. The Office of the President of the United Sates. National drug control strategy. 2015. https://www.whitehouse.gov//sites/default/files/ondcp/policy-and-research/2015_national_drug_control_strategy_0.pdf. Accessed 23 Dec 2016.

96. Spahn V, Massaly N, Temp J, Durmaz V, Sabri P, Reidelbach M, et al. A nontoxic pain killer designed by modeling of pathological receptor conformations. Science (80 —). 2017;355:966–9.

97. Kieffer BL, Gavériaux-ruff C. Exploring the opioid system by gene knockout. Prog Neurobiol. 2002;66:285–306.

98. Oeltjenbruns J, Schäfer M. Peripheral opioid analgesia: clinical applications. Anesth Tech Pain Manag. 2005;9:36–44.

99. Arti H, Mehdinasab SA. The comparison effects of intra-articular injection of different opioids on postoperative pain relieve after arthroscopic anterior cruciate ligament reconstruction: a randomized clinical trial study. J Res Med Sci. 2011;16:1176–82.

100. Reuben SS, Sklar J. Current concepts review pain management in patients who undergo outpatient arthroscopic surgery of the knee. J Bone Jt Surg. 2000;82:1754–66.

101. Ding H, Czoty PW, Kiguchi N, Cami-kobeci G, Sukhtankar DD, Nader MA. A novel orvinol analog, BU08028, as a safe opioid analgesic without abuse liability in primates. Proc Natl Acad Sci USA. 2016;113:5511–8.

102. Emery EC, Luiz AP, Wood JN. Nav1.7 and other voltage-gated sodium channels as drug targets for pain relief. Expert Opin Ther Targets. 2016;20:975–83. https://doi.org/10.1517/14728222.2016.1162295.

103. Hill KP, Palastro MD, Johnson B, Ditre JW. Cannabis and pain: a clinical review. Cannabis Cannabinoid Res. 2017;2:96–104.

104. Ong CKS, Seymour RA, Lirk P, Merry AF. Combining paracetamol (acetaminophen) with nonsteroidal antiinflammatory drugs: a qualitative systematic review of analgesic efficacy for acute postoperative pain. Anesth Analg. 2010;110:1170–9.

105. Hayden JA, Van Tulder MW, Tomlinson G. Systematic review: strategies for using exercise therapy to improve outcomes in chronic low back pain. Ann Intern Med. 2005;142:776–85.

106. Ibrahim MM, Patwardhan A, Gilbraith KB, Moutal A, Yang X, Chew LA. Long-lasting antinociceptive effects of green light in acute and chronic pain in rats. Pain. 2017;158:347–60.

# 10

# Nrf2 signaling increases expression of ATP-binding cassette subfamily C mRNA transcripts at the blood–brain barrier following hypoxia-reoxygenation stress

Kathryn Ibbotson[1], Joshua Yell[2] and Patrick T. Ronaldson[2*]

**Abstract**

**Background:** Strategies to maintain BBB integrity in diseases with a hypoxia/reoxygenation (H/R) component involve preventing glutathione (GSH) loss from endothelial cells. GSH efflux transporters include multidrug resistance proteins (Mrps). Therefore, characterization of Mrp regulation at the BBB during H/R is required to advance these transporters as therapeutic targets. Our goal was to investigate, in vivo, regulation of *Abcc1*, *Abcc2*, and *Abcc4* mRNA expression (i.e., genes encoding Mrp isoforms that transport GSH) by nuclear factor E2-related factor (Nrf2) using a well-established H/R model.

**Methods:** Female Sprague–Dawley rats (200–250 g) were subjected to normoxia (Nx, 21% $O_2$, 60 min), hypoxia (Hx, 6% $O_2$, 60 min) or H/R (6% $O_2$, 60 min followed by 21% $O_2$, 10 min, 30 min, or 1 h) or were treated with the Nrf2 activator sulforaphane (25 mg/kg, i.p.) for 3 h. *Abcc* mRNA expression in brain microvessels was determined using quantitative real-time PCR. Nrf2 signaling activation was examined using an electrophoretic mobility shift assay (EMSA) and chromatin immunoprecipitation (ChIP) respectively. Data were expressed as mean ± SD and analyzed via ANOVA followed by the post hoc Bonferroni *t* test.

**Results:** We observed increased microvascular expression of *Abcc1*, *Abcc2*, and *Abcc4* mRNA following H/R treatment with reoxygenation times of 10 min, 30 min, and 1 h and in animals treated with sulforaphane. Using a biotinylated Nrf2 probe, we observed an upward band shift in brain microvessels isolated from H/R animals or animals administered sulforaphane. ChIP studies showed increased Nrf2 binding to antioxidant response elements on *Abcc1*, *Abcc2*, and *Abcc4* promoters following H/R or sulforaphane treatment, suggesting a role for Nrf2 signaling in *Abcc* gene regulation.

**Conclusions:** Our data show increased *Abcc1*, *Abcc2*, and *Abcc4* mRNA expression at the BBB in response to H/R stress and that *Abcc* gene expression is regulated by Nrf2 signaling. Since these Mrp isoforms transport GSH, these results may point to endogenous transporters that can be targeted for BBB protection during H/R stress. Experiments are ongoing to examine functional implications of Nrf2-mediated increases in *Abcc* transcript expression. Such studies will determine utility of targeting Mrp isoforms for BBB protection in diseases with an H/R component.

**Keywords:** Blood–brain barrier, Endothelial cell, Hypoxia, Multidrug resistance proteins, Nrf2 signaling, Transporters

*Correspondence: pronald@email.arizona.edu
[2] Department of Pharmacology, College of Medicine, University of Arizona, 1501 N. Campbell Avenue, P.O. Box 245050, Tucson, AZ 85724-5050, USA
Full list of author information is available at the end of the article

## Background

Cerebral hypoxia and reoxygenation (H/R) is a component of various diseases including traumatic brain injury, cardiac arrest, and ischemic stroke [1]. Blood–brain barrier (BBB) integrity is modulated by production of reactive oxygen species (ROS) and subsequent oxidative stress in the setting of H/R [2]. For example, studies using bovine brain microvessel endothelial cells subjected to H/R stress reported discrete changes in tight junction protein localization that correlated with increased paracellular permeability to sucrose, a vascular marker that does not cross the intact BBB [3]. Similar observations have been reported in vivo where H/R induced disassembly of occludin oligomers in rat brain microvessels [4, 5]. Furthermore, studies in the same model system showed increased CNS accumulation of sucrose [5, 6] and dextrans [7], evidence indicating BBB dysfunction in response to H/R. Indeed, vascular changes induced by H/R can have deleterious consequences. Enhanced BBB permeabilization can lead to vasogenic edema and cause clinically significant increases in brain volume and intracranial pressure [8, 9]. Additionally, substances that are typically contained within the systemic circulation, including drugs, can leak into brain parenchyma and potentially cause neurotoxicity. Clearly, there is a critical need to preserve BBB integrity in diseases with an H/R component.

In order to develop therapeutic approaches that can confer BBB protection, it is essential to identify specific biological mechanisms that contribute to oxidative stress-induced damage of the brain microvasculature. Indeed, furthering our understanding of the endothelial cell antioxidant defense system will enable advancement of such pharmacological strategies. The endogenous antioxidant glutathione (GSH) is a vital component of this antioxidant defense system. In vivo studies have demonstrated that cerebral GSH levels are significantly decreased in response to reperfusion injury [10] and GSH depletion is associated with increased BBB permeability to both sucrose and sodium fluorescein [11]. Although this does not reflect large-scale BBB disruption, this leak is clinically significant by permitting increased paracellular transport of potentially toxic small molecules. Decreased GSH levels in response to H/R may involve membrane transport processes mediated by multidrug resistance proteins (Mrps). Mrps are members of the ATP-binding cassette (ABC) superfamily of efflux transporters, primarily transport organic anions and conjugated metabolites, and are encoded by genes from ABC subfamily C (i.e., *Abcc* genes) [2]. Both GSH and glutathione disulfide (GSSG) are known transport substrates for Mrp1, Mrp2, and Mrp4. For example, studies in primary cultures of rat astrocytes showed that GSH transport could be blocked using MK571, an established inhibitor of Mrp1 and Mrp2 [12–14]. Similarly, Mrp4 is also believed to be involved in transport of GSH in the brain [15]. Indeed, these observations point towards endogenous transporters that can be targeted to preserve endothelial GSH levels and provide BBB protection in the setting of H/R.

Effective targeting of Mrps to reduce GSH efflux and confer BBB protection requires identification and characterization of regulatory pathways that control expression of these transporters. One such pathway is signaling mediated by nuclear factor E2-related factor (Nrf2). Nrf2 is normally inactive in the cytoplasm and rapidly degraded when associated with Kelch-like ECH-associated protein 1 (Keap1). Under conditions of oxidative stress, Keap1 dissociates and allows Nrf2 to translocate to the nucleus and initiate transcription of genes containing an antioxidant response element (ARE) [16]. Nrf2 has been shown to induce expression of Mrp1, Mrp2, and Mrp4 and the genes that encodes these proteins (i.e., *Abcc1, Abcc2, Abcc4*) at the BBB as well as in other tissues [17–19]. At present, involvement of Nrf2 in regulating Mrp transporter expression at the BBB has not been evaluated under pathophysiological conditions.

In the present study, we show increased expression of *Abcc1, Abcc2, and Abcc4* mRNA transcripts in brain microvessels via Nrf2 signaling in the setting of H/R. Specifically, we show for the first time that H/R activates Nrf2 signaling at the BBB and that Nrf2 binds to an antioxidant response element in the promoter of all three genes that encode GSH transporting Mrp isoforms. These data provide critical information that can inform future studies aimed at targeting Mrp transporters to confer BBB protection in diseases with an H/R component.

## Methods

### Animals and treatments

All animal experiments were approved by the University of Arizona Institutional Animal Care and Use Committee and conform to National Institutes of Health guidelines. Female Sprague–Dawley rats (200–250 g) were obtained from Envigo (Denver, CO), housed under standard 12 h light/12 h dark conditions, and provided with food and water *ad libitum*. Female rats were purposely selected for this study in order to correlate our results with previous data on BBB transporter changes in the setting of H/R [20]. Animals were randomly assigned to treatment groups. Animals were subjected to hypoxic (Hx) insult (i.e., 6% $O_2$) for 1 h as previously described [20]. Using blood-gas analysis, our laboratory has previously demonstrated that these conditions yield a severe, but recoverable, hypoxic insult [20]. Additionally, this model increases CNS expression of apoptotic markers [i.e., ratio of cleaved poly-ADP ribose polymerase (PARP) to uncleaved PARP] [20]. Rats were then euthanized or subjected to reoxygenation (i.e., 21% $O_2$) for 10 min, 30 min, or 1 h. These time points were selected based upon our previous work examining BBB transport mechanisms in the setting of H/R [20]. As shown in Thompson et al. [20], discrete changes in BBB transporters can be observed during reoxygenation as early as 10 min following hypoxic insult. H/R animals were compared with animals subjected to Hx only and with normoxic (Nx) controls. A subset of animals was administered sulforaphane [25 mg/kg (1.0 ml/kg), i.p.; Sigma-Aldrich, St. Louis, MO], an established Nrf2 activator, dissolved in 0.9% saline as a positive control. Following Nx, Hx, H/R or 3 h sulforaphane treatment, animals were euthanized by decapitation and prepared for microvessel isolation.

### Microvessel isolation

Brain microvessels were harvested as previously described by our laboratory [20]. Following anesthesia with sodium pentobarbital [64.8 mg/ml (1.0 ml/kg) i.p.], rats were decapitated and brains were removed. Meninges and choroid plexus were excised and cerebral hemispheres were homogenized in 4 ml of microvessel isolation buffer (103 mM NaCl, 4.7 mM KCl, 2.5 mM $CaCl_2$, 1.2 mM $KH_2PO_4$, 1.2 mM $MgSO_4$, 15 mM HEPES, pH 7.4) containing protease inhibitor cocktail (Sigma-Aldrich). After homogenization, 8 ml of 26% dextran at 4 °C was added and homogenates were vortexed. Homogenates were then centrifuged (5600$g$; 4 °C) for 10 min and the supernatant was aspirated. Pellets were resuspended in 10 ml of microvessel isolation buffer and passed through a 70 μm filter (Becton–Dickinson, Franklin Lakes, NJ). Filtered homogenates were pelleted by centrifugation at 3000×$g$ for 10 min. At this time, the supernatant was aspirated and the pellet, which is enriched in brain microvessels, was collected for use in further experiments.

### Quantitative real-time PCR analysis

Total RNA was extracted from brain microvessels isolated from rats subjected to Nx, Hx, and H/R using the Aurum Total RNA extraction kit (Bio-Rad, Hercules,

CA). Extracted RNA was treated with amplification grade DNase I (Bio-Rad) to remove contaminating genomic DNA. The concentration of RNA in each sample was quantified spectrophotometrically by measuring UV absorbance at 260 nm. The iScript reverse transcriptase kit (Bio-Rad) was used to synthesize first-strand cDNA. Primer pairs were prepared by Integrated DNA Technologies (Coralville, IA) with sequences listed in Table 1. Each set of primers was designed with the use of Primer Express 3 software (Applied Biosystems) and validated for specificity and efficacy by using BioTaq universal rat normal tissue cDNA (BioTaq Inc., Gaithersburg, MD). Primer pairs were designed to be complementary to sequences located on two different exons separated by an intron in order to avoid amplification of genomic DNA. Quantitative PCR was performed using SYBR Green Master Mix (Bio-Rad) on a CFX96 Touch Real-Time PCR Detection System (Bio-Rad). The quantity of the target gene (i.e., Abcc1, Abcc2, Abcc4) was normalized to GAPDH using the comparative $CT$ method ($\Delta\Delta CT$). Results were expressed as mean ± SD of at least three separate experiments.

### Electrophoretic mobility shift assay (EMSA)

EMSA was performed using the LightShift Chemiluminescent EMSA kit (Pierce Biotechnology, Rockford, IL, USA) according to manufacturer's instructions. Briefly, nuclear protein extract was isolated from brain microvessels prepared from Nx, Hx, H/R, and sulforaphane treated rats. Complementary DNA oligonucleotides 5′-CGG TCA CCG TTA CTC AGC ACT TTG-3′ and 5′-CAA AGT GCT GAG TAA CGG TGA CCG-3′ (antioxidant response element recognition sequence highlighted) were purchased from Integrated DNA Technologies, end labeled with biotin, and annealed at 95 °C for 5 min. EMSA samples were prepared using 5 μg of nuclear extract in each Nrf2/ARE binding reaction. The binding reaction was incubated at room temperature for 15 min and DNA–protein complexes were resolved on a precast 6% native polyacrylamide gel in 0.5% TBE buffer. The gel was removed from the electrophoresis unit, blotted onto a nitrocellulose membrane, and incubated with

### Table 1 Quantitative real-time PCR primer sequences

| PCR primer sequences | | |
| --- | --- | --- |
| Gene | Forward primer | Reverse primer |
| Abcc1 (rat) | 5′-TGC-CAG-AGA-TCA-GTT-CAC-ACC-AAG-CC-3′ | 5′-ACC-ATC-CGG-ACG-CAG-TTT-GAA-GAC-AG-3′ |
| Abcc2 (rat) | 5′-GAA-GGC-ATT-GAC-CCT-ATC-T-3′ | 5′-CCA-CTG-AGA-ATC-TCA-TTC-ATG-3′ |
| Abcc4 (rat) | 5′-TGG-AAC-TTC-TGG-AGG-ACG-GGG-ATC-TG-3′ | 5′-CCC-CTT-CTG-CAC-CAT-TTC-CGG-ATC-TT-3′ |
| GAPDH (rat) | 5′-ATG-GCT-ACA-GCA-ACA-GGG-TGG-TGG-AC-3′ | 5′-ATG-GGG-TCT-GGG-ATG-GAA-TTG-TGA-GG-3′ |

streptavidin-horseradish peroxidase for 30 min. Membranes were developed using enhanced chemiluminescence. Experiments to determine specificity of EMSA reactions for the Nrf2/ARE complex were conducted by incubating binding reactions in the presence of a rabbit monoclonal anti-Nrf2 antibody (EP1808Y; 1/20 dilution; Abcam, Cambridge, MA). Control EMSA experiments were performed by adding an excess (200×) of unlabeled probe to binding reactions.

## Chromatin immunoprecipitation (ChIP)

ChIP was performed using the Imprint Chromatin Immunoprecipitation Kit (Sigma-Aldrich) according to manufacturer's instructions. Briefly, microvessels were isolated from Nx, Hx, H/R, and sulforaphane treated rats and subsequently cross-linked in buffer containing 1% formaldehyde for 10 min at room temperature. Cross-linking was stopped by addition of glycine to a final concentration of 125 mM followed by centrifugation at 180×$g$ for 5 min at room temperature. At this time, the microvessel pellet was resuspended in 50 μl of Nuclei Preparation Buffer and incubated on ice for 10 min. Following centrifugation at 180×$g$ for 10 min at 4 °C, the nuclear pellet was resuspended in shearing buffer and incubated on ice for 10 min. Chromatin was sheared to 200–1000 bp by sonication on ice. Sonicated chromatin was diluted twofold in lysis buffer and 100 μl of diluted sample per immunoprecipitation reaction was used. Each sample was added to individual wells of a 96-well assay plate where each well contained 1 μg of specific rabbit monoclonal anti-Nrf2 antibody (EP1808Y) that has been previously validated in ChIP assays [21]. Assay plates were incubated for 90 min at room temperature on an orbital shaker at 75 rpm. In parallel, a no-antibody sample was run as a negative control. At this time, 40 μl of DNA release buffer was added to each well and samples were incubated in a water bath at 65 °C for 15 min. Following this step, 40 μl of reversing solution was added to each well and samples were incubated in a water bath at 65 °C for 90 min. Washes and elutions were performed in accordance with manufacturer's instructions for the Imprint ChIP assay kit. Eluted and input DNA samples were purified using a spin column to a final volume of 50 μl. Quantitative real-time PCR was performed using 2 μl of template DNA per 25 μl of polymerase chain reaction (PCR) amplification scale as described by Hoque and colleagues [22]. Quantification of Nrf2 occupancy to the ARE within *Abcc* gene promoter by SYBR green real-time PCR was performed using primer sets prepared by Integrated DNA Technologies (Table 2). All measurements were performed in triplicate and results were verified in three separate chromatin preparations.

## Statistical analysis

Data are reported as mean ± SD from at least three separate experiments where each treatment group consists of pooled microvessels from three individual animals (n = 3). This sample size is based upon the ability to detect a 35% difference between treatment groups with 20% variability. To determine statistical significance, a repeated measures ANOVA and post hoc multiple-comparison Bonferroni $t$ test were used. A value of $p < 0.05$ was accepted as statistically significant.

## Results

### H/R increases expression of Abcc mRNA transcripts

In order to evaluate and quantitate mRNA expression of *Abcc* mRNA transcripts at the BBB in the setting of H/R, we performed quantitative PCR. After completion of these experiments, we observed increased expression of *Abcc1*, *Abcc2*, and *Abcc4* mRNA in rat brain microvessels following H/R treatment with reoxygenation times of 10 min, 30 min, and 1 h as compared to Nx controls or animals subjected to Hx insult only (Fig. 1). Expression of mRNA for all three genes was also increased in animals treated with the Nrf2 activator sulforaphane (25 mg/kg i.p.) for 3 h (Fig. 1). These studies demonstrate that H/R can increase expression of *Abcc* mRNA at the BBB.

### H/R induces nuclear translocation of Nrf2 in rat brain microvessels

Since our qPCR data showed increased expression of *Abcc* genes at the BBB in response to H/R, we sought to identify a discrete molecular mechanism that is involved in induced expression of *Abcc* mRNA transcripts. We postulated that the Nrf2 pathway is one such mechanism. Therefore, we utilized an EMSA with a biotinylated probe containing the Nrf2 consensus binding sequence

**Table 2  ChIP primer sequences**

| Primer sequences for ChIP | | |
| --- | --- | --- |
| Gene | Forward primer | Reverse primer |
| *Abcc1* | 5'-GCT-GTG-TTA-CCA-GAA-CTG-CC-3' | 5'-AGC-ACA-AGC-AGA-GTC-AGG-AT-5' |
| *Abcc2* | 5'-CAG-GGC-TTT-GGA-GAA-GTG-ATA-3' | 5'-GGA-AGC-AGA-TGT-TAA-GGA-GCA-A-3' |
| *Abcc4* | 5'-CTT-GAG-GCT-GGG-AGT-TCT-AGG-G-3' | 5'-ACT-GAC-AGA-GTG-GTG-TAG-CTG-GT-3' |

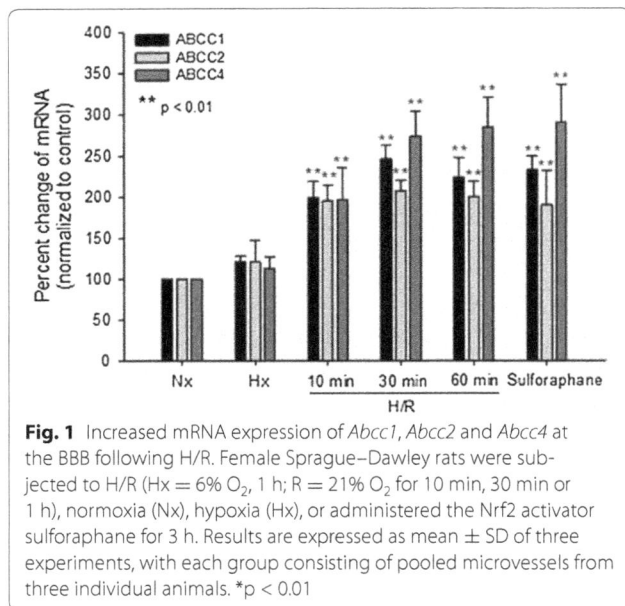

**Fig. 1** Increased mRNA expression of *Abcc1*, *Abcc2* and *Abcc4* at the BBB following H/R. Female Sprague–Dawley rats were subjected to H/R (Hx = 6% $O_2$, 1 h; R = 21% $O_2$ for 10 min, 30 min or 1 h), normoxia (Nx), hypoxia (Hx), or administered the Nrf2 activator sulforaphane for 3 h. Results are expressed as mean ± SD of three experiments, with each group consisting of pooled microvessels from three individual animals. *p < 0.01

to demonstrate activation of Nrf2 signaling in rat brain microvessels following H/R. We observed a shift of the probe band to a higher molecular weight and an increase in intensity of the probe band in microvessels isolated from H/R animals or administered sulforaphane (25 mg/kg i.p.) for 3 h (Fig. 2). This shift was not observed when 200-fold excess unlabeled probe was added to EMSA reactions (Fig. 2). Incubation of EMSA reactions in the presence of the specific rabbit anti-Nrf2 monoclonal

antibody EP1808Y caused an increase in the shift of the probe band, an observation that further indicates nuclear translation of Nrf2 under H/R conditions (Fig. 3). Taken together, these data provide evidence that H/R can activate Nrf2 signaling in brain microvessels.

### Nrf2 is involved in regulation of Abcc mRNA transcripts in rat brain microvessels following H/R

Since our EMSA experiments demonstrated increased Nrf2 nuclear translocation in rat brain microvessels following H/R, we hypothesized that this pathway may be involved in transcriptional regulation of *Abcc* genes. To test this hypothesis, we used ChIP to study Nrf2 recruitment to promoter regions on Abcc genes that contain the Nrf2 consensus binding sequence [i.e., (a/g)TGA(C/T/G)nnnGC(a/g)] within the ARE. In H/R animals or in animals administered the Nrf2 activator sulforaphane, increased Nrf2 binding was determined for *Abcc1*, *Abcc2*, and *Abcc4* (Fig. 4). No difference in Nrf2 binding was observed in a non-specific region of the same promoter (data not shown). These data show that Nrf2 can bind to the promoter of Abcc genes in brain microvessels under H/R conditions, providing evidence for molecular regulation of drug efflux transporters (i.e., Mrps) at the BBB.

### Discussion

The mammalian Mrp family belongs to the ABCC group of proteins, which contains 13 members including one ion channel (i.e., CFTR), two surface receptors (i.e., SUR1 and 2) and a truncated protein that does not mediate transport (i.e., ABCC13) [2, 23]. Several functionally

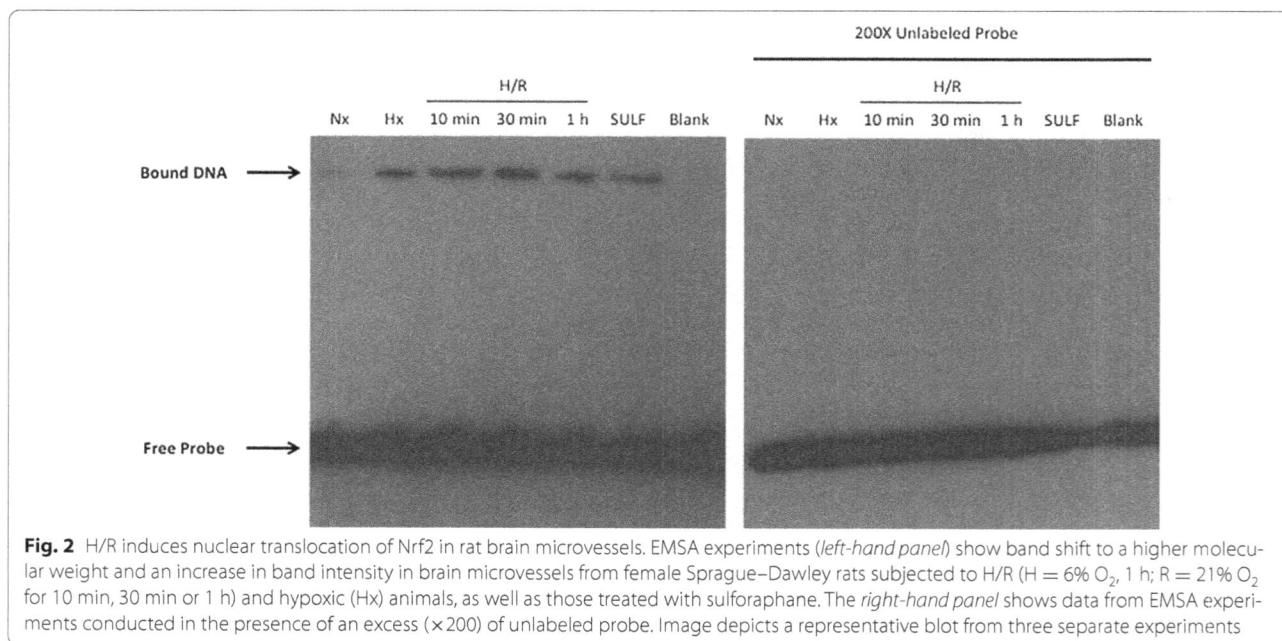

**Fig. 2** H/R induces nuclear translocation of Nrf2 in rat brain microvessels. EMSA experiments (*left-hand panel*) show band shift to a higher molecular weight and an increase in band intensity in brain microvessels from female Sprague–Dawley rats subjected to H/R (H = 6% $O_2$, 1 h; R = 21% $O_2$ for 10 min, 30 min or 1 h) and hypoxic (Hx) animals, as well as those treated with sulforaphane. The *right-hand panel* shows data from EMSA experiments conducted in the presence of an excess (×200) of unlabeled probe. Image depicts a representative blot from three separate experiments

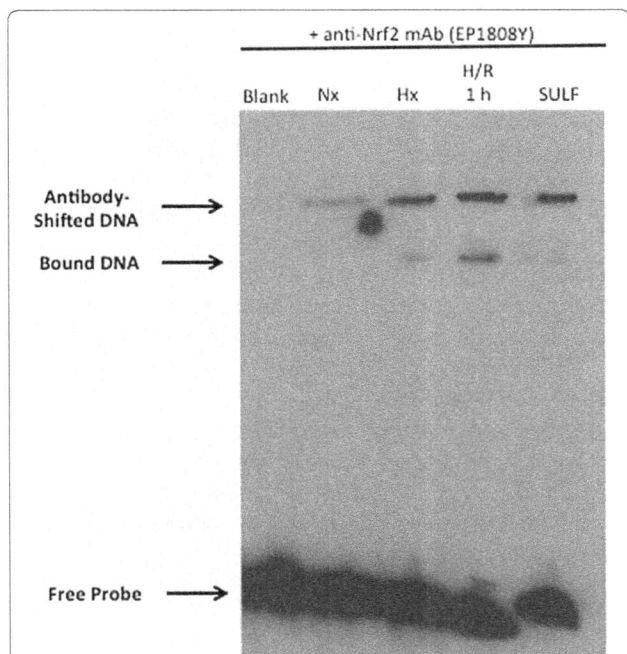

**Fig. 3** H/R induces nuclear translocation of Nrf2 in rat brain microvessels. EMSA experiments using a specific Nrf2 monoclonal antibody (EP1808Y) show a "supershift" of bands corresponding to the nuclear Nrf2/ARE complex in brain microvessels from female Sprague–Dawley rats subjected to H/R (H = 6% $O_2$, 1 h; R = 21% $O_2$ for 10 min, 30 min or 1 h) and hypoxic (Hx) animals, as well as those treated with sulforaphane. Image depicts a representative blot from three separate experiments

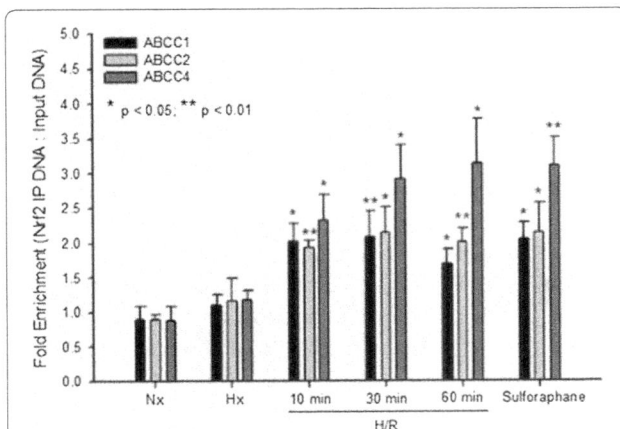

**Fig. 4** Involvement of Nrf2 in regulation of *Abcc* mRNA transcripts in rat brain microvessels following H/R. ChIP was performed on brain microvessels isolated from rats subjected to H/R (H = 6% $O_2$, 1 h; R = 21% $O_2$ for 10 min, 30 min or 1 h), Nx, Hx, or treated with sulforaphane for 3 h. Results are expressed as mean ± SD of three experiments, with each group consisting of pooled microvessels from three individual animals. *p < 0.05; **p < 0.01

characterized Mrp isoforms have been localized to the mammalian BBB. These include Mrp1, Mrp2, Mrp4, Mrp5 and Mrp6 [24–30]. The presence of multiple Mrp isoforms at the BBB is a critical determinant in controlling delivery of therapeutic agents to the brain. Additionally, the ability of Mrp isoforms to actively efflux the endogenous antioxidant glutathione (GSH) has significant implications for diseases with an H/R component. GSH is responsible for maintenance of cellular redox balance and antioxidant defense in the brain. It has been previously demonstrated that various Mrps are upregulated in response to oxidative stress conditions, which leads to enhanced cellular efflux of GSH [14]. Increased functional expression of Mrp isoforms at the BBB could cause reduced endothelial cell concentrations of GSH, an alteration in cellular redox status, and increased potential for cell injury and death. Therefore, biological mechanisms that can modulate Mrp expression at the BBB in response to oxidative stress require further investigation.

A thorough understanding of signaling pathways involved in Mrp regulation in the setting of H/R will enable development of pharmacological approaches to target Mrp-mediated efflux (i.e., GSH transport) for the purpose of preventing BBB dysfunction. One intriguing pathway is signaling mediated by Nrf2, a sensor of oxidative stress [19, 31]. In the presence of ROS, the cytosolic Nrf2 repressor Keap1 undergoes structural alterations that cause dissociation from the Nrf2-Keap1 complex. This enables Nrf2 to translocate to the nucleus and induce transcription of genes that possess an antioxidant response element at their promoter [32, 33]. It has been demonstrated that activation of Nrf2 signaling induces expression of Mrp1, Mrp2, and Mrp4 [17–19, 32, 34, 35]. Our data expands upon these previous studies by showing Nrf2-mediated increases in mRNA transcript expression for *Abcc1*, Abcc2, and *Abcc4* in rat brain microvessels. We also show increased Nrf2 nuclear translocation in the setting of H/R and that Nrf2 binds to the ARE in the respective promoter for *Abcc1*, *Abcc2*, and *Abcc4*. Our findings are novel and highly significant because we have shown, for the first time, that H/R-induced activation of Nrf2 leads to increased expression of mRNA transcripts for transporters endogenously expressed at the BBB. This is a rapid response, which may indicate that genes involved in the H/R stress response may be available for immediate activation in an effort to protect the vasculature from dysfunction and subsequent leak of circulating solutes. It is also intriguing that changes in *Abcc* mRNA transcript expression occur following H/R but are not apparent in the setting of hypoxia despite activation of Nrf2 signaling under both conditions. Such changes may be reflective of the dramatic increase in ROS production following H/R. For example, Fabian and Kent demonstrated increased production of superoxide anions by neutrophils following reperfusion, an event that can greatly exacerbate BBB dysfunction [8, 36]. Such dramatic increases in ROS production can certainly induce cellular changes independent of signaling pathways that are activated in response to hypoxia [37].

Recent evidence has shown that Nrf2 is a component of a complex signaling pathway, which involves additional factors for promoter activation and subsequent modulation of transport mechanisms at the BBB. For example, sulforaphane-induced increases in ABC transporter functional expression at the BBB can be abolished using pifithrin, an inhibitor of p53 signaling, or in p53 null mice [19]. In contrast, nutlin-3, a p53 activator, increased P-gp transport activity in mouse brain capillaries [19]. Of particular note, this study also demonstrated that pharmacological inhibitors of p38 MAPK signaling (i.e., SB203580) and nuclear factor-κB (NF-κB) signaling (i.e., N4-[2-(4-phenoxyphenyl)ethyl]-4,6-quinazolinediamine, SN50) blocked effects of sulforaphane and nutlin-3 on P-gp activity [19]. Taken together, the work of Wang and colleagues suggests that effects of Nrf2 signaling on ABC transporters at the BBB requires involvement of p53, p38 MAPK, and NF-κB signaling.

An emerging concept is that Nrf2 acts as a double-edged sword [33]. Activation of Nrf2 signaling at the BBB is generally considered to be protective owing to its activation of cytoprotective pathways; pre- and post-treatment administration of Nrf2 activators confer BBB protection in animal models of stroke and traumatic brain injury [38–40]. A subset of Nrf2 target genes are involved in the synthesis and metabolism of GSH, including GCLC and GCLM (subunits of glutamate–cysteine ligase), glutathione peroxidase, and glutathione reductase [33]. Indeed, increased expression of GSH synthetic genes can lead to increased cellular production of this critical antioxidant. However, oxidative stress increases the functional expression of Mrp1 [14], and oxidative stress induced by metals or $H_2O_2$ has been previously shown to increase Mrp1-mediated export of GSH and GSSG [13, 41–43]. Upregulation of Mrp isoforms in glial cells may have neuroprotective effects in the setting of oxidative stress through release of GSH into brain parenchyma where it can be readily accessed by neurons [41, 44]. However, an alteration in the balance of Mrp isoforms via activation of Nrf2 signaling may have considerably different effects than in brain parenchyma. Indeed, efflux of GSH by Mrp isoforms expressed at the abluminal membrane of the BBB may provide some neuroprotection; however, increased GSH efflux due to enhanced

Mrp-mediated transport can adversely affect redox balance and antioxidant defense at the brain microvascular endothelium and contribute to barrier dysfunction in the setting of H/R. This indicates that studies designed to develop pharmacological approaches based on targeting Mrp isoforms at the BBB must consider both neuroprotective and vascular protective effects associated with these transporters. Additionally, increased functional expression of Mrp isoforms at the BBB can negatively affect endothelial cell inflammation and repair pathways. Endogenous mediators involved in such pathways include leukotriene C4, a known Mrp1/Mrp2 substrate [45, 46], and prostaglandin $E_2$ [47].

In order to fully comprehend the implications of Nrf2-mediated upregulation of Abcc gene expression at the BBB, future studies must be undertaken to assess Mrp localization in the brain microvasculature. Expression and localization of Mrp isoforms at the BBB is species-dependent and remains highly controversial [48, 49]. Localization of Mrp1 is thought to be at the abluminal plasma membrane in brain microvascular endothelial cells in rodents, but at the luminal membrane in humans [50, 51]. Mrp4 has been detected on the luminal surface of the BBB in rat; however, abluminal expression has not been confirmed [50, 51]. Based on qPCR and proteomic analysis, Mrp4 is the most abundant of the three GSH-transporting isoforms in human brain microvessels [29, 50]. Mrp2 is likely localized to the luminal aspect of the BBB, but several studies have failed to detect Mrp2 at the protein level [49, 51]. This may be due to low basal expression of Mrp2, which may be increased in response to cellular stressors such as oxidative stress [28, 52]. In mice, there are notable differences in Mrp expression between strains and between vessels of different diameters. For example, FVB mice appear to lack Mrp2 in brain vessels, but it is present in C57BL/6 and Swiss mice [53]. This same study also showed that Mrp1is most abundant in vessels 20–50 μm in diameter [53]. Rigorous assessment of Mrp isoform localization will undoubtedly inform the development of therapeutic strategies to protect the BBB in diseases with an H/R component. Furthermore, these studies should include both male and female experimental animals in order to determine differences in Mrp localization based on sex.

## Conclusion

Our data show increased Abcc1, Abcc2, and Abcc4 mRNA expression at the BBB in response to H/R stress and that Abcc gene expression is regulated by Nrf2 signaling (Fig. 5). This is the first time that Nrf2 signaling has been shown to modulate Abcc genes at the brain microvasculature in the setting of H/R stress. Since Mrp1, Mrp2, and Mrp4 transport GSH, these results have considerable

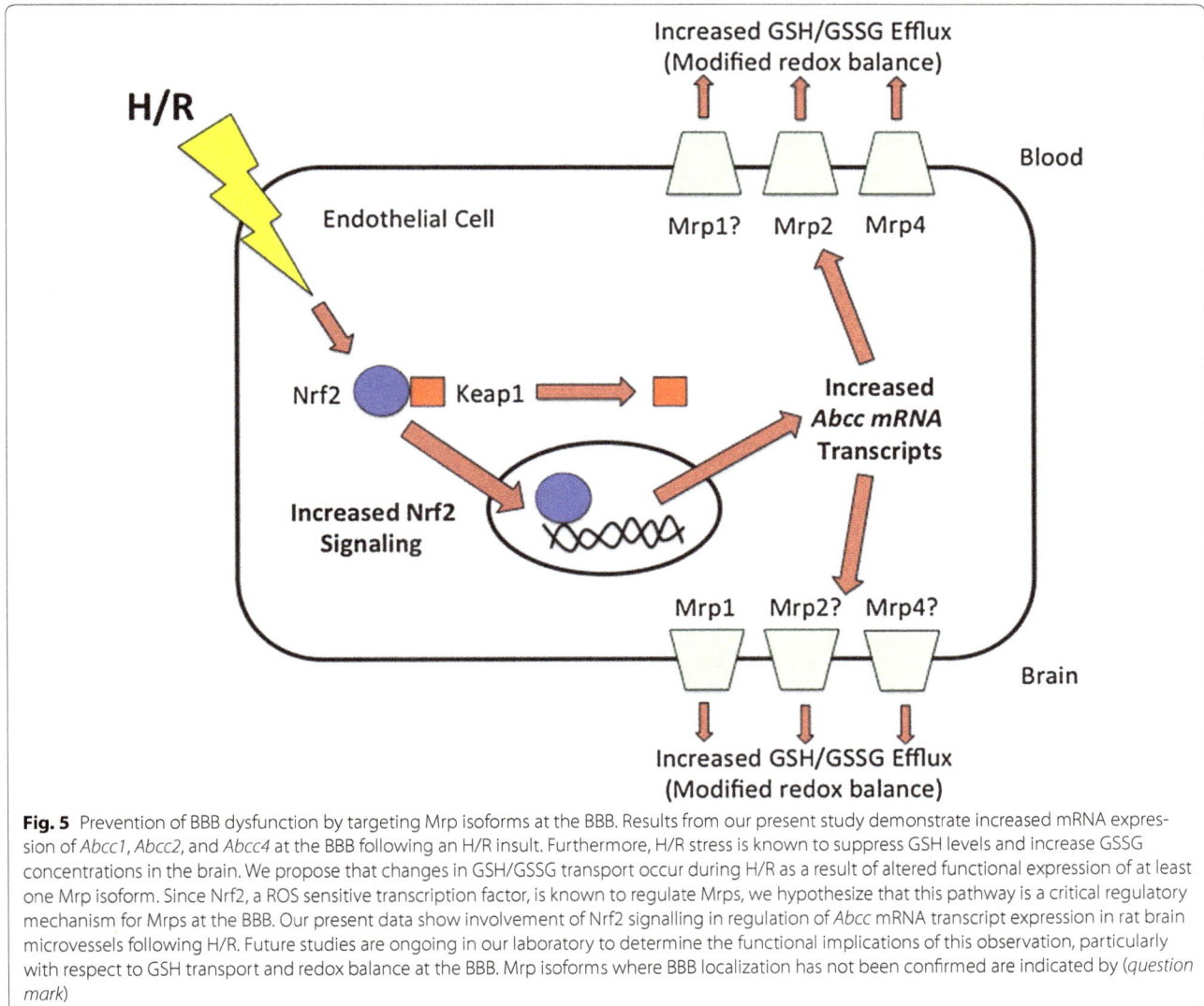

**Fig. 5** Prevention of BBB dysfunction by targeting Mrp isoforms at the BBB. Results from our present study demonstrate increased mRNA expression of *Abcc1*, *Abcc2*, and *Abcc4* at the BBB following an H/R insult. Furthermore, H/R stress is known to suppress GSH levels and increase GSSG concentrations in the brain. We propose that changes in GSH/GSSG transport occur during H/R as a result of altered functional expression of at least one Mrp isoform. Since Nrf2, a ROS sensitive transcription factor, is known to regulate Mrps, we hypothesize that this pathway is a critical regulatory mechanism for Mrps at the BBB. Our present data show involvement of Nrf2 signalling in regulation of *Abcc* mRNA transcript expression in rat brain microvessels following H/R. Future studies are ongoing in our laboratory to determine the functional implications of this observation, particularly with respect to GSH transport and redox balance at the BBB. Mrp isoforms where BBB localization has not been confirmed are indicated by (*question mark*)

pharmacological implications as they point to endogenous transporters that can be targeted for development of novel therapeutic strategies to confer BBB protection. Furthermore, our in vivo H/R treatment does not induce necrotic damage to the endothelium, thus enabling us to study a dynamically regulated and recoverable BBB. Such a model can inform novel strategies to target the penumbra in ischemic stroke, which is subject to hypoxic insult but can be potentially rescued using pharmacological interventions. Future studies are ongoing in our laboratory to examine functional implications of Nrf2-mediated increases in *Abcc* transcript expression, particularly with respect to Mrp protein expression and brain-to-blood transport of GSH, in order to rigorously examine the utility of Mrp isoforms as a therapeutic target in diseases with an H/R component.

**Abbreviations**

ABC: ATP-binding cassette; ARE: antioxidant response element; BBB: blood–brain barrier; ChIP: chromatin immunoprecipitation; GSH: glutathione; GSSG: glutathione disulfide; H/R: hypoxia-reoxygenation; Keap1: Kelch-like ECH-associated protein 1; Mrp: multidrug resistance protein; Nrf2: nuclear factor E2-related factor; PARP: poly-ADP ribose polymerase; ROS: reactive oxygen species.

**Authors' contributions**

KI reviewed experimental data and prepared the manuscript; JY assisted with experimental work. PTR participated in experimental design, performed experiments, performed data analysis, assisted with preparation of the manuscript, and obtained funding via R01-NS084941. All authors read and approved the final manuscript.

**Author details**

[1] Department of Pharmacology and Toxicology, College of Pharmacy, University of Arizona, 1295 N. Martin Avenue, P.O. Box 210202, Tucson 85721, AZ, USA. [2] Department of Pharmacology, College of Medicine, University of Arizona, 1501 N. Campbell Avenue, P.O. Box 245050, Tucson, AZ 85724-5050, USA.

## Competing interests

The authors declare that they have no competing interests.

## Funding

This work was supported by a grant from the National Institute of Neurological Disease and Stroke (NINDS), National Institutes of Health (NIH) (Grant #R01-NS084941) to PTR.

## References

1. Ronaldson PT, Davis TP. Targeted drug delivery to treat pain and cerebral hypoxia. Pharmacol Rev. 2013;65:291–314.
2. Ronaldson PT, Davis TP. Targeting transporters: promoting blood–brain barrier repair in response to oxidative stress injury. Brain Res. 2015;1623:39–52.
3. Mark KS, Davis TP. Cerebral microvascular changes in permeability and tight junctions induced by hypoxia-reoxygenation. Am J Physiol Heart Circ Physiol. 2002;282:H1485–94.
4. McCaffrey G, Willis CL, Staatz WD, Nametz N, Quigley CA, Hom S, Lochhead JJ, Davis TP. Occludin oligomeric assemblies at tight junctions of the blood–brain barrier are altered by hypoxia and reoxygenation stress. J Neurochem. 2009;110:58–71.
5. Lochhead JJ, McCaffrey G, Quigley CE, Finch J, DeMarco KM, Nametz N, Davis TP. Oxidative stress increases blood–brain barrier permeability and induces alterations in occludin during hypoxia-reoxygenation. J Cereb Blood Flow Metab. 2010;30:1625–36.
6. Witt KA, Mark KS, Hom S, Davis TP. Effects of hypoxia-reoxygenation on rat blood–brain barrier permeability and tight junctional protein expression. Am J Physiol Heart Circ Physiol. 2003;285:H2820–31.
7. Willis CL, Meske DS, Davis TP. Protein kinase C activation modulates reversible increase in cortical blood–brain barrier permeability and tight junction protein expression during hypoxia and posthypoxic reoxygenation. J Cereb Blood Flow Metab. 2010;30:1847–59.
8. Witt KA, Mark KS, Sandoval KE, Davis TP. Reoxygenation stress on blood–brain barrier paracellular permeability and edema in the rat. Microvasc Res. 2008;75:91–6.
9. Michinaga S, Koyama Y. Pathogenesis of brain edema and investigation into anti-edema drugs. Int J Mol Sci. 2015;16:9949–75.
10. Al Ahmad A, Gassmann M, Ogunshola OO. Involvement of oxidative stress in hypoxia-induced blood–brain barrier breakdown. Microvasc Res. 2012;84:222–5.
11. Agarwal R, Shukla GS. Potential role of cerebral glutathione in the maintenance of blood–brain barrier integrity in rat. Neurochem Res. 1999;24:1507–14.
12. Hirrlinger J, Dringen R. Multidrug resistance protein 1-mediated export of glutathione and glutathione disulfide from brain astrocytes. Methods Enzymol. 2005;400:395–409.
13. Hirrlinger J, Konig J, Keppler D, Lindenau J, Schulz JB, Dringen R. The multidrug resistance protein MRP1 mediates the release of glutathione disulfide from rat astrocytes during oxidative stress. J Neurochem. 2001;76:627–36.
14. Ronaldson PT, Bendayan R. HIV-1 viral envelope glycoprotein gp120 produces oxidative stress and regulates the functional expression of multidrug resistance protein-1 (Mrp1) in glial cells. J Neurochem. 2008;106:1298–313.
15. Borst P, de Wolf C, van de Wetering K. Multidrug resistance-associated proteins 3, 4, and 5. Pflugers Arch. 2007;453:661–73.
16. Copple IM. The Keap1-Nrf2 cell defense pathway—a promising therapeutic target? Adv Pharmacol. 2012;63:43–79.
17. Aleksunes LM, Slitt AL, Maher JM, Augustine LM, Goedken MJ, Chan JY, Cherrington NJ, Klaassen CD, Manautou JE. Induction of Mrp3 and Mrp4 transporters during acetaminophen hepatotoxicity is dependent on Nrf2. Toxicol Appl Pharmacol. 2008;226:74–83.
18. Maher JM, Dieter MZ, Aleksunes LM, Slitt AL, Guo G, Tanaka Y, Scheffer GL, Chan JY, Manautou JE, Chen Y, et al. Oxidative and electrophilic stress induces multidrug resistance-associated protein transporters via the nuclear factor-E2-related factor-2 transcriptional pathway. Hepatology. 2007;46:1597–610.
19. Wang X, Campos CR, Peart JC, Smith LK, Boni JL, Cannon RE, Miller DS. Nrf2 upregulates ATP binding cassette transporter expression and activity at the blood–brain and blood–spinal cord barriers. J Neurosci. 2014;34:8585–93.
20. Thompson BJ, Sanchez-Covarrubias L, Slosky LM, Zhang Y, Laracuente ML, Ronaldson PT. Hypoxia/reoxygenation stress signals an increase in organic anion transporting polypeptide 1a4 (Oatp1a4) at the blood–brain barrier: relevance to CNS drug delivery. J Cereb Blood Flow Metab. 2014;34:699–707.
21. Chorley BN, Campbell MR, Wang X, Karaca M, Sambandan D, Bangura F, Xue P, Pi J, Kleeberger SR, Bell DA. Identification of novel NRF2-regulated genes by ChIP-Seq: influence on retinoid X receptor alpha. Nucleic Acids Res. 2012;40:7416–29.
22. Hoque MT, Robillard KR, Bendayan R. Regulation of breast cancer resistant protein by peroxisome proliferator-activated receptor alpha in human brain microvessel endothelial cells. Mol Pharmacol. 2012;81:598–609.
23. Dallas S, Miller DS, Bendayan R. Multidrug resistance-associated proteins: expression and function in the central nervous system. Pharmacol Rev. 2006;58:140–61.
24. Miller DS, Nobmann SN, Gutmann H, Toeroek M, Drewe J, Fricker G. Xenobiotic transport across isolated brain microvessels studied by confocal microscopy. Mol Pharmacol. 2000;58:1357–67.
25. Leggas M, Adachi M, Scheffer GL, Sun D, Wielinga P, Du G, Mercer KE, Zhuang Y, Panetta JC, Johnston B, et al. Mrp4 confers resistance to topotecan and protects the brain from chemotherapy. Mol Cell Biol. 2004;24:7612–21.
26. Zhang Y, Schuetz JD, Elmquist WF, Miller DW. Plasma membrane localization of multidrug resistance-associated protein homologs in brain capillary endothelial cells. J Pharmacol Exp Ther. 2004;311:449–55.
27. Bandler PE, Westlake CJ, Grant CE, Cole SP, Deeley RG. Identification of regions required for apical membrane localization of human multidrug resistance protein 2. Mol Pharmacol. 2008;74:9–19.
28. Bauer B, Hartz AM, Lucking JR, Yang X, Pollack GM, Miller DS. Coordinated nuclear receptor regulation of the efflux transporter, Mrp2, and the phase-II metabolizing enzyme, GSTpi, at the blood–brain barrier. J Cereb Blood Flow Metab. 2008;28:1222–34.
29. Uchida Y, Ohtsuki S, Katsukura Y, Ikeda C, Suzuki T, Kamiie J, Terasaki T. Quantitative targeted absolute proteomics of human blood–brain barrier transporters and receptors. J Neurochem. 2011;117:333–45.
30. Sanchez-Covarrubias L, Slosky LM, Thompson BJ, Zhang Y, Laracuente ML, DeMarco KM, Ronaldson PT, Davis TP. P-glycoprotein modulates morphine uptake into the CNS: a role for the non-steroidal anti-inflammatory drug diclofenac. PLoS ONE. 2014;9:e88516.
31. Alfieri A, Srivastava S, Siow RC, Modo M, Fraser PA, Mann GE. Targeting the Nrf2-Keap1 antioxidant defence pathway for neurovascular protection in stroke. J Physiol. 2011;589:4125–36.
32. Hayashi A, Suzuki H, Itoh K, Yamamoto M, Sugiyama Y. Transcription factor Nrf2 is required for the constitutive and inducible expression of multidrug resistance-associated protein 1 in mouse embryo fibroblasts. Biochem Biophys Res Commun. 2003;310:824–9.
33. Ma Q. Role of nrf2 in oxidative stress and toxicity. Annu Rev Pharmacol Toxicol. 2013;53:401–26.
34. Vollrath V, Wielandt AM, Iruretagoyena M, Chianale J. Role of Nrf2 in the regulation of the Mrp2 (ABCC2) gene. Biochem J. 2006;395:599–609.
35. Xu S, Weerachayaphorn J, Cai SY, Soroka CJ, Boyer JL. Aryl hydrocarbon receptor and NF-E2-related factor 2 are key regulators of human MRP4 expression. Am J Physiol Gastrointest Liver Physiol. 2010;299:G126–35.
36. Fabian RH, Kent TA. Superoxide anion production during reperfusion is reduced by an antineutrophil antibody after prolonged cerebral ischemia. Free Radic Biol Med. 1999;26:355–61.
37. Haddad JJ, Land SC. A non-hypoxic, ROS-sensitive pathway mediates TNF-α-dependent regulation of HIF-1α. FEBS Lett. 2001;505:269–74.
38. Zhao J, Moore AN, Redell JB, Dash PK. Enhancing expression of Nrf2-driven genes protects the blood brain barrier after brain injury. J Neurosci. 2007;27:10240–8.
39. Alfieri A, Srivastava S, Siow RC, Cash D, Modo M, Duchen MR, Fraser PA, Williams SC, Mann GE. Sulforaphane preconditioning of the Nrf2/HO-1 defense pathway protects the cerebral vasculature against blood–brain barrier disruption and neurological deficits in stroke. Free Radic Biol Med. 2013;65:1012–22.

40. Zhao Y, Fu B, Zhang X, Zhao T, Chen L, Zhang J, Wang X. Paeonol pretreatment attenuates cerebral ischemic injury via upregulating expression of pAkt, Nrf2, HO-1 and ameliorating BBB permeability in mice. Brain Res Bull. 2014;109:61–7.

41. Hirrlinger J, Schulz JB, Dringen R. Glutathione release from cultured brain cells: multidrug resistance protein 1 mediates the release of GSH from rat astroglial cells. J Neurosci Res. 2002;69:318–26.

42. Scheiber IF, Dringen R. Copper-treatment increases the cellular GSH content and accelerates GSH export from cultured rat astrocytes. Neurosci Lett. 2011;498:42–6.

43. Tadepalle N, Koehler Y, Brandmann M, Meyer N, Dringen R. Arsenite stimulates glutathione export and glycolytic flux in viable primary rat brain astrocytes. Neurochem Int. 2014;76:1–11.

44. Dringen R, Hirrlinger J. Glutathione pathways in the brain. Biol Chem. 2003;384:505–16.

45. Slot AJ, Wise DD, Deeley RG, Monks TJ, Cole SP. Modulation of human multidrug resistance protein (MRP) 1 (ABCC1) and MRP2 (ABCC2) transport activities by endogenous and exogenous glutathione-conjugated catechol metabolites. Drug Metab Dispos. 2008;36:552–60.

46. Cole SP. Targeting multidrug resistance protein 1 (MRP1, ABCC1): past, present, and future. Annu Rev Pharmacol Toxicol. 2014;54:95–117.

47. Tachikawa M, Hosoya K, Terasaki T. Pharmacological significance of prostaglandin E2 and D2 transport at the brain barriers. Adv Pharmacol. 2014;71:337–60.

48. Stieger B, Gao B. Drug transporters in the central nervous system. Clin Pharmacokinet. 2015;54:225–42.

49. Miller DS. Regulation of ABC transporters at the blood–brain barrier. Clin Pharmacol Ther. 2015;97:395–403.

50. Nies AT, Jedlitschky G, Konig J, Herold-Mende C, Steiner HH, Schmitt HP, Keppler D. Expression and immunolocalization of the multidrug resistance proteins, MRP1–MRP6 (ABCC1–ABCC6), in human brain. Neuroscience. 2004;129:349–60.

51. Roberts LM, Black DS, Raman C, Woodford K, Zhou M, Haggerty JE, Yan AT, Cwirla SE, Grindstaff KK. Subcellular localization of transporters along the rat blood–brain barrier and blood–cerebral–spinal fluid barrier by in vivo biotinylation. Neuroscience. 2008;155:423–38.

52. Shawahna R, Uchida Y, Decleves X, Ohtsuki S, Yousif S, Dauchy S, Jacob A, Chassoux F, Daumas-Duport C, Couraud PO, et al. Transcriptomic and quantitative proteomic analysis of transporters and drug metabolizing enzymes in freshly isolated human brain microvessels. Mol Pharm. 2011;8:1332–41.

53 Soontornmalai A, Vlaming ML, Fritschy JM. Differential, strain-specific cellular and subcellular distribution of multidrug transporters in murine choroid plexus and blood–brain barrier. Neuroscience. 2006;138:159–69.

# 11

# Diffusion tensor imaging with direct cytopathological validation: characterisation of decorin treatment in experimental juvenile communicating hydrocephalus

Anuriti Aojula[1,2,5†], Hannah Botfield[1,2,5†], James Patterson McAllister II[3*‡] (iD), Ana Maria Gonzalez[1,5], Osama Abdullah[4], Ann Logan[4,5] and Alexandra Sinclair[1,2,5,6‡]

## Abstract

**Background:** In an effort to develop novel treatments for communicating hydrocephalus, we have shown previously that the transforming growth factor-β antagonist, decorin, inhibits subarachnoid fibrosis mediated ventriculomegaly; however decorin's ability to prevent cerebral cytopathology in communicating hydrocephalus has not been fully examined. Furthermore, the capacity for diffusion tensor imaging to act as a proxy measure of cerebral pathology in multiple sclerosis and spinal cord injury has recently been demonstrated. However, the use of diffusion tensor imaging to investigate cytopathological changes in communicating hydrocephalus is yet to occur. Hence, this study aimed to determine whether decorin treatment influences alterations in diffusion tensor imaging parameters and cytopathology in experimental communicating hydrocephalus. Moreover, the study also explored whether diffusion tensor imaging parameters correlate with cellular pathology in communicating hydrocephalus.

**Methods:** Accordingly, communicating hydrocephalus was induced by injecting kaolin into the basal cisterns in 3-week old rats followed immediately by 14 days of continuous intraventricular delivery of either human recombinant decorin (n = 5) or vehicle (n = 6). Four rats remained as intact controls and a further four rats served as kaolin only controls. At 14-days post-kaolin, just prior to sacrifice, routine magnetic resonance imaging and magnetic resonance diffusion tensor imaging was conducted and the mean diffusivity, fractional anisotropy, radial and axial diffusivity of seven cerebral regions were assessed by voxel-based analysis in the corpus callosum, periventricular white matter, caudal internal capsule, CA1 hippocampus, and outer and inner parietal cortex. Myelin integrity, gliosis and aquaporin-4 levels were evaluated by post-mortem immunohistochemistry in the CA3 hippocampus and in the caudal brain of the same cerebral structures analysed by diffusion tensor imaging.

**Results:** Decorin significantly decreased myelin damage in the caudal internal capsule and prevented caudal periventricular white matter oedema and astrogliosis. Furthermore, decorin treatment prevented the increase in caudal periventricular white matter mean diffusivity (p = 0.032) as well as caudal corpus callosum axial diffusivity (p = 0.004) and radial diffusivity (p = 0.034). Furthermore, diffusion tensor imaging parameters correlated primarily with periventricular white matter astrocyte and aquaporin-4 levels.

*Correspondence: pat.mcallister@wustl.edu
†Anuriti Aojula and Hannah Botfield are co-first authors
‡James Patterson McAllister II and Alexandra Sinclair are co-senior authors
3 Department of Neurosurgery, Division of Pediatric Neurosurgery at the Washington University School of Medicine and the Saint Louis Children's Hospital, St. Louis, MO 63110, USA
Full list of author information is available at the end of the article

**Conclusions:** Overall, these findings suggest that decorin has the therapeutic potential to reduce white matter cytopathology in hydrocephalus. Moreover, diffusion tensor imaging is a useful tool to provide surrogate measures of periventricular white matter pathology in communicating hydrocephalus.

**Keywords:** Hydrocephalus, DTI, Cytopathology, Decorin

## Background

Hydrocephalus is a common paediatric neurosurgical presentation with an incidence of 0.48–0.81 per 1000 live births [1–3]. Communicating hydrocephalus is aetiologically heterogeneous; bacterial meningitis, subarachnoid haemorrhage, trauma, intracranial and intraspinal tumours as well as leptomeningeal metastases can all cause the disorder [4–10]. The incidence of communicating hydrocephalus following subarachnoid haemorrhage is at least 13 % and can be as high as 67 % [11]. In addition to ventriculomegaly, communicating hydrocephalus is accompanied by extensive global cerebral pathology, including widespread reactive gliosis, hydrocephalic oedema and demyelination [10, 12].

Although shunting is the current standard of care for children with hydrocephalus, the procedure is associated with severe complications that contribute to an increased patient morbidity [13–16]. Furthermore, academic attainment and social integration difficulties continue into adulthood for those with the disease [17–19]. Therefore, the development of novel therapeutic strategies to prevent the development of hydrocephalus or promote recovery is of critical importance. Our recent study (Additional file 1: Figure S1) supports the key role of transforming growth factor-beta (TGF-β) in communicating hydrocephalus, as decorin, a TGF-β antagonist [20–23] ameliorated subarachnoid fibrosis and therefore significantly attenuated the enlargement of the ventricular system [12]. However, the effectiveness of decorin to prevent cytopathology in hydrocephalus is yet to be examined thoroughly. Given that cellular pathology is largely responsible for the array of functional deficits observed clinically and contributes to the impairment in patient health-related quality of life, it is important to understand whether decorin can attenuate these alterations in vivo [10, 24, 25].

Greater insight into the cytopathological changes occurring in communicating hydrocephalus can be achieved with the use of advanced non-invasive magnetic resonance diffusion tensor imaging (DTI) [26]. DTI is a specialised magnetic resonance imaging (MRI) technique that examines tissue anisotropic properties and cerebral microstructural integrity [27, 28]. DTI yields a set of quantitative metrics, reflecting the magnitude along the principal axes of water diffusion, which are sensitive to changes in the underlying brain microstructure.

Commonly used scalar DTI parameters such as axial (AD), radial (RD), and mean diffusivities (MD) (equivalent to the speed of motion in the principal axes of diffusion) or the fractional anisotropy (FA) (equivalent to a normalized aspect ratio of the principal axes of diffusion) have been useful in the investigation of cerebral abnormalities; an increase in the AD, RD and MD alongside a decrease in the FA occurs in the cerebral white matter of children with hydrocephalus [29–33]. Furthermore, the specificity of DTI to act as a surrogate measure of cerebral pathology has been highlighted in a variety of conditions, including hypoxic ischaemic injury [34, 35], multiple sclerosis [36–39], spinal cord injury [40], obstructive hydrocephalus [41], temporal lobe epilepsy [42, 43] and for delineating gliomas [44]. However, correlations between DTI parameters and underlying cytopathology in communicating hydrocephalus have yet to be determined (Appendix 1).

Therefore, using immunohistochemistry and clinically relevant neuroimaging we investigated whether decorin is able to attenuate damage-related parameters and if cellular changes in communicating hydrocephalus can be quantitatively characterised by DTI using a juvenile rat model of the disorder.

## Methods

### Experimental animals

Three-week-old Sprague–Dawley rats (Charles River, Massachusetts, USA) were housed in litters in individual cages, kept under a 12 h light/dark cycle with free access to food and water. Animals were monitored for adverse effects of treatments, such as distress, lethargy, weight loss and seizures, and any animals showing severe adverse effects were euthanised. Experiments were conducted at the University of Utah in accordance with the guidelines of the National Institutes of Health Care and Use of Laboratory Animals and approved by the University of Utah Ethics Committee.

### Experimental design and surgical techniques

The experimental design and surgical techniques are described in detail elsewhere [12]. Using a ventral approach, the interval between the occipital bone and the C-1 vertebral body was exposed and a 30 gauge angled needle was inserted into the prepontine (basal cistern) subarachnoid space. 30 µl of 20 % kaolin solution

(200 mg/ml in 0.9 % sterile saline; Fisher Scientific, Massachusetts, USA) was injected to induce communicating hydrocephalus and the rat was either allowed to recover or underwent osmotic pump and intraventricular cannula implantations. The cannulae were inserted into the right lateral ventricle and fixed in place with glue and bone cement (Biomet UK Ltd, Bridgend, UK) to a stabilising screw, and connected to subcutaneously implanted mini osmotic pumps. Osmotic pumps (model 2002 adapted for use in MRI scanners with PEEK tubing, Alzet, Durect Corporation, California, USA) were filled with either 5 mg/ml human recombinant decorin (Galacorin™, Catalent/Pharma Solutions, New Jersey, USA) or 10 mM phosphate buffered saline (PBS) pH 7.4 (Sigma-Aldrich, Missouri, USA). Over the subsequent 14 days, human recombinant decorin was infused at a rate of 2.5 mg/0.5 ml/h.

Rats were randomly assigned to four groups: (1) Intact age-matched controls (Intact group, n = 4); (2) basal cistern kaolin injections only (kaolin group, n = 4); (3) kaolin injection with intraventricular infusion of PBS (kaolin + PBS group; n = 6); and (4) kaolin injection with intraventricular infusion of decorin (kaolin + decorin group; n = 5). Magnetic resonance imaging (MRI) and diffusion tensor imaging (DTI) were conducted after 14 days of treatment to assess the extent of hydrocephalus before sacrifice, then the brains were removed and processed for histology.

**Magnetic resonance imaging and diffusion tensor imaging**
Imaging experiments were conducted 14 days post injury using a 7-Tesla horizontal-bore Bruker Biospec MRI scanner (Bruker Biospin, Ettlingen, MA, USA) interfaced with a 12-cm actively shielded gradient insert capable of producing magnetic field gradient up to 600 mT/m. Animals were anesthetised using 1–3 % Isoflurane and 0.8 L/min $O_2$ and their vital signs (respiration, temperature, heart rate and oxygen saturation percentage) were continuously monitored using a MR-compatible physiological monitoring system (SA Instruments, Stony Brook, NY, USA). Animals were placed in a 72-mm volume coil for signal transmission, and a quadrature surface coil was placed on the head for signal reception. Acquisition of $T_2$-weighted MRI scans and ventricular volume analysis has been described previously [12]. DTI scans were conducted using spin echo diffusion-weighted sequences with single-shot EPI readout, with the following parameters (TR of 3760 ms, TE of 44 ms, 15 coronal 1 mm-thick slices, a field of view of 2.5 × 2.5 cm, and an in-plane resolution of 195 × 195 μm). Thirty uniformly-spaced over unit sphere diffusion-weighted gradient directions and five non-weighted images were acquired with two signal averages and the following diffusion parameters: diffusion gradient duration 7 ms, separation 20 ms, diffusion encoding sensitivity 700 s/mm². Scan time was 4 min. For ventriculomegaly analysis, one MRI scan image was chosen from the rostral cerebrum (−0.36 mm from bregma) and the caudal cerebrum (−3.72 mm from bregma) for each rat, and the ventricular area was determined in each scan using ImageJ.

**DTI voxel based analysis**
Prior to commencing voxel-based analysis, double blinding was introduced to prevent group identification. Using the software, DSI Studio (DSI Studio, Pittsburgh, PA), DTI images were reconstructed and processed to produce voxel based maps, from which regions of interest (ROIs) could be analysed. The seven ROIs selected include: corpus callosum, periventricular white matter, caudal and rostral internal capsule, outer parietal cortex, inner parietal cortex and CA1 hippocampus. DTI parameter values from four serial sections (1.28 mm anterior to Bregma to 3.72 mm posterior to Bregma) of the corpus callosum and periventricular white matter were analysed in a total of 17 rats [Intact (n = 4), kaolin (n = 4), kaolin + PBS (n = 5), kaolin + decorin (n = 4)]. The rostral corpus callosum and periventricular white matter sections were defined as 1.28 and −0.36 mm from Bregma. The caudal corpus callosum and periventricular white matter sections were derived from −2.76 to −3.72 mm from Bregma (Fig. 2a). The remaining five ROIs were analysed in 16 rats, with four animals being examined in each experimental group. Three sections were independently analysed for the CA1, caudal internal capsule, outer and inner parietal cortex from 0.36 to 3.72 mm posterior to Bregma. An average of two sections from 1.28 mm anterior to Bregma to 0.36 mm posterior to Bregma were individually analysed for the rostral internal capsule. ROIs were identified using a FA voxel based map and an analogous DTI image (Fig. 1). The mean FA, MD, AD and RD values were calculated for each ROI of each animal.

**Tissue preparation for histology**
Rats were euthanised and immediately perfused transcardially with PBS followed by 4 % paraformaldehyde (Alfa Aesar, Ward Hill, MA, USA) in PBS. Brains were immersed in 4 % paraformaldehyde overnight at 4 °C, cryoprotected by sequential immersion in 10, 20 and 30 % sucrose solutions in PBS at 4 °C and embedded in optimum cutting temperature embedding matrix (Fisher Scientific). Subsequent sectioning and staining of the tissue was conducted at the University if Birmingham. Coronal sections 15-μm thick were cut on a Bright cryostat

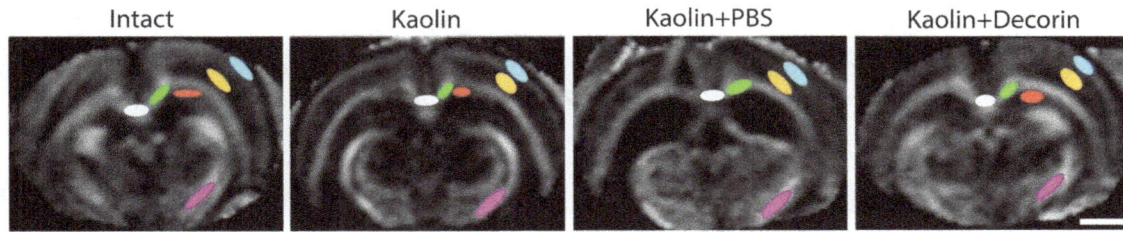

**Fig. 1** Regions of interest (ROIs) for DTI analysis in each experimental group. Representative voxel based map images and analogous diffusion tensor images of the caudal cerebrum at 2.76 mm posterior to Bregma are shown for the four experimental groups. All ROIs selected for analysis, except from the rostral internal capsule, are displayed. ROIs were chosen with the aid of a rat brain atlas [45]; *white* = corpus callosum, *green* = periventricular white matter, *cyan* = outer parietal cortex, *yellow* = inner parietal cortex, *red* = CA1 hippocampus, *magenta* = caudal internal capsule, *scale bar* = 100 µm

(Bright Instrument, Huntingdon, UK), serially mounted and stored at −20 °C before staining.

### Antibodies

Myelin integrity was assessed with an antibody against myelin basic protein (MBP; rat, Merck Millipore, Watford, UK, MAB386). Antibodies against glial fibrillary acidic protein (GFAP; mouse, Sigma-Aldrich, G3893) and OX-42 (CD-11b; mouse, Serotec, Kidlington, UK, MCA527R) were used to assess gliosis and the extent of oedema resolution was examined by aquaporin-4 (AQP4) antibody staining (chicken, Genway, San Diego, CA, USA, 07GA0175-070718).

### Fluorescent immunohistochemistry

Immunohistochemistry was conducted on the caudal cerebrum of 19 rats [Intact (n = 4), kaolin (n = 4), kaolin + PBS (n = 6), kaolin + decorin (n = 5)]. All selected sections were at least −2.5 mm posterior to Bregma and corresponded with the location of the DTI sections. Sections were washed in PBST (10 mM PBS pH 7.4 containing 0.3 % Tween20) and blocked in 2 % bovine serum albumin (BSA) and 15 % normal goat serum in PBST at room temperature for 1 h. Subsequently, sections were washed in PBST, before being incubated at 4 °C overnight in primary antibody diluting buffer containing PBST and 2 % BSA. After washing in PBST the sections were incubated for 1 h in secondary antibody solution (Alexa Fluor® 488 or 594 labelled secondary antibodies (Life Technologies, Paisley, UK) in PBST with 2 % BSA and 1.5 % normal goat serum) at room temperature, in the dark. After further PBST washes, sections were mounted in Vectashield containing DAPI (Vector Laboratories, Peterborough, UK). The Zeiss Axioplan 2 imaging epifluorescent microscope (Carl Zeiss, Germany) and the AxioCam Hrc (Carl Zeiss, Jena, Germany) were used to view and capture images under the same conditions for each antibody at ×400 magnification.

### Pixel based analysis of immunofluorescent staining

Quantitative analysis was undertaken using the software, Image J and all analyses were undertaken with the operator masked to the experimental group. Images for each immunofluorescent stain were processed identically before being analysed. For each image analysed, four randomly placed regions of interest (ROIs) were drawn with each ROI being 2.96 mm wide and 1.57 mm in height. For the corpus callosum, periventricular white matter and CA1 and CA3 hippocampal regions, a mean of 16 ROIs (four regions of interest × four coronal sections) were chosen per rat per stain. An average of 8 ROIs (four regions × two coronal sections) were selected for the internal capsule, caudate-putamen, parietal cortex and occipital cortex. All areas were analysed for GFAP, OX-42 and AQP4 staining however, as MBP is a marker of white matter integrity, only the corpus callosum, periventricular white matter and internal capsule were analysed for this antibody.

GFAP and OX-42 image processing included the conversion of images into a gray scale format prior to spatial filtering, thresholding and despeckling of the images using Image J. Images stained for AQP4 and MBP were identically processed to the GFAP and OX-42 images except thresholding was not performed. The mean percentage area of GFAP, OX-42, AQP4 and MBP positive staining, for each experimental group was calculated.

### Bright field microscopy

In order to assess hippocampal size, one cerebral section, at least 2.5 mm posterior to Bregma from each experimental animal was examined at ×10 magnification using the Nikon SM21500 dissecting microscope (Nikon, Tokyo, Japan). Images were captured with a Nikon ds-2mv high-resolution camera (Nikon). Hippocampal area was assessed by using the Image J software analyze area tool.

## Statistics

Statistical analysis was conducted using SPSS software, version 22 (IBM, Armonk, NY). Normally distributed data were analysed using a one-way ANOVA followed by a post hoc Tukey test. In the absence of normality, data were analysed using the Kruskal–Wallis test and tested for significant pairwise comparisons. Normally distributed data were expressed as the mean ± standard error of the mean (SEM). Correlation analysis was performed using a two-tailed Spearman's correlation test. As immunohistochemistry analysis was performed on caudal sections, mean DTI data from Section 2.76 and 3.72 mm posterior to Bregma were used for correlation analysis. Correlation analysis was not undertaken for the inner parietal cortex, caudate-putamen, occipital cortex or CA3 region of the hippocampus because DTI analysis was not being performed in these areas. Values were considered statistically significant when p values were *p < 0.05, **p < 0.01, ***p < 0.001 and ****p < 0.0001.

## Results

### Decorin reduces hydrocephalus induced DTI changes in the caudal periventricular white matter and corpus callosum

In the caudal periventricular white matter (−2.76 and −3.72 mm from Bregma), compared to Intact controls (0.83 ± 0.00 and 1.20 ± 0.02, respectively; Fig. 2b), the kaolin and kaolin + PBS groups displayed a significant increase in the MD (1.48 ± 0.22, p = 0.023 and 1.56 ± 0.15, p = 0.031 respectively) and AD (2.04 ± 0.27, p = 0.020 and 2.16 ± 0.17, p = 0.018, respectively). By contrast, the MD of decorin treated rats (0.85 ± 0.00) was significantly lower in comparison to kaolin (1.48 ± 0.22, p = 0.032) and kaolin + PBS (1.56 ± 0.15, p = 0.044) rats. No significant differences were observed in any DTI parameters in the rostral periventricular white matter (1.28 and −0.36 mm from Bregma) between the four experimental groups.

In the caudal corpus callosum (−2.76 and −3.72 mm from Bregma), the AD for kaolin (1.80 ± 0.15, p = 0.010) and kaolin + PBS (1.92 ± 0.12, p = 0.001) groups were significantly higher than Intact controls (1.56 ± 0.05; Fig. 2c). Moreover, kaolin + PBS rats displayed a significant elevation in the MD (1.17 ± 0.08, p = 0.030) and RD (1.00 ± 0.06, p = 0.025), compared to Intact animals (0.88 ± 0.02 and

0.54 ± 0.02, respectively). Furthermore, decorin treatment significantly reduced the AD (1.49 ± 0.02, p = 0.004) and RD (0.62 ± 0.03, p = 0.034) compared to the kaolin + PBS animals (1.92 ± 0.12 and 1.00 ± 0.06, respectively) in the caudal corpus callosum. No significant differences existed between decorin treated rats and Intact controls for all DTI parameters in the caudal corpus callosum. Similar to the rostral periventricular white matter, in the rostral corpus callosum (1.28 and −0.36 mm from Bregma), there were no significant differences in the DTI parameters between the experimental groups.

Alongside the corpus callosum and the periventricular white matter, five other regions of interest were examined by DTI voxel based analysis (Additional file 2: Figure S2). Significant differences in the four DTI parameters were not observed in the outer or inner parietal cortex (Additional file 2: Figure S2a, b). However, the FA of the kaolin group was significantly lower (0.11 ± 0.02, p = 0.036) than Intact controls (0.16 ± 0.01) in the CA1 region of the hippocampus (Additional file 2: Figure S2c). Moreover, in the caudal internal capsule (Additional file 2: Figure S2d), decorin (0.83 ± 0.01, p = 0.003) reduced the decrease in the MD observed in kaolin + PBS animals (0.77 ± 0.00). In the rostral internal capsule (Additional file 2: Figure S2e), kaolin + PBS rats displayed significantly greater FA (0.16 ± 0.01, p = 0.022) and AD (1.70 ± 0.28, p = 0.039) compared to Intact controls (0.23 ± 0.00 and 0.68 ± 0.23, respectively).

### Ventriculomegaly is greatest in the caudal hydrocephalic cerebrum and correlates with DTI parameters

As DTI parameter abnormalities were predominantly observed in the caudal cerebrum, we investigated whether non-uniform ventriculomegaly occurs in the basal cistern model of communicating hydrocephalus. In the kaolin and kaolin + PBS groups, the ventricles expanded significantly (p < 0.05) rostrally (8.04 ± 1.74 and 10.12 ± 3.83 mm³, respectively) and caudally (16.22 ± 2.76 and 21.00 ± 5.43 mm³, respectively) compared to the Intact controls (rostral = 1.26 ± 0.11 and caudal = 0.93 ± 0.10 mm³). Furthermore, significant changes in the mean differences between the rostral versus caudal ventricular volume were discovered (Table 1).

Rostrally, ventricular volume significantly correlated with the FA, MD, AD and RD measurements of

---

(See figure on next page.)

**Fig. 2** Decorin reduced hydrocephalus induced abnormalities in the caudal corpus callosum and periventricular white matter as evident from DTI. **a** Representative FA images of the locations at which the corpus callosum and periventricular white matter were analysed. *Section 1* (1.28 mm anterior to Bregma) and *Section 2* (0.36 mm posterior to Bregma) are classified as the rostral periventricular white matter and corpus callosum. *Section 3* (2.76 mm posterior to Bregma) and *Section 4* (3.72 mm posterior to Bregma) refer to the caudal periventricular white matter and corpus callosum. *Line graphs* displaying decorin's ability to reduce abnormalities in the (**b**) corpus callosum and (**c**) periventricular white matter on DTI; *blue* = Intact, *green* = kaolin, *red* = kaolin + PBS, *orange* = kaolin + decorin [Intact (n = 4), kaolin (n = 4), kaolin + PBS (n = 6), kaolin + decorin (n = 5)]. *Error bars* represent the standard error of the mean; *p < 0.05, **p < 0.01, ***p < 0.001

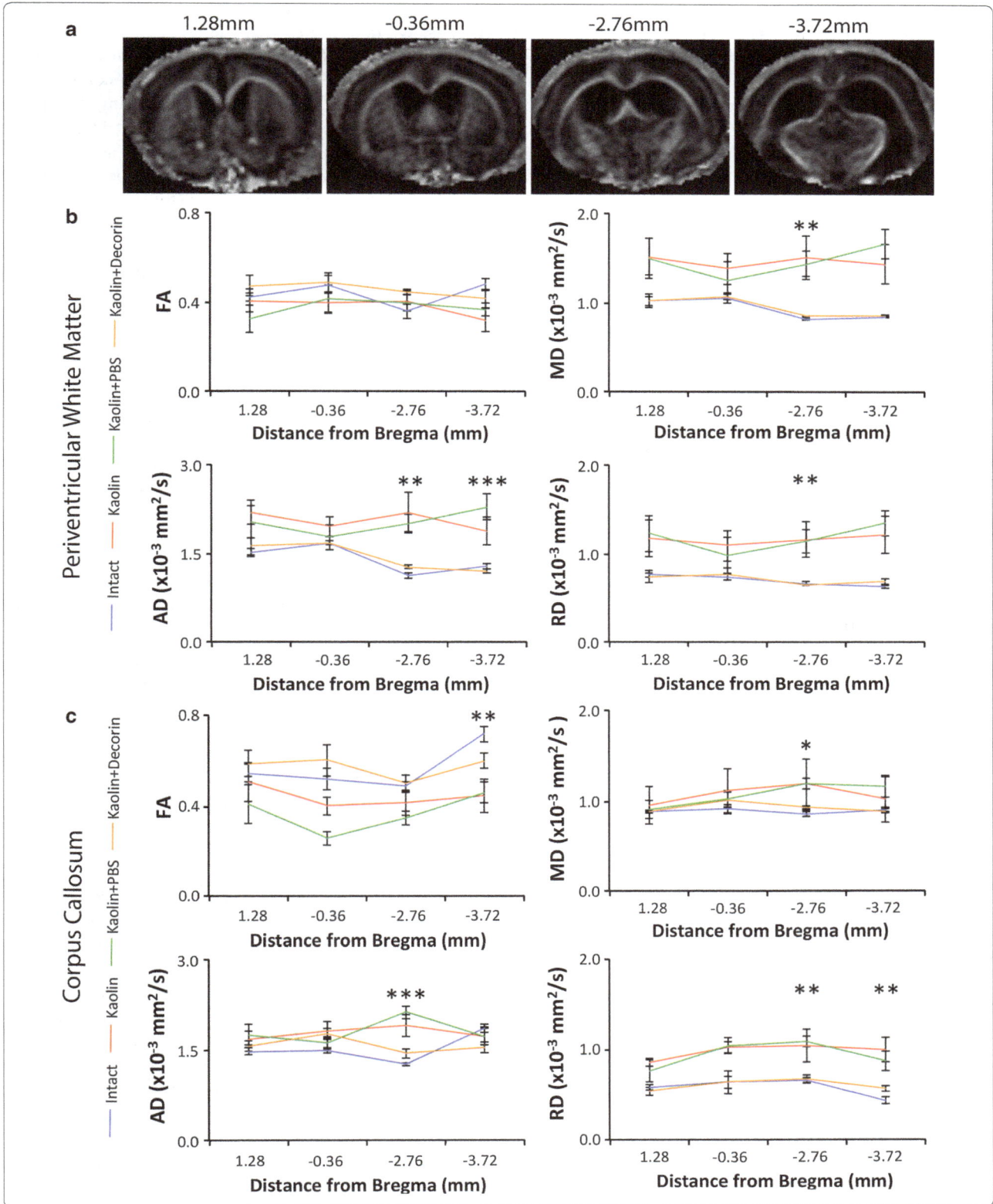

**Table 1 Significant changes in the mean differences between the rostral versus caudal ventricular volumes amongst the four experimental groups**

|  | p |
|---|---|
| Intact vs Kaolin | 0.005 |
| Intact vs Kaolin + PBS | <0.001 |
| Intact vs Kaolin + decorin | 0.946 |
| Kaolin vs Kaolin + PBS | 0.530 |
| Kaolin vs Kaolin + decorin | 0.015 |
| Kaolin + PBS vs Kaolin + decorin | 0.001 |

the corpus callosum and periventricular white matter (Table 2). Likewise, the caudal ventricular volume correlated with all DTI parameter measures in the corpus callosum and all except the AD in the periventricular white matter (Table 2).

### Decorin reduces caudal periventricular white matter cytopathology

As DTI parameter abnormalities were observed in the caudal periventricular white matter, corresponding immunohistochemistry analysis was conducted to aid

**Table 2 DTI parameter values of the corpus callosum and periventricular white matter correlated with rostral and caudal ventricular volume**

| DTI parameter | R (Spearman's rho) | p |
|---|---|---|
| *Rostral ventricular volume* |  |  |
| CC FA | 0.831 | <0.001 |
| CC MD | 0.539 | 0.026 |
| CC AD | 0.527 | 0.030 |
| CC RD | 0.733 | 0.001 |
| PVWM FA | 0.949 | <0.001 |
| PVWM MD | 0.706 | 0.002 |
| PVWM AD | 0.507 | 0.038 |
| PVWM RD | 0.642 | 0.005 |
| *Caudal ventricular volume* |  |  |
| CC FA | −0.676 | 0.003 |
| CC MD | 0.723 | 0.001 |
| CC AD | 0.777 | <0.001 |
| CC RD | 0.838 | <0.001 |
| PVWM FA | −0.520 | 0.033 |
| PVWM MD | 0.537 | 0.026 |
| PVWM AD | 0.441 | 0.076 |
| PVWM RD | 0.547 | 0.023 |

Statistically significant correlations = p < 0.05

*CC* corpus callosum, *PVWM* periventricular white matter, *FA* fractional anisotropy, *MD* mean diffusivity, *AD* axial diffusivity, *RD* radial diffusivity, *R* correlation coefficient (Spearman's rho)

hydrocephalic cytopathology characterisation of these tissues. We determined that the levels of GFAP positive immunostaining (Fig. 3a) were significantly increased in kaolin rats (2.49 ± 0.23 %, p = 0.048) compared to Intact controls (0.82 ± 0.11 %) indicating the presence of astrogliosis in the caudal periventricular white matter. Furthermore, the GFAP positive astrocytes of hydrocephalic animals exhibited features typical of reactive astrocytic morphology; cytoplasmic processes underwent thickening in kaolin and kaolin + PBS rats. The increase in GFAP positive staining observed in the kaolin rats (2.49 ± 0.23 %) was prevented with decorin treatment (0.49 ± 0.11 %, p = 0.002). Additionally, kaolin (1.77 ± 0.14 %, p = 0.040) and kaolin + PBS rats (1.34 ± 0.29 %, p = 0.056) displayed a significant and non-significant increase respectively in periventricular white matter AQP4 positive immunostaining (Fig. 3b) compared to Intact controls (0.80 ± 0.12 %). Importantly, AQP4 immunostaining in kaolin + decorin treated rats was significantly lower (0.56 ± 0.09 %, p = 0.006) than in kaolin animals (1.77 ± 0.14 %). No significant difference existed in periventricular white matter AQP4 immunostaining between decorin treated and Intact control rats (p = 0.860). In contrast, significant differences in OX-42 and MBP levels were not present between the experimental groups in the periventricular white matter (Fig. 3c, d). Furthermore, significant differences in GFAP, OX-42, MBP and AQP4 immunostaining were not present between the experimental groups in the caudal corpus callosum (Additional file 3: Table S1).

### Decorin protects from myelin damage in the caudal internal capsule

Although significant differences in myelin levels were not present in the caudal corpus callosum and caudal periventricular white matter, loss of myelin (assessed by measurement of MBP) in the caudal internal capsule was present in kaolin and kaolin + PBS animals (Fig. 4); compared to Intact controls (8.11 ± 0.49 %), a decrease in MBP immunostaining was present in kaolin (3.13 ± 0.28 %, p < 0.001) and kaolin + PBS (5.15 ± 0.47 %, p = 0.001) rats. Furthermore, decorin treated rats displayed higher MBP levels (5.87 ± 0.29 %) compared to kaolin (3.13 ± 0.28 %, p = 0.002) and kaolin + PBS rats (5.15 ± 0.47 %, p = 0.018), although the levels did not quite reach the same as in intact rats (p = 0.009), indicating some myelin protection. Qualitatively, the longitudinal organisation of myelin was disrupted, with discontinuity present along the length of the myelin fibres in animals receiving kaolin and kaolin + PBS compared to Intact controls. The regular parallel arrangement of MBP staining was protected with decorin treatment.

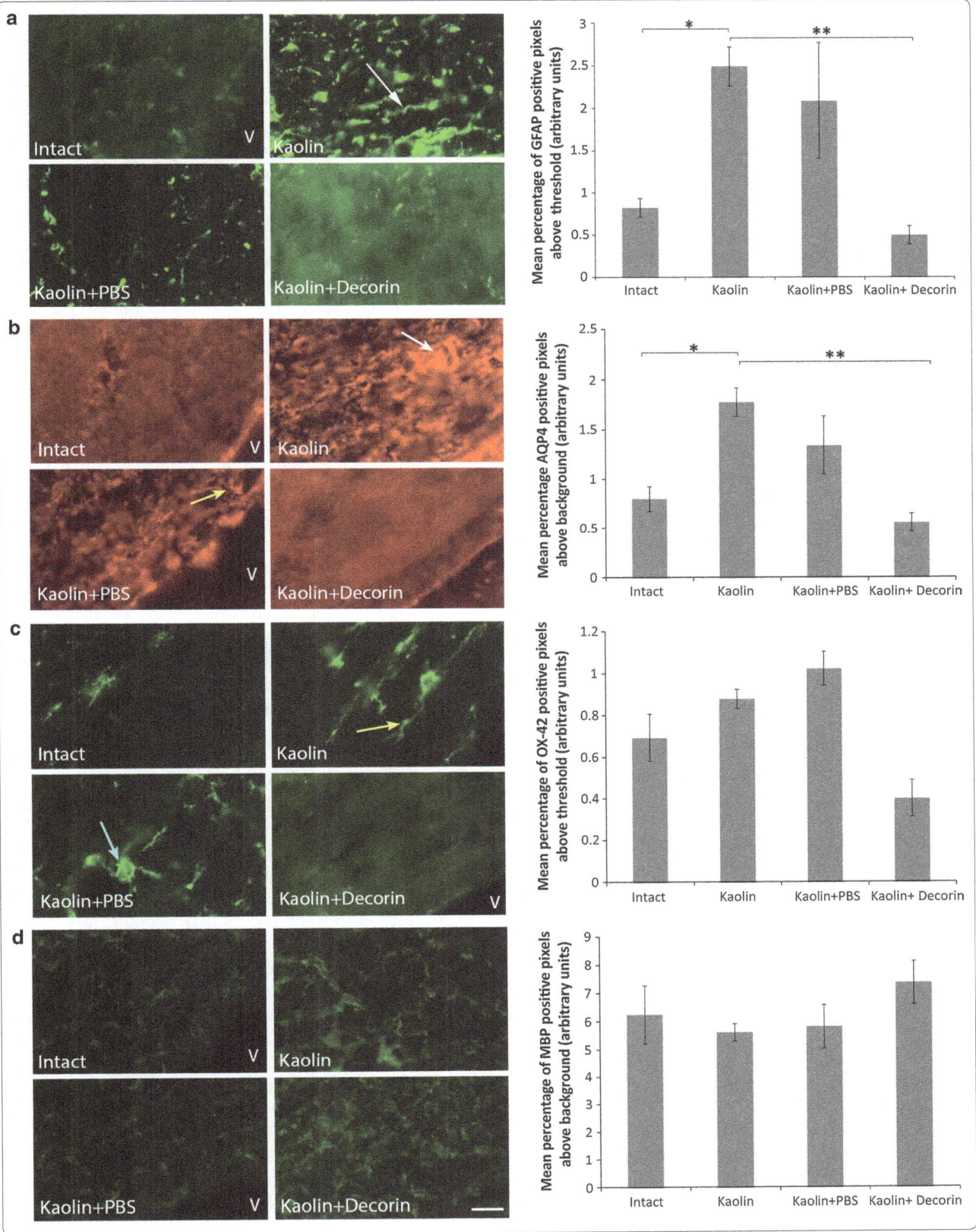

(See figure on previous page.)
**Fig. 3** Decorin prevented an increase in GFAP and AQP4 in the periventricular white matter. Representative images comparing the level of (**a**) GFAP immunostaining (*green*), (**b**) AQP4 immunostaining (*red*), (**c**) OX-42 immunostaining (*green*) and (**d**) MBP immunostaining (*green*) in the periventricular white matter; scale bar = 10 μm. **a** kaolin and kaolin + PBS rats displayed thickening of astrocytic processes (*white arrow*). **b** Accumulation of AQP4 staining was observed in kaolin rats (*white arrow*). AQP4 was further arranged around the circumference of blood vessels (*yellow arrow*). **c** Elongated, amoeboid microglia (*yellow arrow*) were particularly evident in kaolin rats. Microglia of kaolin + PBS rats were captured transitioning from branched resting microglia to activated amoeboid microglia (*blue arrow*). **d** Decorin treatment improved the myelin loss and disorganisation present in kaolin and kaolin + PBS rats (*white arrow*). Each corresponding bar graph displays the mean percentage of GFAP, AQP4, OX-42 or MBP positive pixels above threshold or background in the periventricular white matter across the four experimental groups; V lateral ventricle, *error bars* represent the standard error of the mean, *p < 0.05, **p < 0.01

### Decorin attenuates hippocampal atrophy in communicating hydrocephalus

Upon examining total hippocampal area, significant differences were present between the four experimental groups; a decrease in normalised hippocampal area was identified in the kaolin (47 ± 9 %, p = 0.006) and kaolin + PBS rats (69 ± 9 %, p < 0.001) compared to Intact controls (100 ± 6 %). Decorin treatment attenuated the hippocampal atrophy (89 ± 7 %, p = 0.008) compared to kaolin rats but failed to maintain the hippocampal size to that in Intact controls (100 ± 6 %, p < 0.001). In the CA1 region of the hippocampus, similar levels of GFAP, OX-42 and AQP4 were observed between all the experimental groups. In the CA3 region, GFAP levels were comparable among all four groups however kaolin rats (0.43 ± 0.02 %, p = 0.057) demonstrated a trend towards reduced OX-42 levels compared to Intact controls (0.89 ± 0.03 %), and kaolin + PBS rats (1.04 ± 0.13 %, p = 0.043) displayed a significant increase in AQP4 levels compared to Intact controls (1.60 ± 0.10 %; Additional file 4: Table S2).

### GFAP and AQP4 levels correlate significantly in the corpus callosum, periventricular white matter, caudate-putamen, parietal cortex and occipital cortex

No significant differences in AQP4, OX-42 and GFAP immunostaining were present between the experimental groups in the caudate putamen, parietal cortex and occipital cortex (Additional file 4: Table S2). However, in the corpus callosum, periventricular white matter, caudate-putamen, parietal cortex and occipital cortex, GFAP immunostaining positively correlated with AQP4 levels (Table 3). No significant correlations were present between OX-42 and AQP4 levels in any of the regions of interest.

### Hydrocephalic cytopathology correlates with abnormalities on DTI

In the caudal corpus callosum, increased astrocyte (GFAP) and AQP4 levels positively correlated with the AD (Table 4). Furthermore, in the caudal periventricular white matter (Table 4), GFAP and AQP4 positively correlated with AD, MD and RD. Moreover, the presence of cytopathology discouraged anisotropic water diffusion in the caudal periventricular white matter as the FA negatively correlated with astrocyte (GFAP), microglial (OX-42) and AQP4 immunostaining. A negative correlation was also present between myelin levels (MBP) and the MD of the caudal periventricular white matter.

### Discussion

This study demonstrates that decorin is able to protect and maintain DTI parameter values at normality in the caudal corpus callosum and caudal periventricular white matter. Likewise, decorin prevents astrogliosis and oedema in the caudal periventricular white matter and preserves myelin integrity in the caudal internal capsule. Furthermore, cytopathology in communicating hydrocephalus is predominantly localised to the caudal cerebrum. Moreover, DTI parameters correlate with cytopathology specifically in the caudal periventricular white matter. DTI is therefore a useful tool to act as a surrogate measure of cytopathology in communicating hydrocephalus.

Recent studies in post-haemorrhagic hydrocephalus suggest that occipital horn enlargement is greater and precedes the dilation of the remaining ventricular system [46–48]. This asymmetry is a pattern that is repeated in other types of hydrocephalus including congenital hydrocephalus [49] and idiopathic chronic hydrocephalus [50], although this feature has not been explored in depth or quantitatively. In feline infants [51], neonatal rats [41, 52] and adult dogs [53] with non-communicating hydrocephalus induced by kaolin injections into the cisterna magna, the occipital horns of the lateral ventricles are conspicuously larger than the frontal horns. Our results support these findings, albeit in an experimental model of communicating hydrocephalus, by showing that caudal portions of the lateral ventricles expand more than frontal regions, and DTI abnormalities are largely situated in the caudal white matter.

Asaaf and colleagues [54] suggested that DTI could be used as a marker of white tissue compression in obstructive hydrocephalus. Furthermore there have been no observed DTI changes in the white matter of idiopathic

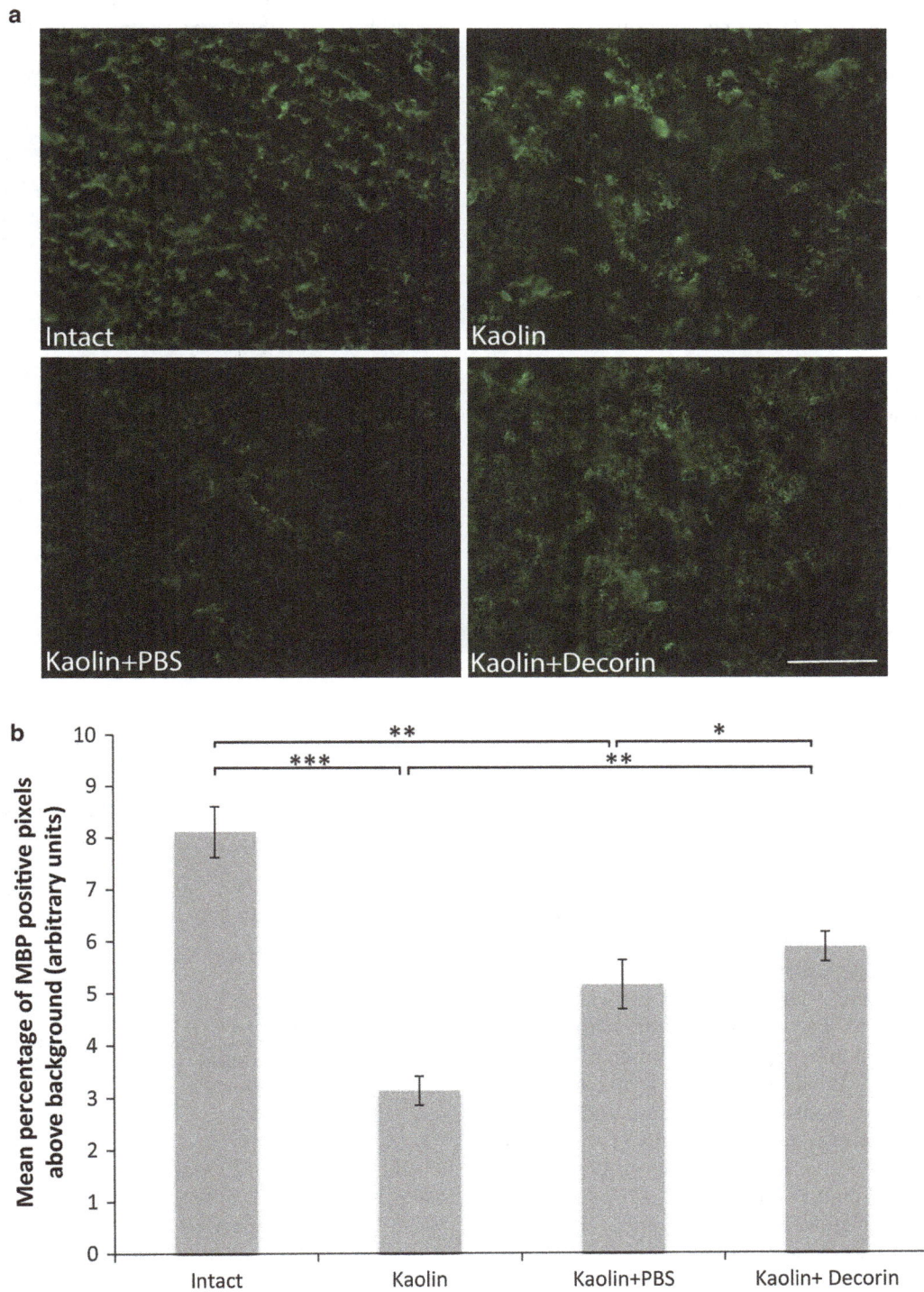

**Fig. 4** Decorin prevented myelin loss in the caudal internal capsule. **a** Representative images comparing caudal internal capsule MBP immunostaining (*green*) across the four experimental groups. Myelin organisation was better maintained with decorin use. **b** A *bar graph* displaying the mean percentage of MBP positive pixels above threshold in the internal capsule across the four experimental groups. Decreased MBP levels were present in kaolin and kaolin + PBS rats which was incompletely attenuated with decorin treatment; *error bars* represent the standard error of the mean, *p < 0.05, **p < 0.01, ***p < 0.001; *scale bar* = 50 μm

**Table 3 AQP4 levels correlated significantly with the marker of gliosis, GFAP, in the corpus callosum, periventricular white matter, caudate-putamen and parietal and occipital cortex**

| Region of interest | R | p |
|---|---|---|
| Corpus callosum | 0.614 | 0.005 |
| Periventricular white matter | 0.854 | <0.001 |
| CA1 hippocampus | 0.332 | 0.166 |
| CA3 hippocampus | 0.446 | 0.056 |
| Internal capsule | 0.291 | 0.226 |
| Caudate-putamen | 0.495 | 0.043 |
| Parietal cortex | 0.528 | 0.020 |
| Occipital cortex | 0.607 | 0.006 |

Statistically significant correlations = p < 0.05

R correlation coefficient

**Table 4 The marker of gliosis, GFAP, and AQP4 levels correlated with DTI parameter values in the periventricular white matter**

| ROI | Immunostain | DTI parameter | R | p |
|---|---|---|---|---|
| Corpus callosum | GFAP | FA | −0.370 | 0.144 |
| | | MD | 0.306 | 0.232 |
| | | AD | 0.600 | 0.011* |
| | | RD | 0.424 | 0.090* |
| | OX-42 | FA | −0.086 | 0.743 |
| | | MD | 0.002 | 0.993 |
| | | AD | 0.352 | 0.165 |
| | | RD | 0.120 | 0.646 |
| | AQP4 | FA | −0.323 | 0.205 |
| | | MD | 0.191 | 0.462 |
| | | AD | 0.566 | 0.018* |
| | | RD | 0.409 | 0.103 |
| | MBP | FA | 0.091 | 0.729 |
| | | MD | −0.031 | 0.903 |
| | | AD | 0.159 | 0.541 |
| | | RD | −0.115 | 0.660 |
| Periventricular white matter | GFAP | FA | −0.485 | 0.048* |
| | | MD | 0.647 | 0.005* |
| | | AD | 0.667 | 0.003* |
| | | RD | 0.680 | 0.003* |
| | OX-42 | FA | −0.495 | 0.043* |
| | | MD | 0.292 | 0.256 |
| | | AD | 0.299 | 0.244 |
| | | RD | 0.213 | 0.411 |
| | AQP4 | FA | −0.640 | 0.006* |
| | | MD | 0.799 | <0.001* |
| | | AD | 0.801 | <0.001* |
| | | RD | 0.829 | <0.001* |
| | MBP | FA | 0.346 | 0.174 |
| | | MD | −0.495 | 0.043* |
| | | AD | −0.360 | 0.155 |
| | | RD | −0.458 | 0.064* |

FA fractional anisotropy, MD mean diffusivity, AD axial diffusivity, RD radial diffusivity, R the correlation coefficient

* Statistically significant correlations = p < 0.05

intracranial hypertension patients (high ICP but no ventriculomegaly [55]) suggesting that compression of tissue impacts DTI parameters. In the caudal periventricular white matter, our findings replicate the abnormalities in the MD, AD and RD observed in hydrocephalic children [29–31]. In contrast to our findings, the MD of the periventricular white matter does not increase in posthaemorrhagic hydrocephalus in adults [56], therefore the maturity of the brain appears to influence DTI alterations. Similar to the findings of Yuan et al. [41] in rats of the same age with obstructive hydrocephalus (blockage of the cisterna magna), our communicating hydrocephalic animals display an increase in MD and reduced FA in the caudal corpus callosum. Our study has also revealed an increase in the AD and RD of the caudal corpus callosum in communicating hydrocephalus, which is additionally preventable by decorin treatment.

The cytopathology observed in our model supports current literature and is largely preventable with decorin treatment [10, 12, 57–64]. Although white matter abnormalities discovered were similar to those in hydrocephalic children [29–34], decorin was only able to protect the internal capsule from myelin damage. TGF-β mediated signaling promotes central nervous system myelination by enhancing oligodendrocyte progenitor cell differentiation and maturation [65, 66]. It is possible that internal capsule oligodendrocyte progenitor cells may be more susceptible to abnormalities in TGF-β signaling than those of the corpus callosum or periventricular white matter, hence explaining the observed result.

The relationship between DTI parameters and cerebral histopathological changes has been discussed extensively in recent literature [27, 31, 32, 67–71]. Events that discourage directional water movement, such as interstitial oedema and neurodegeneration cause a decline in the FA

[27, 28, 72–77]. The AD and RD are two DTI parameters that influence the FA and provide insight into axonal and myelin integrity, respectively [73, 76]. Both the AD and RD are also influenced by gliotic tissue changes [27, 72, 76]. Furthermore, an increase in average amount of diffusion in a given volume of tissue, caused by the presence of interstitial oedema or the loss of cellular barriers, results in a rise in the MD [27, 77, 78].

Consistent with the results of Yuan et al. [41] in juvenile rats with obstructive hydrocephalus, our findings in communicating hydrocephalus show positive correlations between GFAP increases and MD, AD, and RD in caudal periventricular white matter. Likewise, the increased levels of OX-42 (a marker of microglia) correlated negatively with the FA. This result may seem surprising since cytoarchitecturally in the periventricular white matter of kaolin and kaolin + PBS rats, the majority of microglial processes were longitudinally oriented; therefore an increase in FA would have been predicted [58]. However, as others have reported in congenital hydrocephalus [64], the cell bodies of reactive microglia in the periventricular white matter of our kaolin and kaolin + PBS animals were enlarged and widened. This cytopathological characteristic may have obstructed the parallel diffusion of water causing the FA to decrease. Since the pathophysiology of hydrocephalus is extremely multifactorial, it is unlikely that glial alterations alone exert a causative effect on DTI parameters.

The MBP levels of the caudal periventricular white matter correlate with the MD. These results corroborate the current literature; by increasing the volume of the extracellular space, myelin disorganisation and demyelination increases the MD of water molecules [27, 73, 76]. In support of the Tourdias et al. [78] report on communicating hydrocephalus, AQP4 levels positively correlated with the MD measurements in the caudal periventricular white matter. AQP4 levels also positively correlated with the FA, RD and more interestingly the AD measurements. Although sparse literature exists on the relationship between AQP4 and AD, we suggest that the removal of excess interstitial fluid by high levels of AQP4 may promote the unobstructed parallel movement of water through the periventricular white matter, hence resulting in an increase in the AD measurement. Further investigation of this hypothesis needs to be undertaken in order to substantiate such claim.

Here we have used kaolin to induce communicating hydrocephalus to help us determine the therapeutic effects of decorin. It is important to recognize the possibility that some decorin-treated animals may not have developed ventriculomegaly simply because of induction failures. However, it is unlikely that a significant proportion of the decorin-treatment group would not develop ventriculomegaly given the fact that 82 % of kaolin-only or kaolin + PBS animals demonstrated significantly enlarged ventricles [12]. In addition, 79 % of adult rats with identical induction procedures developed ventriculomegaly [79]. Thus, we believe that the improvements in the decorin-treated animals were due primarily to the drug intervention. Another consideration of the study is that the kaolin model of hydrocephalus is not the most clinically relevant model, however it is the best characterised and most widely used, successfully replicating the development and pathophysiological consequence

of acquired hydrocephalus. Kaolin induces an inflammatory response with concomitant deposition of fibrosis in areas of the subarachnoid space close to the injection site [80, 81] which is very similar to that observed in subarachnoid haemorrhage rat models [82]. The next step would be to determine the effects of decorin in a post haemorrhagic model. Recently, Yan et al. [83] demonstrated that pretreating rats with decorin in a subarachnoid haemorrhage model led to a reduction in ventriculomegaly and markers of fibrosis, indicating that decorin may have beneficial effects in subarachnoid haemorrhage. However further work needs to be conducted looking at the changes in cerebral cytopathology and microstructure with decorin treatment in this model.

## Conclusions

Our findings highlight the therapeutic potential of decorin to attenuate hydrocephalus-induced changes in astrogliosis, oedema and demyelination, particularly in the caudal periventricular white matter. Our study also helps to validate the use of DTI as a surrogate marker of cytopathology in communicating hydrocephalus and demonstrates that the caudal region of the brain appears to be the most affected, showing the greatest changes in ventriculomegaly, DTI and cytopathological measures in our experimental model.

## Additional files

**Additional file 1: Figure S1.** Decorin prevents ventriculomegaly assessed by T2 weighted MRI images. A bar graph showing a significant increase in ventricular volume in hydrocephalic rats compared to Intact controls. Furthermore, ventriculomegaly was prevented with 2.5 μg/0.5 μl/h infusion of human recombinant decorin treatment; ***p < 0.001. Corresponding representative T2- weighted MRI images displaying the differences in ventricular volume between the experimental groups in the rostral and caudal brain. Arrows highlight the size of the lateral ventricles (LV) or third ventricle (3V). Ventriculomegaly was evident by MRI in the hydrocephalic rats but not in Intact controls or rats that received decorin. Adapted from [12] with permission.

**Additional file 2: Figue S2.** DTI parameter abnormalities in the CA1 hippocampus, rostral and caudal internal capsule. Mean values + the standard error of the means are displayed for the fractional anisotropy (FA), mean diffusivity (MD), axial diffusivity (AD) and radial diffusivity (RD) in the (A) outer parietal cortex, (B) inner parietal cortex, (C) CA1 hippocampus, (D) caudal internal capsule and (E) rostral internal capsule; significant differences (p < 0.05) in the DTI parameter values from intact (*) or kaolin + PBS (+) levels are presented.

**Additional file 3: Table S1.** In the corpus callosum, no significant cytopathological changes were observed in hydrocephalic animals. The mean values ± the standard error of the means of GFAP, OX-42, AQP4 and MBP immunostaining in the four different experimental groups are expressed.

**Additional file 4: Table S2.** AQP4, GFAP and OX-42 levels in the CA1 and CA3 hippocampus, internal capsule, caudate-putamen, parietal cortex and occipital cortex in the four experimental groups; values represent the mean ± standard error of the means, * = p<0.05.

## Abbreviations

AD: axial diffusivity; AQP4: aquaporin-4; CC: corpus callosum; GFAP: glial acidic fibrillary protein; DTI: diffusion tensor imaging; MBP: myelin basic protein; MD: mean diffusivity; OX-42: part of the C3 complement receptor; PVWM: periventricular white matter; ROI: region of interest; RD: radial diffusivity; TGF-β: transforming growth factor-β.

## Authors' contributions

AA: design, data processing and analysis, interpretation of data, manuscript drafting, revision, and finalising; HB: conception and design, interpretation of data, manuscript drafting, revision, and finalising; JPM: conception and design, interpretation of data, manuscript drafting, revision and finalising; AMG: conception and design, interpretation of data, manuscript drafting, revision and finalising; OA: conception and design, interpretation of data, manuscript revision and finalising; AL: conception and design, manuscript revision and finalising; AS: conception and design, interpretation of data, manuscript drafting, revision, and finalising. All authors read and approved the final manuscript.

## Author details

[1] Institute of Metabolism and Systems Research, University of Birmingham, Edgbaston, Birmingham B15 2TT, UK. [2] Centre for Endocrinology, Diabetes and Metabolism, Birmingham Health Partners, Birmingham B15 2TH, UK. [3] Department of Neurosurgery, Division of Pediatric Neurosurgery at the Washington University School of Medicine and the Saint Louis Children's Hospital, St. Louis, MO 63110, USA. [4] Department of Bioengineering, University of Utah, Salt Lake City, UT 84112, USA. [5] Neurotrauma, College of Medicine and Dentistry, University of Birmingham, Edgbaston, Birmingham B15 2TT, UK. [6] Department of Neurology, University Hospitals Birmingham NHS Foundation Trust, Birmingham B15 2TH, UK.

## Acknowledgements

Anuriti Aojula was funded by the Sir Arthur Thompson Trust. Dr. Hannah Botfield was funded by the BBSRC. Professor James Patterson McAllister II was funded by the Department of Neurosurgery at the University of Utah, the Pediatric Hydrocephalus Association, the University of Utah Vice President for Research and the Department of Neurosurgery, Washington University School of Medicine. Dr. Alexandra Sinclair is funded by an NIHR Clinician Scientist Fellowship (NIHR-CS-011-028) and by the Medical Research Council, UK (MR/K015184/1).

## Competing interests

The authors declare that they have no competing interests.

# Appendix 1

Diffusion tensor imaging (DTI). DTI is a specialised magnetic resonance imaging technique that is used to gain greater appreciation of white matter disease-related pathophysiology via probing the random translational motion of water molecules [26]. The scalar parameters in DTI provide a quantitative method to assess cerebral water motion by specifically examining the magnitude and direction of water diffusion, which is quantified by measuring key parameters such as axial diffusivity (AD), radial diffusivity (RD) and their derivatives mean diffusivity (MD) or fractional anisotropy (FA). The FA values provide insight into the anisotropy of water diffusion. Water may diffuse isotropically, i.e. equally in all directions, or along a specific direction, therefore becoming anisotropic in nature. Moreover, the FA can be influenced by changes in microstructural integrity [27]; neurodegeneration and axonal reorganization hinders isotropic water movement, decreasing the FA. Furthermore, in ventriculomegaly-induced cerebral compression, increased AQP4

levels and gliosis raise the FA [74]. The RD and AD are two parameters that directly influence the FA. In white matter, the proportion of water diffusing perpendicular to neuronal fibres is assessed by RD, whilst the degree of water diffusion parallel to tract orientation is determined by the AD. Increased RD and AD are indicators of myelin and axonal integrity, respectively. Both RD and AD are also reported to increase upon astrogliosis [27]. Quantification of the average magnitude of diffusion in a given volume of tissue is provided by the MD value. MD is decreased by the presence of cellular barriers [80]. In contrast, interstitial edema and greater AQP4 and microglial presence are responsible for a rise in the MD [80].

## References

1. Fernell E, Hagberg G, Hagberg B. Infantile hydrocephalus in preterm, low-birth-weight infants—a nationwide Swedish cohort study 1979–1988. Acta Pediatr. 1993;82:45–8.
2. Simon TD, Riva-Cambrin J, Srivastava R, Bratton SL, Dean JM, Kestle JR, et al. Hospital care for children with hydrocephalus in the United States: utilization, charges, comorbidities, and deaths. J Neurosurg Pediatr. 2008;1:131–7.
3. Blackburn BL, Fineman RM. Epidemiology of congenital hydrocephalus in Utah, 1940–1979: report of an iatrogenically related "epidemic". Am J Med Genet. 1994;52:123–9.
4. Amlashi SF, Riffaud L, Morandi X. Communicating hydrocephalus and papilloedema associated with intraspinal tumours: report of four cases and review of the mechanisms. Acta Neurol Belg. 2006;106:31–6.
5. Cooke RS, Patterson V. Acute obstructive hydrocephalus complicating bacterial meningitis. Hydrocephalus was probably non-obstructive. BMJ. 1999;318:124.
6. Dandy WE. Intracranial tumors and abscesses causing communicating hydrocephalus. Ann Surg. 1925;82:199–207.
7. Groat J, Neumiller JJ. Review of the treatment and management of hydrocephalus. US Pharm. 2013;38:HS8–11.
8. Mirone G, Cinalli G, Spennato P, Ruggiero C, Aliberti F. Hydrocephalus and spinal cord tumors:a review. Childs Nerv Syst. 2011;27:1741–9.
9. Jung TY, Chung WK, Oh IJ. The prognostic significance of surgically treated hydrocephalus in leptomeningeal metastases. Clin Neurol Neurosurg. 2014;119:80–3.
10. McAllister JP. Pathophysiology of congenital and neonatal hydrocephalus. Semin Fetal Neonatal Med. 2012;17:285–94.
11. Yang TC, Chang CH, Liu YT, Chen YL, Tu PH, Chen HC. Predictors of shunt-dependent chronic hydrocephalus after aneurysmal subarachnoid haemorrhage. Eur Neurol. 2013;69:296–303.
12. Botfield H, Gonzalez AM, Abdullah O, Skjolding AD, Berry M, McAllister JP 2nd, et al. Decorin prevents the development of juvenile communicating hydrocephalus. Brain. 2013;136:2842–58.
13. Blegvad C, Skjolding AD, Broholm H, Laursen H, Juhler M. Pathophysiology of shunt dysfunction in shunt treated hydrocephalus. Acta Neurochir (Wien). 2013;155:1763–72.
14. Harris C, McAllister JP. What we should know about the cellular and tissue response causing catheter obstruction in the treatment of hydrocephalus. Neurosurgery. 2012;70:1589–601 **(discussion 1601–1602)**.
15. Lutz BR, Venkataraman P, Browd SR. New and improved ways to treat hydrocephalus: pursuit of a smart shunt. Surg Neurol Int. 2013;4:S38–50.
16. Pople IK. Hydrocephalus and shunts: what the neurologist should know. J Neurol Neurosurg Psychiatry. 2002;73:i17–122.
17. Dennis M, Fitz CR, Netley CT, Sugar J, Harwood-Nash DC, Hendrick EB, et al. The intelligence of hydrocephalic children. Arch Neurol. 1981;38:607–15.

18. Lacy M, Pyykkonen BA, Hunter SJ, Do T, Oliveira M, Austria E, et al. Intellectual functioning in children with early shunted posthemorrhagic hydrocephalus. Pediatr Neurosurg. 2008;44:376–81.

19. Vinchon M, Rekate H, Kulkarni AV. Pediatric hydrocephalus outcomes: a review. Fluids Barriers CNS. 2012;9:18.

20. Douglas MR, Daniel M, Lagord C, Akinwunmi J, Jackowski A, Cooper C, et al. High CSF transforming growth factor beta levels after subarachnoid haemorrhage: association with chronic communicating hydrocephalus. J Neurol Neurosurg Psychiatry. 2009;80:545–50.

21. Kaestner S, Dimitriou I. TGF beta1 and TGF beta2 and their role in posthemorrhagic hydrocephalus following SAH and IVH. J Neurol Surg A Cent Eur Neurosurg. 2013;74:279–84.

22. Kitazawa K, Tada T. Elevation of transforming growth factor-beta 1 level in cerebrospinal fluid of patients with communicating hydrocephalus after subarachnoid hemorrhage. Stroke. 1994;25:1400–4.

23. Tada T, Kanaji M, Kobayashi S. Induction of communicating hydrocephalus in mice by intrathecal injection of human recombinant transforming growth factor-beta 1. J Neuroimmunol. 1994;50:153–8.

24. Del Bigio MR, Wilson MJ, Enno T. Chronic hydrocephalus in rats and humans: white matter loss and behavior changes. Ann Neurol. 2003;53:337–46.

25. Persson EK, Hagberg G, Uvebrant P. Hydrocephalus prevalence and outcome in a population-based cohort of children born in 1989–1998. Acta Paediatr. 2005;94:726–32.

26. Basser PJ, Mattiello J, LeBihan D. MR diffusion tensor spectroscopy and imaging. Biphys J. 1994;66:259–67.

27. Alexander A, Lee J, Lazar M, Field AS. Diffusion tensor imaging of the brain. Neurotherapeutics. 2007;4:316–29.

28. Hagmann P, Jonasson L, Maeder P, Thiran JP, Wedeen VJ, Meuli R. Understanding diffusion MR imaging techniques: from scalar diffusion-weighted imaging to diffusion tensor imaging and beyond. RSNA. 2006;26:S205–23.

29. Hasan KM, Eluvathingal TJ, Kramer LA, Ewing-Cobbs L, Dennis M, Fletcher JM. White matter microstructural abnormalities in children with spina bifida myelomeningocele and hydrocephalus: a diffusion tensor tractography study of the association pathways. J Magn Reson Imaging. 2008;27:700–9.

30. Rajagopal A, Shimony JS, McKinstry RC, Altaye M, Maloney T, Mangano FT, et al. White matter microstructural abnormality in children with hydrocephalus detected by probabilistic diffusion tractography. AJNR Am J Neuroradiol. 2013;34:2379–85.

31. Yuan W, McAllister JPI, Mangano FT. Neuroimaging of white matter abnormalities in pediatric hydrocephalus. J Pediatr Neuroradiol. 2013;2:119–28.

32. Yuan W, McKinstry RC, Shimony JS, Altaye M, Powell SK, Phillips JM, et al. Diffusion tensor imaging properties and neurobehavioral outcomes in children with hydrocephalus. AJNR Am J Neuroradiol. 2013;34:439–45.

33. Cancelliere A, Mangano FT, Air EL, Jones BV, Altaye M, Rajagopal A, et al. DTI values in key white matter tracts from infancy through adolescence. AJNR Am J Neuroradiol. 2013;34:1443–9.

34. Tuor UI, Morgunov M, Sule M, Qiao M, Clark D, Rushforth D, et al. Cellular correlates of longitudinal diffusion tensor imaging of axonal degeneration following hypoxic-ischemic cerebral infarction in neonatal rats. Neuroimage Clin. 2014;6:32–42.

35. Rossi ME, Jason E, Marchesotti S, Dastidar P, Ollikainen J, Soimakallio S. Diffusion tensor imaging correlates with lesion volume in cerebral hemisphere infarctions. BMC Med Imaging. 2010;10:21.

36. Budde MD, Xie M, Cross AH, Song SK. Axial diffusivity is the primary correlate of axonal injury in the EAE spinal cord: a quantitative pixelwise analysis. J Neurosci. 2009;29:2805–13.

37. Elshafey R, Hassanien O, Khalil M. Diffusion tensor imaging for characterizing white matter changes in multiple sclerosis. Egypt J Radiol Nucl Med. 2014;45:881–8.

38. Schmierer K, Wheeler-Kingshott CAM, Boulby PA, Scaravilli F, Altmann DR, Barker GJ, et al. Diffusion tensor imaging of post mortem multiple sclerosis brain. Neuroimage. 2007;35:467–77.

39. Xie M, Tobin JE, Budde MD, Chen CI, Trinkaus K, Cross AH, et al. Rostrocaudal analysis of corpus callosum demyelination and axon damage across disease stages refines diffusion tensor imaging correlations with pathological features. J Neuropathol Exp Neurol. 2010;69:704–16.

40. Brennan FH, Cowin GJ, Kurniawan ND, Ruitenberg MJ. Longitudinal assessment of white matter pathology in the injured mouse spinal cord through ultra-high field (16.4 T) in vivo diffusion tensor imaging. Neuroimage. 2013;82:574–85.

41. Yuan W, Deren KE, McAllister JP 2nd, Holland SK, Lindquist DM, Cancelliere A, et al. Diffusion tensor imaging correlates with cytopathology in a rat model of neonatal hydrocephalus. Cerebrospinal Fluid Res. 2010;7:19.

42. Concha L, Livy DJ, Beaulieu C, Wheatley BM, Gross DW. In vivo diffusion tensor imaging and histopathology of the fimbria-fornix in temporal lobe epilepsy. J Neurosci. 2010;30:996–1002.

43. Goubran M, Hammond RR, de Ribaupierre S, Burneo JG, Mirsattari S, Steven DA, et al. Magnetic resonance imaging and histology correlation in the neocortex in temporal lobe epilepsy. Ann Neurol. 2015;77:237–50.

44. van Eijsden P, Otte WM, van der Hel WS, van Nieuwenhuizen O, Dijkhuizen RM, de Graaf RA, et al. In vivo diffusion tensor imaging and ex vivo histologic characterization of white matter pathology in a post-status epilepticus model of temporal lobe epilepsy. Epilepsia. 2011;52:841–5.

45. Paxinos G, Watson C. The rat brain in stereotaxic coordinates. 7th ed. London: Elsevier Inc; 2013.

46. Brouwer M, de Vries L, Pistorius L. Ultrasound measurements of the lateral ventricles in neonates: why, how and when? A systematic review. Acta Paediatr. 2010;99:1298–306.

47. Brann BS IV, et al. Asymmetric growth of the lateral cerebral ventricle in infants with posthemorrhagic ventricular dilatation. J Pediatr. 1991;118:108–12.

48. O'Hayon BB, et al. Frontal and occipital horn ratio: a linear estimate of ventricular size for multiple imaging modalities in pediatric hydrocephalus. Pediatr Neurosurg. 1998;29(5):245–9.

49. Elgamal E. Natural history of hydrocephalus in children with spinal open neural tube defect. Surg Neurol Int. 2012;3:112.

50. Missori P, Currà A. Progressive cognitive impairment evolving to dementia parallels parieto-occipital and temporal enlargement in idiopathic chronic hydrocephalus: a retrospective cohort study. Front Neurol. 2015;24(6):15.

51. McAllister JP 2nd, et al. Progression of experimental infantile hydrocephalus and effects of ventriculoperitoneal shunts: an analysis correlating magnetic resonance imaging with gross morphology. Neurosurgery. 1991;29(3):329–40.

52. Deren KE, et al. Reactive astrocytosis, microgliosis and inflammation in rats with neonatal hydrocephalus. Exp Neurol. 2010;226(1):110–9.

53. McAllister JP 2nd, et al. Differential ventricular expansion in hydrocephalus. Eur J Pediatr Surg. 1998;8(Suppl 1):39–42.

54. Assaf Y, Ben-Sira L, Constantini S, Chang LC, Beni-Adani L. Diffusion tensor imaging in hydrocephalus: initial experience. AJNR Am J Neuroradiol. 2006;27(8):1717–24.

55. Owler BK, Higgins JN, Péna A, Carpenter TA, Pickard JD. Diffusion tensor imaging of benign intracranial hypertension: absence of cerebral oedema. Br J Neurosurg. 2006;20(2):79–81.

56. Jang SH, Choi BY, Chang CH, Jung YJ, Byun WM, Kim SH, et al. The effects of hydrocephalus on the periventricular white matter in intracerebral hemorrhage: a diffuser tensor imaging study. Int J Neurosci. 2013;123:420–4.

57. Cabuk B, Etus V, Bozkurt SU, Sav A, Ceylan S. Neuroprotective effect of memantine on hippocampal neurons in infantile rat hydrocephalus. Turk Neurosurg. 2011;21:325–58.

58. Del Bigio MR, Khan OH, da Silva Lopes L, Juliet PA. Cerebral white matter oxidation and nitrosylation in young rodents with kaolin-induced hydrocephalus. J Neuropathol Exp Neurol. 2012;71:274–88.

59. Deren KE, Packer M, Forsyth J, Milash B, Abdullah OM, Hsu EW, et al. Reactive astrocytosis, microgliosis and inflammation in rats with neonatal hydrocephalus. Exp Neurol. 2010;226:110–9.

60. Eskandari R, Abdullah O, Mason C, Lloyd KE, Oeschle AN, McAllister JP 2nd. Differential vulnerability of white matter structures to experimental infantile hydrocephalus detected by diffusion tensor imaging. Childs Nerv Syst. 2014;30:1651–61.

61. Eskandari R, Harris C, McAllister J. Reactive astrocytosis in feline neonatal hydrocephalus: acute, chronic, and shunt-induced changes. Childs Nerv Syst. 2011;27:2067–76.

62. Khan OH, Enno TL, Del Bigio MR. Brain damage in neonatal rats following kaolin induction of hydrocephalus. Eep Neural. 2006;200(2):311–20.

63. Klinge PM, Samii A, Mühlendyck A, Visnyei K, Meyer GJ, Walter GF. Cerebral hypoperfusion and delayed hippocampal response after induction of adult kaolin hydrocephalus. Stroke. 2003;1:193–9.

64. Miller JM, McAllister JP 2nd. Reduction of astrogliosis and microgliosis by cerebrospinal fluid shunting in experimental hydrocephalus. Cerebrospinal Fluid Res. 2007;4:5.

65. Palazuelos J, Klingener M, Aguirre A. TGFβ signaling regulates the timing of CNS myelination by modulating oligodendrocyte progenitor cell cycle exit through SMAD3/4/FoxO1/Sp1. J Neurosci. 2014;34:7917–30.

66. Dutta DJ, Zameer A, Mariani JN, Zhang J, Asp L, Huynh J, et al. Combinatorial actions of Tgfβ and Activin ligands promote oligodendrocyte development and CNS myelination. Development. 2014;141:2414–28.

67. Beaulieu C. The basis of anisotropic water diffusion in the nervous system—a technical review. NMR Biomed. 2002;15:435–55.

68. Cheong JL, Thompson DK, Wang HX, Hunt RW, Anderson PJ, Inder TE, et al. Abnormal white matter signal on MR imaging is related to abnormal tissue microstructure. AJNR Am J Neuroradiol. 2009;30:623–8.

69. Klawiter EC, Schmidt RE, Trinkaus K, Liang HF, Budde MD, Naismith RT, et al. Radial diffusivity predicts demyelination in ex vivo multiple sclerosis spinal cords. Neuroimage. 2011;55:1454–60.

70. Neil J, Miller J, Mukherjee P, Huppi PS. Diffusion tensor imaging of normal and injured developing human brain—a technical review. NMR Biomed. 2002;15:543–52.

71. Price SJ, Young AM, Scotton WJ, Ching J, Mohsen LA, Boonzaier NR, et al. Multimodal MRI can identify perfusion and metabolic changes in the invasive margin of glioblastomas. J Magn Reson Imaging. 2016;43(2):487–94 **(Epub ahead of print)**.

72. Budde MD, Janes L, Gold E, Turtzo LC, Frank JA. The contribution of gliosis to diffusion tensor anisotropy and tractography following traumatic brain injury: validation in the rat using Fourier analysis of stained tissue sections. Brain. 2011;134:2248–60.

73. Concha L, Kim H, Bernasconi A, Bernhardt BC, Bernasconi N. Spatial patterns of water diffusion along white matter tracts in temporal lobe epilepsy. Neurology. 2012;79:455–62.

74. Filippi CG, Cauley KA. Lesions of the corpus callosum and other commissural fibers: diffusion tensor studies. Semin Ultrasound CT MR. 2014;35:445–58.

75. Hong YJ, Yoon B, Shim YS, Cho AH, Lim SC, Ahn KJ, et al. Differences in microstructural alterations of the hippocampus in Alzheimer disease and idiopathic normal pressure hydrocephalus: a diffusion tensor imaging study. AJNR Am J Neuroradiol. 2010;31:1867–72.

76. Hoza D, Vlasák A, Hořínek D, Sameš M, Alfieri A. DTI-MRI biomarkers in the search for normal pressure hydrocephalus aetiology: a review. Neurosurg Rev. 2015;38:239–44.

77. Sotak C. The role of diffusion tensor imaging in the evaluation of ischemic brain injury—a review. NMR Biomed. 2002;15:561–659.

78. Tourdias T, Dragonu I, Fushimi Y, Deloire MS, Boiziau C, Brochet B, et al. Aquaporin 4 correlates with apparent diffusion coefficient and hydrocephalus severity in the rat brain: a combined MRI–histological study. Neuroimage. 2009;47:659–66.

79. Li J, McAllister JP 2nd, Shen Y, Wagshul ME, Miller JM, Egnor MR, Johnston MG, Haacke EM, Walker ML. Communicating hydrocephalus in adult rats with kaolin obstruction of the basal cisterns or the cortical subarachnoid space. Exp Neurol. 2008;211(2):351–61.

80. Hatta J, Hatta T, Moritake K, Otani H. Heavy water inhibiting the expression of transforming growth factor-beta1 and the development of kaolin-induced hydrocephalus in mice. J Neurosurg. 2006;104(4 Suppl):251–8.

81. Slobodian I, Krassioukov-Enns D, Del Bigio MR. Protein and synthetic polymer injection for induction of obstructive hydrocephalus in rats. Cerebrospinal Fluid Res. 2007;25(4):9.

82. Sajanti J, Björkstrand AS, Finnilä S, Heikkinen E, Peltonen J, Majamaa K. Increase of collagen synthesis and deposition in the arachnoid and the dura following subarachnoid hemorrhage in the rat. Biochim Biophys Acta. 1999;1454(3):209–16.

83. Yan H, Chen Y, Li L, Jiang J, Wu G, Zuo Y, Zhang JH, Feng H, Yan X, Liu F. Decorin alleviated chronic hydrocephalus via inhibiting TGF-β1/Smad/CTGF pathway after subarachnoid hemorrhage in rats. Brain Res. 2016;1(1630):241–53.

# 12

# LDL receptor blockade reduces mortality in a mouse model of ischaemic stroke without improving tissue-type plasminogen activator-induced brain haemorrhage: towards pre-clinical simulation of symptomatic ICH

Be'eri Niego[1][*][†] (iD), Brad R. S. Broughton[2][†], Heidi Ho[1], Christopher G. Sobey[3][‡] and Robert L. Medcalf[1][‡]

## Abstract

**Background:** Symptomatic intracerebral haemorrhage (sICH) following tissue-type plasminogen activator (rt-PA) administration is the most feared and lethal complication of thrombolytic therapy for ischaemic stroke, creating a significant obstacle for a broader uptake of this beneficial treatment. rt-PA also undermines cerebral vasculature stability in a multimodal process which involves engagement with LDL receptor-related protein 1 (LRP-1), potentially underlying the development of sICH.

**Aims and methods:** We aimed to simulate rt-PA-induced haemorrhagic transformation (HT) in a mouse model of stroke and to assess if it drives symptomatic neurological deterioration and whether it is attenuated by LDL receptor blockade. rt-PA (10 mg/kg) or its vehicle, with or without the LDL receptor antagonist, receptor-associated protein (RAP; 2 mg/kg), were intravenously injected at reperfusion after 0.5 or 4 h of middle cerebral artery occlusion (MCAo). Albumin and haemoglobin content were measured in the perfused mouse brains 24 h post MCAo as indications of blood–brain barrier (BBB) compromise and HT, respectively.

**Results:** rt-PA did not elevate brain albumin and haemoglobin levels in sham mice or in mice subjected to 0.5 h MCAo. In contrast, administration of rt-PA after prolonged MCAo (4 h) caused a marked increase in HT (but similar changes in brain albumin) compared to vehicle, mimicking the clinical shift from a safe to detrimental intervention. Interestingly, this HT did not correlate with functional deficit severity at 24 h, suggesting that it does not play a symptomatic role in our mouse stroke model. Co-administration of RAP with or without rt-PA reduced mortality and neurological scores but did not effectively decrease brain albumin and haemoglobin levels.

**Conclusion:** Despite the proven causative relationship between severe HT and neurological deterioration in human stroke, rt-PA-triggered HT in mouse MCAo does not contribute to neurological deficit or simulate sICH. Model limitations, such as the long duration of occlusion required, the type of HT achieved and the timing of deficit assessment

*Correspondence: beeri.niego@monash.edu
[†]Be'eri Niego and Brad R. S. Broughton contributed equally to this work
[‡]Christopher G. Sobey and Robert L. Medcalf contributed equally to this work
[1] Molecular Neurotrauma and Haemostasis, Australian Centre for Blood Diseases, Monash University, Level 4 Burnet Building, 89 Commercial Road, Melbourne 3004, VIC, Australia
Full list of author information is available at the end of the article

may account for this mismatch. Our results further suggest that blockade of LDL receptors improves stroke outcome irrespective of rt-PA, blood–brain barrier breakdown and HT.

**Keywords:** Stroke, Tissue-type plasminogen activator, Symptomatic intracerebral haemorrhage, Blood–brain barrier, Receptor-associated protein, MCAo

## Background

Intracranial bleeding episodes, or haemorrhagic transformations (HTs), are common in ischaemic stroke [1]. They can occur spontaneously and, according to large meta-analyses, are present in 24.2% of placebo-treated and 32.5% of recombinant tissue-type plasminogen activator (rt-PA)-treated patients [2]. However, only those bleeding events which lead to worsening of neurological outcomes, so-called symptomatic intracerebral haemorrhages (sICH), have direct impact on the safety assessment of rt-PA treatment.

sICH is the most serious complication of thrombolysis with rt-PA in stroke, often resulting in devastating consequences. It occurs in ∼ 6% of thrombolysed patients and carries 50% mortality rate [1, 3], causing reluctance among some practitioners to employ rt-PA-induced thrombolysis [4, 5]. Furthermore, a lack of research exploring the most appropriate management of sICH prevents the establishment of standardised guidelines for treatment of this condition [6]. There is therefore a need to identify those who are at particular risk and to develop research tools to specifically combat this emergency situation.

HTs during stroke are not uniformly presented but classified radiologically as haemorrhagic infarctions (HI-1 and -2, characterised by petechial bleeding) or parenchymal haematomas (PH-1 or -2, defined as haemorrhage occupying < 30 or > 30% of the ischaemic area with mild or significant space-occupying effect, respectively) [1, 3, 7]. While all types of HTs can be accompanied by neurological decline, it is mainly the PH-2 type that independently predicts neurological deterioration at 24 h and poor outcomes at 3 month post stroke [1, 8], particularly if it coincides with other time and neurological criteria [9].

Notably, many animal studies which assess rt-PA-related HTs do not classify the type of haemorrhage or determine whether it plays a role in functional outcome post-treatment [10–15]. Even in rodent studies that use the clinical HT classification, no correlations are performed to evaluate whether brain haemorrhage actually contributes to neurological decline [16–20]. Taken together, the nature of HTs in current pre-clinical stroke models needs further examination to allow refined simulation of the human rt-PA-related sICH.

Regardless of its outcome, for blood extravasation to occur the blood-brain barrier (BBB) must be compromised. With this in mind, considerable pre-clinical and clinical data suggests that rt-PA disrupts the BBB, potentially contributing to subsequent HT [21]. This occurs via plasmin-dependent or -independent effects of rt-PA on various cellular and acellular components of the BBB [22, 23].

Members of the low-density lipoprotein receptor (LDLR) superfamily, in particular LDLR-related protein 1 (LRP-1) [24], have long been considered to serve as t-PA receptors in the CNS [24, 25]. Many t-PA-associated BBB breakdown processes during stroke involve t-PA engagement with LRP-1, an interaction which drives upregulation of matrix metalloproteinase (MMP)-3 [13], MMP-9 [26, 27] and vascular endothelial growth factor (VEGF) in brain endothelial cells [28] and microglia [29], activation of the platelet-derived growth factor (PDGF)-CC [12] and Rho-kinase pathways [30] as well as direct cleavage of LRP-1 [31] in astrocytes and control of vascular tone [32] via stimulation of smooth-muscle cells [33].

The pan LDLR antagonist, receptor-associated protein (RAP) [34], is a small intracellular chaperone which prevents premature ligand binding to LRP-1 and also to other LDLRs such as megalin (gp330; LRP-2), the very low density lipoprotein (VLDL) receptor and the LDLR itself [34, 35]. RAP improved functional outcome and HT in rats after stroke [36] and reduced rt-PA-mediated BBB disruption [28, 31] and brain haemorrhage [13] in permanent and thrombotic mouse models of middle cerebral artery occlusion (MCAo), respectively. Yet, the efficacy of RAP against rt-PA damage in transient mechanical MCAo, which best enables focusing on off-target effects of rt-PA, has not been reported.

Here, we simulated rt-PA-triggered HT formation and examined its characteristics by appearance (HI or PH) and functional consequences in a mouse MCAo model. We further tested the potential of RAP to reduce rt-PA-induced BBB disruption and bleeding complications. Our results highlight the challenges in pre-clinical simulation of sICH and interestingly suggest that the use of RAP as a sole therapeutic agent might offer benefits in stroke despite being insufficient for effective protection of the BBB from rt-PA during thrombolysis.

## Methods

### Reagents

Human t-PA (rt-PA; Actilyse®) was purchased from Boehringer Ingelheim GmbH (Rhein, Germany) and dialysed against 0.35 M HEPES–NaOH, pH 7.4, to remove the original components of the formulation buffer [37]. Low-endotoxin human RAP was obtained from Molecular Innovations (Novi, MI, USA).

### Mouse stroke model and drug treatment

All animal procedures were undertaken in accordance with the National Health and Medical Research Council (NHMRC) "Code of Practice for the Care and Use of Animals for Experimental Purposes in Australia" and were approved by an Animal Ethics Committee of Monash University. Animal procedures also complied with the ARRIVE guidelines (Animal Research: Reporting in Vivo Experiments).

Middle Cerebral Artery occlusion (MCAo): 93 8–12 week-old C57Bl/6 male mice weighing ~ 25 g underwent MCAo (16 and 63 animals for 0.5 and 4 h occlusion periods, respectively) or sham surgery (12 animals) as described below [38]. 77 mice underwent successful experimental protocol (defined as uncomplicated surgery with successful occlusion and good recovery, complete drug treatment and satisfactory intracardial perfusion as judged by liver colour). 16 additional mice (2 shams and 14 MCAo) failed to meet these criteria and were not analysed. The overall mortality by 24 h after successful surgeries was 6.25% (1 out of 16 mice) or 34.7% (17 out of 49) in mice undergoing 0.5 or 4 h MCAo, respectively.

Focal cerebral ischemia was induced in anesthetized mice (ketamine: 80 mg/kg plus xylazine: 10 mg/kg intraperitoneally) by occlusion of the MCA using a 6.0 silicone-coated monofilament (Doccol Corporation, MA, USA). Occlusion was sustained for either 0.5 or 4 h, and the filament was then retracted to allow reperfusion. Both successful occlusion (> 70% reduction in cerebral blood flow; CBF) and reperfusion (> 90% return of CBF to pre-ischemic levels) was verified by transcranial Laser-Doppler flowmetry (PeriMed, Sweden). Head and neck wounds were stitched closed, covered with Betadine® (Sanofi, Australia) and spray dressing, and the mice were then returned to their cages after regaining consciousness. To restore blood flow in the 4 h occlusion cohort, mice were re-anesthetised 15 min before the end of the occlusion period. The wound was re-opened and the filament was retracted to allow reperfusion. Rectal temperature was monitored and maintained at 37.0 ± 0.5 °C throughout the procedure. Sham-operated mice were anesthetized and the right carotid bifurcation exposed, but no filament was inserted.

Drug treatment: rt-PA (10 mg/kg) or its HEPES vehicle were administered in both 0.5 and 4 h MCAo protocols immediately after reperfusion as a bolus injection via the tail vein (4 ml/kg; 100 µl per 25 g mouse). In selected cohorts of animals undergoing 4 h MCAo, RAP (2 mg/kg) [13, 28] was co-administered with vehicle or rt-PA in the same intravenous injection. Notably, similar studies in mice reported good response to intravenous RAP already at 1 mg/kg and only marginal improvement with dose escalation to 2 mg/kg [13, 28], suggesting that RAP at 2 mg/kg is sufficient to exert its maximal effect in our settings.

End point: 24 h post stroke mice were killed by isoflurane and then transcardially perfused with phosphate-buffered saline supplemented with 0.05 U/ml clexane using a peristaltic pump. Brains were finally removed, divided into ipsilateral and contralateral hemispheres and processed as described below.

### Mortality

Mortality occurring between the time of drug treatment at reperfusion and 24 h post MCAo was reported in a targeted cohort of mice which were operated on exclusively by two experienced operators over a limited 3-month period. In this cohort, rt-PA or its HEPES vehicle were compared head to head with or without RAP. Earlier cohorts of animals treated with rt-PA or vehicle (Fig. 1) were not included in the mortality sum. 31 animals in total underwent surgery at this stage. 4 surgeries were unsuccessful and 1 animal was excluded due to severe bleeding from neck sutures, which was unrelated to drug treatment. 26 animals were therefore included in the mortality analysis. Out of 9 mortality events in this cohort, 1 mouse died 2 h after treatment (with HEPES vehicle + RAP) while all other mortalities occurred overnight (> 6 h post occlusion).

### Functional testing and neurological deficit scoring

23 h after stroke mice were scored for neurological deficit using a 5-point scoring system where 0 = normal motor function, 1 = flexion of torso and contralateral forelimb when mouse is lifted by the tail, 2 = circling to the contralateral side, but normal posture at rest, 3 = leaning to the contralateral side and 4 = no spontaneous motor activity [38]. Mice were then placed for 5 min in a parallel rod floor apparatus of an ANY-maze (Stoelting, IL, USA), an automated behaviour tracking system which records spontaneous movements on a grid of rods and extracts parameters such as distance, speed, immobile episodes, circling behaviour and foot faults. Finally, a grip strength hanging wire test was performed as described [38], averaging three trials with 5 min rest intervals. Scores ranged from 0 for animals which fell immediately to a maximum of 180 s, typically achieved by sham-operated mice.

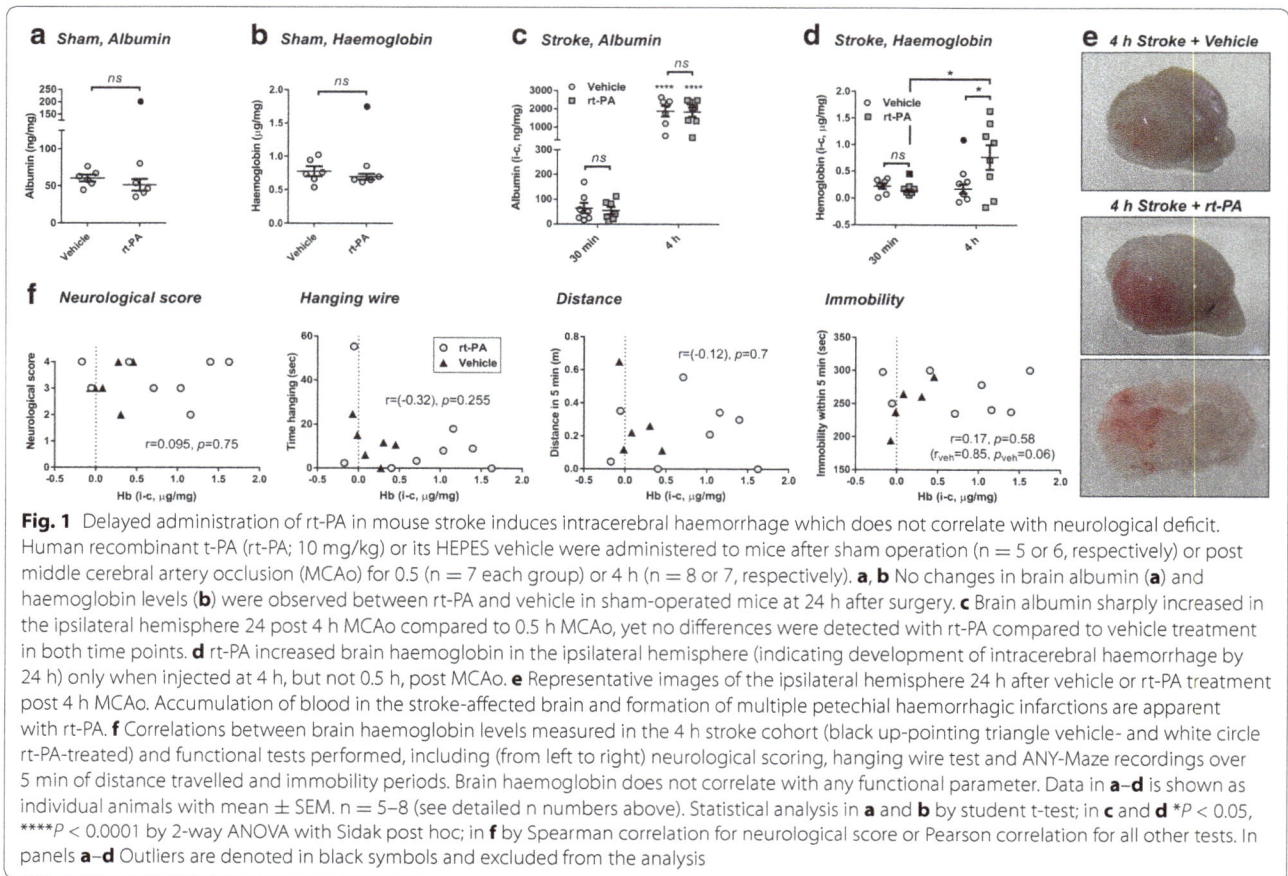

**Fig. 1** Delayed administration of rt-PA in mouse stroke induces intracerebral haemorrhage which does not correlate with neurological deficit. Human recombinant t-PA (rt-PA; 10 mg/kg) or its HEPES vehicle were administered to mice after sham operation (n = 5 or 6, respectively) or post middle cerebral artery occlusion (MCAo) for 0.5 (n = 7 each group) or 4 h (n = 8 or 7, respectively). **a, b** No changes in brain albumin (**a**) and haemoglobin levels (**b**) were observed between rt-PA and vehicle in sham-operated mice at 24 h after surgery. **c** Brain albumin sharply increased in the ipsilateral hemisphere 24 post 4 h MCAo compared to 0.5 h MCAo, yet no differences were detected with rt-PA compared to vehicle treatment in both time points. **d** rt-PA increased brain haemoglobin in the ipsilateral hemisphere (indicating development of intracerebral haemorrhage by 24 h) only when injected at 4 h, but not 0.5 h, post MCAo. **e** Representative images of the ipsilateral hemisphere 24 h after vehicle or rt-PA treatment post 4 h MCAo. Accumulation of blood in the stroke-affected brain and formation of multiple petechial haemorrhagic infarctions are apparent with rt-PA. **f** Correlations between brain haemoglobin levels measured in the 4 h stroke cohort (black up-pointing triangle vehicle- and white circle rt-PA-treated) and functional tests performed, including (from left to right) neurological scoring, hanging wire test and ANY-Maze recordings over 5 min of distance travelled and immobility periods. Brain haemoglobin does not correlate with any functional parameter. Data in **a–d** is shown as individual animals with mean ± SEM. n = 5–8 (see detailed n numbers above). Statistical analysis in **a** and **b** by student t-test; in **c** and **d** *P < 0.05, ****P < 0.0001 by 2-way ANOVA with Sidak post hoc; in **f** by Spearman correlation for neurological score or Pearson correlation for all other tests. In panels **a–d** Outliers are denoted in black symbols and excluded from the analysis

### Intracerebral bleeding assessment

Extravasation of red blood cells into brain parenchyma, indicative of HT following severe malfunction of cerebral blood vessels, was measured in perfused ipsilateral and contralateral brain hemispheres. Hemispheres were first weighed, then homogenised to 300 mg/ml (wet weight) in PBS + 1% Triton X-100 (v/v) and snap-frozen on dry ice. Lysates were thawed before use and spun down at 16,100 g for 10 min. The supernatant was further diluted to 150 mg/ml (wet weight) in equal volume of milli-Q water. Haemoglobin (Hb) concentration in brain supernatants was assessed spectrophotometrically by the QuantiChrom™ Hemoglobin Assay Kit (BioAssay Systems, CA, USA) as per the manufacturer's instructions, incubating samples with the reagent for 15 min [10] before reading absorbance at 405 nm on a microplate reader (VICTOR II, Perkin Elmer, Australia). Hb content in each hemisphere was calculated as µg per mg wet brain tissue using the formula: Hb (µg/mg wet weight) = Hb (µg/ml)/300 mg/ml. In mice which underwent stroke surgery (but not in shams), Hb level obtained in the contralateral hemisphere was subtracted from the ipsilateral hemisphere to account for perfusion efficiency under the assumption that both hemispheres are perfused to a similar degree and that the contralateral value represents the amount of intravascular blood remaining in the brain post perfusion. Importantly, no significant differences were noted in the Hb content of the contralateral hemispheres between vehicle- and rt-PA-treated animals (not shown).

### Evaluation of brain albumin content as a measure of blood–brain barrier disruption

Extravascular albumin is scarcely present in brain parenchyma [39] and its detection at greater levels in perfused brains indicates an increase in BBB permeability. To assess the degree of BBB compromise, brain lysates at 300 mg/ml (wet weight) were thawed and spun down as stipulated above. Supernatants were diluted further in PBS so the final sample concentration in the ELISA plate was 25 or 250 µg/ml (wet weight) for the ipsilateral or contralateral hemisphere, respectively. Brains of sham-operated mice were processed as the contralateral hemispheres. We then quantitated brain albumin concentration in the supernatant by ELISA using a commercial kit (Mouse Albumin ELISA Quantitation Set

#E90-134; Bethyl Laboratories, TX, USA) according to the manufacturer's instructions [40]. Brain albumin content in the perfused brain was calculated according to the formula: Albumin (ng/mg wet weight) = Albumin (ng/ml)/300 mg/ml. As stated above for the analysis of Hb and under the same assumptions, albumin levels obtained in the contralateral hemispheres were subtracted from the ipsilateral hemispheres in stroke mice to account for perfusion efficiency.

## Statistical analysis

Statistical analysis was performed using GraphPad Prism 6 software. Outliers were first determined in all data sets by Grubbs' test with $\alpha \leq 0.1$ and excluded from the analysis. No more than one outlier was identified in any group (see Figs. 1, 2, 3) and its exclusion did not affect the observation. Mortality was analysed by Log-rank (Mantel-Cox) test. Differences between three or more groups were analysed by ordinary one- or two-way ANOVA with Sidak's post hoc analysis (for parametric data) or by Kruskal–Wallis ANOVA with Dunn's multiple comparisons test (for non-parametric data). Differences between two groups were determined using two-tailed unpaired student $t$ test. Correlations were assessed by Spearman correlation for non-parametric data or by Pearson correlation for parametric data. Probability values under 0.05 were considered significant.

## Results

rt-PA administration is approved within 4.5 h from stroke onset. Beyond this time window, its risks, primarily for development of sICH and/or oedema following breach of the BBB, outweigh the potential clinical benefits. In an attempt to mimic these occurrences in the mouse we first characterised the degree of BBB disruption (extravasation of albumin and haemoglobin into the brain) and functional deficit in response to rt-PA under sham conditions and in our MCAo stroke model. In line with other pre-clinical reports [12, 26], intravenous rt-PA (10 mg/kg) administered to uninjured animals did not induce albumin (Fig. 1a) or blood (Fig. 1b) accumulation in the mouse brain 24 h post treatment, suggesting that rt-PA does not affect the mouse BBB under resting conditions (note that no subtraction of the contralateral from the ipsilateral value was performed in shams). In contrast, transient stroke as short as 0.5 h followed by intravenous treatment at reperfusion disrupted the BBB and increased albumin content in the ipsilateral hemisphere by 24 h post MCAo (observed as positive values after subtraction of the contralateral hemisphere) in both vehicle and rt-PA-treated mice, an effect which was dramatically amplified by 29- and 33.1-fold, respectively, when stroke duration was extended to 4 h ($p < 0.0001$, Fig. 1c).

Notably, albumin accumulation at 24 h did not significantly differ between rt-PA and vehicle in both 0.5 and 4 h stroke periods, indicating that a similar degree of BBB permeation to plasma proteins developed with or without the thrombolytic (Fig. 1c) (see "Discussion"). Brain haemoglobin levels, however, were significantly increased by 24 h in mice receiving rt-PA at 4 h, but not at 0.5 h post MCAo or in vehicle-treated animals ($p < 0.05$, Fig. 1d), suggestive of development of significant HTs only during delayed use of rt-PA. Indeed, macroscopic examination of perfused brains 24 after 4 h MCAo revealed no bleeding or sporadic small petechiae in brains of vehicle-treated animals but extended bleeding with multiple sites of haematomas in most rt-PA-treated mice (Fig. 1e). Hence, our stroke model successfully simulated the time-dependent shift of rt-PA from a safe to unsafe intervention as judged by formation of substantial HT.

We then examined whether these extensive bleeding complications were contributing to functional outcome; in other words, if they could be considered 'symptomatic'. Noticeably, none of our functional assessments performed 24 h after MCAo (neurological scoring, hanging wire and ANY-maze tests) correlated with the brain haemoglobin levels measured at this time point, irrespective of vehicle or rt-PA (Fig. 1f). This analysis shows that HTs associated with rt-PA in these experimental stroke settings are not predictive of deficit severity and cannot be considered symptomatic. Importantly, autopsies performed on animals which died before the 24 h end-point (transcardially-perfused where possible) did not reveal consistent HTs, including in rt-PA-treated animals (not shown), suggesting that HT was not playing a major role in their functional deterioration and early death.

LDLR blockade by RAP may provide a unifying solution to a number of rt-PA modes of action which lead to BBB disruption and HT during thrombolysis [22, 23]. We therefore tested the effects of RAP against rt-PA-induced BBB breakdown and formation of HT as well as mortality and functional outcome in our 4 h transient thread occlusion protocol, which to the best of our knowledge has not been attempted before. As observed in our initial characterisation (Fig. 1), rt-PA treatment induced a similar increase in albumin extravasation as seen for vehicle-treated mice (Fig. 2a, b) but caused a significant upsurge in the brain haemoglobin content measured 24 h after stroke ($p < 0.05$, Fig. 2c, d). Administration of RAP (2 mg/kg) at reperfusion with or without rt-PA did not significantly decrease total brain albumin levels (Fig. 2a), yet a trend for reduction of total brain haemoglobin was observed ($p = 0.18$, Fig. 2c). Normalisation of the ipsilateral value to the contralateral baseline for each mouse (i.e. fold increase analysis) revealed near-significant reductions in cerebral albumin ($p = 0.054$, Fig. 2b) and

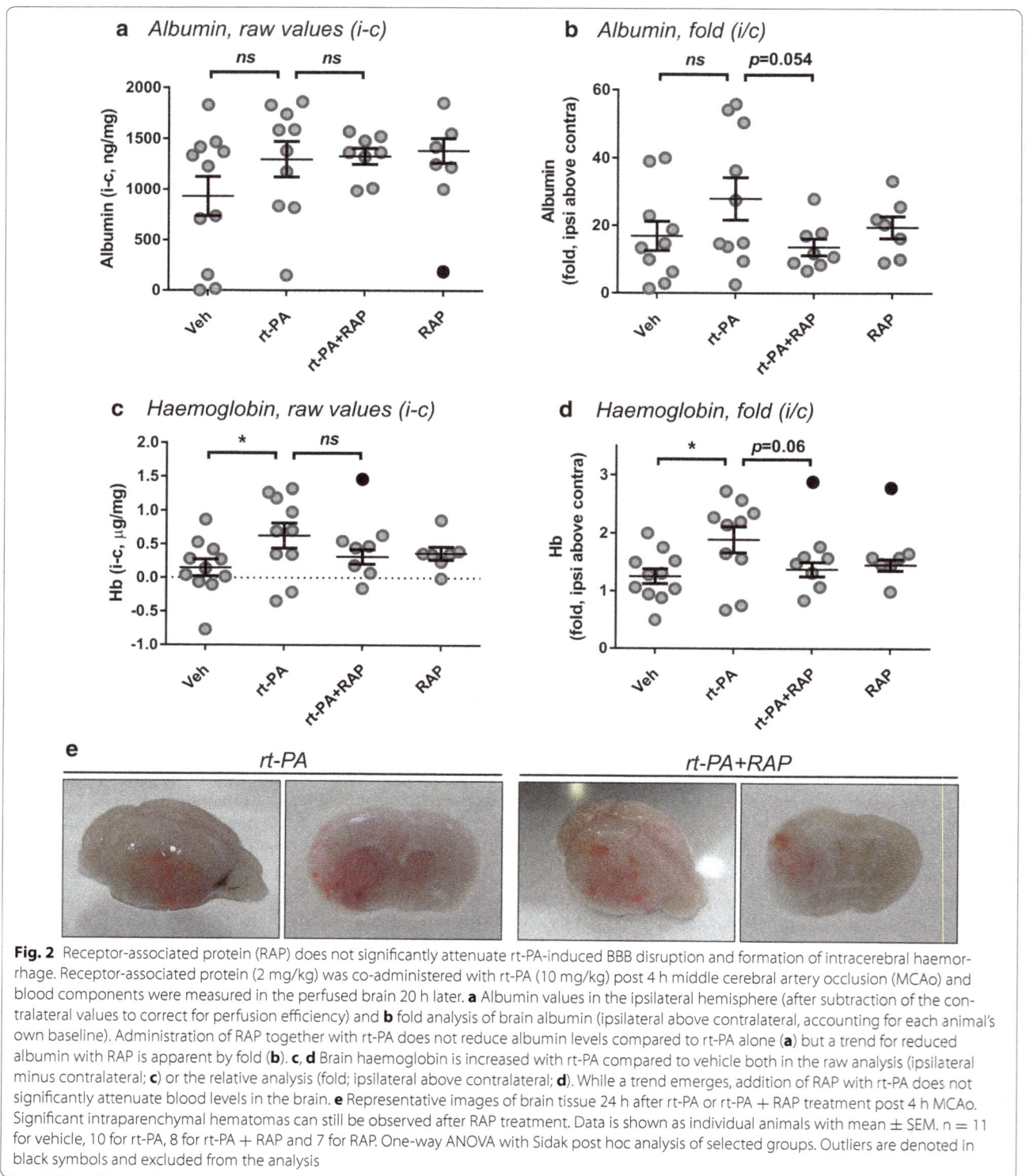

**Fig. 2** Receptor-associated protein (RAP) does not significantly attenuate rt-PA-induced BBB disruption and formation of intracerebral haemorrhage. Receptor-associated protein (2 mg/kg) was co-administered with rt-PA (10 mg/kg) post 4 h middle cerebral artery occlusion (MCAo) and blood components were measured in the perfused brain 20 h later. **a** Albumin values in the ipsilateral hemisphere (after subtraction of the contralateral values to correct for perfusion efficiency) and **b** fold analysis of brain albumin (ipsilateral above contralateral, accounting for each animal's own baseline). Administration of RAP together with rt-PA does not reduce albumin levels compared to rt-PA alone (**a**) but a trend for reduced albumin with RAP is apparent by fold (**b**). **c, d** Brain haemoglobin is increased with rt-PA compared to vehicle both in the raw analysis (ipsilateral minus contralateral; **c**) or the relative analysis (fold; ipsilateral above contralateral; **d**). While a trend emerges, addition of RAP with rt-PA does not significantly attenuate blood levels in the brain. **e** Representative images of brain tissue 24 h after rt-PA or rt-PA + RAP treatment post 4 h MCAo. Significant intraparenchymal hematomas can still be observed after RAP treatment. Data is shown as individual animals with mean ± SEM. n = 11 for vehicle, 10 for rt-PA, 8 for rt-PA + RAP and 7 for RAP. One-way ANOVA with Sidak post hoc analysis of selected groups. Outliers are denoted in black symbols and excluded from the analysis

haemoglobin content ($p = 0.06$, Fig. 2d) by RAP. Indeed, focal haematomas and diffuse bleeding across the infarct could often be observed in rt-PA + RAP-treated brains 24 h post MCAo, as seen with rt-PA alone albeit to a milder extent (Fig. 2e), in line with the biochemical findings. As mentioned above, our autopsies of mice which

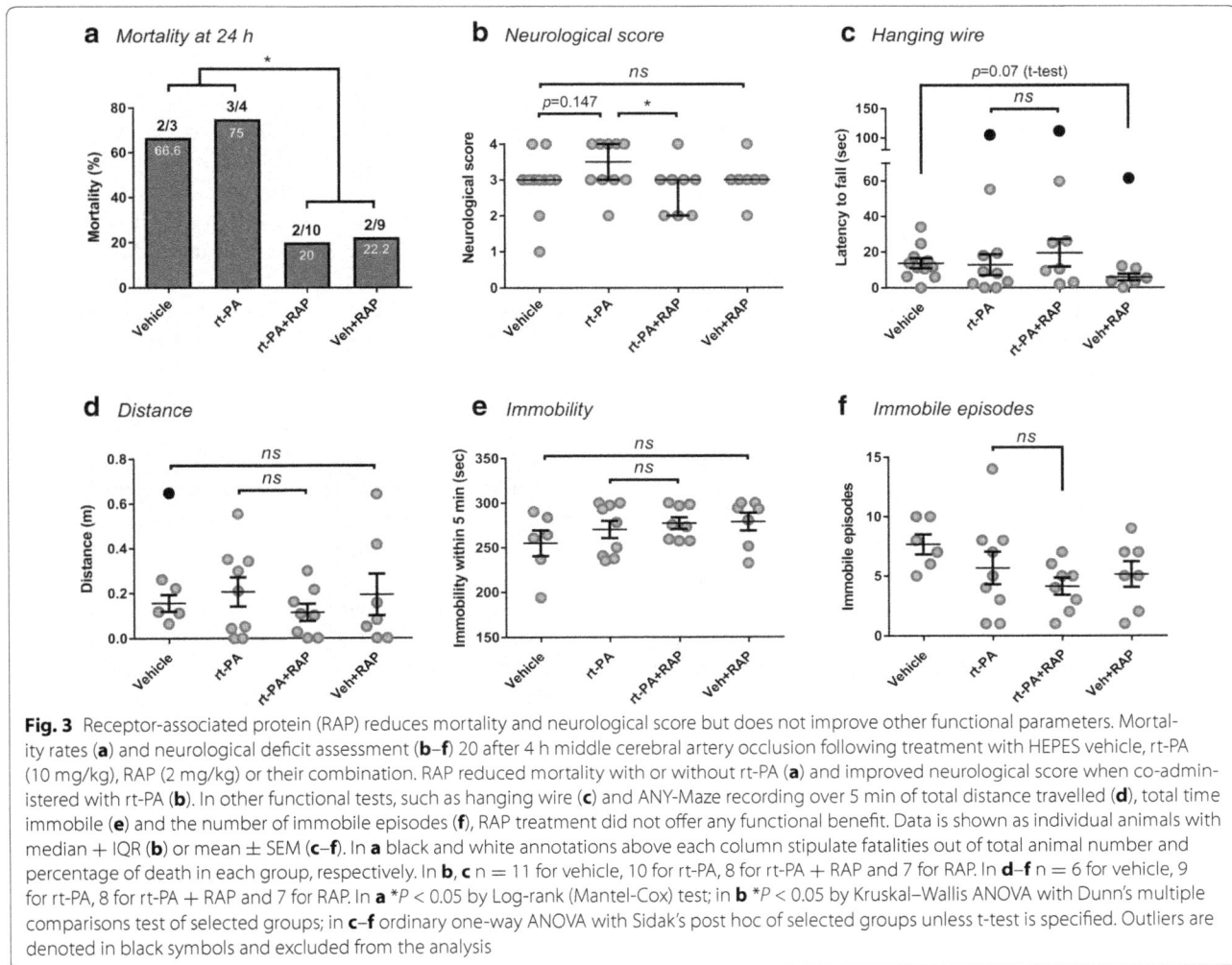

**Fig. 3** Receptor-associated protein (RAP) reduces mortality and neurological score but does not improve other functional parameters. Mortality rates (**a**) and neurological deficit assessment (**b–f**) 20 after 4 h middle cerebral artery occlusion following treatment with HEPES vehicle, rt-PA (10 mg/kg), RAP (2 mg/kg) or their combination. RAP reduced mortality with or without rt-PA (**a**) and improved neurological score when co-administered with rt-PA (**b**). In other functional tests, such as hanging wire (**c**) and ANY-Maze recording over 5 min of total distance travelled (**d**), total time immobile (**e**) and the number of immobile episodes (**f**), RAP treatment did not offer any functional benefit. Data is shown as individual animals with median + IQR (**b**) or mean ± SEM (**c–f**). In **a** black and white annotations above each column stipulate fatalities out of total animal number and percentage of death in each group, respectively. In **b**, **c** n = 11 for vehicle, 10 for rt-PA, 8 for rt-PA + RAP and 7 for RAP. In **d–f** n = 6 for vehicle, 9 for rt-PA, 8 for rt-PA + RAP and 7 for RAP. In **a** *P < 0.05 by Log-rank (Mantel-Cox) test; in **b** *P < 0.05 by Kruskal–Wallis ANOVA with Dunn's multiple comparisons test of selected groups; in **c–f** ordinary one-way ANOVA with Sidak's post hoc of selected groups unless t-test is specified. Outliers are denoted in black symbols and excluded from the analysis

died before the 24 h end-point and were not included in the biochemical analysis did not establish a contributory relationship between HT and mortality, reducing the possibility of underestimation of the RAP effect on the BBB. Overall, these data suggest that RAP does not protect the BBB from rt-PA to an extent where blood cells and blood protein extravasation can be effectively inhibited, but may still harbour a partial capacity to attenuate rt-PA-induced development of HT.

Interestingly, despite its weak activity on the BBB, RAP treatment with or without rt-PA resulted in a marked decrease in mortality within 24 h from stroke onset (from 71.4% overall mortality in vehicle and rt-PA groups to 21% in RAP-treated groups, $p < 0.05$, Fig. 3a). RAP administration also resulted in a functional benefit since rt-PA + RAP-treated animals received on average significantly lower neurological scores than mice treated with rt-PA alone ($p < 0.05$, Fig. 3b). A strong trend for improved grip strength was further demonstrated with

RAP in vehicle-treated ($p = 0.07$ by t-test, Fig. 3c), but not in rt-PA-treated animals. Notably, none of the mobility parameters assessed by ANY-maze at 24 h were influenced by RAP (Fig. 3d–f). Taken together, these observations suggest that LDLR blockade during severe stroke could offer fundamental benefits such as improved (short-term) survival and attenuation of deficit, which may not be related to rt-PA, BBB breakdown or brain haemorrhage.

## Discussion

Because severe intracranial haemorrhage is the main complication limiting thrombolysis with rt-PA in stroke [1, 3, 6], we attempted to simulate rt-PA-driven HT in a mouse stroke model and to test whether LDLR blockade could protect against its occurrence. However, since only symptomatic bleeding episodes (sICH) are pertinent for the safety assessment of rt-PA, we further evaluated if HTs obtained in the mouse actually carry the functional and structural characteristics of the clinical condition, such as neurological deterioration and development of parenchymal haematoma type-2 (PH-2), respectively [8]. This distinction is rarely made in rodent stroke studies but may be important for improvement of research efforts.

In line with pre-clinical reports by others [17, 18, 41], rt-PA caused substantial HTs in our study by 24 h post stroke, but only when given 4 h after stroke initiation. Rodent studies therefore mimic the basic clinical observation showing lower incidence of severe intracranial bleeding at onset to treatment (OTT) $\leq$ 90 min and a shift towards higher risk of dangerous bleeding outcome at later OTTs [2], which usually occurs within 24–36 h [6]. Interestingly, despite the increase in rt-PA-mediated HT after prolonged occlusion, we saw no differences between rt-PA- and vehicle-treated groups in albumin extravasation into the brain within 24 h regardless of stroke duration. These observations provide valuable insight into the most significant activities of rt-PA on the BBB, as they presumably stem from differential opening of the BBB to varying degrees, allowing passage of different sized particles depending on the severity of disruption. Albumin (and other plasma proteins) can penetrate the brain paracellularly through damaged tight junctions or transcellularly via transcytosis [39], while passage of red blood cells into the brain requires complete capillary disintegration. Hence, it seems that the long occlusion duration (4 h) is sufficient to substantially compromise the BBB for extravasation of plasma proteins regardless of rt-PA (or, that the effect of prolonged MCAo on albumin extravasation is robust enough to reach saturation within 24 h—the time of our evaluation—and mask early acceleration in this process by rt-PA). However, only rt-PA seems to drive the vessel further towards final catastrophic breakdown, permitting the passage of whole blood into the brain. Such vessel disintegration must involve mechanical rupture and total loss of key structural elements of brain capillaries like the lumen-forming endothelial cells and the supportive basement membrane; accordingly, robust rt-PA-associated activities such as plasmin- and MMP-dependent proteolytic degradation of basal lamina and tight junctions [22], worsening of cerebral inflammation by reduction of regulatory T-cells [42] and recruitment of other immune cells [21] as well as changes to blood pressure and vascular tone [32] should logically become therapeutic candidates in the context of sICH prevention after thrombolysis.

Despite successful modelling of the temporal bleeding formation which occurs in humans, HTs developing post-rt-PA in the mouse did not resemble clinical sICH in their appearance and functional consequence. These bleeding events, while substantial, appeared more as scattered (HI-1) or more confluent yet heterogeneous petechiae (HI-2) rather than parenchymal hematomas, characterised by a homogenous and dense haemorrhage creating a mass effect and occupying a large area of the infarct [8]. Functionally, no cause-effect relationship could be established between HT and deficit severity. Few possible contributors may account for this outcome, including a lack of sensitivity of the functional assessment methods, the absence of longitudinal HT and deficit monitoring throughout the first 24 h to identify earlier associations (before mortality occurs) or the need to administer rt-PA by infusion rather than a bolus (the latter described in rodent studies with similar outcomes [16, 17]). Nevertheless, as vehicle-treated mice generally suffered from high mortality similar to rt-PA-treated animals (Fig. 3) and displayed severe deficits 24 post 4 h MCAo (Figs. 1, 3), a lead explanation is a 'ceiling' effect, referring to such intense brain damage developing in the mouse as a result of complete MCA shutdown over many hours (required, however, to simulate rt-PA-dependent HT), that it cannot be modified any further when significant haemorrhage occurs [9]. This notion is highly plausible, since a typical infarct size achieved in mice by the suture MCAo model is approximately an order of magnitude larger than the infarct produced by an average human stroke (by percentage of the hemisphere affected). Equivalent massive infarcts in humans are usually accompanied by substantial oedema, progressive infarct expansion, brain herniation or pan-hemispheric destruction, with minimal functional recovery [43]. A prolonged transient mouse stroke might therefore be closer in outcome to a malignant human stroke, where a devastating outcome develops with or without HT [43]. Taken together, our study highlights substantial limitations in pre-clinical modelling of rt-PA-triggered sICH by the popular suture model of transient MCAo in mice. A more suitable protocol to study this phenomena in rodents could consist of transient occlusion of a smaller brain territory for longer periods of time (e.g. 6–9 h) before rt-PA treatment, accompanied by periodic magnetic resonance imaging (MRI). Such approach may reduce baseline deficit but allow the occurrence of substantial bleeding in severely-impaired blood vessels and their progressive monitoring. Worsening of neurological symptoms as HT occurs should be incorporated in models specifically dealing with sICH and its prevention.

A second interesting finding of our study was that LDLR blockade with the pan LDLR antagonist RAP had only a weak capacity to influence BBB-related outcomes of rt-PA treatment, yet it offered marked improvement in short-term survival and more limited attenuation of deficit severity. One might further speculate that RAP-mediated improvements in neurological function is in fact underestimated, since only animals undergoing 4 h MCAo which survived up to 24 h post-occlusion were assessed; earlier functional assessment, before mortality occurred, would have included critically ill animals and may have resulted in better correlation between function and mortality.

Regarding the BBB, while we indeed noticed a non-significant trend of decreased brain albumin with RAP, this observation overall lies in contrast to other studies demonstrating reduction of blood and blood protein extravasation into the brain by intravenous [13, 28] or intracerebroventricular [31, 36] administration of RAP, with or without rt-PA treatment. While differences in stroke models most likely contribute to these discrepancies (i.e. rat [36] vs. mice, thrombotic [13, 36] vs. mechanical or permanent [28, 31] vs. transient), our results can be logically explained by the multifaceted nature of rt-PA actions, some of which are LDLR-independent. In particular, while most plasminogen-independent pathways for rt-PA-induced BBB breakdown identify LRP-1 as a rt-PA receptor (see "Background") [22, 23], more recently-discovered, plasmin-dependent cascades have partial or no reliance on LDLRs, including rt-PA/plasmin-driven activation of plasma kallikrein [11], bradykinin [44], monocyte chemoattractant protein (MCP)-1 [45] and Rho-kinase 2 [46]. The numerous mechanistic avenues by which rt-PA disrupts the BBB during thrombolysis implies that a sole therapeutic agent will probably be unable to achieve sufficient barrier protection. Instead, combination therapy of substances that address multiple pathways simultaneously, for example inhibitors of cell-surface receptors (Imatinib [12], RAP [13, 28], Icatibant [44]) together with plasma and intracellular enzymes antagonists (GM6001 [20], BPCCB [11] and fasudil/KD025 [30, 46], respectively) should be considered, similar to growing approaches in cancer therapy.

Importantly, rt-PA signalling via LDLRs, in particular LRP-1, also plays a key role in neuronal calcium haemostasis via regulation of the N-methyl-D-aspartate receptor function [37, 47], linking rt-PA and endogenous t-PA to pathological brain processes such as excitotoxicity and neurotoxicity [47]. Hence, even in the absence of efficient protection of the BBB, RAP might still reduce neuronal damage and infarct size, as already shown in rats [36]. Together with other effects of LDLR blockade, such as a decrease in t-PA-induced brain MMP-9 levels [29], the net consequence of RAP treatment could be a reduction in brain damage to a level where animal survival and gross neurological deficits improve, in line with our observations.

## Conclusions

In summary, we have shown here that pre-clinical modelling of rt-PA-triggered sICH during stroke only partially correlates with the clinical event, most likely owing to a mismatch between the duration of stroke and severity of outcome between humans and mice. A therapeutic strategy based on a single agent, such as LDLR blockade by RAP, has only a limited chance of success in protecting the barrier due to the diversity of mechanisms employed by rt-PA to disrupt the BBB. RAP, however, should be included since its protective action in the brain may span more than just the BBB. Future studies aiming to reduce the risk of sICH during thrombolysis will benefit from closer simulation of sICH features and from incorporation of a combination therapy to increase the relevance and translation potential of the finding.

### Abbreviations
BBB: blood–brain barrier; HI: haemorrhagic infarctions; HT: haemorrhagic transformation; LRP-1: low-density lipoprotein receptor-related protein 1; MCAo: middle cerebral artery occlusion; MMP: matrix metalloproteinase; PH: parenchymal haematoma; sICH: symptomatic intra-cerebral haemorrhage; RAP: receptor-associated protein; rt-PA: recombinant tissue-type plasminogen activator.

### Authors' contributions
BN formed the concept, designed the experiments and assisted in their execution, analysed data, generated the figures and drafted the manuscript. BRB performed experiments and provided critical technical expertise, analysed data and contributed intellectual input. HH performed experiments and provided critical technical expertise. CGS and RLM supervised the work and provided critical expertise in drafting the manuscript. All authors read and approved the final manuscript.

### Author details
[1] Molecular Neurotrauma and Haemostasis, Australian Centre for Blood Diseases, Monash University, Level 4 Burnet Building, 89 Commercial Road, Melbourne 3004, VIC, Australia. [2] Cardiovascular & Pulmonary Pharmacology Group, Biomedicine Discovery Institute, Department of Pharmacology, Monash University, Clayton, VIC, Australia. [3] Vascular Biology and Immunopharmacology Group, Department of Physiology, Anatomy & Microbiology, School of Life Sciences, La Trobe University, Bundoora, VIC, Australia.

### Acknowledgements
B.N. is supported by a postdoctoral fellowship from the National Heart Foundation of Australia (Award Number 100906). C.G.S and R.L.M are Senior and Principal Research Fellows, respectively, of the NHMRC of Australia. The authors wish to thank Ms Volga Tarlac for her guidance and expertise on the ANY-maze system.

### Competing interests
The authors declare that they have no competing interests.

**Funding**
This study was funded by grants awrded to R.L.M and C.G.S by the NHMRC of Australia (Grant Number APP1045756). B.N. is supported by a postdoctoral fellowship from the National Heart Foundation of Australia (Award Number 100906). The funding bodies had no roles in the design of the study and collection, analysis, and interpretation of data and in writing the manuscript.

**References**

1.  Balami JS, Sutherland BA, Buchan AM. Complications associated with recombinant tissue plasminogen activator therapy for acute ischaemic stroke. CNS Neurol Disord Drug Targets. 2013;12(2):155–69.

2.  Lees KR, Bluhmki E, von Kummer R, Brott TG, Toni D, Grotta JC, et al. Time to treatment with intravenous alteplase and outcome in stroke: an updated pooled analysis of ECASS, ATLANTIS, NINDS, and EPITHET trials. Lancet. 2010;375(9727):1695–703. https://doi.org/10.1016/S0140-6736(10)60491-6.

3.  Yaghi S, Eisenberger A, Willey JZ. Symptomatic intracerebral hemorrhage in acute ischemic stroke after thrombolysis with intravenous recombinant tissue plasminogen activator: a review of natural history and treatment. JAMA Neurol. 2014;71(9):1181–5. https://doi.org/10.1001/jamaneurol.2014.1210.

4.  Bambauer KZ, Johnston SC, Bambauer DE, Zivin JA. Reasons why few patients with acute stroke receive tissue plasminogen activator. Arch Neurol. 2006;63(5):661–4. https://doi.org/10.1001/archneur.63.5.661.

5.  Caplan LR. Stroke thrombolysis: slow progress. Circulation. 2006;114(3):187–90. https://doi.org/10.1161/CIRCULATIONAHA.106.638973.

6.  O'Carroll CB, Aguilar MI. Management of postthrombolysis hemorrhagic and orolingual angioedema complications. Neurohospitalist. 2015;5(3):133–41. https://doi.org/10.1177/1941874415587680.

7.  Hacke W, Kaste M, Fieschi C, von Kummer R, Davalos A, Meier D, et al. Randomised double-blind placebo-controlled trial of thrombolytic therapy with intravenous alteplase in acute ischaemic stroke (ECASS II). Second European-Australasian Acute Stroke Study Investigators. Lancet. 1998;352(9136):1245–51.

8.  Berger C, Fiorelli M, Steiner T, Schabitz WR, Bozzao L, Bluhmki E, et al. Hemorrhagic transformation of ischemic brain tissue: asymptomatic or symptomatic? Stroke. 2001;32(6):1330–5.

9.  Seet RC, Rabinstein AA. Symptomatic intracranial hemorrhage following intravenous thrombolysis for acute ischemic stroke: a critical review of case definitions. Cerebrovasc Dis. 2012;34(2):106–14. https://doi.org/10.1159/000339675.

10. Ishiguro M, Kawasaki K, Suzuki Y, Ishizuka F, Mishiro K, Egashira Y, et al. A Rho kinase (ROCK) inhibitor, fasudil, prevents matrix metalloproteinase-9-related hemorrhagic transformation in mice treated with tissue plasminogen activator. Neuroscience. 2012;https://doi.org/10.1016/j.neuroscience.2012.06.015.

11. Simao F, Ustunkaya T, Clermont AC, Feener EP. Plasma kallikrein mediates brain hemorrhage and edema caused by tissue plasminogen activator therapy in mice after stroke. Blood. 2017;129(16):2280–90. https://doi.org/10.1182/blood-2016-09-740670.

12. Su EJ, Fredriksson L, Geyer M, Folestad E, Cale J, Andrae J, et al. Activation of PDGF-CC by tissue plasminogen activator impairs blood-brain barrier integrity during ischemic stroke. Nat Med. 2008;14(7):731–7. https://doi.org/10.1038/nm1787.

13. Suzuki Y, Nagai N, Yamakawa K, Kawakami J, Lijnen HR, Umemura K. Tissue-type plasminogen activator (t-PA) induces stromelysin-1 (MMP-3) in endothelial cells through activation of lipoprotein receptor–related protein. Blood. 2009;114(15):3352–8. https://doi.org/10.1182/blood-2009-02-203919.

14. Won S, Lee JH, Wali B, Stein DG, Sayeed I. Progesterone attenuates hemorrhagic transformation after delayed tPA treatment in an experimental model of stroke in rats: involvement of the VEGF-MMP pathway. J Cereb Blood Flow Metab. 2014;34(1):72–80. https://doi.org/10.1038/jcbfm.2013.163.

15. Yagi K, Kitazato KT, Uno M, Tada Y, Kinouchi T, Shimada K, et al. Edaravone, a free radical scavenger, inhibits MMP-9-related brain hemorrhage in rats treated with tissue plasminogen activator. Stroke. 2009;40(2):626–31. https://doi.org/10.1161/STROKEAHA.108.520262.

16. Copin JC, Gasche Y. Effect of the duration of middle cerebral artery occlusion on the risk of hemorrhagic transformation after tissue plasminogen activator injection in rats. Brain Res. 2008;1243:161–6. https://doi.org/10.1016/j.brainres.2008.09.025.

17. Garcia-Culebras A, Palma-Tortosa S, Moraga A, Garcia-Yebenes I, Duran-Laforet V, Cuartero MI, et al. Toll-like receptor 4 mediates hemorrhagic transformation after delayed tissue plasminogen activator administration in in situ thromboembolic stroke. Stroke. 2017;https://doi.org/10.1161/STROKEAHA.116.015956.

18. Garcia-Yebenes I, Sobrado M, Zarruk JG, Castellanos M, Perez de la Ossa N, Davalos A, et al. A mouse model of hemorrhagic transformation by delayed tissue plasminogen activator administration after in situ thromboembolic stroke. Stroke. 2011;42(1):196–203. https://doi.org/10.1161/STROKEAHA.110.600452.

19. Lapchak PA. Effect of internal carotid artery reperfusion in combination with Tenecteplase on clinical scores and hemorrhage in a rabbit embolic stroke model. Brain Res. 2009;1294:211–7. https://doi.org/10.1016/j.brainres.2009.07.058.

20. Suzuki Y, Nagai N, Umemura K, Collen D, Lijnen HR. Stromelysin-1 (MMP-3) is critical for intracranial bleeding after t-PA treatment of stroke in mice. J Thromb Haemost JTH. 2007;5(8):1732–9. https://doi.org/10.1111/j.1538-7836.2007.02628.x.

21. Shi Y, Zhang L, Pu H, Mao L, Hu X, Jiang X, et al. Rapid endothelial cytoskeletal reorganization enables early blood-brain barrier disruption and long-term ischaemic reperfusion brain injury. Nat Commun. 2016;7:10523. https://doi.org/10.1038/ncomms10523.

22. Niego B, Medcalf RL. Plasmin-dependent modulation of the blood-brain barrier: a major consideration during tPA-induced thrombolysis? J Cereb Blood Flow Metab. 2014;34(8):1283–96. https://doi.org/10.1038/jcbfm.2014.99.

23. Suzuki Y, Nagai N, Umemura K. A review of the mechanisms of blood-brain barrier permeability by tissue-type plasminogen activator treatment for cerebral ischemia. Front Cell Neurosci. 2016;10:2. https://doi.org/10.3389/fncel.2016.00002.

24. Lillis AP, Van Duyn LB, Murphy-Ullrich JE, Strickland DK. LDL receptor-related protein 1: unique tissue-specific functions revealed by selective gene knockout studies. Physiol Rev. 2008;88(3):887–918. https://doi.org/10.1152/physrev.00033.2007.

25. Herz J, Strickland DK. LRP: a multifunctional scavenger and signaling receptor. J Clin Invest. 2001;108(6):779–84. https://doi.org/10.1172/JCI13992.

26. Cheng T, Petraglia AL, Li Z, Thiyagarajan M, Zhong Z, Wu Z, et al. Activated protein C inhibits tissue plasminogen activator-induced brain hemorrhage. Nat Med. 2006;12(11):1278–85. https://doi.org/10.1038/nm1498.

27. Wang X, Lee SR, Arai K, Tsuji K, Rebeck GW, Lo EH. Lipoprotein receptor-mediated induction of matrix metalloproteinase by tissue plasminogen activator. Nat Med. 2003;9(10):1313–7. https://doi.org/10.1038/nm926nm926.

28. Suzuki Y, Nagai N, Yamakawa K, Muranaka Y, Hokamura K, Umemura K. Recombinant tissue-type plasminogen activator transiently enhances blood-brain barrier permeability during cerebral ischemia through vascular endothelial growth factor-mediated endothelial endocytosis in mice. J Cereb Blood Flow Metab. 2015;35(12):2021–31. https://doi.org/10.1038/jcbfm.2015.167.

29. Zhang C, An J, Haile WB, Echeverry R, Strickland DK, Yepes M. Microglial low-density lipoprotein receptor-related protein 1 mediates the effect of tissue-type plasminogen activator on matrix metalloproteinase-9 activity in the ischemic brain. J Cereb Blood Flow Metab Off J Int Soc Cereb Blood Flow Metab. 2009;29(12):1946–54. https://doi.org/10.1038/jcbfm.2009.174.

30. Niego B, Freeman R, Puschmann TB, Turnley AM, Medcalf RL. t-PA-specific modulation of a human BBB model involves plasmin-mediated activation of the Rho-kinase pathway in astrocytes. Blood. 2012;https://doi.org/10.1182/blood-2011-07-369512.

31. Polavarapu R, Gongora MC, Yi H, Ranganthan S, Lawrence DA, Strickland D, et al. Tissue-type plasminogen activator-mediated shedding of astrocytic low-density lipoprotein receptor-related protein increases the permeability of the neurovascular unit. Blood. 2007;109(8):3270–8. https://doi.org/10.1182/blood-2006-08-043125.

32. Nassar T, Akkawi S, Shina A, Haj-Yehia A, Bdeir K, Tarshis M, et al. In vitro and in vivo effects of tPA and PAI-1 on blood vessel tone. Blood. 2004;103(3):897–902. https://doi.org/10.1182/blood-2003-05-1685.

33. Se Akkawi, Nassar T, Tarshis M, Cines DB, Higazi AAR. LRP and αvβ3 mediate tPA activation of smooth muscle cells. Am J Physiol Heart Circulatory Physiol. 2006;291(3):H1351–9. https://doi.org/10.1152/ajpheart.01042.2005.

34. Bu G, Geuze HJ, Strous GJ, Schwartz AL. 39 kDa receptor-associated protein is an ER resident protein and molecular chaperone for LDL receptor-related protein. EMBO J. 1995;14(10):2269–80.

35. Willnow TE, Armstrong SA, Hammer RE, Herz J. Functional expression of low density lipoprotein receptor-related protein is controlled by receptor-associated protein in vivo. Proc Natl Acad Sci USA. 1995;92(10):4537–41.

36. Li DD, Pang HG, Song JN, Zhao YL, Zhang BF, Ma XD, et al. Receptor-associated protein promotes t-PA expression, reduces PAI-1 expression and improves neurorecovery after acute ischemic stroke. J Neurol Sci. 2015;350(1–2):84–9. https://doi.org/10.1016/j.jns.2015.02.022.

37. Samson AL, Nevin ST, Croucher D, Niego B, Daniel PB, Weiss TW, et al. Tissue-type plasminogen activator requires a co-receptor to enhance NMDA receptor function. J Neurochem. 2008;107(4):1091–101. https://doi.org/10.1111/j.1471-4159.2008.05687.x.

38. Broughton BR, Brait VH, Kim HA, Lee S, Chu HX, Gardiner-Mann CV, et al. Sex-dependent effects of G protein-coupled estrogen receptor activity on outcome after ischemic stroke. Stroke. 2014;45(3):835–41. https://doi.org/10.1161/STROKEAHA.113.001499.

39. Abbott NJ, Patabendige AA, Dolman DE, Yusof SR, Begley DJ. Structure and function of the blood-brain barrier. Neurobiol Dis. 2010;37(1):13–25. https://doi.org/10.1016/j.nbd.2009.07.030.

40. Sashindranath M, Sales E, Daglas M, Freeman R, Samson AL, Cops EJ, et al. The tissue-type plasminogen activator-plasminogen activator inhibitor 1 complex promotes neurovascular injury in brain trauma: evidence from mice and humans. Brain. 2012;135(Pt 11):3251–64. https://doi.org/10.1093/brain/aws178.

41. Ishiguro M, Mishiro K, Fujiwara Y, Chen H, Izuta H, Tsuruma K, et al. Phosphodiesterase-III inhibitor prevents hemorrhagic transformation induced by focal cerebral ischemia in mice treated with tPA. PLoS ONE. 2010;5(12):e15178. https://doi.org/10.1371/journal.pone.0015178.

42. Mao L, Li P, Zhu W, Cai W, Liu Z, Wang Y, et al. Regulatory T cells ameliorate tissue plasminogen activator-induced brain haemorrhage after stroke. Brain. 2017;140(7):1914–31. https://doi.org/10.1093/brain/awx111.

43. Carmichael ST. Rodent models of focal stroke: size, mechanism, and purpose. NeuroRx. 2005;2(3):396–409. https://doi.org/10.1602/neurorx.2.3.396.

44. Marcos-Contreras OA, Martinez de Lizarrondo S, Bardou I, Orset C, Pruvost M, Anfray A, et al. Hyperfibrinolysis increases blood-brain barrier permeability by a plasmin- and bradykinin-dependent mechanism. Blood. 2016;128(20):2423–34. https://doi.org/10.1182/blood-2016-03-705384.

45. Yao Y, Tsirka SE. Truncation of monocyte chemoattractant protein 1 by plasmin promotes blood-brain barrier disruption. J Cell Sci. 2011;124(Pt 9):1486–95. https://doi.org/10.1242/jcs.082834.

46. Niego B, Lee N, Larsson P, De Silva TM, Au AE, McCutcheon F, et al. Selective inhibition of brain endothelial Rho-kinase-2 provides optimal protection of an in vitro blood-brain barrier from tissue-type plasminogen activator and plasmin. PLoS ONE. 2017;12(5):e0177332. https://doi.org/10.1371/journal.pone.0177332.

47. Samson AL, Medcalf RL. Tissue-type plasminogen activator: a multifaceted modulator of neurotransmission and synaptic plasticity. Neuron. 2006;50(5):673–8. https://doi.org/10.1016/j.neuron.2006.04.013.

# 13

# Cerebrospinal fluid abnormalities in meningeosis neoplastica

Marija Djukic[1,2]*, Ralf Trimmel[1,2], Ingelore Nagel[3], Annette Spreer[3,4], Peter Lange[3], Christine Stadelmann[2] and Roland Nau[1,2]

## Abstract

**Background:** Meningeosis neoplastica is a diffuse metastatic spread of tumor cells in the subarachnoid space. Although first recognized in 1870, systematic investigations regarding cerebrospinal fluid (CSF) constituents in this condition are scarce.

**Methods:** Routine CSF samples analyzed from 2001 to 2012 at the Laboratory of Clinical Neurochemistry, University of Göttingen, were re-evaluated. Patients, whose CSF contained malignant cells were included in this study.

**Results:** Patients (n = 132, age $59.1 \pm 29.1$, 58% women) were identified, whose CSF contained malignant cells. The most frequent primary tumor was breast cancer (32.6%), followed by lung cancer (25.0%) and hematologic malignancies (21.2%). The most frequent clinical symptoms were affections of cranial nerves (41.7%), psychiatric abmormalities (32.6%) and radicular lesions of the lower extremities (20.5%). CSF cell counts ranged from 0 to 4692 cells/µl (median 4 cells/µl) and were elevated in 50%. The CSF-to-serum albumin ratio was abnormal in 69.4%. It ranged from 1.8 to $330 \times 10^{-3}$ (median $17.5 \times 10^{-3}$). Total CSF protein ranged from 166 to 15,840 mg/l (median 1012 mg/l). CSF lactate was elevated (>2.4 mmol/l) in 65.2% [3.6 mmol/l (1.3/15.6 mmol/l); median (minimum/maximum)]. In 50% of all patients CSF lactate was ≥3.5 mmol/l. The CSF cell counts correlated significantly with the CSF lactate levels and the CSF protein contents. In 56 of 118 CSF samples (47.5%) ferritin was elevated, and in 25 of 65 carcinoma patients (38.5%) an intrathecal production of carcinoembryonic antigen (CEA) was detected. Granulocytes were found in 52.7% of the CSF samples. The percentages of granulocytes and lymphocytes were higher in samples with an elevated cell count.

**Conclusion:** In approximately 50% of CSF samples with meningeosis neoplastica the CSF cell count is not elevated. Diagnosis may be missed when only CSF samples with elevated cell counts are subjected to cytological analysis. CSF lactate and protein and the CSF-to-serum albumin ratio are frequently increased in meningeosis neoplastica. The differential diagnosis between meningeosis neoplastica and central nervous infections, in particular tuberculous or fungal meningitis, can be difficult.

**Keywords:** Meningeosis neoplastica, Meningeosis carcinomatosa, Meningeosis lymphomatosa, Lactate, Carcinoembryonic antigen (CEA), CSF/serum albumin ratio

## Background

Meningeosis neoplastica, the infiltration of the meninges and the subarachnoid space by malignant cells as a consequence of metastatic cancer, was first described by Karl Joseph Eberth as early as 1870 [1]. Meningeosis neoplastica is the generic term for all infiltrations of the meninges by malignancies including (1) Meningeosis carcinomatosa as the metastatic spread of a carcinoma to the meninges, (2) Meningeosis lymphomatosa with leptomeningeal involvement by hematologic malignancies and (3) dissemination to the meninges of primary

*Correspondence: mdjukic@gwdg.de
[2] Institute of Neuropathology, University Medical Center Göttingen (UMG), Robert-Koch-Strasse 40, 37075 Göttingen, Germany
Full list of author information is available at the end of the article

tumors of the central nervous system, e.g. germinomas, medulloblastomas, primitive neuroectodermal tumors, ependymomas and malignant gliomas. Meningeosis carcinomatosa occurs in 3–8% of all cancer patients. Among solid tumors, the most frequent tumor types associated with meningeosis carcinomatosa are carcinomas of the lung and breast, and melanoma. Meningeosis lymphomatosa can be observed in approximately 5–15% of patients with hematologic malignancies. Meningeal involvement is most common with high-risk lymphomas and acute lymphocytic leukemia [2, 3]. Tumor cells migrate into the meninges either hematogeneously via small meningeal arteries and veins or by direct infiltration from the vicinity, i.e., from metastases or primary tumors in the skull, spinal cord or brain [4, 5]. After entry into the subarachnoid space or ventricles, malignant cells spread with the cerebrospinal fluid (CSF) along the whole CSF space. These cells frequently accumulate in regions with a reduced circulation velocity of the CSF, i.e., in the basal cisterns, the cauda equina or the hippocampal fissure [2].

Frequent clinical symptoms suggesting meningeosis neoplastica are headache, changes in mental status, difficulty in walking, nausea, vomiting, diplopia, lower motor weakness, limb paresthesia, back or neck pain, and radiculopathy [6]. Many antineoplastic drugs do not readily cross the blood–CSF and blood–brain barrier, but the doses of antineoplastic drugs necessary to produce effective CSF concentrations after direct injection into the CSF space are comparatively low (e.g., 10–15 mg for methotrexate, 40 mg for cytosine–arabinoside) [7]. For this reason, high antineoplastic drug concentrations in the CSF with low systemic toxicity can be reached by intrathecal chemotherapy. The magnetic resonance tomographic and CSF findings in meningeosis neoplastica can be confounded with infectious diseases of the CNS, particularly CNS tuberculosis and fungal meningoencephalitis.

An early diagnosis of meningeosis neoplastica, before persisting neurologic deficits have developed, permits earlier and potentially more effective treatment, thereby leading to a better quality of life in affected patients [6]. Since the indication for intrathecal chemotherapy relies on the detection of malignant cells in the CSF, all efforts must be undertaken to firmly establish the diagnosis. The present study aims at characterizing the CSF findings in a large group of patients with meningeosis neoplastica. Special emphasis was placed on the possible contribution of routine parameters for the differential diagnosis between meningeosis neoplastica and infectious or autoimmune diseases of the CNS.

## Methods

### Patients

The medical files including lumbar or ventricular CSF of patients with meningeosis neoplastica, who were treated

between January 1, 2001, and December 31, 2012, with different clinical symptoms in the University Hospital Göttingen, in the Protestant Hospital Göttingen-Weende and other regional hospitals, were retrospectively analyzed. The inclusion criterion was the presence of tumor cells as assessed by morphological criteria. Clinical symptoms were assessed by review of the patients' medical files. We also assessed the results, when cranial computer tomography (CCT) or magnetic resonance imaging (CMRI) was performed. The study was approved by the Ethics Committee of the Medical Faculty of the Georg-August University Göttingen, Germany.

### CSF analysis

After lysis of the erythrocytes, CSF cells were counted manually in a Fuchs-Rosenthal chamber. A cell count of $\leq 4/\mu l$ was considered normal. CSF cell differentiation was performed after cell sedimentation by means of a cytocentrifuge (Omnifuge 2.0 ORS, Thermo Scientific, Darmstadt, Germany) and May-Grünwald-Giemsa (MGG) staining (Merck, Darmstadt, Germany). Cytology was performed on MGG-stained cytospins. The appearance of tumor cells depended on the origin of the primary tumor. Tumor cells were in general larger than mononuclear hematopoietic cells. Furthermore, they frequently showed a marked increase in the nuclear/cytoplasmic ratio, basophilic cytoplasm, hyperchromasia, irregular nuclear membrane, pseudopodia and increased number of nucleoli. Especially in the case of epithelial cancer, tumor cells frequently lay in clusters and occasionally, in part atypical, mitotic figures were observed. Depending on the primary tumor, tumor cells occasionally showed evidence for mucus production or pigmentation. The CSF protein content was measured by nephelometry after precipitation with trichloroacetic acid in a Dosascat nephelometer (Dosatec, Gilching, Germany) using Gesamteiweiß UC Standard FS (DiaSys Diagnostic Systems, Holzheim, Germany) [8]. CSF and serum albumin, and immunoglobulins IgG, IgA and IgM were determined by nephelometry (BN ProSpec, Siemens Healthcare Diagnostics, Tarrytown, NY, USA), and the respective albumin and immunoglobulin CSF/serum quotients (IgG, IgA, IgM) were calculated and plotted in Reiber-Felgenhauer nomograms [9]. CSF oligoclonal IgG bands were detected by isoelectric focusing in polyacrylamide gels; for the comparison of CSF and serum bands samples were blotted at equalized IgG concentrations and, after immobilization on a nitrocellulose membrane, stained with anti-human IgG antibodies [9–11]. CSF lactate was determined enzymatically using the lactate oxidase reaction cleaving lactate into pyruvate and hydrogen peroxide. The resulting chinonimine concentration, which was proportional to the CSF lactate concentration, was quantified in an ELISA reader at 620 nm. CSF lactate concentrations $\leq 2.4$ mmol/l were considered normal; CSF lactate concentrations $\geq 3.5$ mmol/l are generally considered an indicator of CNS bacterial infection.

In addition to cytology, protein biomarkers were established especially for carcinomas invading the CNS and the leptomeninges [12]. Carcinoembryonic antigen (CEA), an oncofetal antigen and tumor marker particularly for gastrointestinal, breast or lung adenocarcinoma, was found to be secreted into the CSF of patients with meningeosis carcinomatosa [13]. Carcinoembryonic antigen (CEA) in CSF and serum was measured by enzyme immunoassay using antibody-coated beads and a CSF volume of 3 ml in order to increase the sensitivity of the assay [10, 14]. Since the molecular mass of CEA and IgA is approximately equal, intrathecal secretion of CEA was quantified by using the Reiber-Felgenhauer nomogram for the immunoglobulin IgA [14].

The CSF concentration of ferritin was measured by nephelometry (BN ProSpec, Siemens Healthcare Diagnostics, Tarrytown, NY, USA).

### Statistics

Statistical calculations were performed with GraphPad Prism software (GraphPad Software, La Jolla, USA). Data was described by means $\pm$ standard deviations (SD), when normally distributed. In the absence of normal distribution data was described by medians and interquartile ranges or as medians and ranges (minima/maxima). For univariate analyses, we used Mann–Whitney U test in the absence of normal distribution. The relation between CSF cell count and CSF lactate concentration and CSF protein was assessed by Spearman's rank correlation coefficient, $r_S$. p values $\leq 0.05$ were considered statistically significant.

### Results

A group of 132 patients with meningeosis neoplastica [age 16–97 years ($59.1 \pm 29.1$ years; mean $\pm$ SD), 77 women, 55 men)] was included in this study. In 128 patients lumbar CSF and in four patients ventricular CSF was studied.

Clinical symptoms of the patients studied are depicted in Table 1. Cranial nerve palsies were most frequent, followed by psychiatric abnormalities (mainly fluctuating level of consciousness and confusion) and radicular symptoms of the lower extremities and headache. In 32.6% breast carcinoma was the primary malignoma, followed by bronchial carcinomas (25.0%), hematologic malignancies (21.2%), gastrointestinal tumors (8.3%) and neoplasias of the skin (3.8%). All other malignancies including primary brain and spinal tumors accounted for 9.1% of the cases (Fig. 1).

**Table 1** Clinical symptoms of the patients studied (n = 132) upon admission

| Symptoms in the order of decreasing frequency | All patients n (%) |
|---|---|
| Cranial nerve palsy | 55 (41.7%) |
| Psychiatric abnormalities | 43 (32.6) |
| Radicular motor symptoms of the lower extremities | 27 (20.5) |
| Headache | 25 (18.9) |
| Hemiparesis | 23 (17.4) |
| Nausea/vomiting | 22 (16.7) |
| Radicular sensory symptoms of the lower extremities | 21 (15.9) |
| Non-radicular sensory abnormalities | 18 (13.6) |
| Para- or tetraparesis | 17 (12.9) |
| Aphasia | 14 (11.4) |
| Nuchal rigidity | 12 (9.1) |
| Cognitive decline | 11 (8.3) |
| Radicular motor symptoms of the upper extremities | 11 (8.3) |
| Epileptic seizures | 10 (7.6) |
| Radicular sensory symptoms of the upper extremities | 5 (3.8) |
| Fever | 2 (1.5) |

Cranial nerve palsies were most frequent, followed by psychiatric abnormalities (mainly fluctuating level of consciousness and confusion)

97 patients with cytologically proven meningeosis neoplastica received cranial imaging [CCT (n = 19), CMRI (n = 24) or both (n = 54)] within a short time period before or after the diagnostic lumbar or ventricular CSF analysis. In 50 of these patients (51.5%), typical signs of meningeosis neoplastica were present on CCT or CMRI.

The results of CSF analysis in patients with meningeosis neoplastica are presented in Table 2. The CSF cell count (leukocytes and tumor cells cannot be distinguished reliably in the Fuchs-Rosenthal cytometer, and erythrocytes were lysed before counting) was elevated (>4 cells/µl) in the CSF samples of 66 patients and normal ($\leq$4 cells/µl) in the other 66 patients. CSF pleocytosis $\geq$100 cells/µl was present in 18 patients (13.6%), and four patients had a CSF pleocytosis $\geq$500 cells/µl. Malignant cells were detected in all CSF samples (inclusion criterion). Differentiation into lymphocytes, monocytes and granulocytes was carried out in the CSF of 55 patients (28 of them with normal cell count and 27 with pleocytosis).

Overall, lymphocytes were the most abundant cell population. Granulocytes were found in 52.7% of the CSF samples, in only two patients was the percentage of granulocytes >50%. Both of them had more than 500 cells/µl. In the CSF of patients with >4 cells/µl, lymphocytes and granulocytes were significantly more frequent than in the CSF with $\leq$4 cells/µl [lymphocytes 92% (72/94%) versus 77.5% (67/87.8% ), median (25th/75th quartile) (Mann-WhitneyU test: p < 0.01); granulocytes 19% (2/31%) versus 3.5% (0/8.3%) (Mann–Whitney U test: p = 0.013).

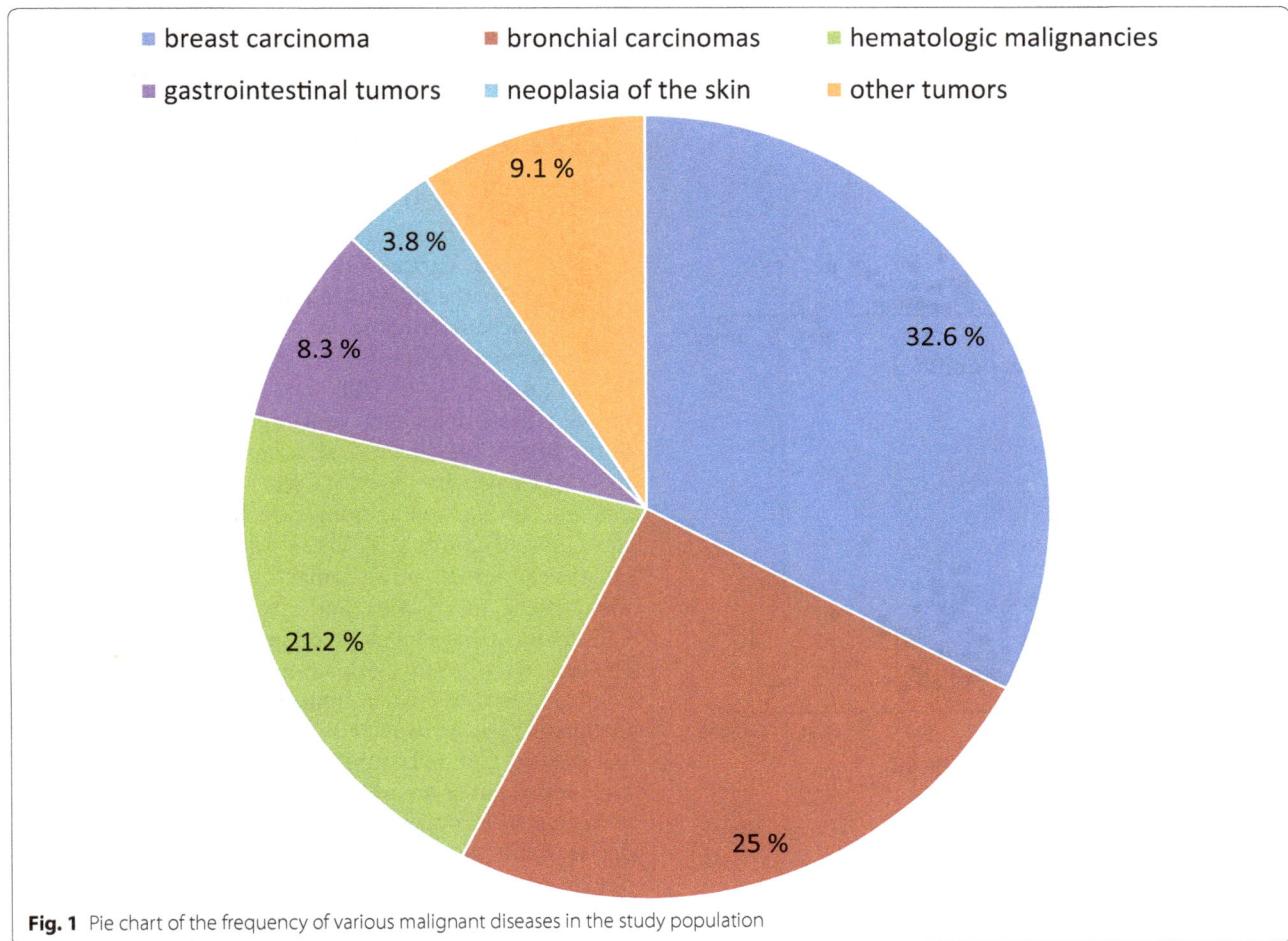

**breast carcinoma** ■ **bronchial carcinomas** ■ **hematologic malignancies**
■ **gastrointestinal tumors** ■ **neoplasia of the skin** ■ **other tumors**

- 9.1 %
- 3.8 %
- 8.3 %
- 21.2 %
- 32.6 %
- 25 %

**Fig. 1** Pie chart of the frequency of various malignant diseases in the study population

### Table 2 Cerebrospinal fluid analysis in patients with meningeosis neoplastica

| Parameter | Normal findings n (%) | Abnormal findings n (%) | Median (minimum; maximum) |
|---|---|---|---|
| CSF cells (/µl) excluding erythrocytes | 66 (50) | 66 (50) | 4 (0/4692) |
| CSF protein (mg/l) | 28 (21.5) | 102 (78.5) | 1012 (166/15,840) |
| $Q_{Albumin} \times 10^{-3}$ | 37 (30.6) | 84 (69.4) | 17.5 (1.8/330) |
| CSF lactate (mmol/l) | 46 (34.8) | 86 (65.2) | 3.6 (1.3/15.6) |

In 50% of CSF samples with meningeosis neoplastica the CSF cell count was not elevated. The CSF-to-serum albumin ratio was abnormal in 69.4%, and total CSF protein was elevated (>450 mg/l) in 102 of 130 patients (78.5%). CSF lactate was elevated (>2.4 mmol/l) in 65.2%

In 32.6% breast cancer was the primary malignoma, followed by bronchial carcinomas (25.0%), hematologic malignancies (21.2%), gastrointestinal tumors (8.3%) and neoplasias of the skin (3.8%). All other malignancies including primary brain and spinal tumors accounted for 9.1% of the cases

Conversely, monocytes were less frequent in CSF samples with pleocytosis than in those with a normal cell count [8% (6/14%) versus 12% (10/20%), p < 0.01].

Total CSF protein was elevated (>450 mg/l) in 102 of 130 patients (78.5%). The CSF protein was positively correlated with the CSF cell count (n = 130, Spearman's rank correlation coefficient $r_S = 0.45$, p < 0.001) (Fig. 2a). The CSF-to-serum albumin ratio was abnormal in 84 of 121 patients (69.4%). Intrathecal synthesis of IgG or IgA or IgM antibodies as assessed by the Reiber–Felgenhauer nomograms was detected in the CSF of 13 patients: four showed an isolated intrathecal synthesis of IgG, two synthesis of IgA, and nine synthesis of IgM. In two patients, nephelometry suggested synthesis of more than one class

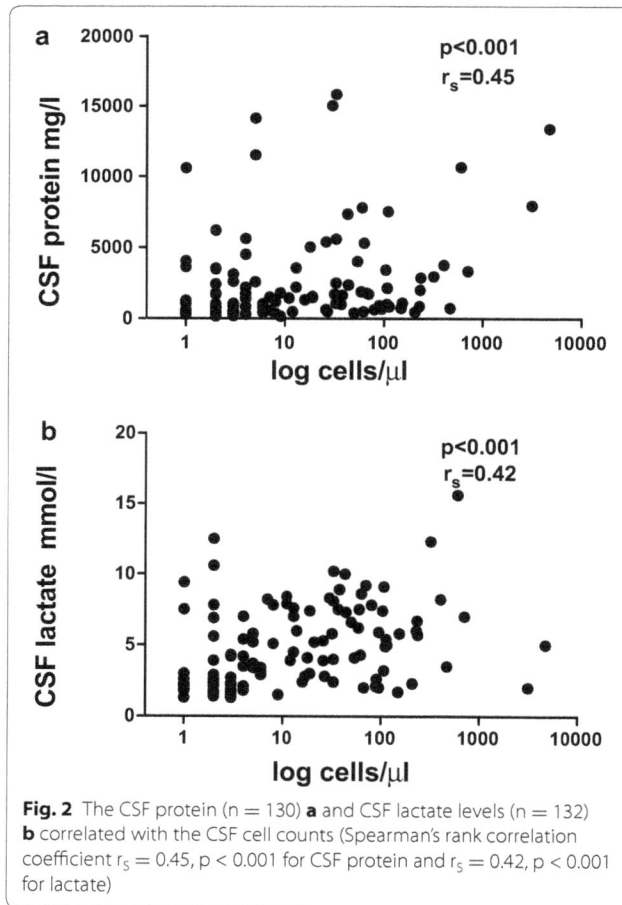

Fig. 2 The CSF protein (n = 130) a and CSF lactate levels (n = 132) b correlated with the CSF cell counts (Spearman's rank correlation coefficient $r_S$ = 0.45, p < 0.001 for CSF protein and $r_S$ = 0.42, p < 0.001 for lactate)

of antibodies (one patient: IgG plus IgM; one patient: IgG plus IgA). Nephelometry detected intrathecal immunoglobulin synthesis in 10 lymphoma and three carcinoma patients. By isoelectric focusing, intrathecal IgG synthesis was detected in the CSF of 25 of 62 patients (40.3%), i.e., isoelectric focusing was by far more sensitive than nephelometry in detecting intrathecal IgG synthesis.

Cerebrospinal fluid lactate was elevated (>2.4 mmol/l) in 65.2% [3.6 mmol/l (1.3/15.6 mmol/l); median (minimum/maximum)]. In 66 of 132 patients (50%), CSF lactate was strongly elevated (≥3.5 mmol/l). The CSF lactate concentration was correlated with the CSF cell count (n = 132, Spearman's rank correlation coefficient $r_S$ = 0.42, p < 0.001) (Fig. 2b).

Ferritin and CEA were not measured in all samples, but only upon request of the clinician in charge of the patient. In 56 of 118 CSF samples (47.5%) ferritin was elevated, and in 25 of 81 cases (30.9%) an intrathecal production of CEA was detected. No intrathecal CEA production was detected in lymphoma patients. Of the 65 patients with meningeosis carcinomatosa, 25 patients (38.5%) had intrathecal CEA synthesis.

## Discussion

Clinical signs and symptoms of the patients included in this study were very similar to those reported by others [6]. CSF analysis is the key laboratory investigation to diagnose/confirm meningeosis neoplastica. If this diagnosis is suspected, repeated analyses of CSF may be necessary to prove the presence of malignant cells in the CSF, as this is the diagnostic cornerstone of meningeosis neoplastica. Furthermore, the detection of malignant cells in CSF is the prerequisite for the start of intrathecal therapy, and one criterion for successful treatment is the disappearance of tumor cells. In our study the presence of malignant cells in CSF was the inclusion criterion, i.e., all CSF samples evaluated contained malignant cells. Surprisingly, 50% of the CSF samples included had normal cell counts. In a previous study, 32% of patients with cytologically-proven meningeosis neoplastica had normal CSF cell counts [15]. These studies illustrate that clinicians cannot rely on a normal CSF cell count to exclude meningeosis neoplastica, and cytological examination of CSF should always be included in the routine work-up of CSF analysis. Careful cytopathologic analysis is necessary in all CSF samples, when infiltration of the CSF space by malignant cells is suspected.

When the CSF cell count is elevated and malignant cells are not present or are overlooked, differentiation between meningeosis neoplastica and infections or autoimmune diseases affecting the CSF space can be difficult. In particular, tuberculous meningitis can be confounded with meningeosis neoplastica, because the clinical symptoms and CSF abnormalities can be similar. Moreover, many patients suffering from malignant diseases are immunosuppressed either by chemotherapy or the underlying disease. They, therefore, are prone to develop CNS infections with M. tuberculosis, fungi and other opportunistic pathogens, which also can cause CSF alterations similar to those observed in meningeosis neoplastica.

Elevated CSF lactate is not specific for certain diseases. Meningeosis neoplastica can cause a CSF lactate elevation [16], but a concentration ≥3.5 mmol/l is considered an indicator of bacterial or fungal meningoencephalitis [11]. Most of the CSF lactate originates from host cells, in particular, leukocytes and neurons. Even in bacterial meningitis, ≥95% of the CSF lactate originates from anaerobic glycolysis of host cells and not from bacteria in the CSF [17]. In the present study, CSF lactate was correlated with the CSF cell count. In a recent receiver operating characteristic (ROC) curve analysis, CSF lactate had the highest accuracy for discriminating bacterial from viral meningitis with a cutoff set at 3.5 mmol/l [18]. Using a cutoff of 3.5 mmol/l, CSF lactate was also very useful to discriminate between cryptococcal or tuberculous meningitis and HIV chronic meningitis [19]. In acute Lyme neuroborreliosis, an atypical bacterial CNS infection with low pathogen concentrations in CSF and symptoms, which may resemble meningeosis carcinomatosa (in particular, radicular lesions and cranial nerve involvement), only 5 of 118 patients (4%) had a CSF lactate $\geq$3.5 mmol/l, and the mean CSF lactate level was not elevated [20]. This implies that CSF lactate concentrations $\geq$3.5 mmol/l can help in discriminating meningeosis neoplastica from viral meningitis, neuroborreliosis, mitochondriopathy and many other conditions, but not from neurotuberculosis and fungal meningoencephalitis.

Meningeosis neoplastica frequently is associated with an inflammatory response. The presence of intrathecal IgG, IgA and IgM synthesis as well as the high proportion of lymphocytes in the CSF of patients with meningeosis neoplastica indicate a strong involvement of the adaptive immune system. As in neuroborreliosis, isoelectric focusing was more sensitive for detecting an intrathecal IgG synthesis than the Reiber–Felgenhauer nomogram [20]. The presence of granulocytes in the CSF in neoplastic meningeosis suggests a contribution of the innate immune system to the inflammatory reaction. In tuberculous meningitis which also is characterized by a strong elevation of CSF lactate and total protein and a moderate elevation of cell counts (10–500 cells/µl), neutrophil predominance (>50%) [21] was a strong predictor of tuberculous meningitis with a sensitivity of 54% and a specificity of 98% [22]. Since only two of the 55 CSF samples in our study, where differential cell counts were carried out, contained >50% granulocytes, neutrophilic predominance in CSF is an argument against the diagnosis of meningeosis neoplastica. However, in nearly 50% of patients with tuberculous meningitis, neutrophil predominance is absent, and the differentiation between these two diseases relies on bacteriologic exams (Ziehl-Neelsen stain, culture, polymerase chain reaction) and on the cytological identification of tumor cells.

The CSF protein concentration correlated positively with the CSF cell count. One explanation for this is an abnormal blood–CSF barrier function with increased permeability for leukocytes and serum-derived proteins. In particular, the leptomeningeal structures and the epithelial cells of the choroid plexus can be infiltrated by neoplastic cells, resulting in an increased permeability for serum compounds [23]. Another explanation for this correlation is a decreased CSF flow rate due to the obstruction of the sites of CSF absorption, especially arachnoid granulations and the perineural spaces of the cranial and spinal nerves by malignant cells or leukocytes. As a consequence of the CSF flow reduction, the protein gradient between serum and CSF can decrease [24].

Ferritin CSF concentrations were elevated in 56 of 118 patients (47.5%). CSF ferritin concentrations are elevated after intracranial bleeding and in neoplastic and meningitic CNS diseases, but this parameter is neither specific nor sensitive. An elevated CSF ferritin reliably, but non-specifically indicates severe CNS disease [25].

Carcinoembryonic antigen was measured in 81 patients. In patients with metastatic CEA-producing tumors, diffusion of CEA across the blood–CSF and blood–brain barrier cannot be neglected. The CSF concentrations depend on the respective serum concentration, and absolute cut-off values are not appropriate. Because of the similar molecular mass of CEA and IgA, the Reiber–Felgenhauer nomogram for IgA can be used to detect intrathecal CEA synthesis [10, 14, 26]. In 25 patients of 65 carcinomas cases (38.5%) the Reiber–Felgenhauer nomogram indicated intrathecal CEA synthesis. Using the IgA nomogram, the detection of intrathecal CEA is considered a very specific, but not very sensitive indicator of meningeosis carcinomatosa or cerebral metastases. A normal or undetectable CSF-to-serum ratio of CEA does not exclude infiltration of CNS compartments by carcinoma cells, lymphomas and primary brain tumors do not produce CEA [14]. Another method to detect intracranial synthesis of CEA compares the CSF-to-serum ratio of CEA with the CSF-to-serum albumin ratio and assumes intrathecal synthesis when the CSF-to-serum ratio of CEA is greater than the CSF-to-serum albumin ratio determined on the same day. Since the molecular mass of CEA is larger than albumin, this method is less sensitive than the use of the IgA nomogram [10]. We doubt that CEA CSF concentrations without knowledge of the corresponding serum levels are of value for the detection of meningeosis carcinomatosa. Others, however, have reported that the combination of CSF concentrations of CEA, neuron specific enolase (NSE) and cytokeratin 19 fragments (CYFRA21-1) using cut-off values without consideration of the respective serum levels appears to be useful for the detection of meningeal carcinomatosis of lung cancer [27].

## Conclusions

The two main findings of this study are: (1) In half of the CSF samples with meningeosis neoplastica the CSF cell count is not elevated. Therfore, diagnosis can be missed when only CSF samples with elevated cell counts are subjected to cytological analysis. (2) CSF lactate and protein and the CSF-to-serum albumin ratio are frequently increased in meningeosis neoplastica. The differential diagnosis between meningeosis neoplastica and central nervous infections, in particular tuberculous or fungal meningitis, can be difficult. For the detection or exclusion of malignant cells in the CSF, cytology performed by an experienced pathologist is necessary.

## Abbreviations

CEA: carcinoembryonic antigen; CCT: cranial computer tomography; CMRI: cranial magnetic resonance imaging; CSF: cerebrospinal fluid; CYFRA21-1: cytokeratin 19 fragments; MGG: May-Grünwald-Giemsa; NSE: neuron specific enolaseMGG May-Grünwald-Giemsa.

## Authors' contributions

MD and RN planned the study. MD, RT, IN, AS and PL analyzed the data and participated in the study design and manuscript preparation. CS participated in the study design and preparation of the manuscript and, together with IN, was responsible for the cytopathology. RT and RN wrote the first draft of the manuscript. All authors read and approved the final manuscript.

## Author details

[1] Department of Geriatrics, Evangelisches Krankenhaus Göttingen-Weende, Göttingen, Germany. [2] Institute of Neuropathology, University Medical Center Göttingen (UMG), Robert-Koch-Strasse 40, 37075 Göttingen, Germany. [3] Department of Neurology, University Medical Center Göttingen (UMG), Göttingen, Germany. [4] Department of Neurology, University Medical Centre Mainz, Mainz, Germany.

## Competing interests

The authors declare that they have no competing interests.

## Funding

The study was supported by Sparkasse Göttingen and Evangelisches Krankenhaus Göttingen-Weende. The funding bodies did not influence the design of the study and collection, analysis, and interpretation of data.

## References

1. Eberth CJ. Zur Entwicklung des Epitheliomas (Cholesteatomas) der Pia und der Lunge. Virchow's Arch. 1870;49:51–63.
2. Grossman SA, Krabak MJ. Leptomeningeal carcinomatosis. Cancer Treat Rev. 1999;25:103–19.
3. Kaplan JG, DeSouza TG, Farkash A, Shafran B, Pack D, Rehman F, Fuks J, Portenoy R. Leptomeningeal metastases: comparison of clinical features and laboratory data of solid tumors, lymphomas and leukemias. J Neurooncol. 1990;9:225–9.
4. Rosen ST, Aisner J, Makuch RW, Matthews MJ, Ihde DC, Whitacre M, Glatstein EJ, Wiernik PH, Lichter AS, Bunn PA Jr. Carcinomatous leptomeningitis in small cell lung cancer: a clinicopathologic review of the national cancer institute experience. Medicine (Baltimore). 1982;61:45–53.
5. http://www.dgn.org/leitlinien/2979-ll-77-metastasen-und-meningeosneoplastica Accessed 15 Dec 2016.
6. Le Rhun E, Taillibert S, Chamberlain MC. Carcinomatous meningitis: leptomeningeal metastases in solid tumors. Surg Neurol Int. 2013;4(Suppl 4):265–88.
7. Morikawa N, Mori T, Kawashima H, Fujiki M, Abe T, Kaku T, Konisi Y, Takeyama M, Hori S. Pharmacokinetics of nimustine, methotrexate, and cytosine arabinoside during cerebrospinal fluid perfusion chemotherapy in patients with disseminated brain tumors. Eur J Clin Pharmacol. 1998;54:415–20.
8. Reiber H. Eine schnelle und einfache nephelometrische Bestimmungsmethode für Protein im Liquor cerebrospinalis. J Clin Chem Clin Biochem. 1980;18:123–7.
9. Reiber H, Felgenhauer K. Protein transfer at the blood cerebrospinal fluid barrier and the quantitation of the humoral immune response within the central nervous system. Clin Chim Acta. 1987;163:319–28.
10. Wick M Ausgewählte Methoden der Liquordiagnostik und klinichen Neurochemie, 2004. https://www.uke.de/extern/dgln/pdf/Methodenkatalog.pdf. Accessed 12 Dec 2016
11. Wildemann B, Oschmann P, Reiber H. Neurologische Labordiagnostik. Stuttgart: Georg Thieme Verlag; 2006.
12. Weston CL, Glantz MJ, Connor JR. Detection of cancer cells in the cerebrospinal fluid: current methods and future directions. Fluids Barriers CNS. 2011;8(1):14.
13. Jacobi C, Reiber H, Felgenhauer K. The clinical relevance of locally produced carcinoembryonic antigen in cerebrospinal fluid. J Neurol. 1986;233:358–61.
14. Petereit HF, Sindern E, Wick M. Leitlinien der Liquordiagnostik und Methodenkatalog der Deutschen Gesellschaft für Liquordiagnostik und Klinische Neurochemie. Heidelberg: Springer; 2007.
15. Liu J, Jia H, Yang Y, Dai W, Su X, Zhao G. Cerebrospinal fluid cytology and clinical analysis of 34 cases with leptomeningeal carcinomatosis. J Int Med Res. 2009;37:1913–20.
16. Hornig CR, Busse O, Kaps M. Importance of cerebrospinal fluid lactate determination in neurological diseases. Klin Wochenschr. 1983;61:357–61.
17. Wellmer A, Prange J, Gerber J, Zysk G, Lange P, Michel U, Eiffert H, Nau R. D- and L-lactate in rabbit and human bacterial meningitis. Scand J Infect Dis. 2001;33:909–13.
18. Giulieri S, Chapuis-Taillard C, Jaton K, Cometta A, Chuard C, Hugli O, Du Pasquier R, Bille J, Meylan P, Manuel O, Marchetti O. CSF lactate for accurate diagnosis of community-acquired bacterial meningitis. Eur J Clin Microbiol Infect Dis. 2015;34:2049–55.
19. de Almeida SM, Boritza K, Cogo LL, Pessa L, França J, Rota I, Muro M, Ribeiro C, Raboni SM, Vidal LR, Nogueira MB, Ellis R. Quantification of cerebrospinal fluid lactic acid in the differential diagnosis between HIV chronic meningitis and opportunistic meningitis. Clin Chem Lab Med. 2011;49:891–6.
20. Djukic M, Schmidt-Samoa C, Lange P, Spreer A, Neubieser K, Eiffert H, Nau R, Schmidt H. Cerebrospinal fluid findings in adults with acute Lyme neuroborreliosis. J Neurol. 2012;259:630–6.
21. Thwaites GE, Chau TT, Stepniewska K, Phu NH, Chuong LV, Sinh DX, White NJ, Parry CM, Farrar JJ. Diagnosis of adult tuberculous meningitis by use of clinical and laboratory features. Lancet. 2002;360:1287–92.
22. Zou Y, He J, Guo L, Bu H, Liu Y. Prediction of cerebrospinal fluid parameters for tuberculous meningitis. Diagn Cytopathol. 2015;43:701–4.
23. Schumacher M, Orszagh M. Imaging techniques in neoplastic meningiosis. J Neurooncol. 1998;38(2–3):111–20.
24. Reiber H. Flow rate of cerebrospinal fluid (CSF)–a concept common to normal blood–CSF barrier function and to dysfunction in neurological diseases. J Neurol Sci. 1994;122(2):189–203.
25. Kolodziej MA, Proemmel P, Quint K, Strik HM. Cerebrospinal fluid ferritin—unspecific and unsuitable for disease monitoring. Neurol Neurochir Pol. 2014;48:116–21.
26. Reiber H. Cerebrospinal fluid data compilation and knowledge-based interpretation of bacterial, viral, parasitic, oncological, chronic inflammatory and demyelinating diseases. Diagnostic patterns not to be missed in neurology and psychiatry. Arq Neuropsiquiatr. 2016;74:337–50.
27. Wang P, Piao Y, Zhang X, Li W, Hao X. The concentration of CYFRA 21-1, NSE and CEA in cerebro-spinal fluid can be useful indicators for diagnosis of meningeal carcinomatosis of lung cancer. Cancer Biomark. 2013;13:123–30.

# 14

# Directional cerebrospinal fluid movement between brain ventricles in larval zebrafish

Ryann M. Fame[1], Jessica T. Chang[1,2], Alex Hong[2], Nicole A. Aponte-Santiago[2] and Hazel Sive[1,2]*

## Abstract

**Background:** Cerebrospinal fluid (CSF) contained within the brain ventricles contacts neuroepithelial progenitor cells during brain development. Dynamic properties of CSF movement may limit locally produced factors to specific regions of the developing brain. However, there is no study of in vivo CSF dynamics between ventricles in the embryonic brain. We address CSF movement using the zebrafish larva, during the major period of developmental neurogenesis.

**Methods:** CSF movement was monitored at two stages of zebrafish development: early larva [pharyngula stage; 27–30 h post-fertilization (hpf)] and late larva (hatching period; 51–54 hpf) using photoactivatable Kaede protein to calculate average maximum CSF velocity between ventricles. Potential roles for heartbeat in early CSF movement were investigated using $tnnt2a$ mutant fish ($tnnt2a^{-/-}$) and chemical [2,3 butanedione monoxime (BDM)] treatment. Cilia motility was monitored at these stages using the Tg($\beta act{:}Arl13b$–GFP) transgenic fish line.

**Results:** In wild-type early larva there is net CSF movement from the telencephalon to the combined diencephalic/mesencephalic superventricle. This movement directionality reverses at late larval stage. CSF moves directionally from diencephalic to rhombencephalic ventricles at both stages examined, with minimal movement from rhombencephalon to diencephalon. Directional movement is partially dependent on heartbeat, as indicated in assays of $tnnt2a^{-/-}$ fish and after BDM treatment. Brain cilia are immotile at the early larval stage.

**Conclusion:** These data demonstrate directional movement of the embryonic CSF in the zebrafish model during the major period of developmental neurogenesis. A key conclusion is that CSF moves preferentially from the diencephalic into the rhombencephalic ventricle. In addition, the direction of CSF movement between telencephalic and diencephalic ventricles reverses between the early and late larval stages. CSF movement is partially dependent on heartbeat. At early larval stage, the absence of motile cilia indicates that cilia likely do not direct CSF movement. These data suggest that CSF components may be compartmentalized and could contribute to specialization of the early brain. In addition, CSF movement may also provide directional mechanical signaling.

**Keywords:** Cerebrospinal fluid, Brain ventricular system, Fluid dynamics, Zebrafish

## Background

Cerebrospinal fluid (CSF) is contained in the brain ventricles (chambers derived from the brain lumen) and contacts neuroepithelial progenitor cells during brain development and in adulthood. The CSF contains a unique composition of proteins (CSF proteome) [1–6], small molecules [5, 7] and lipid particles [8] for which limited studies have demonstrated function during brain development [1–5, 7–9]. Since the brain lumen forms before the choroid plexus (CP), ventricles exist with no requirement for a CP to be associated with each ventricle. In some cases early pre-CP fluid is called ependymal fluid [10]. The cohort of proteins in zebrafish CSF is largely overlapping with early amniote CSF prior to

*Correspondence: sive@wi.mit.edu
[2] Massachusetts Institute of Technology, 77 Massachusetts Avenue, Cambridge, MA 02139-4307, USA
Full list of author information is available at the end of the article

CP development [7] and this conservation has not been investigated at later stages. Once the CPs have become functional they secrete most of the ventricular fluid, although there is clear data that fluid continues to be produced from ependymal cells even after CP differentiation is complete [11–14]. The ventricular fluid is thus always a mix from different sources and the term CSF is most general and appropriate to refer to the ventricular fluid at all stages.

Restricted or directional CSF movement, either during production and drainage or coupled to heartbeat [15–19], could limit locally-produced factors to specific regions of the developing brain. Studies in *Xenopus* have investigated local intraventricular CSF dynamics in the developing brain [19, 20], but there has been no direct study of in vivo CSF movement dynamics between ventricles. Recent studies have suggested that cilia on neuroepithelial cells may detect a mechanical signal to regulate neuronal progenitor differentiation [21]. The nature of this signal is unknown but could be CSF movement. CSF fluid dynamics have been examined in zebrafish after CP formation [22], but have not been studied earlier in development during the major period of developmental neurogenesis. To address these deficits, we investigate CSF movement in the accessible larval zebrafish brain, prior to CP formation. Our data demonstrate directional movement of CSF, which may function during brain development.

## Methods

### Fish lines and maintenance

*Danio rerio* fish were raised and bred according to standard methods [23]. Embryos were kept at 28.5 °C and staged according to Kimmel et al. [24]. Times of development are expressed as hours post-fertilization (hpf) or days post-fertilization (dpf). Analyses were performed at early larva (pharyngula stage; 27–30 hpf) stage, late larva (hatching period; 51–54 hpf) stage, and some at 5 dpf. Lines used were: AB; Tg(*βact:Arl13b*–GFP) transgenic line [25]; *troponin T type 2a* (cardiac) mutants *tnnt2a*$^{-/-}$ (R14GBT0031/silent heart; obtained from The Zebrafish International Resource Center (ZIRC; Eugene, USA)) [26]. Larvae were incubated in 3 μg/mL 1-phenyl-2-thiourea (PTU) starting between 22 and 24 hpf to inhibit maturation of melanocytes and allow for clear visualization. All experimental procedures on live animals and embryos were reviewed and approved by the Institutional Animal Care and Use Committee of the Massachusetts Institute of Technology (Protocol# 0414-026-17) and were carried out in accordance with the recommendations in the National Institutes of Health (NIH) Guide for the Care and Use of Laboratory Animals.

### Multiview SPIM brain ventricle imaging

Larvae were anesthetized in 0.1 mg/mL (0.38 mM) Tricaine (Sigma, St. Louis, USA) dissolved in embryo medium [23] prior to injection and imaging. At high doses, Tricaine can induce death or stop the heart [27–29], but these effects have not been shown at the concentration used here. Direct effects of Tricaine on CSF movement have not been investigated.

The rhombencephalic ventricle was microinjected with 2 nL of 2000 kDa dextran conjugated to fluorescein (ThermoFisher/Invitrogen Molecular Probes, Waltham, USA; D7137) diluted to 25 mg/mL in sterile ddH$_2$O. Embryos were embedded in 1 % low-melting point agarose in a glass capillary, and selective plane illumination microscopy (SPIM) was performed using a Zeiss LightsheetZ.1 microscope within 60 min of injection. Six multi-view images were acquired (60° apart), and were processed using ZEN software (Zeiss, Oberkochen, Germany), FIJI [30, 31], and the Multiview reconstruction plugin [32, 33]. Images were analyzed using Imaris software (Bitplane, Belfast, UK) to visualize 3-D images and to generate volume measurements for ventricles at each age. The image threshold was set so that both the ventricle outline and the spinal canal were detected. For rhombencephalic ventricular volume measurements, the same threshold as above was used, but only the rhombencephalon was included in the region of interest. Injection does not affect development, survival or ventricle size over the time period studied ([34] and Additional file 1: Fig. S1).

### Tissue histology and hematoxylin and eosin staining

Larvae were anesthetized as described above and fixed overnight in aqueous Bouin's fixative (RICCA Chemical, Pokomoke City, USA). Larvae were washed in 70 % EtOH until supernatant was clear (at least six washes of 1 h each at room temperature). Larvae were oriented in Richard Allan Scientific HistoGel (ThermoFisher, Waltham, USA). The HistoGel discs containing oriented larvae were fixed for 1 h in Bouin's fixative, and subsequently washed in 70 % EtOH until supernatant was clear. Samples were infiltrated with paraffin using a Tissue-Tek VIP5 Vacuum Infiltration Processor (Sakura Finetek, Torrance, USA; model 5215). Sections were cut at 4–5 μm and slides were stained with Harris acidified hematoxylin (3 min) and eosin Y (10 s) using the "standard" H&E protocol [35] on a Shandon Varistain Gemini Slide Stainer (ThermoFisher, Waltham, USA). Slides were imaged using an Axioplan 2 (Zeiss, Oberkochen, Germany) equipped with a Q-Capture MicroPublisher 5.0 RTV camera/software (QImaging Scientific, Surrey, Canada) using 10× and 40× air objectives and 63× and 100× oil-immersion objectives.

### Live time-lapse confocal imaging

Larvae were anesthetized as described above and the rhombencephalic ventricle was microinjected with 2 nL of Kaede, a photoactivatable protein with fluorescence that changes from green to red upon illumination with UV light [36, 37]. After injection, larvae recovered from injection and anesthesia for at least 30 min prior to imaging, mitigating any immediate effects of dye injection. Embryos were then anesthetized as described above and placed in wells of 1 % agarose (early larva), or embedded in 1 % low-melting point agarose on a coverslip (late larva) for confocal microscopy [37]. Confocal imaging and photoconversion was performed using an inverted Zeiss LSM710 laser-scanning microscope equipped with a 25× (0.8 NA) LD LCI Plan Apochromat water-immersion objective (Fig. 1a). Kaede photoconversion was performed on a circle (diameter of 8 pixels) in the center of the ventricle of interest using the 405 nm laser at 85–95 % strength (for 700 iterations at scan speed = 7, ~20 s per stack). Stacks were collected using simultaneous activation of green and red channels and continuous acquisition for 10–15 min (Fig. 1a).

### Image processing and fluid movement quantification

Confocal time-lapse images were analyzed using Imaris software (Bitplane, Belfast, UK) to create thresholded volumetric surfaces of photoconverted Kaede. The red threshold was set for each image such that no signal was detected before photoconversion, and no signal was detected in the unconverted target ventricle at time = 0 (first scan after photoconversion) (Fig. 1b). Imaris generated volume (V) data from each time point. From these volume readings, the volumetric flow rate at time t ($Q_t$) was calculated for each time point using Eq. (1):

$$Q_t = \frac{V_t - V_{t-1}}{T_t - T_{t-1}} = \frac{\Delta V}{\Delta T} \tag{1}$$

Q was then smoothed to negate technical noise using a 9-point moving window average. To control for individual variations in ventricle shape, $Q_t$ was converted to linear velocity (v) by dividing Q by the cross-sectional area of the aqueduct. Cross-sectional areas were measured using Imaris software (Bitplane, Belfast, UK) by creating surfaces of the unconverted (green) Kaede signal in the first scan (before photoconversion) at the narrowest point between the two ventricles being analyzed. The maximum velocity number ($v_{max}$) was used to analyze brain ventricle CSF movement (see Fig. 1c).

### Acute inhibition of heartbeat

Heartbeat was acutely inhibited by soaking ventricle-injected embryos in 40 mM 2,3 butanedione monoxime (BDM; Sigma, St. Louis, USA) solubilized in embryo medium [23] for 10–30 min prior to imaging as previously shown [38]. This treatment stops heartbeat, but does not change the gross ventricular anatomy within 2 h of incubation (Additional file 1: Fig. S2). BDM prevents action of all muscles (and can alter activities of connexins [39], potassium channels [40, 41], and L-type calcium channels [42]) and is therefore less precise for disruption of heartbeat than the $tnnt2a^{-/-}$ mutant.

### Cilia imaging

The Tg($\beta act$:Arl13b–GFP) transgenic line was used for visualization of cilia. Embryos were treated with 40 mM BDM, as described above for 10 min to stop heartbeat and enable completely steady, immotile embryos suitable for high-speed imaging. They were prepared for SPIM as described above and incubated in 20 mM BDM and 0.1 mg/mL Tricaine (Sigma, St. Louis, USA) in embryo medium during imaging. Images were collected at 57.22 frames per second (fps) in the telencephalon, diencephalon/mesencephalon, rhombencephalon and spinal canal. Time-lapse movies were registered using FIJI [30, 31] and the StackReg plugin [43]. The ciliary beat frequency (CBF) was calculated using the following formula: [CBF = (number of frames per second)/(average number of frames for single beat)] [44]. Images were processed by overlaying sequential frames in pseudocolor using Photoshop (Adobe).

## Results

### The early zebrafish brain ventricular system is complex and dynamic

In order to obtain detailed structure of the zebrafish brain ventricular system, we filled the ventricles with 2000 kDa dextran conjugated to fluorescein and used SPIM to acquire images at 30 hpf (pharyngula or early larval stage; Fig. 2a, b) and 54 hpf (hatching period or late larval stage; Fig. 2d, e), prior to CP maturation but after ventricle inflation and spinal canal (SC) formation. We also examined ventricle anatomy at 5 dpf (Fig. 2g, h) after CP formation. Since the brain is still developing, the early ventricle anlagen are dynamic over these times. The telencephalic (T) ventricle is the most rostral. Early, the combined diencephalic/mesencephalic (D/M) superventricle is caudal to the T ventricle while later this middle ventricle subdivides into the diencephalic (D) and the tectal (Te) ventricles. The rhombencephalic (R) ventricle is at the most caudal aspect of the brain [22, 45] (Fig. 2). At these stages, the SC branches off from the ventral aspect of the D ventricle (Fig. 2b′, c–c″, e, f–f′). This is the first demonstration of early connection from the diencephalon to the spinal canal in any species.

Ventricular shape changes over the first 2 days of development; with the combined diencephalic/tectal (D/Te)

**a  Kaede Injection and Photoconversion**

**b  Image Processing**

**c  Computing Maximum Velocity**

**Fig. 1** Experimental workflow. **a** Schematic representation of rhombencephalic ventricle Kaede injection and confocal photoconversion and imaging of zebrafish ventricles. **b** Workflow for image processing. Raw images were collected and then thresholded in Imaris (Bitplane) software so that red (photoconverted) Kaede was only detected after photoconversion and was not detected in the unconverted target ventricle immediately after photoconversion. Then the volume of the unconverted target ventricle was calculated over time by Imaris (Bitplane) software. *Dashed line* indicates telencephalic-to-mesencephalic/diencephalic boundary. **c** Workflow for data analysis. From volume measurements of the target ventricle, volumetric flow rate (Q) was calculated using Eq. (1) (see "Methods" section). Q was smoothed using a 9-point moving-window average. Q was then converted to linear velocity by dividing by the cross-sectional area of the smallest part of the aqueduct between the two ventricles. These CSF dynamics were reported as the maximum velocity between the two ventricles ($v_{max}$). *T* telencephalic ventricle, *D/M* diencephalic/mesencephalic ventricle, *R* rhombencephalic ventricle, *hpf* hours post-fertilization, *V* volume, *Q* volumetric flow rate, *v* velocity. *Scale bar*: 50 μm

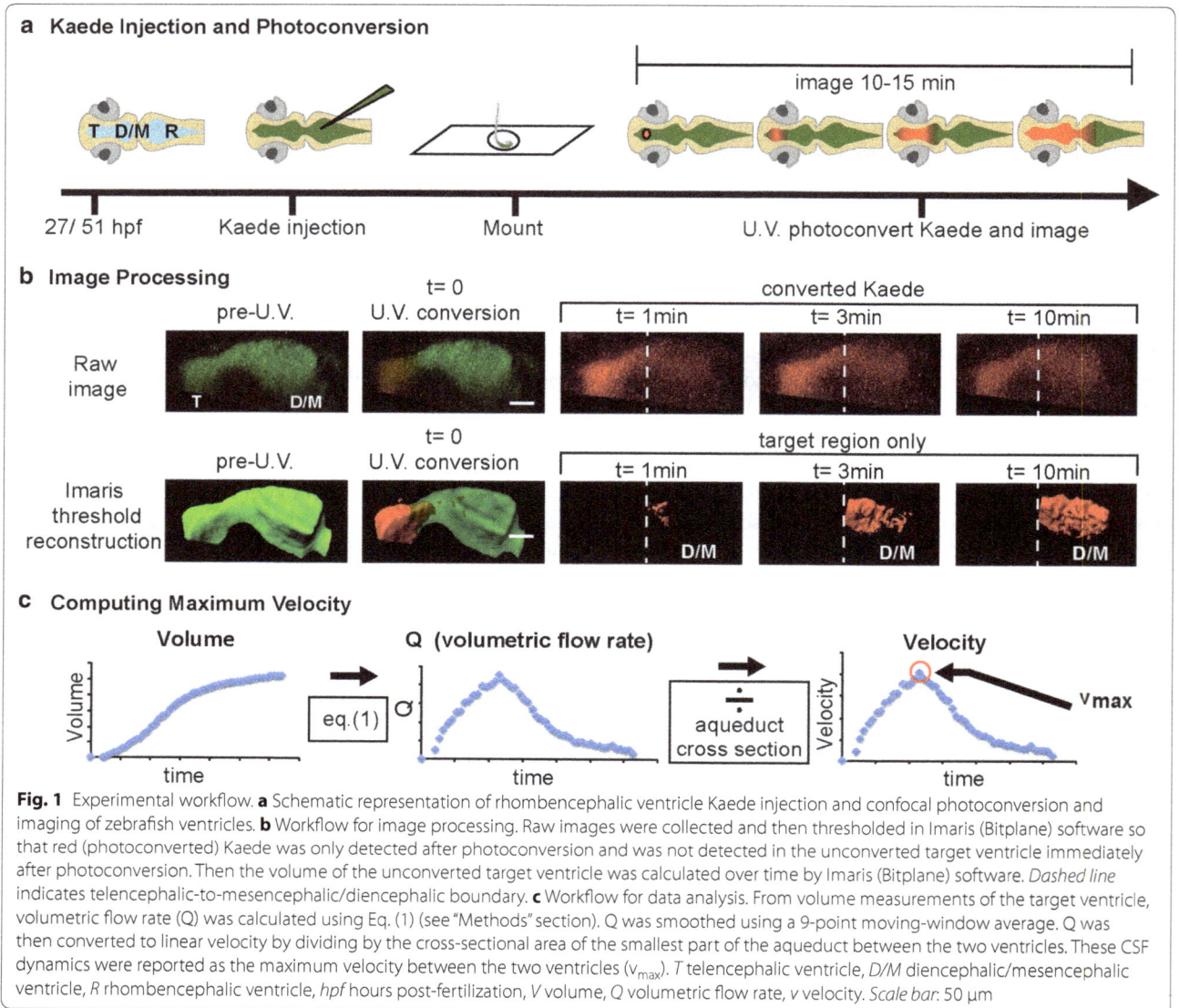

ventricle developing a more complex shape as development proceeds allowing the two regions to be discernible (Fig. 2d, e). The ventricular volume increases over development and the total volume of the ventricular system is ~4 nL at early larval stage, ~5.5 nL at late larval stage and ~6.5 nL at 5 dpf. The rhombencephalic ventricular volume increases from ~1.5 to ~3.5 nL from 30 to 54 hpf, but stabilizes at ~3.5 nL from 2 to 5 dpf. At the early larval stage, the isthmic (D/M-to-R) canal is significantly narrower than the anterior (T-to-D/M) canal (cross-sectional area: anterior: $1667 \pm 131.3$ μm$^2$; n = 18 vs. isthmic: $1159 \pm 61.9$ μm$^2$; p = 0.0016). At the late larval stage, the isthmic (D-to-R) and anterior (T-to-D) canals are smaller than at early larval stage, but are equal to one another (cross-sectional area: anterior:

$665.3 \pm 118.0$ μm$^2$; n = 17 vs. isthmic: $716.2 \pm 129.5$ μm$^2$; n = 21; p = 0.78). By 5 dpf, the adult connection from the R ventricle to the SC is forming (Fig. 2g–i'). These data add detail to the anatomical understanding of the developing ventricular system and ventricular dimensions may also play a role in influencing CSF movement.

## CSF moves from anterior to posterior in early larval zebrafish brain ventricles, but partially reverses direction at late larval stages

To quantify CSF movement during the major period of developmental neurogenesis, we filled the ventricles with photoactivatable Kaede protein. Kaede was injected into zebrafish brain ventricles and activated by a local UV pulse at 405 nm in the T, D (D/M) or R ventricle at early

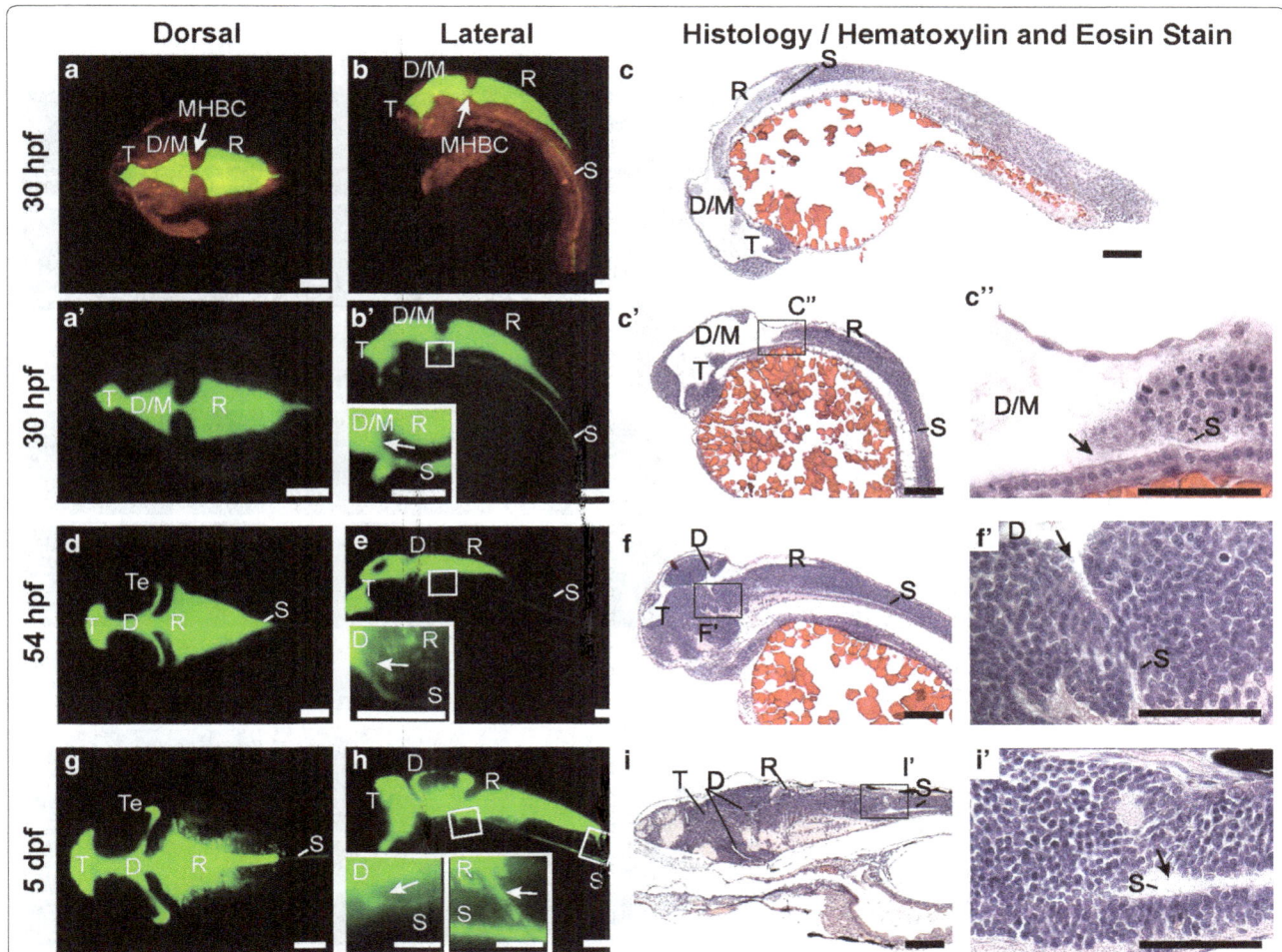

**Fig. 2** Zebrafish brain ventricle anatomy at early and late larval stages. Using 2 nL rhomencephalic ventricular injections of fluorescein-labeled dextran and imaging by Selective Plane Illumination Microscopy (SPIM, or Lightsheet Microscopy), ventricular system anatomy, volume, and connectivity was visualized in three dimensions. **a** Dorsal, **b** lateral view, 30 hpf zebrafish larvae with neuroepithelium labeled in *red* (mApple-caax) and the ventricular system labeled in *green* (fluorescein dextran injection). **c** H&E stain of 4 μm thick parasagittal section of 30 hpf zebrafish. **a′** Dorsal, **b′** Lateral view, 30 hpf larval zebrafish ventricular system. **b′** *inset* Magnification of *boxed* region in **b′** to show spinal canal (S) branching from the ventral aspect of the D/M ventricle (*arrow*). **c′** H&E stain of 4 μm thick section of 30 hpf zebrafish. **c″** magnification of *boxed* region in **c′** to show spinal canal (S) branching from D/M ventricle. **d** Dorsal, **e** Lateral view, 54 hpf larval zebrafish ventricular system. **e** *inset* Magnification of *boxed* region in **d** to show SC branching from the ventral aspect of the diencephalon (*arrow*). **f** H&E stain of 4 μm thick section of 54 hpf zebrafish. **f′** magnification of *boxed* region in **f** to show spinal canal (S) branching from diencephalon. **g** Dorsal, **h** Lateral view of the 5 dpf larval zebrafish ventricular system. **h** *insets* Magnification of *boxed* regions in **h** to show SC branching from the ventral aspect of the diencephalon (*arrow*) and rhombencephalon (*arrow*). **i** H&E stain of 4 μm thick section of 5 dpf zebrafish. **i′** magnification of *boxed* region in **i** to show spinal canal (S) branching from rhombencephalon. *T* telencephalic ventricle, *D/M* diencephalic/mesencephalic ventricle, *D* diencephalic ventricle, *Te* tectal ventricle, *R* rhombencephalic ventricle, *S* spinal canal, *hpf* hours post-fertilization, *dpf* days post-fertilization. *Scale bar*: **b′**, **e**, **h** *insets*, **c″**, **f′**, **i′**: 50 μm; all others: 100 μm

or late larval stages. CSF movement was subsequently determined and $v_{max}$ calculated (see "Methods" section, Fig. 1). At 27–30 hpf (early larva), the average $v_{max}$ for CSF movement from T to D/M ventricle is significantly greater than for CSF movement in the reverse direction, from D/M to T ventricle (Fig. 3a–c). Preferential anterior-to-posterior movement is also observed in the D/M to R ventricle direction in early larvae (Fig. 3d–f).

However, at late larval stages (51–54 hpf) the average $v_{max}$ for CSF movement from T to D/Te ventricle is less than that of CSF movement in the D to T ventricular direction (Fig. 3g–i), indicating a reversed direction of movement between these two ventricles comparing the stages examined. The anterior-to-posterior directionality is still observed between D and R ventricles at these later stages (Fig. 3j–l).

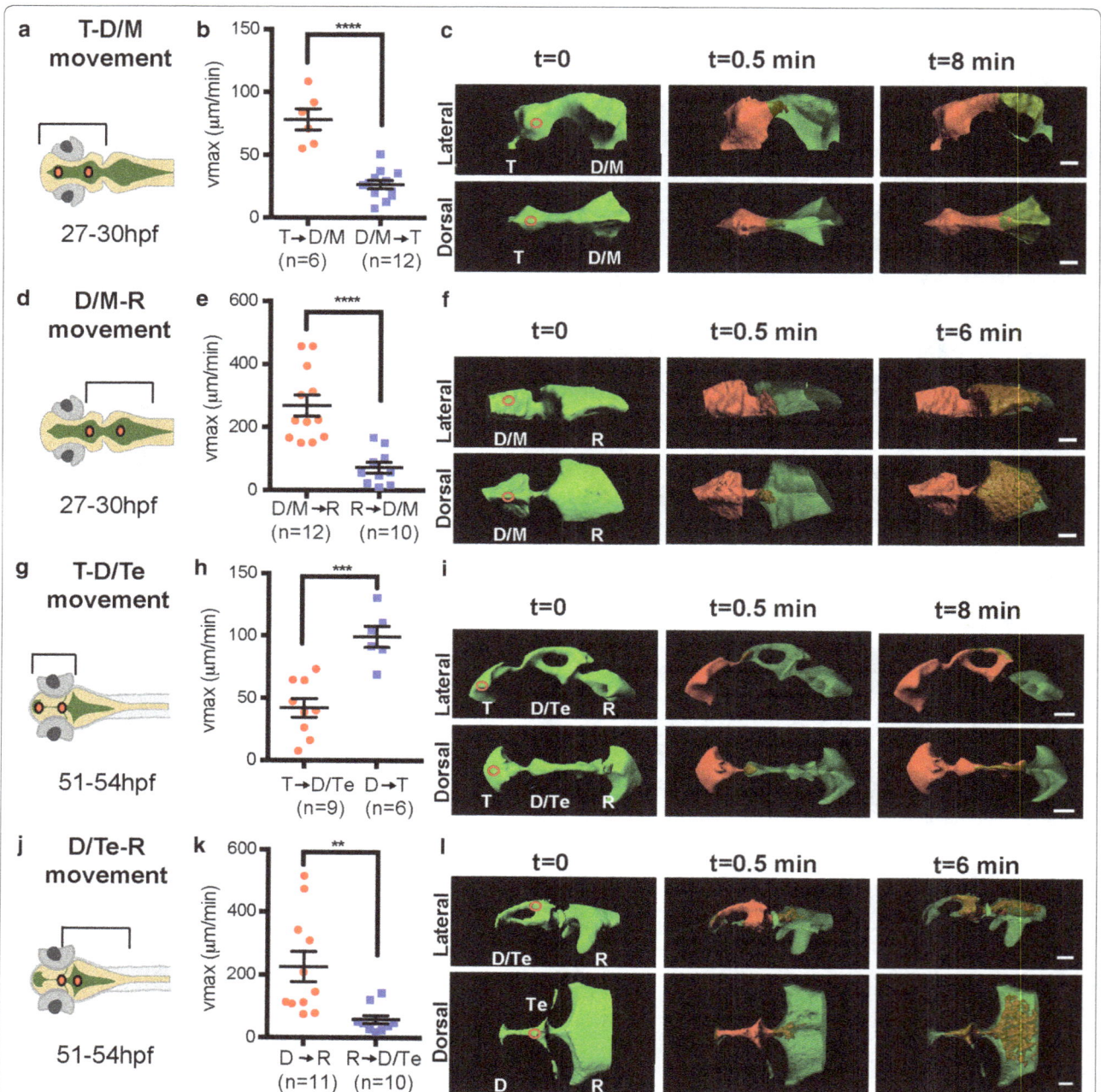

**Fig. 3** Bulk movement of CSF at early and late larval stages. **a**, **d**, **g**, **j** Schematics of brain ventricular regions analyzed. **b** At 27–30 hpf, the average $v_{max}$ is significantly higher in the anterior to posterior (*red*) direction through the telencephalic-to-diencephalic/mesencephalic aqueduct than in the posterior to anterior direction (*blue*). **c** Overlaid thresholded volumes generated by Imaris (Bitplane) software of a representative 27–30 hpf T → D/M dataset. **e** At 27–30 hpf, the average $v_{max}$ is significantly higher in the anterior to posterior (*red*) direction through the diencephalic/mesencephalic-to-rhombencephalic aqueduct than in the posterior to anterior direction (*blue*). **f** Overlaid thresholded volumes generated by Imaris (Bitplane) software of a representative 27–30 hpf D/M → R dataset. **h** At 51–54 hpf, through the telencephalic-to-diencephalic aqueduct, directionality is reversed such that the $v_{max}$ is significantly higher in the posterior to anterior (*blue*) direction through the telencephalic-to-diencephalic aqueduct than in the anterior to posterior direction (*red*). **i** Overlaid thresholded volumes generated by Imaris (Bitplane) software of a representative 51–54 hpf T → D dataset. **k** At 51–54 hpf, the average $v_{max}$ is significantly higher in the anterior to posterior (*red*) direction through the diencephalic-to-rhombencephalic aqueduct than in the posterior to anterior direction (*blue*). **l** Overlaid thresholded volumes generated by Imaris (Bitplane) software of a representative 51–54 hpf D → R dataset. *Red circles* indicate photoconversion region. *Lines* represent average $v_{max}$ and *error bars* denote SEM. p value calculated using unpaired Student's t test, **p < 0.001; ***p < 0.0005; ****p < 0.0001. *T* telencephalic ventricle, *D/M* diencephalic/mesencephalic ventricle, *Te* tectal ventricle, *R* rhombencephalic ventricle, *hpf* hours post-fertilization. *Scale bar*: 50 μm

## CSF directional movement is dependent on heartbeat at early larval stages

Adult CSF pulses and mixes during the cardiac cycle and with breathing [15–18], zebrafish ventricle expansion and early *Xenopus* CSF movement is dependent on heartbeat [19, 34]. We therefore investigated whether directionality of CSF movement is dependent on heartbeat at early larval stages (27–30 hpf). Heartbeat was prevented genetically using the *tnnt2a*$^{-/-}$ fish that never develop a heartbeat. In *tnnt2a*$^{-/-}$ fish, directionality was maintained (albeit with a less significant difference), but $v_{max}$ from D/M → T ventricle in *tnnt2a*$^{-/-}$ animals is significantly higher than in WT and is unchanged from T → D/M ventricle (Fig. 4a). However, loss of *tnnt2a* function eliminated directional movement between the D/M and R ventricles and $v_{max}$ was significantly lower from D/M → R ventricle than in WT, but unchanged from R → D/M (Fig. 4b). To acutely disrupt heartbeat, we treated WT fish with 40 mM 2,3 butanedione monoxime (BDM). In BDM-treated animals $v_{max}$ directionality was eliminated in both T → D/M and D/M → R ventricular directions (Additional file 1: Fig. S3). BDM has a wide variety of targets that are not associated with heartbeat disruption (see "Methods" and "Discussion" sections), which might account for differences observed in CSF movement between BDM-treated and *tnnt2a*$^{-/-}$ animals. These data suggest that the heartbeat is partially required to maintain directional CSF movement, specifically between D/M and R. In *tnnt2a*$^{-/-}$ fish, the ventricles develop normally until 27 hpf but do not fully inflate at 36 hpf [34], suggesting brain abnormalities that could be attributed to disruption in CSF movement.

## Brain ventricle cilia are non-motile at 27 hpf and cannot contribute to directional CSF movement

It has been suggested that ciliary beating in the neuroepithelium bordering the brain ventricular lumen drives CSF movement [46]. Monociliated cells are present in the zebrafish neuroepithelium at the stages examined [25], so we investigated whether these cilia beat in a concerted fashion. Early central nervous system cilia in the zebrafish spinal canal beat at ~12 Hz [38], but motility of the cilia in the early zebrafish brain has not been characterized. Using the Tg(*βact:Arl13b*–GFP) transgenic line (Fig. 5a, c) to visualize CNS cilia, we confirmed that a subset of spinal canal cilia beat at early (27 hpf) and late (51 hpf) larval stages (Fig. 5; Additional file 2: Movie S1, Additional file 3: Movie S2). At the early larval stage, cilia in the neuroepithelium do not beat (Fig. 5b, e; Additional file 2: Movie S1). However in late larvae, motile brain cilia are observed in telencephalon and are

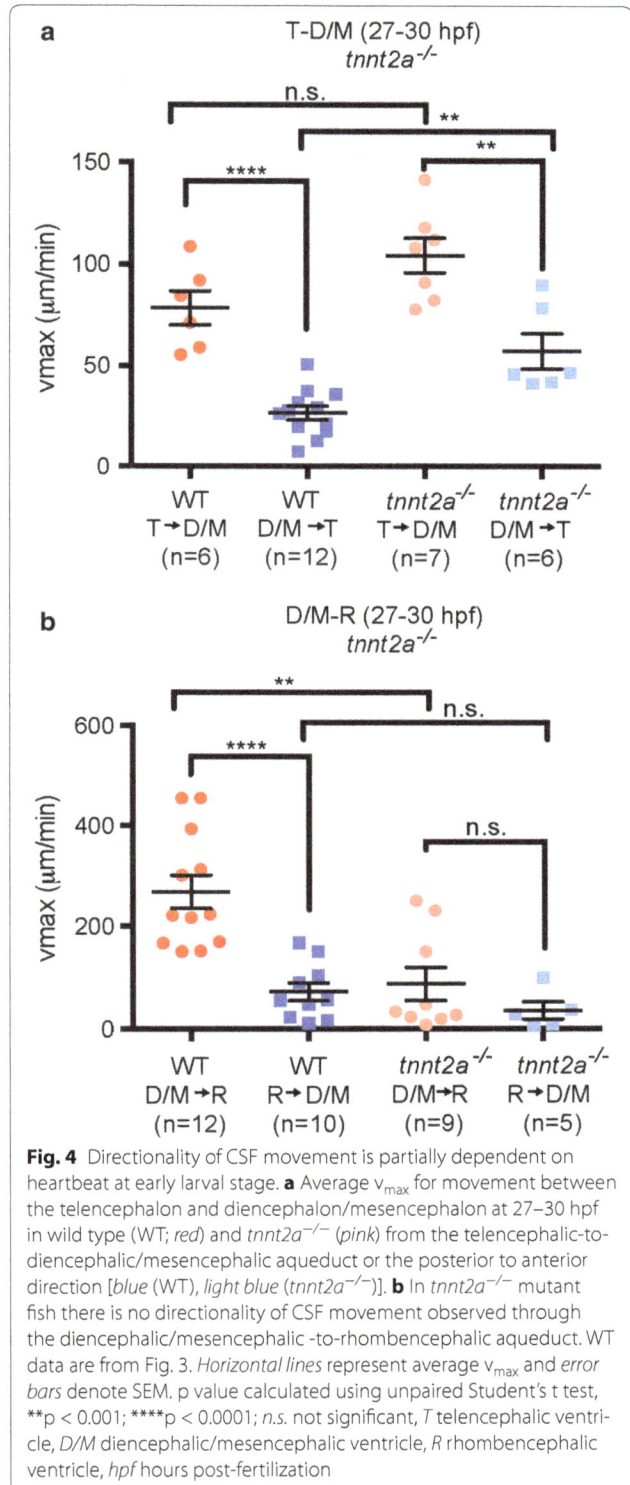

**Fig. 4** Directionality of CSF movement is partially dependent on heartbeat at early larval stage. **a** Average $v_{max}$ for movement between the telencephalon and diencephalon/mesencephalon at 27–30 hpf in wild type (WT; *red*) and *tnnt2a*$^{-/-}$ (*pink*) from the telencephalic-to-diencephalic/mesencephalic aqueduct or the posterior to anterior direction [*blue* (WT), *light blue* (*tnnt2a*$^{-/-}$)]. **b** In *tnnt2a*$^{-/-}$ mutant fish there is no directionality of CSF movement observed through the diencephalic/mesencephalic -to-rhombencephalic aqueduct. WT data are from Fig. 3. *Horizontal lines* represent average $v_{max}$ and *error bars* denote SEM. p value calculated using unpaired Student's t test, **p < 0.001; ****p < 0.0001; *n.s.* not significant, *T* telencephalic ventricle, *D/M* diencephalic/mesencephalic ventricle, *R* rhombencephalic ventricle, *hpf* hours post-fertilization

especially active in the diencephalon (Fig. 5d, f; Additional file 3: Movie S2). We conclude that at early larval stages it is unlikely that the immotile cilia contribute to CSF movement.

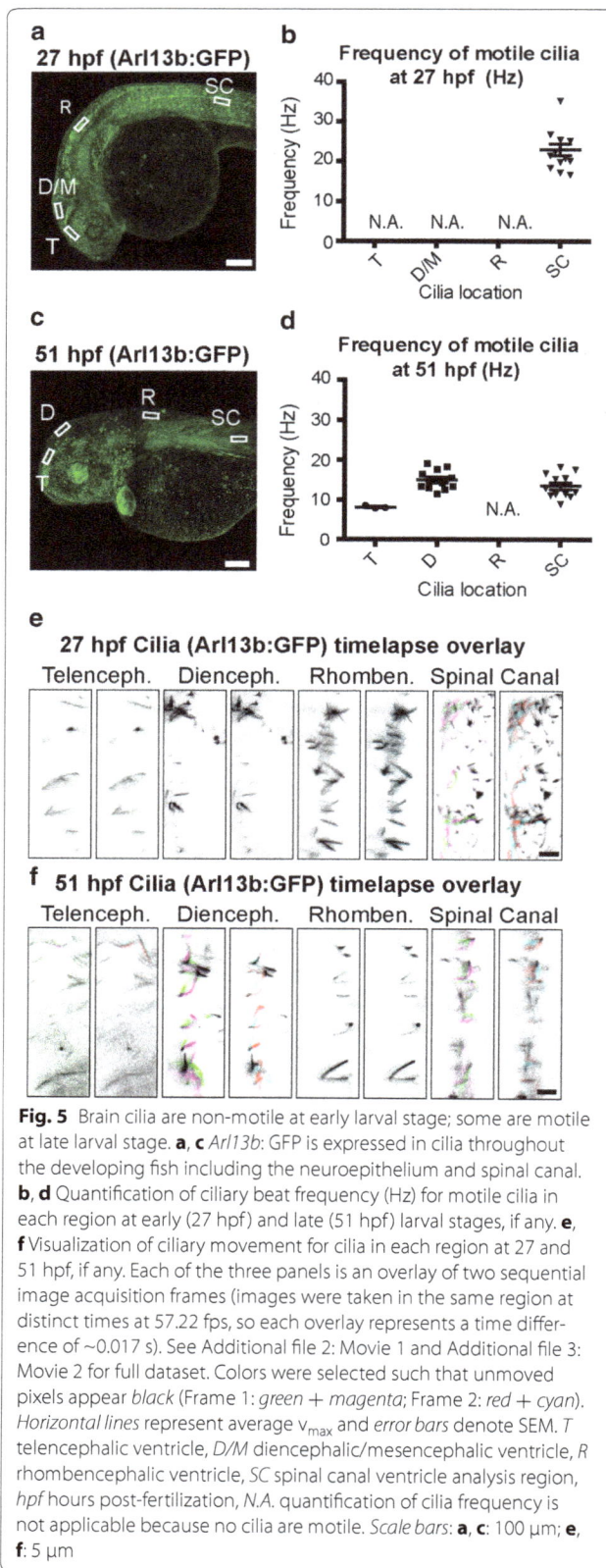

**Fig. 5** Brain cilia are non-motile at early larval stage; some are motile at late larval stage. **a, c** *Arl13b*: GFP is expressed in cilia throughout the developing fish including the neuroepithelium and spinal canal. **b, d** Quantification of ciliary beat frequency (Hz) for motile cilia in each region at early (27 hpf) and late (51 hpf) larval stages, if any. **e, f** Visualization of ciliary movement for cilia in each region at 27 and 51 hpf, if any. Each of the three panels is an overlay of two sequential image acquisition frames (images were taken in the same region at distinct times at 57.22 fps, so each overlay represents a time difference of ~0.017 s). See Additional file 2: Movie 1 and Additional file 3: Movie 2 for full dataset. Colors were selected such that unmoved pixels appear *black* (Frame 1: *green + magenta*; Frame 2: *red + cyan*). *Horizontal lines* represent average $v_{max}$ and *error bars* denote SEM. *T* telencephalic ventricle, *D/M* diencephalic/mesencephalic ventricle, *R* rhombencephalic ventricle, *SC* spinal canal ventricle analysis region, *hpf* hours post-fertilization, *N.A.* quantification of cilia frequency is not applicable because no cilia are motile. *Scale bars*: **a, c**: 100 μm; **e, f**: 5 μm

## Discussion

In this study, we expanded understanding of CSF dynamics through quantification of CSF movement. Using the zebrafish model, we focused on the major period of developmental neurogenesis at two stages: early larva [pharyngula stage; 27–30 h post-fertilization (hpf)] and late larva (hatching period; 51–54 hpf). Our study leads to four conclusions: (1) CSF moves preferentially anterior to posterior from the diencephalic (D) (or combined diencephalic/mesencephalic superventricle (D/M)) to rhombencephalic (R) ventricles. (2) Direction of CSF movement between the telencephalic (T) and diencephalic (D) ventricles reverses from early to late larval stages. (3) Directional CSF movement is partially dependent on heartbeat. (4) At early larval stages no motile cilia are present in the brain and therefore are not likely to direct the CSF movement observed. Together these data indicate that locally restricted CSF factors or physical signals associated with fluid movement may contribute to specialization of the early brain.

The primarily unidirectional CSF movement observed between D (or D/M) and R ventricles was associated with a large $v_{max}$ from D (D/M) to R ventricles. Reverse movement was present, but with about 25 % of the observed forward $v_{max}$. This raises two questions: (1) where does the excess volume of CSF entering the R ventricle go and (2) what mechanisms underlie directional CSF movement? First, with respect to CSF "destination", the brain-CSF barrier is quite tight at early developmental stages [47], however small molecules (<70 kDa) can pass between the ventricles and the neuroepithelium [36]. Water is also likely selectively transported since aquaporins 1a.1, 3a, 7 are expressed by the neuroepithelium [48]. Therefore some CSF components could pass in or out of the ventricular system. Additionally, we note that R ventricle volume more than doubles over this timeframe of development, perhaps due to CSF influx from more anterior ventricles as movement proceeds from D → R ventricles. Second, with respect to potential mechanisms of directional CSF movement at the stages examined, the choroid plexuses (CP) are not yet mature and there is unlikely to be active secretion from CP precursors. It is not known at what stage the CPs become mature and secrete CSF in zebrafish. Ventricles inflate at approximately 20 hpf [34] with no evidence of CPs. Henson et al. [49] claim that the zebrafish CP are mostly mature by 3 dpf, but Garcia-Lecea et al. [50] report more complete maturation and coalescing of the CP in the R ventricle by 5 dpf. However, even without secretory CP, different regions of the neuroepithelium could produce CSF at different rates to drive directional movement. Alternately, osmolarity differences between the ventricles could drive directional CSF movement, a mechanism that contributes to diffusion gradients in adult brain [51].

Directional CSF movement from D (D/M) to R ventricles could result in factors from the D (D/M) ventricle entering the R ventricle, but factors unique to the R ventricle may remain largely distinct from those of D (D/M). The stages examined encompass a major period of neurogenesis, when the detailed patterns of the diencephalon, mesencephalon, and rhombencephalon begin to read out as distinct neuronal and glial differentiation programs. Thus differentially localized CSF factors could modulate differentiation of the optic tectum (which is derived from the mesencephalic epithelium) or the cerebellum and medulla (which is derived from the rhombencephalic epithelium). At the stages examined, the spinal canal connects to the D (D/M) ventricle. We observed no converted Kaede protein in the spinal canal (data not shown), indicating that the vast majority of D (D/M) CSF movement is into the R ventricle, consistent with the smaller diameter of the spinal canal connector relative to the isthmic canal.

A surprising contrast to the consistent direction of movement between D (D/M) and R ventricles was the reversal of direction between T and D (D/M) ventricles when early and late larval stages were examined. What would lead to this reversal? One possibility is that at late larval stages, CP cells present along the D ventricle, which arise later but complete differentiation first, have begun to coalesce and are producing CSF, while the CP cells in the R and T ventricles have not yet completed differentiation [50, 52]. This could lead to greater pressure from in the D ventricle from more mature CP cells and promote CSF entry into the T ventricle, where the CP is the last to form [31]. Therefore, posterior-to-anterior CSF movement between D and T ventricles could result from active CSF secretion and greater D ventricular CSF pressure. The strong ciliary movement in D neuroepithelium relative to T neuroepithelium at late larva stage may also contribute to reversal of flow. Another possibility is that the reverse flow could result from gradually increasing pressure in the D ventricle as result of ventricular shape change and the subsequent reduction in D ventricular volume as development proceeds. Whatever the mechanism, the outcome of this change in direction would be that at early larval stages CSF in the D ventricle would contain factors derived from the T, whereas at late larval stages CSF in the T ventricle would contain some components derived from the D. Thus distinct cohorts of factors in T or D ventricles could be present at each stage.

Heartbeat plays a role in CSF dynamics early in brain development, as has also been shown in *Xenopus* [19]. After *tnnt2a* loss of function, a mechanism independent of heartbeat, perhaps CSF production, maintains directional CSF movement from T and D/M ventricles, but not for D/M to R ventricular movement, although there is a trend toward less significant directionality.

Consistently, acute loss of heartbeat with BDM treatment disrupts all directional CSF movement. However, BDM prevents action of all muscles (and can alter activities of connexins [39], potassium channels [40, 41] and L-type calcium channels [42]) and some of these side effects may contribute to the phenotypes observed.

At early larval stages no motile cilia are present in the neuroepithelium and are therefore unlikely to contribute to the CSF movement observed. The non-motile cilia at this time may be able to detect CSF movement, potentially to activate planar cell polarity signaling described by Ohata and colleagues [21], or to guide migrating neurons or extending axons [54]. At late larval stages, cilia along the D ventricle are highly motile and may indicate differentiating CP, as CP cells have motile cilia [52]. As discussed above, these ciliary movements or CSF production may drive CSF movement from D to T ventricles. Mutants that disrupt the primary cilia present with hydrocephalus [53], which would preclude clear comparison of CSF movement. However, future studies acutely disrupting cilia are needed to fully address potential roles of cilia in CSF movement.

In summary, this study demonstrates directional CSF movement during early brain development. One outcome of this may be differential concentrations of CSF factors in different ventricles, which may contribute to regional specialization of the brain. Directional CSF movement may also act as a physical signal to modulate neuroepithelial fates. The zebrafish offers an excellent system with which to address these intriguing possibilities.

## Conclusion

Embryonic CSF in the zebrafish model moves directionally during the major period of developmental neurogenesis. Specifically, CSF moves preferentially from the diencephalic into the rhombencephalic ventricle. In addition, direction of CSF movement between telencephalic and diencephalic ventricles reverses from early [pharyngula stage; 27–30 h post-fertilization (hpf)] to late (hatching period; 51–54 hpf) larval stages. CSF movement is partially dependent on heartbeat. At early larval stages, the absence of motile cilia indicates that cilia likely do not direct CSF movement. These data suggest that CSF components may be compartmentalized and could contribute to specialization of the early brain and CSF movement may also provide directional mechanical cues.

## Abbreviations

BDM: 2,3 butanedione monoxime; CP: choroid plexus; CSF: cerebrospinal fluid; D: diencephalon; D/M: combined diencephalic/mesencephalic superventricle; dpf: days post-fertilization; hpf: hours post-fertilization; Q: volumetric flow rate; R: rhombencephalon; SC: spinal canal; SPIM: Selective Plane Illumination Microscopy; T: telencephalon; v: velocity; V: volume; WT: wild-type animals.

## Authors' contributions

RMF completed all experimental components and wrote the paper. AH contributed to experimental data collection. JTC and NAS contributed to the design and feasibility of experiments and produced the Kaede protein. HLS contributed to experimental design, interpretation of results, and to writing the paper. All authors read and approved the final manuscript.

## Author details

[1] Whitehead Institute for Biomedical Research, Nine Cambridge Center, Cambridge, MA 02142, USA. [2] Massachusetts Institute of Technology, 77 Massachusetts Avenue, Cambridge, MA 02139-4307, USA.

## Acknowledgements

The Tg(βact:Arl13b–GFP) transgenic fish line was a kind gift from Brian Ciruna (Sick Kids/University of Toronto). The authors would also like to thank Rotem Gura, Jeremy England, and Mark Bathe (MIT) for thoughtful discussions about fluid dynamics; the Koch Institute Swanson Biotechnology Center, specifically the Hope Babette Tang Histology Facility, for technical support; Wendy Salmon (The Whitehead Institute W. M. Keck Microscopy Facility) and Douglas Richardson (The Harvard Center for Biological Imaging) for valuable insight into appropriate imaging methods; members of the Sive lab for helpful comments; and Olivier Paugois for expert fish husbandry.

## Competing interests

The authors declare they have no competing interests.

## Funding

This work was supported by NSF IOS-1258087 (H. Sive PI), the HHMI-funded MIT Biology Summer internship program (NAS), and by the Balkin-Markell-Weinberg Postdoctoral Fellowship (RMF).

## References

1. Martín C, Bueno D, Alonso MI, Ja Moro, Callejo S, Parada C, et al. FGF2 plays a key role in embryonic cerebrospinal fluid trophic properties over chick embryo neuroepithelial stem cells. Dev Biol. 2006;297:402–16. doi:10.1016/j.ydbio.2006.05.010.
2. Huang X, Liu J, Ketova T, Fleming JT, Grover VK, Cooper MK, et al. Transventricular delivery of Sonic hedgehog is essential to cerebellar ventricular zone development. Proc Natl Acad Sci USA. 2010;107(18):8422–7. doi:10.1073/pnas.0911838107.
3. Lehtinen MK, Zappaterra MW, Chen X, Yang YJ, Hill AD, Lun M, et al. The cerebrospinal fluid provides a proliferative niche for neural progenitor cells. Neuron. 2011;69:893–905. doi:10.1016/j.neuron.2011.01.023.
4. Parada C, Gato A, Bueno D. All-trans retinol and retinol-binding protein from embryonic cerebrospinal fluid exhibit dynamic behaviour during early central nervous system development. NeuroReport. 2008;19(9):945–50. doi:10.1097/WNR.0b013e3283021c94.
5. Chau KF, Springel MW, Broadbelt KG, Park HY, Topal S, Lun MP, et al. Progressive differentiation and instructive capacities of amniotic fluid and cerebrospinal fluid proteomes following neural tube closure. Dev Cell. 2015;35(6):789–802. doi:10.1016/j.devcel.2015.11.015.
6. Zappaterra MD, Lisgo SN, Lindsay S, Gygi SP, Walsh CA, Ballif BA. A comparative proteomic analysis of human and rat embryonic cerebrospinal fluid. J Proteome Res. 2007;6(9):3537–48. doi:10.1021/pr070247w.
7. Chang JT, Lehtinen MK, Sive H. Zebrafish cerebrospinal fluid mediates cell survival through a retinoid signaling pathway. Dev Neurobiol. 2016;76(1):75–92. doi:10.1002/dneu.22300.
8. Feliciano DM, Zhang S, Nasrallah CM, Lisgo SN, Bordey A. Embryonic cerebrospinal fluid nanovesicles carry evolutionarily conserved molecules and promote neural stem cell amplification. PLoS One. 2014;9:1–10. doi:10.1371/journal.pone.0088810.
9. Gato Á, Moro JA, Alonso MI, Bueno D, De La Mano A, Martín C. Embryonic cerebrospinal fluid regulates neuroepithelial survival, proliferation, and neurogenesis in chick embryos. Anat Rec A Discov Mol Cell Evol Biol. 2005;284:475–84. doi:10.1002/ar.a.20185.
10. O'Rahilly R, Muller F. Ventricular system and choroid plexuses of the human brain during the embryonic period proper. Am J Anat. 1990;189(4):285–302. doi:10.1002/aja.1001890402.
11. Brinker T, Stopa E, Morrison J, Klinge P. A new look at cerebrospinal fluid circulation. Fluids and Barriers CNS. 2014;11:10. doi:10.1186/2045-8118-11-10.
12. Pollay M, Curl F. Secretion of cerebrospinal fluid by the ventricular ependyma of the rabbit. Am J Physiol. 1967;213(4):1031–8.
13. Sonnenberg H, Solomon S, Frazier DT. Sodium and chloride movement into the central canal of cat spinal cord. Proc Soc Exp Biol Med. 1967;124(4):1316–20.
14. Davson H. The physiology of the cerebrospinal fluid. London: Churchill; 1967.
15. Bakshi R, Caruthers SD, Janardhan V, Wasay M. Intraventricular CSF pulsation artifact on fast fluid-attenuated inversion-recovery MR images: analysis of 100 consecutive normal studies. AJNR Am J Neuroradiol. 2000;21(3):503–8.
16. Bradley WG Jr, Scalzo D, Queralt J, Nitz WN, Atkinson DJ, Wong P. Normal-pressure hydrocephalus: evaluation with cerebrospinal fluid flow measurements at MR imaging. Radiology. 1996;198(2):523–9. doi:10.1148/radiology.198.2.8596861.
17. Sherman JL, Citrin CM, Gangarosa RE, Bowen BJ. The MR appearance of CSF flow in patients with ventriculomegaly. AJR Am J Roentgenol. 1987;148(1):193–9. doi:10.2214/ajr.148.1.193.
18. Brinker T, Ludemann W, Berens von Rautenfeld D, Samii M. Dynamic properties of lymphatic pathways for the absorption of cerebrospinal fluid. Acta Neuropathol. 1997;94(5):493–8.
19. Miskevich F. Imaging fluid flow and cilia beating pattern in Xenopus brain ventricles. J Neurosci Methods. 2010;189:1–4. doi:10.1016/j.jneumeth.2010.02.015.
20. Hagenlocher C, Walentek P, Ller C, Thumberger T, Feistel K. Ciliogenesis and cerebrospinal fluid flow in the developing Xenopus brain are regulated by foxj1. Cilia. 2013;2:12. doi:10.1186/2046-2530-2-12.
21. Ohata S, Herranz-Perez V, Nakatani J, Boletta A, Garcia-Verdugo JM, Alvarez-Buylla A. Mechanosensory genes Pkd1 and Pkd2 contribute to the planar polarization of brain ventricular epithelium. J Neurosci. 2015;35(31):11153–68. doi:10.1523/JNEUROSCI.0686-15.2015.
22. Turner MH, Ullmann JF, Kay AR. A method for detecting molecular transport within the cerebral ventricles of live zebrafish (Danio rerio) larvae. J Physiol. 2012;590(Pt 10):2233–40. doi:10.1113/jphysiol.2011.225896.
23. Westerfield M. The zebrafish book. a guide for the laboratory use of zebrafish (Danio rerio). 3rd ed. Eugene: University of Oregon Press; 1995.
24. Kimmel CB, Ballard WW, Kimmel SR, Ullmann B, Schilling TF. Stages of embryonic development of the zebrafish. Dev Dyn. 1995;203:253–310. doi:10.1002/aja.1002030302.
25. Borovina A, Superina S, Voskas D, Ciruna B. Vangl2 directs the posterior tilting and asymmetric localization of motile primary cilia. Nat Cell Biol. 2010;12(4):407–12. doi:10.1038/ncb2042.
26. Clark KJ, Balciunas D, Pogoda HM, Ding Y, Westcot SE, Bedell VM, et al. In vivo protein trapping produces a functional expression codex of the vertebrate proteome. Nat Methods. 2011;8(6):506–15. doi:10.1038/nmeth.1606.
27. Muntean BS, Horvat CM, Behler JH, Aboualaiwi WA, Nauli AM, Williams FE, et al. A comparative study of embedded and anesthetized zebrafish in vivo on myocardial calcium oscillation and heart muscle contraction. Front Pharmacol. 2010;1:139. doi:10.3389/fphar.2010.00139.

28. Strykowski JL, Schech JM. Effectiveness of recommended euthanasia methods in larval zebrafish (Danio rerio). J Am Assoc Lab Anim Sci. 2015;54(1):81–4.

29. Denvir MA, Tucker CS, Mullins JJ. Systolic and diastolic ventricular function in zebrafish embryos: influence of norepenephrine, MS-222 and temperature. BMC Biotechnol. 2008;8:21. doi:10.1186/1472-6750-8-21.

30. Schneider CA, Rasband WS, Eliceiri KW. NIH Image to ImageJ: 25 years of image analysis. Nat Methods. 2012;9(7):671–5.

31. Schindelin J, Arganda-Carreras I, Frise E, Kaynig V, Longair M, Pietzsch T, et al. Fiji: an open-source platform for biological-image analysis. Nat Methods. 2012;9(7):676–82. doi:10.1038/nmeth.2019.

32. Preibisch S, Amat F, Stamataki E, Sarov M, Singer RH, Myers E, et al. Efficient Bayesian-based multiview deconvolution. Nat Methods. 2014;11(6):645–8. doi:10.1038/nmeth.2929.

33. Preibisch S, Saalfeld S, Schindelin J, Tomancak P. Software for bead-based registration of selective plane illumination microscopy data. Nat Methods. 2010;7(6):418–9. doi:10.1038/nmeth0610-418.

34. Lowery LA, Sive H. Initial formation of zebrafish brain ventricles occurs independently of circulation and requires the nagie oko and snakehead/atp1a1a.1 gene products. Development. 2005;132:2057–67. doi:10.1242/dev.01791.

35. Sheehan DC, Hrapchak BB. Theory and practice of histotechnology. 2nd ed. Columbus: Battelle Press; 1980.

36. Chang JT, Sive H. An assay for permeability of the zebrafish embryonic neuroepithelium. J Vis Exp. 2012;68:e4242. doi:10.3791/4242.

37. Gutzman JH, Sive H. Zebrafish brain ventricle injection. J Vis Exp. 2009. doi:10.3791/1218.

38. Kramer-Zucker AG, Olale F, Haycraft CJ, Yoder BK, Schier AF, Drummond IA. Cilia-driven fluid flow in the zebrafish pronephros, brain and Kupffer's vesicle is required for normal organogenesis. Development. 2005;132:1907–21. doi:10.1242/dev.01772.

39. Verrecchia F, Herve JC. Reversible blockade of gap junctional communication by 2,3-butanedione monoxime in rat cardiac myocytes. Am J Physiol. 1997;272(3 Pt 1):C875–85.

40. Schlichter LC, Pahapill PA, Chung I. Dual action of 2,3-butanedione monoxime (BDM) on K+ current in human T lymphocytes. J Pharmacol Exp Ther. 1992;261(2):438–46.

41. Lopatin AN, Nichols CG. 2,3-Butanedione monoxime (BDM) inhibition of delayed rectifier DRK1 (Kv2.1) potassium channels expressed in Xenopus oocytes. J Pharmacol Exp Ther. 1993;265(2):1011–6.

42. Ferreira G, Artigas P, Pizarro G, Brum G. Butanedione monoxime promotes voltage-dependent inactivation of L-type calcium channels in heart. Effects on gating currents. J Mol Cell Cardiol. 1997;29(2):777–87.

43. Thevenaz P, Ruttimann UE, Unser M. A pyramid approach to subpixel registration based on intensity. IEEE Trans Image Process. 1998;7(1):27–41. doi:10.1109/83.650848.

44. Chilvers MA, O'Callaghan C. Analysis of ciliary beat pattern and beat frequency using digital high speed imaging: comparison with the photomultiplier and photodiode methods. Thorax. 2000;55(4):314–7.

45. Butler AB, Hodos W. Comparative vertebrate neuroanatomy: evolution and adaptation. 2nd ed. Hoboken: Wiley-Interscience; 2005.

46. Narita K, Takeda S. Cilia in the choroid plexus: their roles in hydrocephalus and beyond. Front Cell Neurosci. 2015;9:39. doi:10.3389/fncel.2015.00039.

47. Stolp HB, Liddelow SA, Sa-Pereira I, Dziegielewska KM, Saunders NR. Immune responses at brain barriers and implications for brain development and neurological function in later life. Front Integr Neurosci. 2013;7:61. doi:10.3389/fnint.2013.00061.

48. Thisse B, Heyer V, Lux A, Alunni V, Degrave A, Seiliez I, et al. Spatial and temporal expression of the zebrafish genome by large-scale in situ hybridization screening. Methods Cell Biol. 2004;77:505–19.

49. Henson HE, Parupalli C, Ju B, Taylor MR. Functional and genetic analysis of choroid plexus development in zebrafish. Front Neurosci. 2014;8:364. doi:10.3389/fnins.2014.00364.

50. Garcia-Lecea M, Kondrychyn I, Fong SH, Ye ZR, Korzh V. In vivo analysis of choroid plexus morphogenesis in zebrafish. PLoS One. 2008;3(9):e3090. doi:10.1371/journal.pone.0003090.

51. Bito LZ, Davson H. Local variations in cerebrospinal fluid composition and its relationship to the composition of the extracellular fluid of the cortex. Exp Neurol. 1966;14(3):264–80.

52. Lun MP, Monuki ES, Lehtinen MK. Development and functions of the choroid plexus-cerebrospinal fluid system. Nat Rev Neurosci. 2015;16(8):445–57. doi:10.1038/nrn3921.

53. Choksi SP, Babu D, Lau D, Yu X, Roy S. Systematic discovery of novel ciliary genes through functional genomics in the zebrafish. Development. 2014;141(17):3410–9. doi:10.1242/dev.108209.

54. Sawamoto K, Wichterle H, Gonzalez-Perez O, Cholfin JA, Yamada M, Spassky N, et al. New neurons follow the flow of cerebrospinal fluid in the adult brain. Science. 2006;311:629–32. doi:10.1126/science.1119133.

# 15

# Effect of shear stress on iPSC-derived human brain microvascular endothelial cells (dhBMECs)

Jackson G. DeStefano[1,2†], Zinnia S. Xu[1,3†], Ashley J. Williams[1], Nahom Yimam[1] and Peter C. Searson[1,2*] ⓘ

## Abstract

**Background:** The endothelial cells that form the lumen of capillaries and microvessels are an important component of the blood–brain barrier. Cell phenotype is regulated by transducing a range of biomechanical and biochemical signals in the local microenvironment. Here we report on the role of shear stress in modulating the morphology, motility, proliferation, apoptosis, and protein and gene expression, of confluent monolayers of human brain microvascular endothelial cells derived from induced pluripotent stem cells.

**Methods:** To assess the response of derived human brain microvascular endothelial cells (dhBMECs) to shear stress, confluent monolayers were formed in a microfluidic device. Monolayers were subjected to a shear stress of 4 or 12 dyne cm$^{-2}$ for 40 h. Static conditions were used as the control. Live cell imaging was used to assess cell morphology, cell speed, persistence, and the rates of proliferation and apoptosis as a function of time. In addition, immunofluorescence imaging and protein and gene expression analysis of key markers of the blood–brain barrier were performed.

**Results:** Human brain microvascular endothelial cells exhibit a unique phenotype in response to shear stress compared to static conditions: (1) they do not elongate and align, (2) the rates of proliferation and apoptosis decrease significantly, (3) the mean displacement of individual cells within the monolayer over time is significantly decreased, (4) there is no cytoskeletal reorganization or formation of stress fibers within the cell, and (5) there is no change in expression levels of key blood–brain barrier markers.

**Conclusions:** The characteristic response of dhBMECs to shear stress is significantly different from human and animal-derived endothelial cells from other tissues, suggesting that this unique phenotype that may be important in maintenance of the blood–brain barrier. The implications of this work are that: (1) in confluent monolayers of dhBMECs, tight junctions are formed under static conditions, (2) the formation of tight junctions decreases cell motility and prevents any morphological transitions, (3) flow serves to increase the contact area between cells, resulting in very low cell displacement in the monolayer, (4) since tight junctions are already formed under static conditions, increasing the contact area between cells does not cause upregulation in protein and gene expression of BBB markers, and (5) the increase in contact area induced by flow makes barrier function more robust.

**Keywords:** Shear stress, Brain microvascular endothelial cells (BMECs), Human endothelial cell line, Blood–brain barrier, Endothelial turnover, Cell morphology, Cell motility, Stem cells

---

*Correspondence: searson@jhu.edu
†Jackson G. DeStefano and Zinnia S. Xu contributed equally to this work
[1] Institute for Nanobiotechnology, Johns Hopkins University, 100 Croft Hall, 3400 North Charles Street, Baltimore, MD 21218, USA
Full list of author information is available at the end of the article

# Background

The blood–brain barrier (BBB) is a dynamic interface that separates the brain from the circulatory system and protects the central nervous system from potentially harmful chemicals while regulating transport of essential nutrients [1, 2]. Endothelial cells in the brain are highly specialized with tight junctions that effectively block paracellular transport and an array of transporters and efflux pumps that control entry into the brain. A reliable source of human, brain-specific cells has been a major barrier to developing BBB models [3], however, stem cell technology provides a solution to this problem [4–6]. Human iPSC-derived BMECs (dhBMECs) show expression and localization of tight junction proteins, very high transendothelial electrical resistance (TEER > 2000 Ω cm$^2$), low permeability, and polarized expression of P-gp efflux pumps [4–6].

Previous studies have been performed under static conditions, and hence the goal of this study is to assess the influence of shear stress on dhBMECs in confluent monolayers. Shear stress can play a profound role on endothelial morphology and function, regulating signaling and transport between blood and surrounding tissues [7–9]. In straight sections of large vessels under laminar flow, endothelial cells (ECs) are elongated and aligned in the direction of flow [10–13]. In 2D cell culture, confluent monolayers of many ECs elongate and align in the direction of flow [7, 8, 10–21], recapitulating EC morphology in larger vessels. As a result of the similarity in morphology in large vessels and in 2D monolayers, elongation and alignment under shear stress is thought to be a hallmark of ECs [10, 11, 14, 16, 19, 22–24]. In previous work we have shown that immortalized brain microvascular endothelial cells do not exhibit this characteristic elongation and alignment in response to shear stress [19] or in response to curvature [25], suggesting that hBMECs have a unique phenotype.

Here we assess the morphology, cell motility, rates of proliferation and apoptosis, and protein and gene expression of dhBMECs in 2D confluent monolayers under shear stress in comparison to static conditions. We show that dhBMECs exhibit a unique phenotype in response to shear stress: (1) they do not elongate and align, (2) the rates of proliferation and apoptosis decrease, (3) the mean displacement of individual cells within the monolayer over time is significantly decreased, (4) there is no cytoskeletal reorganization or formation of stress fibers within the cell, and (5) there is no change in expression levels of key blood–brain barrier markers. This phenotype is significantly different from human and animal derived endothelial cells from other tissues, indicating that dhBMEC have a unique phenotype that may be important in maintenance of the blood–brain barrier.

# Methods

## Cell culture

Human brain microvascular endothelial cells (dhBMECs) were differentiated from the BC1 human induced pluripotent cell (hiPSC) line (provided by Dr. Linzhao Cheng, Johns Hopkins University). Details of the differentiation and characterization of the hBMECs have been reported elsewhere [4]. Briefly, all cells were cultured in T25 and T75 flasks (Falcon, Tewksbury, MA, USA) with daily media changes. BC1-hiPSCs were cultured in colonies on 40 µg mL$^{-1}$ Matrigel-treated tissue culture dishes (Corning, Tewksbury, MA, USA) and maintained in TeSR-E8 media, changed daily (Stem Cell Technologies, Vancouver, Canada). BC1-hiPSCs were passaged using StemPro® Accutase® solution (Life Technologies, Waltham, MA, USA). 10 µM ROCK inhibitor Y27632 (ATCC, Manassas, VA, USA) was included in the TeSR-E8 culture media for the first 24 h after passaging. After culture for 3–4 days in TeSR-E8, the media was switched to unconditioned media without basic fibroblast growth factor (bFGF) (UM/F- media) to induce the differentiation. The cells were maintained in this media for 6 days with daily media replacement. The UM/F- media is composed of DMEM/F12 (Life Technologies) supplemented with 20% KnockOut Serum Replacement (Life Technologies), 1% non-essential amino acids (Life Technologies), 0.5% L-glutamine (Sigma-Aldrich, St. Louis, MO, USA), and 0.84 µM beta-mercaptoethanol (Life Technologies). The media was then switched to endothelial cell media (EC) for 2 days to promote growth of the endothelial cells. The EC media is composed of endothelial cell serum-free media (Life Technologies), supplemented with 1% human platelet poor derived serum (Sigma-Aldrich), 20 ng mL$^{-1}$ bFGF (R&D Systems), and 10 µM all-trans retinoic acid (Sigma-Aldrich). After 2 days in EC media, the cells were sub-cultured into the microfluidic devices.

## Microfluidic platform

The microfluidic device and flow loop were fabricated as reported previously (Fig. 1a, b) [19]. Briefly, polydimethylsiloxane (PDMS, Sylgard 184 silicon elastomer kit, Dow Corning, Midland, MI, USA) was cast in an aluminum mold to create four rectangular channels with different heights to allow simultaneous measurements at different shear stresses. The PDMS channels were plasma bonded to a 50 mm × 75 mm glass microscope slide (Corning). The flow loop included a custom-machined Teflon media reservoir connected via 1/8″ ID silicon tubing to a peristaltic pump (NE-9000, New Era Pump Systems, Farmingdale, NY, USA) that was programmed to steadily ramp up flow and obtain final shear stresses of 4 and 12 dyne cm$^{-2}$ in respective channels of the device. Channels under static conditions (0 dyne cm$^{-2}$) were not connected to the flow loop.

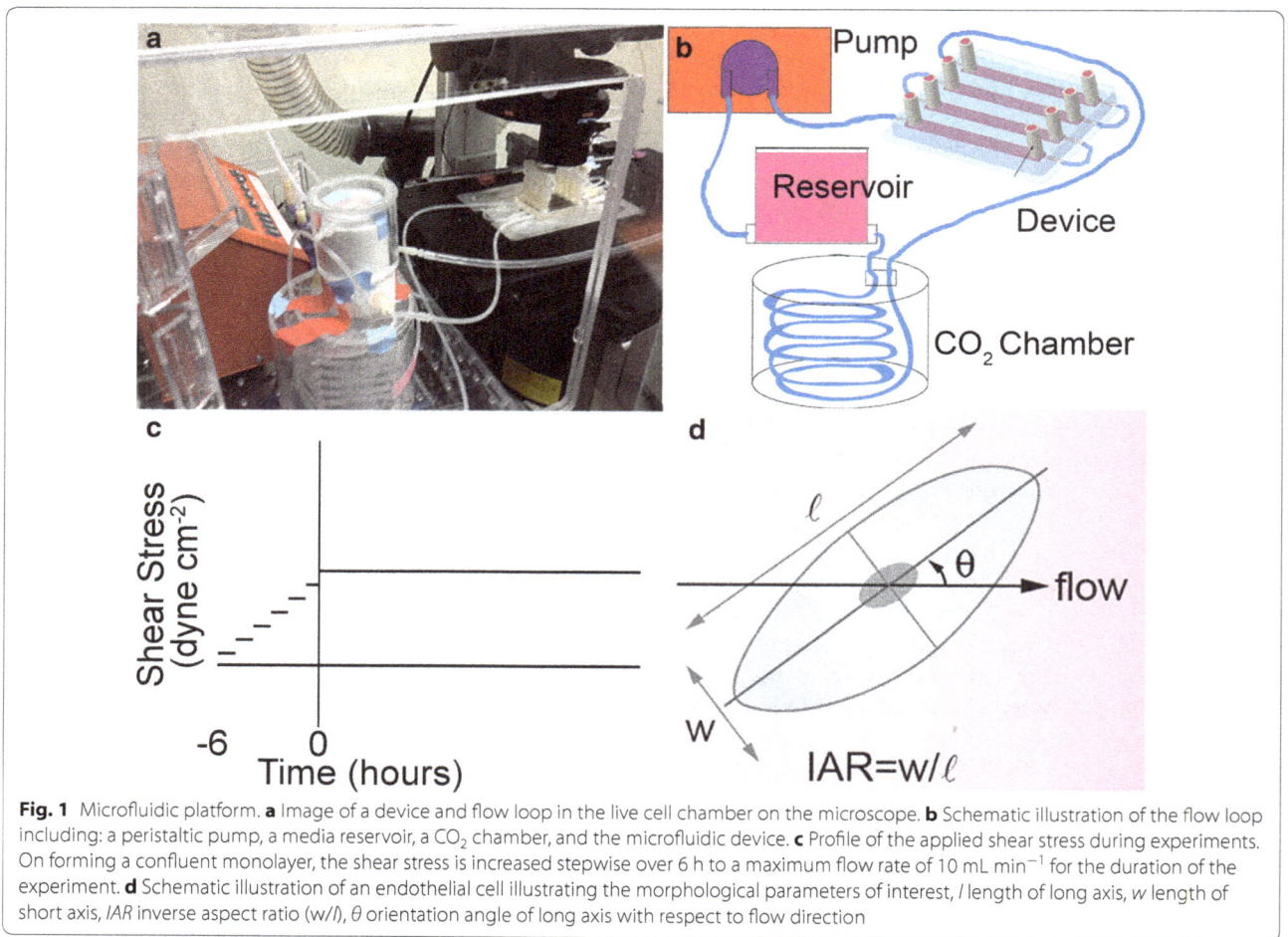

**Fig. 1** Microfluidic platform. **a** Image of a device and flow loop in the live cell chamber on the microscope. **b** Schematic illustration of the flow loop including: a peristaltic pump, a media reservoir, a $CO_2$ chamber, and the microfluidic device. **c** Profile of the applied shear stress during experiments. On forming a confluent monolayer, the shear stress is increased stepwise over 6 h to a maximum flow rate of 10 mL $min^{-1}$ for the duration of the experiment. **d** Schematic illustration of an endothelial cell illustrating the morphological parameters of interest, *l* length of long axis, *w* length of short axis, *IAR* inverse aspect ratio (w/l), $\theta$ orientation angle of long axis with respect to flow direction

The dhBMECs were seeded into the microfluidic devices after 48 h sub-culture. Each microfluidic device has four channels: two static (0 dyne $cm^{-2}$) channels, a 4 dyne $cm^{-2}$ channel, and a 12 dyne $cm^{-2}$ channel. All channels were coated with a 1:1 mixture of 50 μg $mL^{-1}$ fibronectin (Sigma-Aldrich) and 100 μg $mL^{-1}$ collagen IV (Sigma-Aldrich) for 12 h prior to cell seeding. A confluent T25 of sub-cultured dhBMECs was washed three times with PBS without $Ca^{2+}$ and $Mg^{2+}$, followed by a prolonged wash, approximately 7 min, with TrypLE™ Express (Life Technologies) at 37 °C to gently dissociate the cells from the culture flask. Two to three million cells were collected and then spun down to a pellet and the excess media aspirated away. 400 μL of EC media was then added to the pellet and mixed using a pipette such that all the cells from one T25 are suspended in 400 μL. Each channel was seeded with 100 μL of cell suspension corresponding to approximately 500,000 cells per channel. Additional media was added to fill each channel (54 μL in the 4 dyne $cm^{-2}$ channel and 122 μL in the 12 dyne $cm^{-2}$ channel). The cell density is relatively high

to ensure the formation of a confluent monolayer since non-adherent cells are washed away with the addition of media. To demonstrate that the seeding density does not play a significant role in cell behavior, experiments were also performed with 250,000 cells and 125,000 cells seeded per channel. Cells were allowed to settle and attach to the fibronectin/collagen IV coated glass slide for about 2 h at which point 1 mL of media was added to each channel to wash away cells that did not attach, and the monolayers were allowed to grow to confluence, approximately 24 h, at 37 °C and 5% $CO_2$. We aimed to start experiments at an average cell area of between 800 and 1000 $μm^2$. If after 24 h, the average cell area was outside this range, the experiment was not performed. For static experiments (0 dyne $cm^{-2}$), cells were seeded using the same protocol but not connected to the flow loop.

After formation of a confluent monolayer, the microfluidic device was connected to a peristaltic pump, gas exchange chamber, and media reservoir for live-cell imaging. The channels requiring flow (4 and 12 dyne $cm^{-2}$ channels) were connected in series via tubing to the peristaltic pump, whereas the 0 dyne $cm^{-2}$ channels were not connected to the flow loop. The peristaltic pump was programmed to increase flow from 1.25 to 10 mL $min^{-1}$ over 6 h. The flow rate was then maintained at 10 mL $min^{-1}$ for 40 h unless otherwise stated. The time at which the maximum flow rate was reached (after the 6 h conditioning period) is designated as the zero time point. Experiments were performed in EC media, composed of endothelial cell serum free media (Life Technologies), supplemented with 1% human platelet poor derived serum (Sigma-Aldrich), 20 ng $mL^{-1}$ bFGF (R&D Systems, Minneapolis, MN, USA), and 10 μM all-trans retinoic acid (Sigma-Aldrich). For cell maintenance and to avoid overgrowth and formation of mounds, media was replaced every 24 h in the static channels. To assess the role of vasomodulators on dhBMEC monolayers, some experiments were performed in EC media containing either (1) 400 μM DB-cAMP or (2) 10 μM ROCK inhibitor. The flow system was maintained at 37 °C and humidified with 5% $CO_2$ for the duration of the experiments. After 6 h conditioning and 40 h under the designated shear stress, the monolayers were either immediately fixed for immunofluorescence staining or prepared for genetic or proteomic analysis.

### Live-cell imaging

To assess the response of dhBMECs to flow, confluent monolayers were imaged under static conditions (0 dyne $cm^{-2}$) or under a shear stress of 4 or 12 dyne $cm^{-2}$ for 40 h in a custom microfluidic device (Fig. 1). A shear stress of 4 dyne $cm^{-2}$ is representative of the average shear stress in the venous system (typically 1–4 dyne $cm^{-2}$) and 12 dyne $cm^{-2}$ is representative of the average shear stress in capillaries (typically 10–20 dyne $cm^{-2}$) [26–32].

Live-cell time lapse imaging was performed using a Nikon TE-2000U inverted microscope controlled by NIS Elements Software (Nikon, Tokyo, Japan) with a 10× Nikon Plan Fluor objective. Imaging was performed at three locations in each channel: in the center of the channel and at points 10 mm from either end of the channel. The locations were centered approximately 2 mm from either side wall, to avoid edge effects. Time lapse images were recorded for 46 h with images taken every 20 min. Autofocus adjustment was performed before each image capture to correct for any z-drift. The number of cells in each imaging region (1.5 mm × 1.2 mm) was about 2000. All experiments were performed in triplicate (three microfluidic devices with three imaging locations per device) and hence all parameters represent an average of about 18,000 cells at each time point.

### Morphological analysis

Quantitative analysis of cell morphology was performed using ImageJ (NIH, Bethesda, MD, USA) and techniques previously developed in our lab [19]. Images of the cell monolayers from time-lapse movies were imported into ImageJ and the cell borders were delineated automatically using a custom macro [19]. Morphological parameters (inverse aspect ratio, orientation angle, and cell area) of individual cells were obtained as long as more than 85% of the monolayer could be traced by this method. The automated analysis of cell monolayers from phase contrast images was validated by comparison to analysis by manually tracing cell boundaries in immunofluorescence images at the same time point [19].

### Turnover analysis

Quantitative analysis of cell proliferation and apoptosis was performed using ImageJ. Proliferation events were identified visually from cell division and the formation of daughter cells. Apoptosis and cell loss from the monolayer was apparent from pronounced cell contraction and detachment events. Both proliferation and apoptosis events are readily identified in phase contrast time-lapse images (Additional files 1, 2 and 3). Individual division and apoptosis events occur over 20–40 min spanning 1–3 frames. Proliferation and apoptosis events were identified and quantified under both static and shear flow conditions. Time-lapse videos of cell monolayers were imported as stacks of image sequences and cell division and apoptotic events counted manually every 20 min. Proliferation and apoptosis rates are reported as % $h^{-1}$. Analysis was performed at each of the three imaging locations in respective channels to obtain the rates of cell division and apoptosis for each shear stress and media condition. To determine the net rate of change in cell number (% $h^{-1}$), the apoptosis rate was subtracted from the division rate. Identification of apoptosis and proliferation events from phase contrast movies allows quantitative analysis of the dynamic behavior of the monolayer as a function of time [33, 34]. Furthermore, direct observation ensures that we include apoptosis events associated with cell loss and removal from the monolayer by shear flow, which may not be detected by labeling methods. To ensure that proliferation and apoptosis event counting was reproducible, analysis was performed by five different observers. Post-evaluation analysis revealed that less than 5% of the events were misidentified or not counted, and there was no statistical difference between independent analysis of the same time lapse images.

### Cell motility analysis

To assess cell motility we measured three parameters: cell speed, root mean square (RMS) displacement, and directionality. Cell speed, a measure of the average velocity of cells moving within the monolayer, is a directionless velocity with units of $\mu m$ $min^{-1}$. RMS displacement is a measure of how far a cell moves from its original position in a monolayer as a function of time. Finally, directionality is a measure of the direction of cell motion with respect to the flow direction. Quantitative analysis of cell speed was performed using OpenPIV [35] using methods reported previously [19]. Image sequences of cell monolayers from time-lapse movies were imported into OpenPIV and analyzed using particle image velocimetry (PIV). Reproducible approximations of monolayer speed were obtained between each successive image and reported over time as averages of triplicate experiments. The cell speed obtained from PIV was validated by manual tracking of individual cells (Additional file 4: Figure S1).

Root mean square displacement and directionality were quantified by manually tracking the location of the center of cell nuclei throughout an experiment. RMS displacement is quantified as the magnitude of the vector from the starting location of a cell to the current location, and is a measure of how far a cell in a confluent monolayer moves over time. The displacement is measured for at least 10 cells in each of the three imaging locations. Directionality is quantified as the change in x- or y-direction between two frames and is reported in microns. RMS displacement and directionality were obtained for at least 100 cells over three independent experiments.

### Immunofluorescence imaging

After time-lapse live-cell imaging, monolayers were immediately fixed for immunofluorescence staining and imaging. Cell monolayers were first washed twice in $1\times$ PBS with $Ca^{2+}$ and $Mg^{2+}$, and fixed in 3.7% formaldehyde (Fisher Scientific Hampton, NH, USA) in PBS for 5 min. Next, the samples were washed three times with PBS and permeabilized with 0.1% Triton-X 100 (Sigma-Aldrich Aldrich). The samples were subsequently washed three times in PBS and blocked with 10% donkey serum in PBS for 1 h. The samples were then incubated with primary antibodies overnight at 4 °C. Primary antibodies include claudin-5 (Thermo Fisher Scientific, #35-2500), occludin (Thermo Fisher Scientific, #40-4700), and ZO-1 (Thermo Fisher Scientific, #40-2200). The samples were washed three times with PBS for 5 min each on a rocker. The samples were then incubated with DAPI nuclear stain (Roche Applied Science), Alexa Fluor 488 phalloidin (F-actin, Thermo Fisher Scientific), and secondary antibodies. Immunofluorescence images were taken using a Nikon Eclipse Ti-E inverted microscope controlled by NIS Elements Software (Nikon). Images were obtained from similar locations to the phase contrast

images to minimize possible edge effects. Immunofluorescence images were quantified for claudin-5, occludin, and ZO-1 expression, and F-actin orientation. To assess junctional expression, cell–cell boundaries were traced using ImageJ (from one edge of the image field to the other edge three times per image) and the average pixel intensity minus the background was collected and averaged [36]. To assess F-actin orientation, FibrilTool was used to find the average orientation of the fibers within each cell [37].

### Protein analysis

Confluent monolayers of cells were lysed immediately after time-lapse imaging experiments using RIPA buffer (Sigma-Aldrich) containing protease inhibitor cocktail (Sigma-Aldrich). Samples were centrifuged at 25,000 RPM for 25 min at 4 °C, and stored at −20 °C. Western blots were performed on 4–15% pre-cast polyacrylamide gels (Bio-Rad, Hercules, CA, USA). The bands were transferred from the gels onto nitrocellulose membranes (Bio-Rad), and blocked with 5% fat-free skim milk (Bio-Rad) in TBS (Corning) with 0.05% TWEEN-20 (Sigma-Aldrich) for 1 h at room temperature. Primary antibodies (Additional file 4: Table S1) were added to the milk cocktail and incubated overnight at 4 °C. Membranes were washed three times for 5 min each with TBS with 0.05% TWEEN-20. Secondary HRP antibodies (Bio-Rad) were added to milk and incubated for 1 h at room temperature before imaging (Bio-Rad molecular imager ChemiDoc XRS+) using ImageLab 5.1 software. β-actin was used as a loading control. Western blots were performed in quadruplicate for CLDN-5 and LAT-1 and triplicate for ZO-1 using lysate from three or four independent experiments. Analysis of relative intensities of the bands was performed using imageJ. Each lane was normalized and compared against the intensity of the 0 dyne $cm^{-2}$ lane to reduce the influence of the background.

### Gene analysis

Quantitative PCR (qPCR) was performed using an Applied Biosystems StepOnePlus Real-time PCR system to assess changes in mRNA expression in the following genes: ABCB1, CDH5, CLDN5, OCLN, SLC2A1, and TJP1, with ACTB and GAPDH as the housekeeping genes. PCR samples were prepared using the TaqMan® Gene Expression Cells-to-CT™ Kit (Life Technologies). Cells were washed twice in PBS, dissociated with StemPro® Accutase® solution (Life Technologies) and lysed with the cells-to-CT lysing solution (Life Technologies). Fold changes were analyzed using the comparative $C_T$ method ($\Delta\Delta C_T$) [38] normalizing to ACTB and GAPDH expression and comparing to static conditions (0 dyne $cm^{-2}$) as a reference.

## Statistics

To determine statistical significance, we use a two-tailed Student's $t$ test to compare two samples with unequal variances, with a p value of 0.05 being the threshold for significance ($p \leq 0.05$ = *; $p \leq 0.01$ = **; $p \leq 0.001$ = ***).

## Results

### Morphology

From phase contrast images, the dhBMECs initially show a cobblestone morphology with well-defined cell nuclei and subtle cell–cell junctions under all conditions (Fig. 2). At longer times the nuclei become less well-defined and the cell–cell junctions become more distinct due to increased overlap and flattening of the cells. At higher magnification it is also evident that organelles and other intracellular vesicles become more pronounced. Despite these changes in appearance, the cells maintain their cobblestone morphology under shear stress (the average IAR and orientation angle remain the same). The key results, described below, are summarized in Table 1.

To quantitatively characterize cell morphology, we measured the inverse aspect ratio (IAR), orientation angle, and cell area as a function of shear stress and time (Fig. 3). The IAR for dhBMEC monolayers under static conditions was about 0.65 and did not change with time (Fig. 3a). Under static and flow conditions, the average orientation angle of the dhBMEC monolayers remained close to 45°, corresponding to a random orientation of cells and showing that there was no cell alignment in response to shear stress (Fig. 3b). These results show that the dhBMECs do not elongate in response to physiological shear stress.

Changes in cell area reflect gross changes in cell turnover. Histograms of cell area (Additional file 4: Figure S2) show a log-normal distribution with a well-defined peak and a small number of cells that are considerably larger. Under 4 dyne cm$^{-2}$, the average cell area was about 800 μm$^2$ and remained approximately constant throughout the experiment (Fig. 3c). At 12 dyne cm$^{-2}$, the average cell area was about 750 μm$^2$ and also remained constant throughout the experiment. Under static conditions, the cell area decreased to a steady state value of about 750 μm$^2$ after about 5 h. Despite these differences, there is no statistically significant difference in average area at 40 h between 0, 4, and 12 dyne$^{-2}$ across all experiments analyzed.

Morphological changes to endothelial cells in response to shear flow are usually observed within 12–24 h [10, 13,

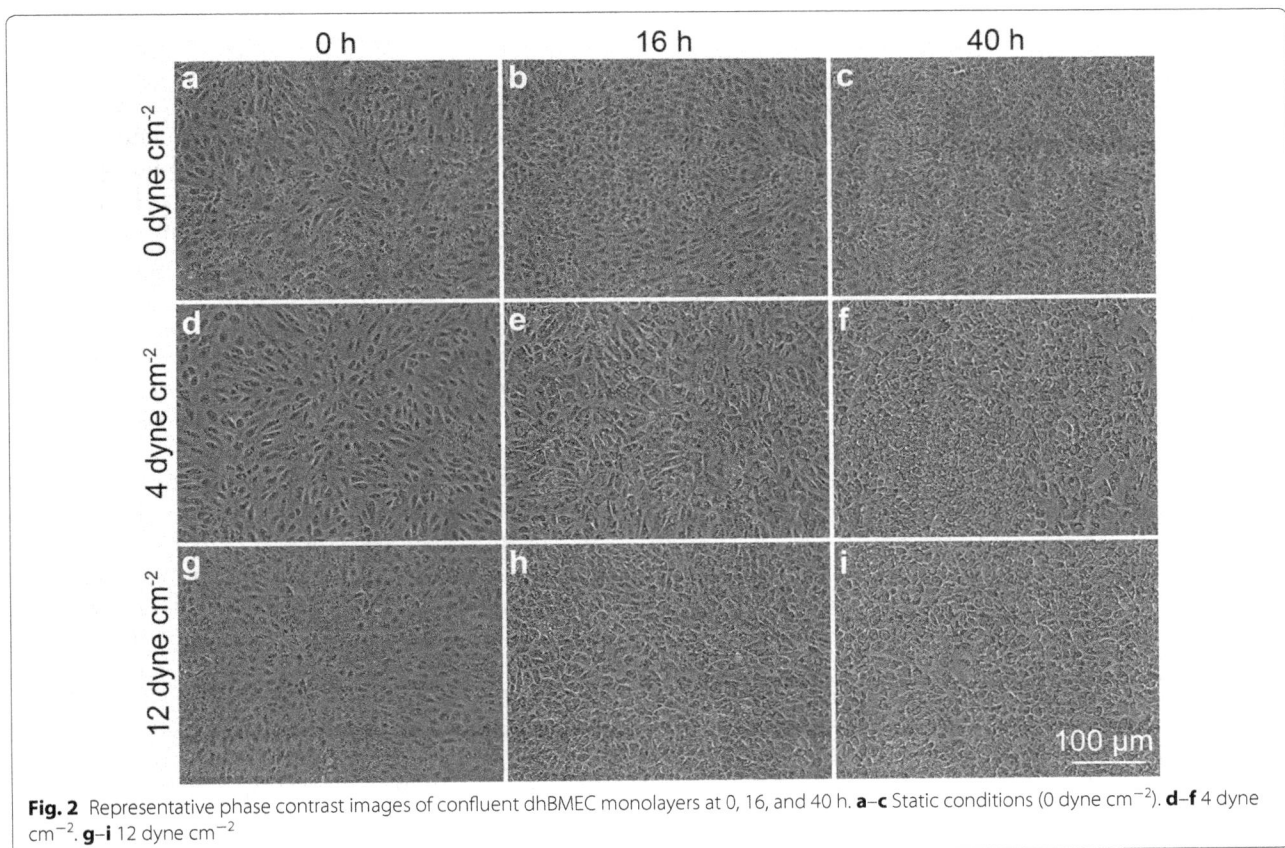

**Fig. 2** Representative phase contrast images of confluent dhBMEC monolayers at 0, 16, and 40 h. **a–c** Static conditions (0 dyne cm$^{-2}$). **d–f** 4 dyne cm$^{-2}$. **g–i** 12 dyne cm$^{-2}$

**Table 1  Summary of steady state results from this study (dhBMECs) and previous studies (Other ECs)**

| dhBMEC | | | Other EC | | |
|---|---|---|---|---|---|
| Steady state | Static | Flow | HUVEC | BAEC | In vivo |
| Morphology | Small cell area Random orientation Cobblestone morphology | Moderate cell area Random orientation Cobblestone morphology | Large cell area Aligned to flow Spindle-like morphology [14, 16, 17] | Large cell area Aligned to flow Spindle-like morphology [18, 20, 64, 67] | Moderate cell area Aligned to flow Spindle-like morphology [12, 13, 21, 22] |
| Motility | Small displacement | Small displacement | Large displacement | N/A | N/A |
| Proliferation rate | High | Moderate | Moderate | N/A | Low-moderate [4, 66] |
| Apoptosis rate | High | Low | Moderate | N/A | N/A |
| Protein and gene expression | No change | No change in transporters ZO-1↓ (WB, 4 dyne cm$^{-2}$) | OCLN (no change) | ZO-1 (no change) [14] OCLN ↓ (WB, 10 & 20 dyne cm$^{-2}$) [77] | N/A |

Morphological analysis is quantified as cell area, inverse aspect ratio, and orientation angle with respect to the flow direction. Cell area: small (<700 μm$^2$), moderate (700–1200 μm$^2$), large (>1200 μm$^2$). Orientation: random/cobblestone (IAR ~ 0.6, orientation ~ 45°), aligned to flow/spindle-like (IAR < 0.4, orientation < 20°). Displacement is defined as the distance between the current location and its original position: small (<50 μm), large (>50 μm). Proliferation rate is defined as the percent of all cells that divide per hour: low (<0.1% h$^{-1}$), moderate (0.1–0.3% h$^{-1}$), high (>0.3% h$^{-1}$). Apoptosis rate is defined as the percent of all cells that divide per hour: low (<0.05% h$^{-1}$), moderate (0.05–0.1% h$^{-1}$), high (>1% h$^{-1}$)

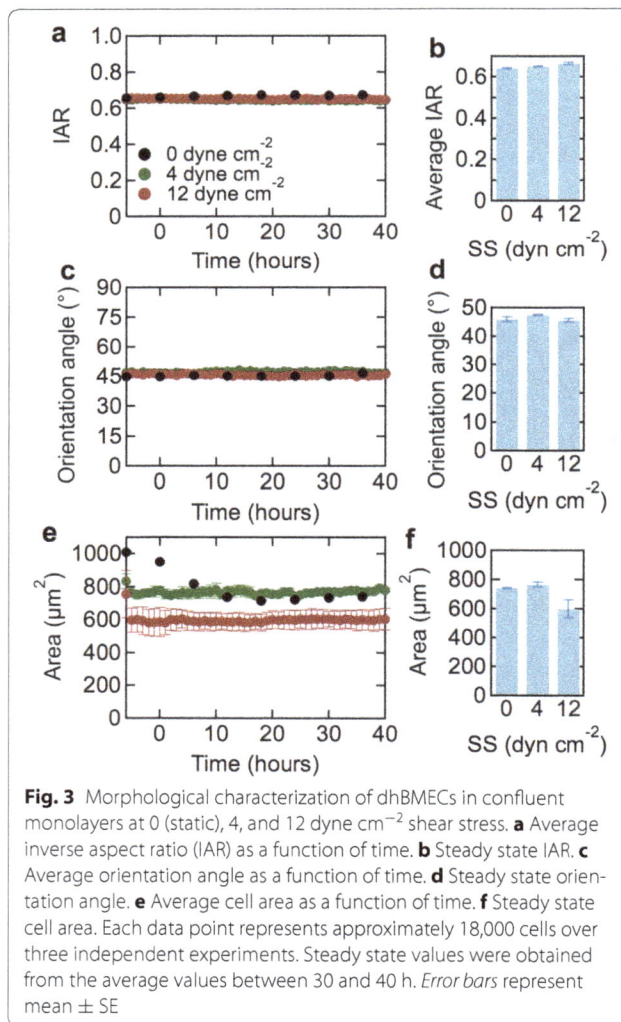

**Fig. 3** Morphological characterization of dhBMECs in confluent monolayers at 0 (static), 4, and 12 dyne cm$^{-2}$ shear stress. **a** Average inverse aspect ratio (IAR) as a function of time. **b** Steady state IAR. **c** Average orientation angle as a function of time. **d** Steady state orientation angle. **e** Average cell area as a function of time. **f** Steady state cell area. Each data point represents approximately 18,000 cells over three independent experiments. Steady state values were obtained from the average values between 30 and 40 h. *Error bars* represent mean ± SE

14, 16, 23, 24], therefore the experiments reported here were performed for 40 h. To verify the lack of a morphological response of dhBMECs at longer times, selected experiments were performed for 60 h under shear stress confirming that there is no further change in cell morphology (Additional file 4: Figure S3, Table S2).

In these experiments, cells were seeded at a density of 500,000 cells per channel. To ensure that seeding density did not influence steady state morphology, we also performed experiments at seeding densities of 250,000 and 125,000 cells per channel. Seeding at 250,000 cells per channel resulted in a longer time reach confluence, however, there was no difference in cell morphology (Additional file 4: Figure S4, Table S3). Seeding at 125,000 cells per channel did not result in the formation of a confluent monolayer.

### Rates of proliferation and apoptosis

To assess the effect of shear stress on turnover, we visually detected proliferation and apoptosis events in phase contrast, time-lapse videos (Fig. 4). Relative turnover rates are usually measured using labeling probes (e.g. thymidine, EdU) that incorporate into the cell nucleus upon cell division [39–42]. Direct visualization provides direct, quantitative measurement of both proliferation and apoptosis rates, and enables monitoring in real time. The proliferation and apoptosis rates are reported as a percentage of the total number of cells per hour (Fig. 5). Under static conditions, the proliferation rate is around 1.0% h$^{-1}$ (Fig. 5a, b). Under 4 dyne cm$^{-2}$, the proliferation rate reaches a maximum of about 0.4% h$^{-1}$ during the conditioning phase and gradually decreases to a steady state value of 0.35 ± 0.02% h$^{-1}$. Similar results are

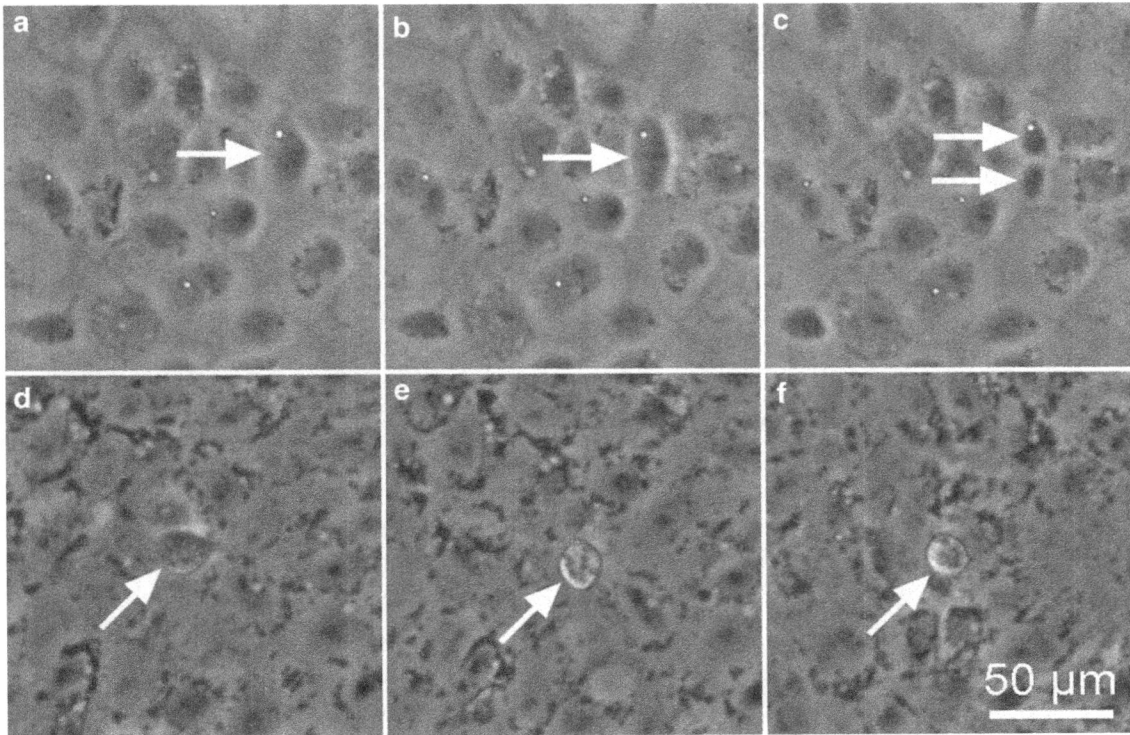

**Fig. 4** Representative phase contrast images of cell division and apoptosis events in confluent dhBMEC monolayers. **a–c** dhBMEC undergoing division over the course of 1 h. **d–f** dhBMEC undergoing apoptosis over an hour. Images were captured at 20 min intervals

obtained at 12 dyne $cm^{-2}$, although the steady state value is somewhat smaller ($0.27 \pm 0.01\%$ $h^{-1}$).

The apoptosis rate under static conditions has a steady state value of $0.12\%$ $h^{-1}$ (Fig. 5c, d). Under shear stress at both 4 and 12 dyne $cm^{-2}$, the apoptosis rate remained constant throughout the experiment with a steady state value of $0.01\%$ $h^{-1}$, an order of magnitude lower than under static conditions (Fig. 5c, d). The net rate of change in the number of cells within a monolayer, defined as the difference between the proliferation and apoptosis rates (Fig. 5e, f), is dominated by the larger proliferation rate.

To determine the effects of vascular modulators on steady state proliferation and apoptosis rates, we performed additional experiments at 12 dyne $cm^{-2}$ where the endothelial cell media was supplemented with DB-cAMP or ROCK inhibitor (Fig. 6a, b). Cyclic-AMP (DB-cAMP) is an intracellular secondary messenger that has a variety of functions, and has been shown to increase barrier function and decrease proliferation and apoptosis rates in endothelial cells [42]. The addition of DB-cAMP had no effect on the steady state rates of proliferation and apoptosis, suggesting that the dhBMEC monolayers are already in a relatively quiescent state. The ROCK pathway mainly regulates cell shape and motility by acting on the cytoskeleton [43], but is commonly used to promote

survival of iPSCs [44]. The addition of ROCK inhibitor significantly increased the proliferation rate from 0.27 to $0.57\%$ $h^{-1}$ and increased the apoptosis rate from 0.012 to $0.033\%$ $h^{-1}$. The increase in proliferation rate is larger than the increase in apoptosis rate, resulting in an increase in the net change in cell number on exposure to ROCK inhibitor from 0.26 to $0.54\%$ $h^{-1}$, consistent with increased survival.

**Cell motility**

To assess cell motility, we measured the average cell speed, the RMS displacement, and the directionality. The average cell speed, a measure of cell activity [11, 26, 33], was calculated by automated particle image velocimetry (PIV) analysis [19]. The average speed within the monolayers decreased from a maximum of approximately 0.2 μm $min^{-1}$ during the 6-h conditioning period, to a steady state value of about 0.1 μm $min^{-1}$ under static conditions and under 4 and 12 dyne $cm^{-2}$ shear stress (Fig. 7a).

The RMS displacement is a measure of translation within the monolayer and is calculated as the distance of the center of mass of the cell nucleus from an initial reference point. Under static conditions, the displacement increases monotonically with a slope of about

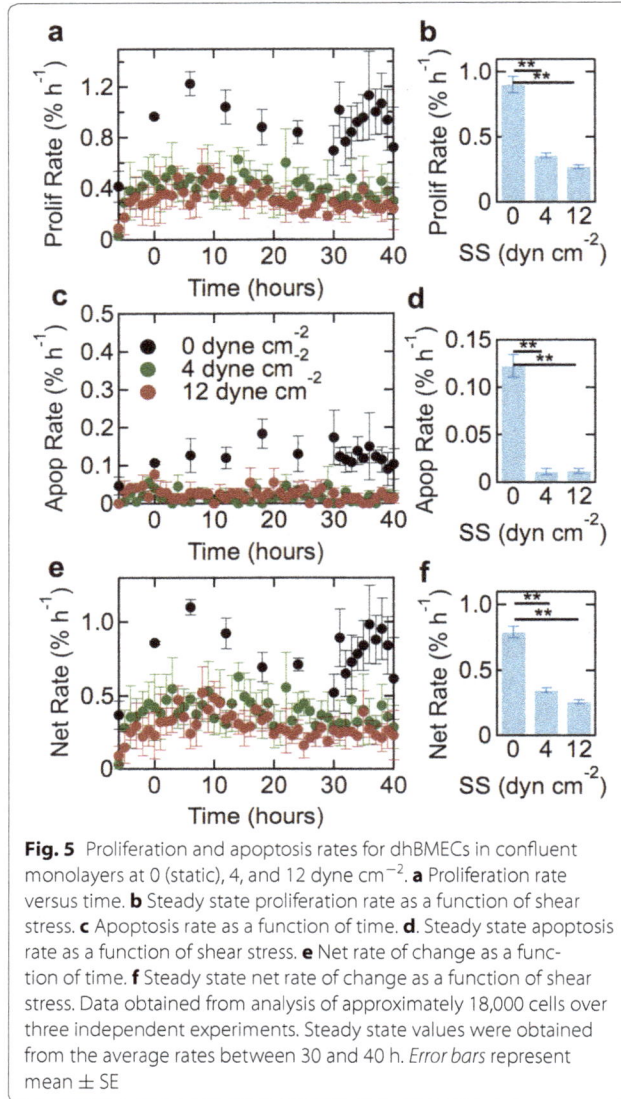

**Fig. 5** Proliferation and apoptosis rates for dhBMECs in confluent monolayers at 0 (static), 4, and 12 dyne cm$^{-2}$. **a** Proliferation rate versus time. **b** Steady state proliferation rate as a function of shear stress. **c** Apoptosis rate as a function of time. **d**. Steady state apoptosis rate as a function of shear stress. **e** Net rate of change as a function of time. **f** Steady state net rate of change as a function of shear stress. Data obtained from analysis of approximately 18,000 cells over three independent experiments. Steady state values were obtained from the average rates between 30 and 40 h. *Error bars* represent mean ± SE

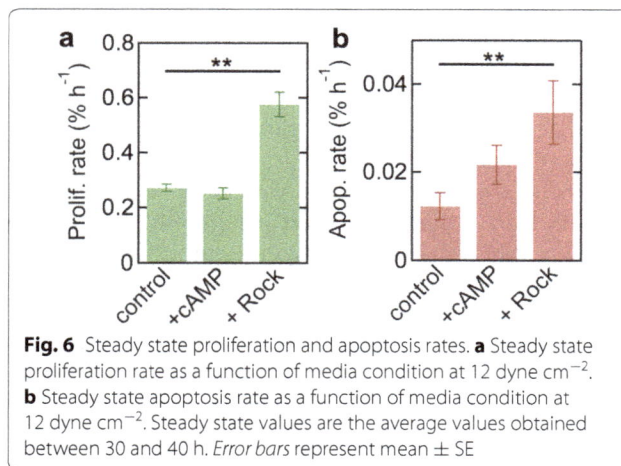

**Fig. 6** Steady state proliferation and apoptosis rates. **a** Steady state proliferation rate as a function of media condition at 12 dyne cm$^{-2}$. **b** Steady state apoptosis rate as a function of media condition at 12 dyne cm$^{-2}$. Steady state values are the average values obtained between 30 and 40 h. *Error bars* represent mean ± SE

0.01 µm min$^{-1}$, corresponding to 30 µm over the course of the experiment (Fig. 7b). Under shear stress, the displacement was about 15 µm during the initial 6-h conditioning period, but then increased very slowly during experiment (Fig. 7b). At both 4 and 12 dyne cm$^{-2}$, the displacement under shear stress was about 10 µm over 40 h (Fig. 7c). We confirmed that there is no influence of flow on displacement within the monolayer by measuring the x- and y- components of the directionality (Fig. 7d, e).

### Expression of BBB markers

To assess changes in protein and gene expression of dhBMECs in confluent monolayers in response to shear stress, immunofluorescence staining, western blot and qPCR were performed after 40 h under static conditions (0 dyne cm$^{-2}$) and at 4 and 12 dyne cm$^{-2}$.

### Immunofluorescence imaging

To evaluate the expression and localization of tight junction and cytoskeletal proteins, monolayers were stained for claudin-5, occludin, zonula occludens 1 (ZO-1), and F-actin (Fig. 8). Claudin-5 and occludin are transmembrane tight junction proteins that bind to the PDZ domain and associate with the actin cytoskeleton [45]. ZO-1 is a peripheral junctional protein that is part of the PDZ domain and links occludin directly to the cortical actin skeleton [45, 46]. Under static conditions, claudin-5, occludin, and ZO-1 are localized to cell–cell junctions (Fig. 8a–c). The cell boundaries are generally straight resulting in a well-defined polygonal network, consistent with previous reports of dhBMEC monolayers [4–6, 47–49]. In contrast, tight junction stains for immortalized and primary BMECs from humans and animals often show elongated cells with junctions that are often serrated [50–52]. There are no clear differences between claudin-5, occludin, and ZO-1 stains under static and flow conditions, suggesting that tight junction networks are already well established under static conditions. The junctional network also shows that there is no elongation and alignment under flow, as described previously.

F-actin is a cytoskeletal protein that plays an important role in cell motility, cell shape, and the maintenance of cell junctions [53]. After 40 h at 0, 4, or 12 dyne cm$^{-2}$, F-actin is highly localized to the peripheral regions of the cell, near the cell–cell junctions and few stress fibers were seen within the cell (Fig. 8d, h, l). F-actin remained randomly oriented in all conditions and did not align parallel to flow. Quantitative analysis of the intensity of claudin-5, occludin, ZO-1, and F-actin expression at the cell–cell junctions revealed no significant differences between static and flow conditions (Additional file 4: Figure S5). The endothelial cell nuclei maintain an oval shape under all conditions (Additional file 4: Figure S6).

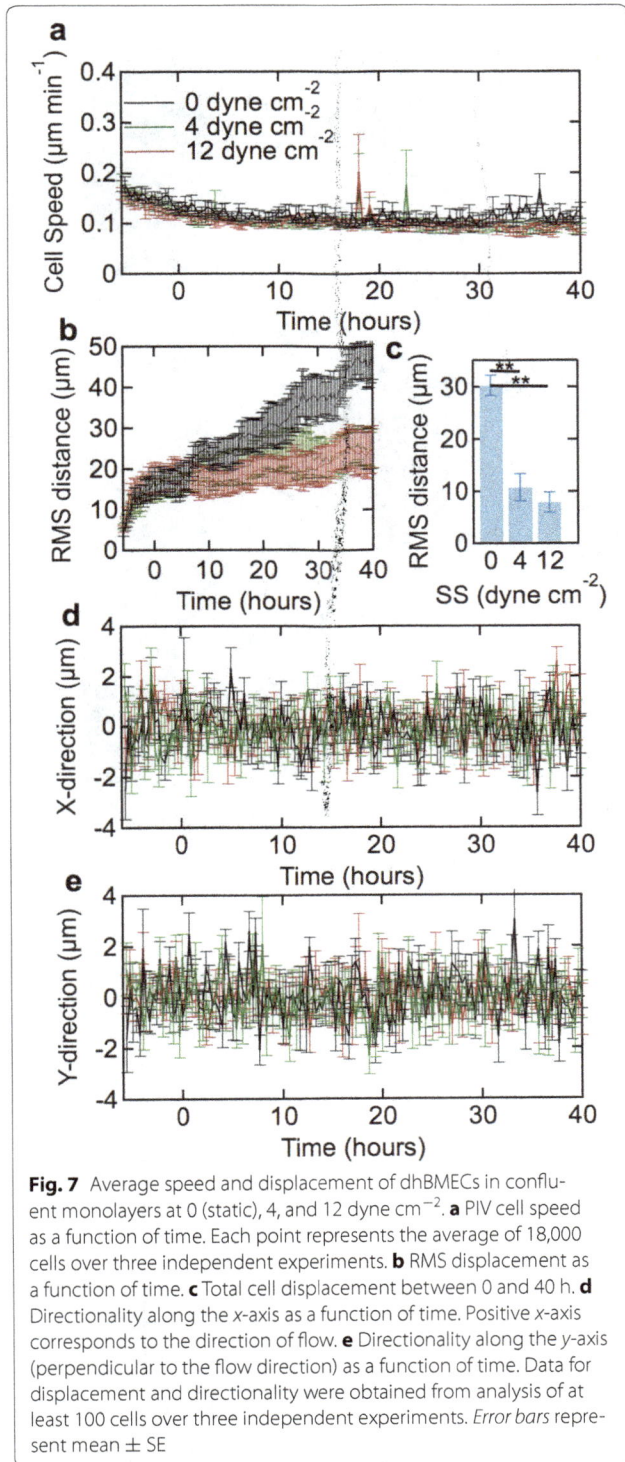

**Fig. 7** Average speed and displacement of dhBMECs in confluent monolayers at 0 (static), 4, and 12 dyne cm$^{-2}$. **a** PIV cell speed as a function of time. Each point represents the average of 18,000 cells over three independent experiments. **b** RMS displacement as a function of time. **c** Total cell displacement between 0 and 40 h. **d** Directionality along the x-axis as a function of time. Positive x-axis corresponds to the direction of flow. **e** Directionality along the y-axis (perpendicular to the flow direction) as a function of time. Data for displacement and directionality were obtained from analysis of at least 100 cells over three independent experiments. *Error bars* represent mean ± SE

## Western blot

To determine whether protein level expression of key BBB proteins changes in response to shear stress, western blots were performed for claudin-5 (CLDN-5), large amino acid transporter 1 (LAT-1), and ZO-1 after 40 h at 0, 4, or 12 dyne cm$^{-2}$ (Fig. 9a; Additional file 4: Figure S7). Claudin-5 is a tight junction protein that is highly expressed in the brain and responsible for maintaining proper blood–brain barrier function [54]. LAT-1 is a large neutral amino acid transporter that is highly expressed in the brain [55]. There were no significant differences in CLDN-5 or LAT-1 expression levels under shear stress compared to static conditions, and no difference between low and high shear stress. Although the mean expression of claudin-5 increased almost twofold at 4 dyne cm$^{-2}$ compared to static conditions, the difference is not statistically significant (p > 0.05). The level of LAT-1 expression at 4 dyne cm$^{-2}$ is lower than under static conditions but also not statistically significant (p > 0.05). ZO-1 expression at 4 dyne cm$^{-2}$ is statistically lower than static conditions (0 dyne cm$^{-2}$), but there is no statistical difference between ZO-1 expression at 4 and 12 dyne cm$^{-2}$.

## Gene expression

To examine the impact of shear stress on gene expression of important blood–brain barrier proteins, we determined the relative expression of several transporters (*ABCB1*, *SLC2A1*) and tight junction and junctional proteins (*CDH5*, *CLDN5*, *OCLN*, *TJP1*) (Fig. 9b). *ABCB1* (P-gp) is the gene for the P-glycoprotein efflux pump [56]. *SLC2A1* is the gene for the GLUT-1 transporter that transports glucose across the blood–brain barrier, and is highly expressed in brain capillary endothelium [57]. *CDH5* (VE-cad) is the gene for vascular endothelial cadherin (VE-cadherin), an endothelial-specific cadherin and adherens junction protein that links adjacent cells together and plays an important role in vascular homeostasis [58]. *CLDN5* encodes for the tight junction protein claudin-5 that is highly expressed in BMECs [54]. *OCLN* encodes occludin, a membrane-spanning tight junction protein that connects adjacent cells to each other and is highly expressed in the brain [59]. *TJP1* is the gene for ZO-1, a tight junction protein that is localized to tight junctions and links the transmembrane tight junction protein occludin to the cytoskeleton [60].

There were no significant differences in gene expression of transporters (*ABCB1*, *SLC2A1*) or junctional proteins (*CDH5*, *CLDN5*, *OCLN*, *TJP1*) at 4 and 12 dyne cm$^{-2}$ compared to static conditions (0 dyne cm$^{-2}$). *CDH5* and *CLDN5* exhibit high standard error in fold change due to batch-to-batch variability between different differentiations (Additional file 4: Figure S8). These differences may originate from differential expression of these proteins due to variations in tight junction formation between differentiations (Additional file 4: Figure S8). Changes in gene expression of *CDH5* and *CLDN5* due to shear stress within individual differentiations also revealed no trend.

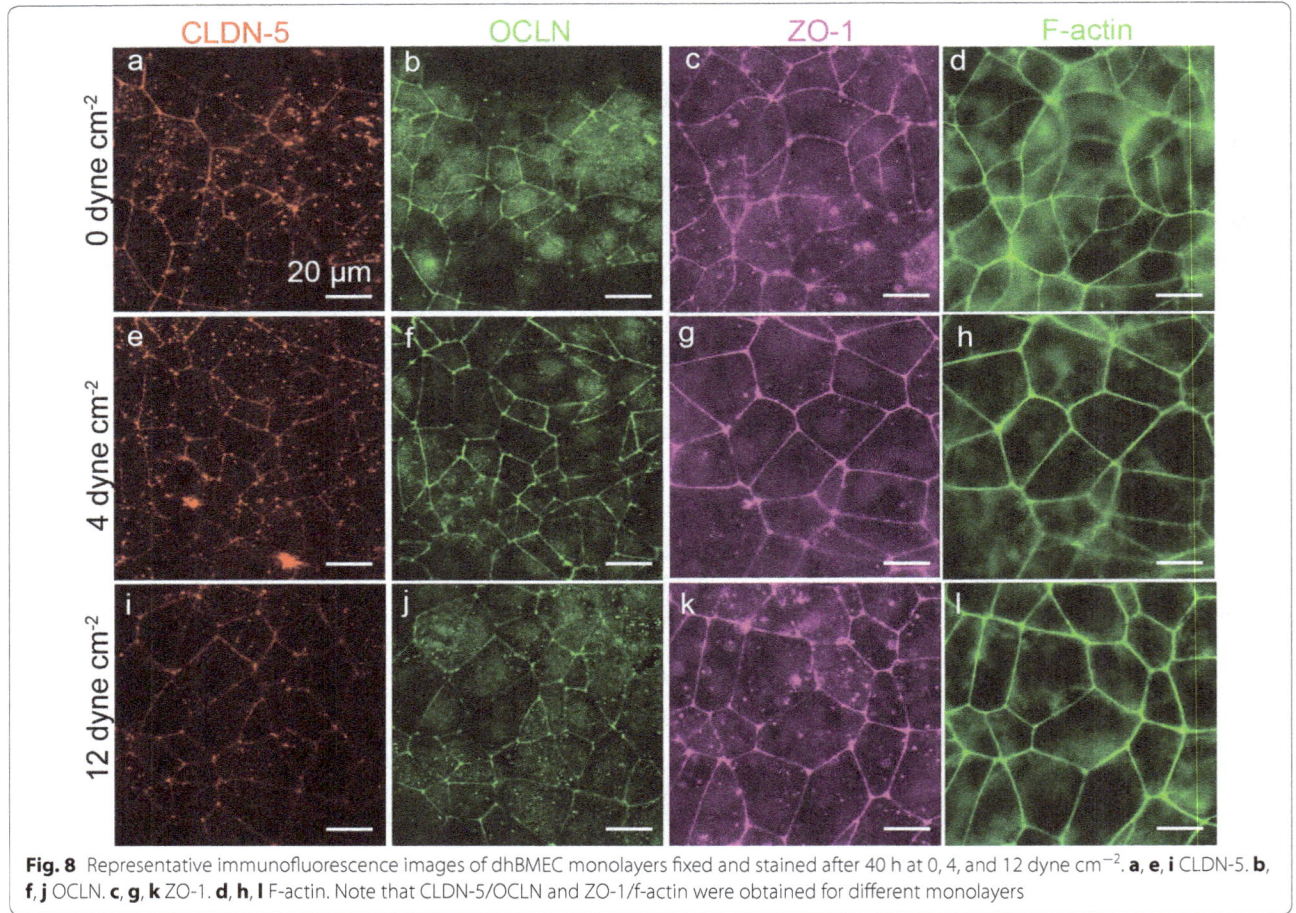

**Fig. 8** Representative immunofluorescence images of dhBMEC monolayers fixed and stained after 40 h at 0, 4, and 12 dyne cm$^{-2}$. **a, e, i** CLDN-5. **b, f, j** OCLN. **c, g, k** ZO-1. **d, h, l** F-actin. Note that CLDN-5/OCLN and ZO-1/f-actin were obtained for different monolayers

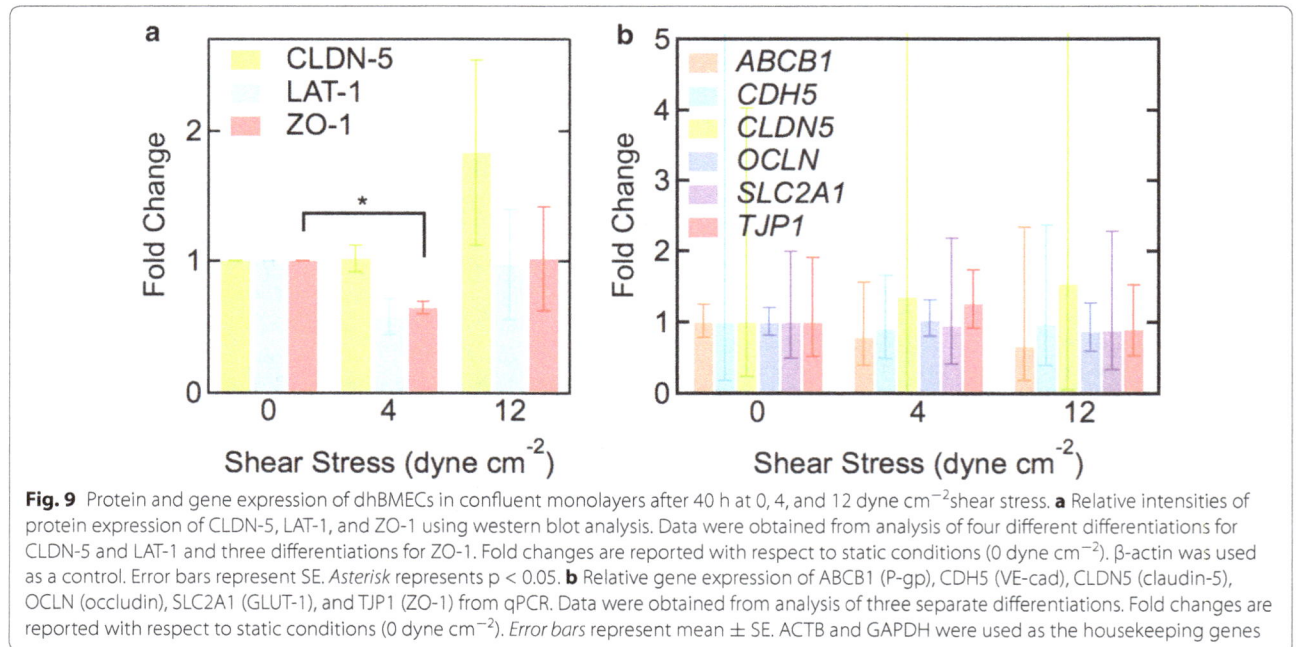

**Fig. 9** Protein and gene expression of dhBMECs in confluent monolayers after 40 h at 0, 4, and 12 dyne cm$^{-2}$ shear stress. **a** Relative intensities of protein expression of CLDN-5, LAT-1, and ZO-1 using western blot analysis. Data were obtained from analysis of four different differentiations for CLDN-5 and LAT-1 and three differentiations for ZO-1. Fold changes are reported with respect to static conditions (0 dyne cm$^{-2}$). β-actin was used as a control. Error bars represent SE. *Asterisk* represents p < 0.05. **b** Relative gene expression of ABCB1 (P-gp), CDH5 (VE-cad), CLDN5 (claudin-5), OCLN (occludin), SLC2A1 (GLUT-1), and TJP1 (ZO-1) from qPCR. Data were obtained from analysis of three separate differentiations. Fold changes are reported with respect to static conditions (0 dyne cm$^{-2}$). *Error bars* represent mean ± SE. ACTB and GAPDH were used as the housekeeping genes

## Discussion

### Cell morphology

Elongation and alignment in response to shear stress is a hallmark of endothelial cells in large vessels [8, 14, 16, 23, 24, 61–63]. In 2D cell culture, confluent monolayers of human umbilical vein endothelial cells (HUVECs), bovine aortic endothelial cells (BAECs), porcine pulmonary artery ECs, and primary baboon arterial endothelial cells (pBAECs) under physiological shear stress undergo a transition from a cobblestone morphology to an elongated spindle-like morphology and align in the direction of flow, recapitulating EC morphology in larger vessels [7, 8, 10, 11, 14–19]. In previous work, we have shown that immortalized hBMECs do not elongate or align in response to physiological shear stress [19]. Here we show that, similarly, iPSC-derived hBMECs do not elongate and align in response to shear stress, providing further evidence that this is a unique phenotype of brain microvascular endothelial cells. The average cell area for dhBMECs is considerably smaller than for HUVECs, which is in the range 1500–2000 $\mu m^2$ [19], and around 1200 $\mu m^2$ for BAECs [64]. In previous work we have shown that the area for immortalized hBMECs is 800–1500 $\mu m^2$ and increases with increasing shear stress [19].

### Proliferation and apoptosis

The rates of proliferation and apoptosis for dhBMECs decrease significantly under shear stress. The proliferation rate decreases by about threefold and the apoptosis rate by more than tenfold compared to static conditions. The net turnover rate (proliferation rate–apoptosis rate) under steady state conditions is 0.8% $h^{-1}$ under static conditions, but decreases with increasing shear stress, to 0.3% $h^{-1}$ at 4 dyne $cm^{-2}$ and 0.2% $h^{-1}$ at 12 dyne $cm^{-2}$.

The net turnover rate reflects any significant changes in cell area and hence is a measure of stress on the monolayer. For example, large positive values can lead to the formation of mounds or overgrowth, while large negative values can lead to gaps in the monolayer. The positive net turnover rate corresponds to an increase in the number of cells over time, however, this increase is not sufficiently large to cause a measurable change in the average cell area. Under steady state conditions (30–40 h) we can expect the monolayer to increase the number of cells by 8, 3, and 2% at 0, 4, and 12 dyne $cm^{-2}$, respectively. Therefore, the expected decrease in average cell area is within the variation and is not detected.

The net turnover rate of 0.2–0.3% $h^{-1}$ under shear stress is similar to values for HUVEC monolayers (0.1% $h^{-1}$), and 3D microvessels (0.25–0.6% $h^{-1}$; labeling index) [65]. Surprisingly little is known about the turnover of hBMECs in vivo, however, results from thymidine labeling in mice suggest rates of about 0.04% $h^{-1}$, about an order of magnitude lower than endothelial cells in other tissues [39–41, 66, 67].

### Cell motility and displacement

The average speed of dhBMECs under shear stress is around 0.1 $\mu m\ min^{-1}$, lower than values for both HUVECs and immortalized hBMECs, typically around is 0.2 $\mu m\ min^{-1}$ [19]. More importantly, the average cell displacement in dhBMEC monolayers is extremely low, around 15 $\mu m$ over 40 h. In contrast, HUVECs under the same conditions show a displacement of 200–500 $\mu m$ over 40 h under shear stress, an increase of more than 100-fold compared to the dhBMECs. The very small displacement observed for dhBMECs could arise from increased adhesion to the substrate or increased cell–cell adhesion. Since dhBMEC monolayers are relatively easy to displace from the substrate as sheets of cells, the low displacement is likely due to increased cell–cell adhesion. As described previously, dhBMECs in confluent monolayers cells appear to flatten under shear stress. There is no change in cell area and hence if the cell volume remains constant, then the flattening must be a result of increased overlap between cells. Increased cell–cell overlap would increase the strength of cell–cell junctions and explain the very low cell displacement. Ultrastructural studies of capillaries in animal models show substantial cell–cell overlap at tight junctions which may be important for maintaining low blood–brain barrier permeability [68, 69]. These results suggest that an important role of flow may be in increasing the contact area between cells which in turn enhances barrier function.

### Protein and gene expression

Immunofluorescence images revealed no difference in the expression and localization of claudin-5, occludin, ZO-1, or F-actin in response to flow, suggesting that tight junctions are established under static conditions [70]. In contrast, bovine brain microvascular endothelial cells under 10 dyne $cm^{-2}$ shear stress for 24 h showed increased localization of tight junction proteins to the cell–cell borders [71].

The ability of cells to sense and adapt to their environment is crucial, and the mechanosensing responses to shear stress and other mechanical forces are mediated by the actin cytoskeleton [72]. In dhBMEC monolayers, F-actin is localized to the cell–cell junctions and we do not see any significant stress fibers within the cell body. In contrast, other ECs such as HUVECs and BAECs, show significant cytoskeleton reorganization with alignment of stress fibers parallel to the direction of flow [73–75]. Stress fibers formed in vivo in cardiac vascular endothelial cells are also aligned parallel to the direction of flow and are thought to be necessary to withstand high hemodynamic stresses [76]. These results suggest that elongation and alignment is coupled with cytoskeleton reorganization, neither of which are observed in dhB-MEC monolayers.

Shear stress did not induce any changes in expression of several BBB markers at the protein or gene level. The fact that there were no changes in expression of BBB markers with shear stress is coupled with the fact that there is no morphological transition (cobblestone to spindle-like). Previous in vitro studies with bovine and human brain microvascular endothelial cells have shown up-regulation of various junctional and transporter genes in response to shear stress [77, 78]. In contrast to other cell lines, dhBMECs under static conditions exhibit transendothelial electrical resistance values in excess of 2000 $\Omega$ cm$^2$ [5, 6, 79], comparable to values reported in vivo in rat brains (1000–1500 $\Omega$ cm$^2$) [80]. These results suggest that the tight junction architecture in dhBMECs is already established during monolayer formation under static conditions, and that flow is not necessary for this process. This conclusion is supported by the fact that very high TEER vales are obtained for confluent monolayers on transwell supports under static conditions [5, 6, 79]. As described previously, we hypothesize that flow serves to increase the contact area between cells, resulting in very low cell displacement and preventing the morphological transition that is thought to be a hallmark of ECs.

## Conclusions

Shear stress plays an important role in modulating endothelial cell morphology, structure and function. Here we show that dhBMECs exhibit a unique phenotype in response to shear stress: (1) they do not elongate and align, (2) the displacement of individual cells within the monolayer over time is significantly decreased, (3) the rates of proliferation and apoptosis decrease, (4) there is no cytoskeletal reorganization or formation of stress fibers within the cell, and (5) there is no change in expression levels of key blood–brain barrier markers. This response is very different to the response of endothelial cells from other tissues, indicating that the dhBMEC have a unique phenotype in response to shear stress that may be important in maintenance of the blood–brain barrier. Since the blood–brain barrier has specialized endothelial cells with tight junctions that minimize paracellular transport and specialized transporters to regulate transport across the brain, our results suggest that these endothelial cells may also have a unique response to shear stress. The implications of this work are that: (1) in confluent monolayers of dhBMECs, tight junctions are well formed under static conditions, (2) the formation of tight junctions decreases cell motility, compared to other

ECs, and hence prevents any morphological transitions, (3) flow serves to increase the contact area between cells, resulting in very low cell displacement in the monolayer, (4) since tight junctions are already formed under static conditions, increasing the contact area between cells does not cause upregulation in protein and gene expression of BBB markers, and (5) the increase in contact area induced by flow makes barrier function more robust. These unique features of dHBMECs as compared to other endothelial cell lines may contribute to the unique tightness and highly selective permeability of the blood–brain barrier. Shear stress is one of many parameters that influence endothelial phenotype. Therefore, this work contributes to the emerging understanding of factors that are important in developing accurate in vitro models of the blood–brain barrier.

### Abbreviations

ABCB1: ATP binding cassette subfamily B member 1; ACTB: beta actin; BAEC: bovine aortic endothelial cell; BBB: blood–brain barrier; BBMvEC: bovine brain microvascular endothelial cell; BC1-hBMEC: BC1-derived human brain microvascular endothelial cell; bFGF: basic fibroblast growth factor; BMEC: brain microvascular endothelial cell; CDH5: cadherin 5/VE-cadherin; CLDN5: claudin-5; DAPI: 4′,6-diamidino-2-phenylindole fluorescent stain; EC: endothelial cell; GAPDH: glyceraldehyde 3-phosphate dehydrogenase; GLUT1: glucose transporter 1; hBMEC: human brain microvascular endothelial cell; hiPSC: human induced pluripotent stem cell; HUVEC: human umbilical vein endothelial cell; IAR: inverse aspect ratio; ID: inner diameter; OCLN: occludin; pBAEC: primary baboon artery endothelial cell; PBS: phosphate buffered saline; PDMS: polydimethylsiloxane; P-gp: p-glycoprotein; PIV: particle image velocimetry; qPCR: quantitative polymerase chain reaction; RIPA: radio immunoprecipitation assay; ROCK: rho-associated protein kinase; SLC2A1: solute carrier family 2 member 1; TEER: transendothelial electrical resistance; TJP1: tight junction protein 1/gene for ZO-1; UM/F-: unconditioned media without bFGF; VECAD: VE-cadherin; ZO1: zonula occludens 1.

### Authors' contributions

JD and ZX performed the experiments. JD, ZX, AW, NY, and PS analyzed the data. JD, ZX, and PS wrote the manuscript. All authors read and approved the final manuscript.

### Author details

[1] Institute for Nanobiotechnology, Johns Hopkins University, 100 Croft Hall, 3400 North Charles Street, Baltimore, MD 21218, USA. [2] Department of Materials Science and Engineering, Johns Hopkins University, Baltimore, MD 21218, USA. [3] Department of Biomedical Engineering, Johns Hopkins University, 720 Rutland Avenue, Baltimore, MD 21205, USA.

### Acknowledgements

AW and NY gratefully acknowledge support from the Institute for Nanobiotechnology at Johns Hopkins University through the NSF-funded research experience for undergraduates program.

### Competing interests

The authors declare that they have no competing interests.

### Funding

The authors gratefully acknowledge support from DTRA (HDTRA1-15-1-0046) and the American Heart Association (15GRNT25090122).

# References

1. Abbott NJ, Patabendige AA, Dolman DE, Yusof SR, Begley DJ. Structure and function of the blood–brain barrier. Neurobiol Dis. 2010;37(1):13–25.
2. Wong AD, Ye M, Levy AF, Rothstein JD, Bergles DE, et al. The blood–brain barrier: an engineering perspective. Front Neuroeng. 2013;6:7.
3. Neuwelt EA, Bauer B, Fahlke C, Fricker G, Iadecola C, et al. Engaging neuroscience to advance translational research in brain barrier biology. Nat Rev Neurosci. 2011;12(3):169–82.
4. Katt ME, Xu ZS, Gerecht S, Searson PC. Human brain microvascular endothelial cells derived from the BC1 iPS cell line exhibit a blood–brain barrier phenotype. PLoS ONE. 2016;11(4):e0152105.
5. Lippmann ES, Al-Ahmad A, Azarin SM, Palecek SP, Shusta EV. A retinoic acid-enhanced, multicellular human blood–brain barrier model derived from stem cell sources. Sci Rep. 2014;4:4160.
6. Lippmann ES, Azarin SM, Kay JE, Nessler RA, Wilson HK, et al. Derivation of blood–brain barrier endothelial cells from human pluripotent stem cells. Nat Biotechnol. 2012;30(8):783–91.
7. Chien S. Mechanotransduction and endothelial cell homeostasis: the wisdom of the cell. Am J Physiol Heart Circ Physiol. 2007;292(3):H1209–24.
8. Davies PF. Flow-mediated endothelial mechanotransduction. Physiol Rev. 1995;75(1):519–60.
9. Burnstock G. Release of vasoactive substances from endothelial cells by shear stress and purinergic mechanosensory transduction. J Anat. 1999;194(Pt 3):335–42.
10. Levesque MJ, Nerem RM. The elongation and orientation of cultured endothelial cells in response to shear stress. J Biomech Eng. 1985;107(4):341–7.
11. Levesque MJ, Nerem RM. The study of rheological effects on vascular endothelial cells in culture. Biorheology. 1989;26(2):345–57.
12. Reidy MA, Langille BL. The effect of local blood flow patterns on endothelial cell morphology. Exp Mol Pathol. 1980;32(3):276–89.
13. Nerem RM, Levesque MJ, Cornhill J. Vascular endothelial morphology as an indicator of the pattern of blood flow. J Biomech Eng. 1981;103(3):172–6.
14. Blackman BR, Garcia-Cardena G, Gimbrone MA Jr. A new in vitro model to evaluate differential responses of endothelial cells to simulated arterial shear stress waveforms. J Biomech Eng. 2002;124(4):397–407.
15. Galbraith CG, Skalak R, Chien S. Shear stress induces spatial reorganization of the endothelial cell cytoskeleton. Cell Motil Cytoskelet. 1998;40(4):317–30.
16. Simmers MB, Pryor AW, Blackman BR. Arterial shear stress regulates endothelial cell-directed migration, polarity, and morphology in confluent monolayers. Am J Physiol Heart Circ Physiol. 2007;293(3):H1937–46.
17. Chiu JJ, Wang DL, Chien S, Skalak R, Usami S. Effects of disturbed flow on endothelial cells. J Biomech Eng. 1998;120(1):2–8.
18. Malek AM, Izumo S. Mechanism of endothelial cell shape change and cytoskeletal remodeling in response to fluid shear stress. J Cell Sci. 1996;109:713–26.
19. Reinitz A, DeStefano J, Ye M, Wong AD, Searson PC. Human brain microvascular endothelial cells resist elongation due to shear stress. Microvasc Res. 2015;99:8–18.
20. Eskin S, Ives C, McIntire L, Navarro L. Response of cultured endothelial cells to steady flow. Microvasc Res. 1984;28(1):87–94.
21. Silkworth J, Stehbens W. The shape of endothelial cells in en face preparations of rabbit blood vessels. Angiology. 1975;26(6):474–87.
22. Levesque MJ, Liepsch D, Moravec S, Nerem RM. Correlation of endothelial cell shape and wall shear stress in a stenosed dog aorta. Arteriosclerosis. 1986;6(2):220–9.
23. DePaola N, Gimbrone MA Jr, Davies PF, Dewey CF Jr. Vascular endothelium responds to fluid shear stress gradients. Arterioscler Thromb. 1992;12(11):1254–7.
24. Dewey C, Bussolari S, Gimbrone M, Davies PF. The dynamic response of vascular endothelial cells to fluid shear stress. J Biomech Eng. 1981;103(3):177–85.
25. Ye M, Sanchez HM, Hultz M, Yang Z, Bogorad M, et al. Brain microvascular endothelial cells resist elongation due to curvature and shear stress. Sci Rep. 2014;4:4681.
26. Guntheroth WG, Gould R, Butler J, Kinnen E. Pulsatile flow in pulmonary artery, capillary, and vein in the dog. Cardiovasc Res. 1974;8(3):330–7.
27. Milnor WR. Pulsatile blood flow. N Engl J Med. 1972;287(1):27–34.
28. Fronek K, Zweifach BW. Microvascular blood flow in cat tenuissimus muscle. Microvasc Res. 1977;14(2):181–9.
29. Ivanov KP, Kalinina MK, Levkovich YuI. Blood flow velocity in capillaries of brain and muscles and its physiological significance. Microvasc Res. 1981;22(2):143–55.
30. Morkin E. Analysis of pulsatile blood flow and its clinical implications. N Engl J Med. 1967;277(3):139–46.
31. Cheng C, Helderman F, Tempel D, Segers D, Hierck B, et al. Large variations in absolute wall shear stress levels within one species and between species. Atherosclerosis. 2007;195(2):225–35.
32. Koutsiaris AG, Tachmitzi SV, Batis N, Kotoula MG, Karabatsas CH, et al. Volume flow and wall shear stress quantification in the human conjunctival capillaries and post-capillary venules in vivo. Biorheology. 2007;44(5–6):375–86.
33. DeStefano J, Williams A, Wnorowski A, Yimam N, Searson P, et al. Real-time quantification of endothelial response to shear stress and vascular modulators. Integr Biol. 2017;9:362–74.
34. Bogorad MI, DeStefano J, Wong AD, and Searson PC. Tissue-engineered 3D microvessel and capillary network models for the study of vascular phenomena. Microcirc. 2017;4:e12360.
35. Taylor ZJ, Gurka R, Kopp GA, Liberzon A. Long-duration time-resolved PIV to study unsteady aerodynamics. IEEE Trans Instrum Meas. 2010;59(12):3262–9.
36. McNeil E, Capaldo CT, Macara IG. Zonula occludens-1 function in the assembly of tight junctions in Madin-Darby canine kidney epithelial cells. Mol Biol Cell. 2006;17(4):1922–32.
37. Boudaoud A, Burian A, Borowska-Wykret D, Uyttewaal M, Wrzalik R, et al. FibrilTool, an ImageJ plug-in to quantify fibrillar structures in raw microscopy images. Nat Protocol. 2014;9(2):457–63.
38. Schmittgen TD, Livak KJ. Analyzing real-time PCR data by the comparative C(T) method. Nat Protocols. 2008;3(6):1101–8.
39. Hobson B, Denekamp J. Endothelial proliferation in tumours and normal tissues: continuous labelling studies. Br J Cancer. 1984;49(4):405–13.
40. Spaet TH, Lejnieks I. Mitotic activity of rabbit blood vessels. Proc Soc Exp Biol Med. 1967;125(4):1197–201.
41. Tannock IF, Hayashi S. The proliferation of capillary endothelial cells. Cancer Res. 1972;32(1):77–82.
42. Wong KH, Truslow JG, Tien J. The role of cyclic AMP in normalizing the function of engineered human blood microvessels in microfluidic collagen gels. Biomaterials. 2010;31(17):4706–14.
43. Amano M, Nakayama M, Kaibuchi K. Rho-kinase/ROCK: a key regulator of the cytoskeleton and cell polarity. Cytoskeleton (Hoboken). 2010;67(9):545–54.
44. Watanabe K, Ueno M, Kamiya D, Nishiyama A, Matsumura M, et al. A ROCK inhibitor permits survival of dissociated human embryonic stem cells. Nat Biotechnol. 2007;25(6):681–6.
45. Chiba H, Osanai M, Murata M, Kojima T, Sawada N. Transmembrane proteins of tight junctions. Biochim Biophys Acta. 2008;1778(3):588–600.
46. Fanning AS, Jameson BJ, Jesaitis LA, Anderson JM. The tight junction protein ZO-1 establishes a link between the transmembrane protein occludin and the actin cytoskeleton. J Biol Chem. 1998;273(45):29745–53.
47. Patel R, Alahmad AJ. Growth-factor reduced Matrigel source influences stem cell derived brain microvascular endothelial cell barrier properties. Fluids Barriers CNS. 2016;13:6.
48. Mantle JL, Min L, Lee KH. Minimum transendothelial electrical resistance thresholds for the study of small and large molecule drug transport in a human in vitro blood-brain barrier model. Mol Pharm. 2016;13(12):4191–8.
49. Wilson HK, Canfield SG, Hjortness MK, Palecek SP, Shusta EV. Exploring the effects of cell seeding density on the differentiation of human pluripotent stem cells to brain microvascular endothelial cells. Fluids Barriers CNS. 2015;12:13.
50. Weksler BB, Subileau EA, Perriere N, Charneau P, Holloway K, et al. Blood–brain barrier-specific properties of a human adult brain endothelial cell line. FASEB J. 2005;19(13):1872–4.

51. Nakagawa S, Deli MA, Kawaguchi H, Shimizudani T, Shimono T, et al. A new blood-brain barrier model using primary rat brain endothelial cells, pericytes and astrocytes. Neurochem Int. 2009;54(3–4):253–63.

52. Sano Y, Kashiwamura Y, Abe M, Dieu LH, Huwyler J, et al. Stable human brain microvascular endothelial cell line retaining its barrier-specific nature independent of the passage number. Clin Exp Neuroimmunol. 2013;4:92–103.

53. Clarke M, Spudich JA. Nonmuscle contractile proteins: the role of actin and myosin in cell motility and shape determination. Annu Rev Biochem. 1977;46:797–822.

54. Nitta T, Hata M, Gotoh S, Seo Y, Sasaki H, et al. Size-selective loosening of the blood-brain barrier in claudin-5-deficient mice. J Cell Biol. 2003;161(3):653–60.

55. Tsuji A. Small molecular drug transfer across the blood–brain barrier via carrier-mediated transport systems. NeuroRx. 2005;2(1):54–62.

56. Tatsuta T, Naito M, Oh-hara T, Sugawara I, Tsuruo T. Functional involvement of P-glycoprotein in blood–brain barrier. J Biol Chem. 1992;267(28):20383–91.

57. Pardridge WM, Boado RJ, Farrell CR. Brain-type glucose transporter (GLUT-1) is selectively localized to the blood-brain barrier. Studies with quantitative western blotting and in situ hybridization. J Biol Chem. 1990;265(29):18035–40.

58. Giannotta M, Trani M, Dejana E. VE-cadherin and endothelial adherens junctions: active guardians of vascular integrity. Dev Cell. 2013;26(5):441–54.

59. Bolton SJ, Anthony DC, Perry VH. Loss of the tight junction proteins occludin and zonula occludens-1 from cerebral vascular endothelium during neutrophil-induced blood–brain barrier breakdown in vivo. Neuroscience. 1998;86(4):1245–57.

60. Fischer S, Wobben M, Marti HH, Renz D, Schaper W. Hypoxia-induced hyperpermeability in brain microvessel endothelial cells involves VEGF-mediated changes in the expression of zonula occludens-1. Microvasc Res. 2002;63(1):70–80.

61. Kibria G, Heath D, Smith P, Biggar R. Pulmonary endothelial pavement patterns. Thorax. 1980;35(3):186–91.

62. Schnittler HJ, Schneider SW, Raifer H, Luo F, Dieterich P, et al. Role of actin filaments in endothelial cell–cell adhesion and membrane stability under fluid shear stress. Pflugers Arch Eur J Physiol. 2001;442(5):675–87.

63. Seebach J, Dieterich P, Luo F, Schillers H, Vestweber D, et al. Endothelial barrier function under laminar fluid shear stress. Lab Investig. 2000;80(12):1819–31.

64. Li S, Bhatia S, Hu YL, Shiu YT, Li YS, et al. Effects of morphological patterning on endothelial cell migration. Biorheology. 2001;38(2–3):101–8.

65. Price GM, Wong KH, Truslow JG, Leung AD, Acharya C, et al. Effect of mechanical factors on the function of engineered human blood microvessels in microfluidic collagen gels. Biomaterials. 2010;31(24):6182–9.

66. Engerman RL, Pfaffenbach D, Davis MD. Cell turnover of capillaries. Lab Investig. 1967;17(6):738–43.

67. Gospodarowicz D, Mescher AL, Birdwell CR. Stimulation of corneal endothelial cell-proliferation invitro by fibroblast and epidermal growth-factors. Exp Eye Res. 1977;25(1):75–89.

68. Nag S. Morphological and molecular properties of cellular components of normal cerebral vessels. In: Nag S, editor. The blood–brain barrier: biological and research protocols. New Jersey: Humana Press; 2003. p. 3–36.

69. Begley DJ, Brightman MW. Structural and functional aspects of the blood brain barrier. In: Prokai-Tatrai LPaK, editor. Progress in drug research. Basel: Birkhauser Verlag; 2003. p. 39–78.

70. Rubin LL, Staddon JM. The cell biology of the blood–brain barrier. Annu Rev Neurosci. 1999;22:11–28.

71. Walsh TG, Murphy RP, Fitzpatrick P, Rochfort KD, Guinan AF, et al. Stabilization of brain microvascular endothelial barrier function by shear stress involves VE-cadherin signaling leading to modulation of pTyr-occludin levels. J Cell Physiol. 2011;226(11):3053–63.

72. Shao X, Li Q, Mogilner A, Bershadsky AD, Shivashankar GV. Mechanical stimulation induces formin-dependent assembly of a perinuclear actin rim. Proc Natl Acad Sci USA. 2015;112(20):E2595–601.

73. Barbee KA, Davies PF, Lal R. Shear stress-induced reorganization of the surface topography of living endothelial cells imaged by atomic force microscopy. Circ Res. 1994;74(1):163–71.

74. Franke RP, Grafe M, Schnittler H, Seiffge D, Mittermayer C, et al. Induction of human vascular endothelial stress fibres by fluid shear stress. Nature. 1984;307(5952):648–9.

75. Wechezak AR, Viggers RF, Sauvage LR. Fibronectin and F-actin redistribution in cultured endothelial cells exposed to shear stress. Lab Investig. 1985;53(6):639–47.

76. Wong AJ, Pollard TD, Herman IM. Actin filament stress fibers in vascular endothelial cells in vivo. Science. 1983;219(4586):867–9.

77. DeMaio L, Chang YS, Gardner TW, Tarbell JM, Antonetti DA. Shear stress regulates occludin content and phosphorylation. Am J Physiol Heart Circ Physiol. 2001;281(1):H105–13.

78. Colgan OC, Ferguson G, Collins NT, Murphy RP, Meade G, et al. Regulation of bovine brain microvascular endothelial tight junction assembly and barrier function by laminar shear stress. Am J Physiol Heart Circ Physiol. 2007;292(6):H3190–7.

79. Katt ME, Placone AL, Wong AD, Xu ZS, Searson PC. In vitro tumor models: advantages, disadvantages, variables, and selecting the right platform. Front Bioeng Biotechnol. 2016;4:12.

80. Butt AM, Jones HC, Abbott NJ. Electrical-resistance across the blood–brain barrier in anesthetized rats: a developmental study. J Physiol Lond. 1990;429:47–62.

# 16

# Small cisterno-lumbar gradient of phosphorylated Tau protein in geriatric patients with suspected normal pressure hydrocephalus

Marija Djukic[1,2†], Annette Spreer[3,4†], Peter Lange[3], Stephanie Bunkowski[2], Jens Wiltfang[5,6] and Roland Nau[1,2*]

## Abstract

**Background:** The composition of the cerebrospinal fluid (CSF) is not homogeneous, and concentrations of proteins from different origins diverge among ventricular, cisternal and lumbar CSF fractions. Concentrations of blood-derived proteins increase and of brain-derived proteins decrease from ventricular to lumbar fractions. We studied whether the origin of the CSF portion analysed may affect results in CSF analysis for dementia.

**Methods:** In 16 geriatric patients with suspected normal pressure hydrocephalus [age 82.5 (76/87) years; median (25th/75th percentile)] a lumbar spinal tap of 40 ml was performed. The CSF was sequentially collected in 8 fractions of 5 ml with the 1st fraction corresponding to lumbar CSF, the 8th to cisterna magna-near CSF. Fractions were analysed for total protein, albumin, Tau protein (Tau), phosphorylated Tau (pTau), Amyloid beta 1–42 (Aβ1–42), Amyloid beta 1–40 (Aβ1–40), and the Aβ1–42/Aβ1–40 ratio.

**Results:** The concentrations of total protein and albumin increased from cisternal to lumbar fractions due to diffusion-related accumulation from blood to CSF with significantly higher concentrations in fraction 1 compared to fraction 8. The concentrations of Tau showed a non-significant trend towards decreased values in lumbar samples, and pTau was slightly, but significantly decreased in the lumbar fraction 1 [26.5 (22.5/35.0) pg/ml] compared to the cistern-near fraction 8 [27.0 (24.2/36.3) pg/ml] (p = 0.02, Wilcoxon signed rank test). Aβ1-42, Aβ1-40, and the Aβ1-42/Aβ1-40 ratio remained almost constant.

**Conclusions:** According to the flow-related diverging dynamics of blood-derived and brain-derived proteins in CSF, the concentrations of Tau and pTau tended to be lower in lumbar compared to cisternal CSF fractions after a spinal tap of 40 ml. The differences reached statistical significance for pTau only. The small differences will not affect clinical interpretation of markers of dementia in the vast majority of cases.

**Keywords:** Cerebrospinal fluid, Amyloid beta 1–40, Amyloid beta 1–42, Tau protein, Phosphorylated Tau protein

## Background

Normal pressure hydrocephalus (NPH) is characterized clinically by the triad of gait disturbance, bladder incontinence, and later dementia. Cerebral imaging shows ventricular dilation, whereas the subarachnoid space on both sides of the superior sagittal sinus is comparatively small [1]. Unlike in acute or subacute obstructive hydrocephalus, response to surgical shunt treatment in NPH is difficult to predict [2]. At autopsy, many of these patients display pathological findings suggesting neurodegenerative disease. Morphological findings of Alzheimer's dementia (AD) were detected in 30 to 75 % of patients with clinically diagnosed NPH where a biopsy was available suggesting a large subgroup of patients with overlapping clinical features

*Correspondence: rnau@gwdg.de
†Marija Djukic and Annette Spreer contributed equally to this work
2 Institute of Neuropathology, University Medical Center Goettingen (UMG), Robert-Koch-Strasse 40, D-37075 Göttingen, Germany
Full list of author information is available at the end of the article

of both AD and NPH [1–5]. A spinal tap of 40 ml is a relatively insensitive, minimally-invasive procedure to assess which patients may benefit from ventriculoperitoneal shunting.

Many compounds do not distribute homogeneously in the CSF spaces, but have ventriculo-lumbar or lumbo-ventricular gradients. Compounds originating in the brain (e.g., Tau protein, neuron-specific enolase, S-100 protein) generally have higher ventricular than lumbar CSF concentrations, whereas compounds originating from the meninges (e.g., β-trace protein and cystatin C) have higher lumbar than ventricular levels, and the concentrations of blood-derived proteins such as albumin increase from the ventricular to the lumbar CSF space [6–8]. In pathological conditions with decreased CSF flow or in central nervous system bacterial infections, where the CSF spaces can be, in part, obstructed by pus, the distribution of leukocytes and proteins can be particularly inhomogeneous, whereas the small molecule lactate is distributed homogeneously even in this condition [9]. Amyloid beta 1–42 (Aβ1–42, molecular mass 4514 Da), Amyloid beta 1–40 (Aβ1–40, molecular mass 4330 Da), Tau protein (Tau) and Tau protein phosphorylated at position 181 (pTau) (molecular mass 36800–45900 Da) are proteins originating from the brain and the myelon which help to discriminate AD from other types of dementia [4]. In a usual diagnostic lumbar puncture, approximately 5–10 ml of CSF is removed, and CSF analysis is performed on this fraction. Here, we collected 40 ml of CSF in fractions of 5 ml, to assess whether the markers are evenly distributed in these CSF fractions, or whether a ventriculo-lumbar concentration gradient can be also detected between the cistern-near and lumbar fractions, a situation which may affect the interpretation of these markers in the differential diagnosis of dementia.

## Methods

A diagnostic or therapeutic lumbar spinal tap of 40 ml was performed on 16 patients with suspected or documented normal pressure hydrocephalus [11 women, 5 men, age 82.5 (76/87) years; median (25th/75th percentile)]. All patients suffered from cognitive impairment. In 15 of the 16 patients an abnormal gait, and in 10 patients bladder incontinence were documented. All patients had an abnormal cranial computer tomography (CCT) scan with wide ventricles compared to the width of the sulci. Moreover, 14 patients had crowding of the gyri at the vertex with small sulci close to the superior sagittal sinus, and 14 patients had a corpus callosum angle below 90°. Four patients (including a patient who received three lumbar punctures) clearly improved after the spinal taps, and in three patients a small clinically non-significant

improvement of either gait or cognition were noted. None of the patients studied had a ventriculoperitoneal shunt or external ventriculostomy. The treating physicians recommended ventriculoperitoneal shunting to the 4 patients with clear clinical improvement after the spinal tap. Because of their advanced age, these patients and/or their relatives refused surgery, as they feared the risks.

The CSF was sequentially collected in eight fractions of 5 ml in polypropylene tubes and was transported to the laboratory within 1 h for analysis. One set of CSF fractions was available from 15 patients. Three sets of CSF fractions were available from one patient with documented normal pressure hydrocephalus, who underwent repeated lumbar punctures as part of his therapy.

Albumin, immunoglobulins IgG, IgA and IgM were determined by nephelometry, and CSF leukocytes were counted manually in a Fuchs-Rosenthal chamber. Albumin and immunoglobulin CSF/serum quotients (IgG, IgA, IgM) were calculated in fraction 1. The CSF protein contents were measured by nephelometry using Gesamteiweiß UC Standard FS (DiaSys Diagnostic Systems, Holzheim, Germany). After centrifugation at $200 \times g$, aliquots of each fraction were stored at −80 °C for the determination of markers of dementia, protein and albumin concentrations.

Tau protein (Tau), tau protein phosphorylated at threonine 181 (pTau), Amyloid beta 1–42 and Amyloid beta 1–40 (Aβ1–42 and Aβ1–40) were measured by commercially-available immunoassays (Innotest hTAU Ag, Innotest PHOSPHO-TAU 181P, Innotest β-AMYLOID 1–42, Fujirebio, Gent, Belgium; Amyloid-beta 1–40 CSF ELISA, IBL, Hamburg, Germany), and the Aβ1–42/Aβ1–40 ratio was calculated. The raw data were uploaded as Additional file 1 on Aug 6th, 2016.

Correlation of measured values between fraction 1 and fraction 8 of each individual patient was assessed by Spearman's rank correlation coefficient $r_S$. The concentrations of the compounds measured in fractions 1 and 8 were compared by the two-tailed non-parametric paired Wilcoxon signed rank test using Gaph Pad Prism software, as most parameters were not normally distributed. $P$ values <0.05 were considered statistically significant. The study was approved by the Ethics Committee of the Medical Faculty of the Georg-August University Göttingen, Germany, and each participant gave written informed consent to participate in this study.

## Results

The CSF leukocyte counts were normal in all patients studied, and the Reiber–Felgenhauer diagrams of albumin- and immunoglobulin-CSF/serum quotients (IgG, IgA, IgM) indicated absence of inflammation in all patients studied. Three patients had an elevated CSF-serum albumin ratio (10.2, 14.9 and 15.4 $\times$ 10$^{-3}$) probably because of an impaired circulation of the CSF in the spinal canal: one of these patients had prior surgery because of stenosis of the lumbar spinal canal, one had a history of two fractures of lumbar vertebrae, and one suffered from lower back pain with hardening of muscles, suggesting degenerative spine disease. The concentrations of the parameters measured in fractions 1 and 8 of each individual patient were strongly correlated ($r_S \geq 0.81$, $p < 0.0001$). The CSF protein contents were lower in the cistern-near fraction 8 than in the lumbar fraction 1 ($p < 0.0001$, Wilcoxon signed rank test) (Table 1). Albumin as a strictly blood-derived protein showed a rostro-caudal increase of concentration with significantly lower values in the cistern-near fraction 8 than in the lumbar fraction 1 ($p < 0.0001$, Wilcoxon signed rank test).

pTau concentrations in the CSF fraction 8 were slightly, but significantly higher than in lumbar CSF (medians 27.0 versus 26.5 pg/ml, $p = 0.02$) indicating a small decrease of pTau from cisternal to lumbar CSF. Tau concentrations also were slightly higher in CSF fraction 8 than in lumbar CSF, the difference, however, failed to reach statistical significance (Table 1). No differences among fractions 8 and 1 were found for Aβ1–40, Aβ1–42 and the Aβ1–42/Aβ1–40 ratio. Only one patient had an elevated CSF Tau concentration (893 pg/ml in fraction 1 and 884 pg/ml in fraction 8). No patient had an elevated pTau (>61 pg/ml) or an abnormal CSF Aβ1–42 concentration (<450 pg/ml).

In the patient with 3 consecutive spinal taps in 11 months the intra-individual variation of the determined markers of neurodegenerative disease was low. Concentrations of Tau in the lumbar fraction 1 ranged from 148 to 176 pg/ml, of pTau from 25.5 to 28.0 pg/ml, of Aβ1–42 from 859 to 933 pg/ml, of Aβ1–40 from 8815 to 9731 pg/ml, and the Aβ1–42/Aβ1–40 ratio ranged from 0.088 to 0.106.

## Discussion

The total volume of CSF in adults is approximately 140 ml with a wide variation dependent on age, and volume of the brain and medulla spinalis in relation to the size of the cranial cavity and the spinal canal. The volume of the spinal subarachnoid fluid is 30–80 ml [6, 10], i.e., the first 5 ml fraction in our study represents lumbar CSF, whereas the 8th 5 ml fraction contains a large proportion of CSF from regions close to the cisterna magna and cisterna pontis.

In agreement with flow-related diverging dynamics of blood-derived and brain-derived proteins in CSF [7], we found an increase in the blood-derived protein albumin from cisternal to lumbar fractions and correspondingly an increase in total protein. In the analysis of markers of degenerative disorders, we found a small, statistically significant decrease in pTau from cisternal to lumbar fractions and a similar, yet not significant, decrease of Tau in fraction 1 (lumbar CSF) compared to fraction 8 (predominantly cisternal CSF), i.e. median pTau and Tau concentrations were higher in the cistern-near than in the lumbar CSF. In the patient receiving three spinal taps, the intra-individual variance between the different sampling points of pTau and Tau in lumbar CSF was higher (25.5–28.0 and 148–176 pg/ml, respectively) than the difference at group level between fraction 8 and 1 (27.0 versus 26.5 pg/ml and 210 versus 188 pg/ml). It has to be considered that these samples from one individual patient were drawn in an interval of 11 months. In two of these three samples from this patient, the pTau and Tau concentrations in cistern-near were higher than in lumbar CSF supporting our concept of a small cisterno-lumbar gradient of pTau and Tau. Similar rostro-caudal gradients have been found for α-synuclein and NSE in 5 patients with NPH [8]. In contrast to the small cisterno-lumbar concentration differences for pTau and Tau found in fractions 8 and 1 in the present study, the ventriculo-lumbar concentration

**Table 1  Markers of dementia and protein concentrations in lumbar (fraction 1) and cistern-near cerebrospinal fluid (fraction 8) (n = 16 pairs of samples)**

|  | CSF protein (mg/l) | | Albumin (mg/l) | | Tau (pg/ml) | | PTau (pg/ml) | | Aβ1–42 (pg/ml) | | Aβ1–40 (pg/ml) | | Aβ1–42/Aβ1–40 | |
|---|---|---|---|---|---|---|---|---|---|---|---|---|---|---|
| Fraction | 1 | 8 | 1 | 8 | 1 | 8 | 1 | 8 | 1 | 8 | 1 | 8 | 1 | 8 |
| Median | 433 | 353 | 253 | 202 | 188 | 210 | 26.5 | 27.0 | 985 | 955 | 12567 | 12576 | 0.077 | 0.075 |
| 25th percentile | 309 | 240 | 177 | 138 | 145 | 151 | 22.5 | 24.2 | 765 | 783 | 11215 | 11045 | 0.065 | 0.065 |
| 75th percentile | 513 | 427 | 288 | 234 | 280 | 265 | 35.0 | 36.3 | 1279 | 1191 | 15691 | 15465 | 0.088 | 0.087 |
| Correlation between fraction 1 and 8 ($r_S$) | 0.95* | | 0.91* | | 0.94* | | 0.98* | | 0.97* | | 0.93* | | 0.81* | |
| Fraction 1 versus 8, $p$ value; Wilcoxon signed rank test | <0.0001 | | <0.0001 | | NS | | 0.02 | | NS | | NS | | NS | |

*NS* difference not significant

* $p < 0.0001$

ratios in NPH patients for Tau and pTau were previously found to be approximately five and twofold, respectively [11–13]. The existence of a ventriculo-lumbar Tau and pTau gradient was shown to depend on the diagnosis: it was large in NPH, but apparently absent in post-traumatic hydrocephalus [11]. The ventriculo-lumbar gradient observed previously and the cisterno-lumbar gradient observed by us suggests that Tau and pTau are mainly brain-derived, and that the fluids entering the spinal CSF from blood (interstitial fluid of the medulla spinalis and of the meninges) contain lower Tau and pTau concentrations than the interstitial fluid of the brain. This compares well with immunohistochemical findings demonstrating that in the spinal cord and the peripheral nervous system Tau immuno-reactivity is less abundant than in the brain [14]. Conversely, in previous studies lumbar Aβ1–40 and Aβ1–42 concentrations were slightly higher than the respective ventricular levels [12, 13]. In the present study, no clear gradients of Aβ1–40 and Aβ1–42 concentrations were observed, possibly as a consequence of their lower molecular mass compared to Tau proteins facilitating a more homogeneous distribution [9].

The median total protein content and the albumin concentrations were 1.23- and 1.25-fold higher, respectively, in fraction 1 than in fraction 8. This reflects a relevant influx of proteins from non-neuronal sources into the CSF in the spinal canal. In a previous study of 21 patients with NPH, 10 fractions of approximately 3 ml were drawn, and the albumin concentrations were 1.5-fold higher in fraction 1 than in fraction 10 [15]. Since the CSF flow dynamics are altered in NPH, these gradients of 1.25 or 1.5 in a spinal tap of 30–40 ml may not represent the gradients in healthy persons or patients with other diseases. Because high volumes of CSF can only be drawn with a clear clinical indication, it would be very difficult to obtain similar data in healthy adults or patients with other diseases. Patients with other forms of dementia, in particular those with Alzheimer`s disease, also develop brain atrophy (hydrocephalus ex vacuo) altering the dynamics of CSF flow, and many elderly patients suffer from degenerative spine disease impairing the circulation of the CSF in the spinal canal. For these reasons, we suggest that the cisterno-lumbar gradients of protein, albumin and markers of neurodegenerative diseases in the spinal canal may be similar in elderly patients with dementia irrespective of its cause. Lumbar (fraction 1) and cisternal (fraction 8) Tau, pTau, Aβ1–40 and Aβ1–42 concentrations and the Aβ1–40/Aβ1–42 ratios were closely correlated (Table 1) suggesting that these concentrations strongly depend on each other as a consequence of CSF bulk flow and diffusion.

## Conclusions

The rostro-caudal gradient of pTau and Tau in this and other studies on NPH suggests that both proteins are mainly brain-derived. This gradient, however, may not be present in all diseases. The differences between pTau and Tau concentrations in lumbar and cistern-near CSF were small, and the Aβ1–42 and Aβ1–40 concentrations and Aβ1–40/Aβ1–42 ratios in lumbar and cistern-near CSF were almost equal. Therefore, all fractions of CSF after a spinal tap of 40 ml appear to be equally suitable for the assessment of markers of dementia in CSF.

### Abbreviations

Tau: Tau protein; pTau: phosphorylated Tau protein; Aβ1-42: Amyloid beta 1-42; Aβ1-40: Amyloid beta 1-40; Aβ1-42/Aβ1-40 ratio: ratio of Amyloid beta 1–42 and Amyloid beta 1–40.

### Authors' contributions

MD, AS, SB and PL obtained informed consent from the participants, collected and analyzed the samples, and participated in the study design and manuscript preparation. AS performed the biometric calculations. JW participated in the study design, discussion of the data and preparation of the manuscript. RN planned the study and wrote the first draft of the manuscript. All authors read and approved the final manuscript.

### Author details

[1] Department of Geriatrics, Evangelisches Krankenhaus Göttingen-Weende, Göttingen, Germany. [2] Institute of Neuropathology, University Medical Center Goettingen (UMG), Robert-Koch-Strasse 40, D-37075 Göttingen, Germany. [3] Department of Neurology, University Medical Center Goettingen (UMG), Göttingen, Germany. [4] Department of Neurology, University Medical Centre Mainz, Mainz, Germany. [5] Department of Psychiatry and Psychotherapy, University Medical Center Goettingen (UMG), Göttingen, Germany. [6] German Center for Neurodegenerative Diseases (DZNE), Georg August University Göttingen, Göttingen, Germany.

### Competing interests

The authors declare that they have no competing interests.

### Funding

The study was supported by Sparkasse Göttingen and Evangelisches Krankenhaus Göttingen-Weende. The funding bodies did not influence the design of the study and collection, analysis, and interpretation of data.

## References

1. Silverberg GD, Mayo M, Saul T, Rubenstein E, McGuire D. Alzheimer's disease, normal-pressure hydrocephalus, and senescent changes in CSF circulatory physiology: a hypothesis. Lancet Neurol. 2003;2:506–11.
2. Hiraoka K, Narita W, Kikuchi H, Baba T, Kanno S, Iizuka O, Tashiro M, Furumoto S, Okamura N, Furukawa K, Arai H, Iwata R, Mori E, Yanai K. Amyloid deposits and response to shunt surgery in idiopathic normal-pressure hydrocephalus. J Neurol Sci. 2015;356:124–8.
3. Golomb J, Wisoff J, Miller DC, Boksay I, Kluger A, Weiner H, Salton J, Graves W. Alzheimer's disease comorbidity in normal pressure hydrocephalus: prevalence and shunt response. J Neurol Neurosurg Psychiatr. 2000;68:778–81.
4. Ott BR, Cohen RA, Gongvatana A, Okonkwo OC, Johanson CE, Stopa EG, Donahue JE, Silverberg GD. Alzheimer's disease neuroimaging initiative. brain ventricular volume and cerebrospinal fluid biomarkers of Alzheimer's disease. J Alzheimers Dis. 2010;20:647–57.
5. Malm J, Graff-Radford NR, Ishikawa M, Kristensen B, Leinonen V, Mori E, Owler BK, Tullberg M, Williams MA, Relkin NR. Influence of comorbidities in idiopathic normal pressure hydrocephalus—research and clinical care.a report of the ISHCSF task force on comorbidities in INPH. Fluids Barriers CNS. 2013;10(1):1.
6. Davson H, Welch K, Segal MB. Physiology and pathophysiology of the cerebrospinal fluid. Edinburgh: Churchill Livingstone; 1987.
7. Reiber H. Dynamics of brain-derived proteins in cerebrospinal fluid. Clin Chim Acta. 2001;310(2):173–86.
8. Mollenhauer B, Trautmann E, Otte B, Ng J, Spreer A, Lange P, Sixel-Döring F, Hakimi M, Vonsattel JP, Nussbaum R, Trenkwalder C, Schlossmacher MG. α-Synuclein in human cerebrospinal fluid is principally derived from neurons of the central nervous system. J Neural Transm (Vienna). 2012;119:739–46.
9. Gerber J, Tumani H, Kolenda H, Nau R. Lumbar and ventricular CSF protein, leukocytes, and lactate in suspected bacterial CNS infections. Neurology. 1998;51:1710–4.
10. Carpenter RL, Hogan QH, Liu SS, Crane B, Moore J. Lumbosacral cerebrospinal fluid volume is the primary determinant of sensory block extent and duration during spinal anesthesia. Anesthesiology. 1998;89:24–9.
11. Brandner S, Thaler C, Lelental N, Buchfelder M, Kleindienst A, Maler JM, Kornhuber J, Lewczuk P. Ventricular and lumbar cerebrospinal fluid concentrations of Alzheimer's disease biomarkers in patients with normal pressure hydrocephalus and posttraumatic hydrocephalus. J Alzheimers Dis. 2014;41:1057–62.
12. Pyykkö OT, Lumela M, Rummukainen J, Nerg O, Seppälä TT, Herukka SK, Koivisto AM, Alafuzoff I, Puli L, Savolainen S, Soininen H, Jääskeläinen JE, Hiltunen M, Zetterberg H, Leinonen V. Cerebrospinal fluid biomarker and brain biopsy findings in idiopathic normal pressure hydrocephalus. PLoS ONE. 2014;9:e91974.
13. Seppälä TT, Nerg O, Koivisto AM, Rummukainen J, Puli L, Zetterberg H, Pyykkö OT, Helisalmi S, Alafuzoff I, Hiltunen M, Jääskeläinen JE, Rinne J, Soininen H, Leinonen V, Herukka SK. CSF biomarkers for Alzheimer disease correlate with cortical brain biopsy findings. Neurology. 2012;78:1568–75.
14. Trojanowski JQ, Schuck T, Schmidt ML, Lee VM. Distribution of tau proteins in the normal human central and peripheral nervous system. J Histochem Cytochem. 1989;37:209–15.
15. Seyfert S, Faulstich A. Is the blood-CSF barrier altered in disease? Acta Neurol Scand. 2003;108:252–6.

# 17

# Do patients with schizophreniform and bipolar disorders show an intrathecal, polyspecific, antiviral immune response?

Dominique Endres[1]* [iD], Daniela Huzly[2], Rick Dersch[3], Oliver Stich[3], Benjamin Berger[3], Florian Schuchardt[3], Evgeniy Perlov[1], Nils Venhoff[4], Sabine Hellwig[1], Bernd L. Fiebich[1], Daniel Erny[5,6], Tilman Hottenrott[3†] and Ludger Tebartz van Elst[1†]

## Abstract

**Background:** We previously described inflammatory cerebrospinal fluid (CSF) alterations in a subgroup of patients with schizophreniform disorders and the synthesis of polyspecific intrathecal antibodies against different neurotropic infectious pathogens in some patients with bipolar disorders. Consequently, we have measured the prevalence of a positive MRZ reaction (MRZR)—a marker for a polyspecific, antiviral, intrathecal, humoral immune response composed of three antibody indices for the neurotropic viruses of measles (M), rubella (R), and varicella zoster (Z)—in these patients.

**Methods:** We analyzed paired CSF and serum samples of 39 schizophreniform and 39 bipolar patients. For comparison, we used a group of 48 patients with other inflammatory neurological disorders (OIND) and a cohort of 203 multiple sclerosis (MS) patients.

**Results:** We found a positive MRZR in two patients with schizophreniform disorders (5.1%); both suffered from schizodepressive disorders without any other signs suggestive of MS. None of the bipolar patients (0%) and four members of the OIND group (8.3%) showed a positive MRZR. In the MS cohort, a positive MRZR was found significantly more frequently [in 99 patients (48.8%)] than in the other patient groups (p > 0.001). In summary, we did not find a positive MRZR in a relevant subgroup of patients with schizophreniform or bipolar disorders.

**Conclusions:** Our results indicate that the MRZR is highly specific to MS. Nevertheless, two schizodepressive patients also had a positive MRZR. This finding corresponds to the few MRZR-positive patients with OIND or other autoimmune disorders with central nervous involvement, implicating that the MRZR specificity for MS is high, but not 100%.

**Keywords:** Schizophrenia, Bipolar disorder, Antibody index, MRZ reaction, Immunological encephalopathy

## Background

Schizophreniform and bipolar disorders are common psychiatric axis I disorders, with prevalence rates of at least 1% [1, 2]. Schizophreniform disorders are characterized by dysexecutive, amotivational, disorganized, affective, delusional, hallucinatory, or catatonic symptoms [3]. Bipolar disorders present with depressive, (hypo)manic, or mixed episodes. From a pathophysiological perspective, the primary idiopathic forms of these disorders and secondary forms with a recognizable cause can be distinguished. The primary idiopathic forms often display a familial liability associated with polygenetic vulnerability. Secondary forms can be due to different brain

---

*Correspondence: dominique.endres@uniklinik-freiburg.de
†Tilman Hottenrott and Ludger Tebartz van Elst senior authors contributed equally
[1] Section for Experimental Neuropsychiatry, Department of Psychiatry and Psychotherapy, Medical Center-University of Freiburg, Faculty of Medicine, University of Freiburg, Freiburg, Germany
Full list of author information is available at the end of the article

disorders caused by immunological (limbic encephalitis, anti-NMDA-R-encephalitis, Hashimoto's encephalopathy, etc.), infectiological (neuroborreliosis, neurosyphilis, etc.), epileptic (paraepileptic psychosis, etc.), metabolic (Niemann Pick type c, etc.), vascular (vasculitis, etc.), traumatic (traumatic brain injury), or neurodegenerative (Huntington's chorea, etc.) factors [3, 4]. Interest in immunological encephalopathies has increased in the last decade. Paraneoplastic limbic encephalitis (e.g., associated with anti-Hu antibodies), idiopathic autoimmune encephalitis (e.g., associated with anti-NMDAR- or anti-VGKC-LG1 antibodies), or Hashimoto encephalopathy (in the context of Hashimoto thyroiditis) can mimic schizophreniform and, in single cases, bipolar disorders, as well [3, 5–7]. These observations are highly relevant in understanding the etiology of psychiatric disorders because they show the necessity for a broad, organic diagnostic workup and for new treatment strategies with immunomodulatory medications, such as corticosteroids, intravenous immunoglobulins, or plasmapheresis [3, 8].

## Cerebrospinal fluid (CSF) characteristics in schizophreniform and bipolar disorders

Changes in the composition of cerebrospinal fluid (CSF) are detected frequently in patients with schizophreniform disorders [9–11]. We previously found mild pleocytosis in 3.4%, increased albumin quotients in 21.8%, elevated protein levels in 42.2%, and intrathecal immunoglobulin syntheses in 7.2% of a cohort with schizophreniform disorders [11]. Basic diagnostic CSF alterations were less frequent in bipolar patients; increased white blood cell counts were found in 1.6% of our bipolar cohort, increased albumin quotients in 12.8%, and intrathecal immunoglobulin synthesis in 4.8% [12]. Another study found increased lactate levels in 5 out of 15 patients with bipolar disorder [13]. In an earlier study, we detected a synthesis of polyspecific, intrathecal antibodies against different neurotropic infectious pathogens (*Toxoplasma gondii*, Herpes simplex virus types 1/2, cytomegalovirus, and Epstein–barr virus) in some patients with bipolar disorders [14].

## The MRZ reaction

The MRZ reaction (MRZR) is a marker for a polyspecific, antiviral, intrathecal, humoral immune response calculated as the antibody index (AI) directed against three neurotropic viruses of measles (M), rubella (R), and varicella zoster (Z) most commonly found in MS [15]. A positive MRZR was reported to be quite specific to multiple sclerosis (MS) [16, 17]. Elevated AIs (i.e., $\geq 1.5$) usually occur due to intrathecal synthesis of antibodies against intrathecal pathogens. For example, in patients with Lyme neuroborreliosis, increased AIs demonstrate an intrathecal antibody synthesis against the pathogen *Borrelia burgdorferi* [18]. However, in case of a positive MRZR in MS patients, no causal virus DNA was detectable [19]; therefore, the MRZR has been interpreted as an autoimmune epiphenomenon of polyspecific B cell activation within the central nervous system [17, 20].

### Rationale for our study

Our recent findings of a potential polyspecific, antiviral, intrathecal, humoral synthesis against different neurotropic agents other than MRZ in bipolar patients, as well as frequent chronic inflammatory CSF alterations in schizophreniform patients, led to the question of whether a positive MRZR might be a marker of immunological encephalopathy in bipolar or schizophreniform disorders, similar to MS. We thus analyzed the MRZR in these patient cohorts and compared the findings with previously published data derived from two patient cohorts with MS and other inflammatory neurological disorders (OIND) [16, 21]. We hypothesized a positive MRZR in a subgroup of patients with potentially autoimmune-mediated schizophreniform and bipolar disorders.

## Participants and methods

This study was a part of a larger CSF project that received approval from the local ethics committee of the University of Freiburg (EK-Fr 609/14). CSF analysis was part of the routine clinical workup. As a screening procedure, lumbar punctures were routinely offered to patients with schizophreniform disorders. Bipolar patients were investigated unsystematically (i.e., in the case of signs of inflammation or neurodegeneration). Only those patients who provided written consent for lumbar puncture were included in the study.

### Study sample

We included 39 patients with schizophreniform syndromes and 39 patients with bipolar disorders. The schizophreniform cohort consisted of consecutively identified patients with schizophrenia, organic schizophrenia-like disorders, and schizoaffective [i.e. with (schizo)depressive or (schizo)manic episodes] disorders from which CSF was collected between 2016 and 2017. The bipolar cohort comprised bipolar or manic patients (i.e., with hypomanic, manic, depressive, mixed, or remitted episodes and organic bipolar disorders) in whom CSF was collected between 2006 and 2017. The patients were only one-time lumbar punctured in the course of the diagnostic routine examination, and single samples were analyzed retrospectively. Lumbar puncture was done using a sterile technique between the 3rd and 5th lumbar vertebrae (mostly between 4 and 5). The serum samples were taken on the same day. All samples were stored at $-80\,°C$ after routine laboratory testing. The patient selection was unsystematic; only those patients with completed instrument-based diagnostics [i.e., electroencephalography (EEG), cerebral magnetic resonance imaging, laboratory, and CSF data] and those with sufficient residual serum/CSF material were included. Organic forms of schizophreniform or bipolar disorders were diagnosed after different serological tests, CSF, EEG and cerebral magnetic resonance imaging analyses. All patients with drug-induced schizophreniform and bipolar disorders were excluded. For comparison, we used a group of 48 patients with OIND (22 with neurosarcoidosis, 19 with autoimmune encephalitis, 7 with acute disseminated encephalomyelitis) and a group of 203 MS patients (100 with primary progressive MS, 103 with relapsing–remitting MS). The OIND and MS samples were reported in previous publications [21].

## MRZR measurement

The MRZR analyses were carried out at the Institute for Virology of the University of Freiburg. For the MRZR, the virus-specific AIs were determined for M, R, and Z. The M, R, and Z immunoglobulin (Ig) G (IgGspecific$_{(for\ M/R/Z)}$) concentrations in the serum and CSF were measured with enzyme-linked immunosorbent assays (Serion classic, Würzburg, Germany) following the manufacturer's instructions. The total Ig levels in the CSF and serum were analyzed nephelometrically (ProSpect System, Siemens, Munich, Germany) with the use of the same procedure established in previous studies [16, 21].

The virus-specific AIs for M, R, and Z were calculated with the quotient from CSF to serum antibody titers (QIgG[specific$_{(for\ M/R/Z)}$]) and the reference to the relevant quotient of the total CSF/serum IgG (QIgG[total]) in relation to the age-corrected albumin quotient [22]. The calculation was performed using Reiber's formula: $AI = QIgG_{[specific]}/QIgG_{[total]}$, if $QIgG_{[total]} < Qlim$, or $AI = QIgG_{[specific]}/Qlim$, if $QIgG_{[total]} > Qlim$ [23]. AIs $\geq 1.5$ were defined as positive [16, 21, 23]. MRZR-1, which requires one positive AI, is less specific and of unclear significance. Therefore, a positive MRZR was defined by two or three increased AIs [16, 17, 21].

## Data handling and statistical analysis

All necessary information on our study cohort was transferred into the Statistical Package for the Social Sciences, version 22 database. Categorical variables (gender, MRZR) were compared with Pearson's Chi squared test. The continuous variable of participants' age was compared with two-sided independent sample t tests. A $p < 0.05$ was considered statistically significant.

## Results
### Demographic data of patients (Table 1)

The demographic parameters of our study cohort are summarized in Table 1. The patients with schizophreniform disorders differed significantly in age, but not in gender, from those in the OIND and MS groups. The bipolar patients differed in age and gender from those in the OIND group, but not from the MS cohort in either of these parameters.

**Table 1  Demographic data of the study cohort**

|  | Schizophreniform cohort (N = 39) | Bipolar cohort (N = 39) | Other inflammatory neurological disorders (N = 48[c]) | Multiple sclerosis (N = 203[c]) | Statistics |
|---|---|---|---|---|---|
| Mean age ± SD (Range in years) | 32.3 ± 11.3 (18–75) | 44.3 ± 14.7 (19–73) | 51.8 ± 18.6 (4–84) | 45.73 ± 12.128 (19–78) | $p_1 < 0.001$ $p_2 < 0.001$ $p_3 = 0.044$ $p_4 =$ n.s. |
| Gender | 19M: 20F | 14M: 25F | 29M: 19F | 68M: 135F | $p_1 =$ n.s. $p_2 =$ n.s. $p_3 = 0.023$ $p_4 =$ n.s. |
| Disorder catego-rization | Schizophrenia-like: 30[a] Schizoaffective-like: 9 | Hypomanic/manic episode[b]: 14 Depressive episode[b]: 20 Mixed episode: 4 Remitted: 1 | Neurosarcoidosis: 22 Autoimmune encephalitis: 19 Acute disseminated encephalomyelitis: 7 | Primary-progressive MS: 103 Relapsing–remitting MS: 100 |  |

MS, multiple sclerosis; SD, standard deviation; M, male; f, female; $p_1$, schizophreniform vs. OIND; $p_2$, schizophreniform vs. multiple sclerosis; $p_3$, bipolar vs. OIND cohort; $p_4$, bipolar vs. MS cohort

[a] Six patients were diagnosed with organic schizophrenia-like disorders after diagnostic work-up

[b] Three patients turned out to have organic bipolar disorders after diagnostic work-up

[c] According to Hottenrott et al. [21]

## Frequency of MRZR in the study cohorts (Table 2)

Two patients with schizophreniform disorders showed a positive MRZR (5.1%; 2.6% in the whole psychiatric patient cohort). In four of the schizophreniform patients, one isolated AI (MRZR-1) was positive, which consisted of a specific reaction against varicella zoster. None of the bipolar controls showed a positive MRZR. Two bipolar patients had positive AIs for varicella zoster (MRZR-1). Four of the OIND patients had a positive MRZR, whereas 7 of these patients had one isolated positive AI (2 against rubella, 5 against varicella zoster). No relevant statistical differences were found between the frequency of positive MRZR in patients with schizophreniform and in those with bipolar disorders and OIND. The MS cohort showed a more frequently positive MRZR (99 of 203 patients: 48.8%) when compared to all other study groups (OIND, bipolar, and schizophreniform patients), and this difference was highly significant (p $\leq$ 0.001, Table 2). Focusing on only idiopathic psychiatric disorders (after the exclusion of organic schizophreniform or bipolar disorders) leads to increased overall prevalence rate in both patient groups of 2.9% (2 patients with positive MRZR out of 69 patients) and 6.1% of schizophreniform patients (2 patients with positive MRZR out of 33 patients). The exact findings of the MS subgroups were published in an earlier paper [21].

## Characteristics of the MRZR-positive psychiatric patients (Table 3)

Two psychiatric patients showed a positive MRZR; both patients suffered from schizodepressive disorders. Neither of these two MRZR-positive patients displayed any neurological symptoms, and both had a normal CSF cell count without oligoclonal bands. Cerebral magnetic resonance imaging did not fulfill the MS criterion for dissemination in time and space, according to the 2010 revision of the McDonald diagnostic criteria [24]. The detailed characteristics of the MRZR-positive patients are presented in Table 3. Four schizophreniform patients had only one increased AI; these patients all suffered from isolated schizophrenia syndromes. One of these four patients (25%) was ultimately diagnosed with an organic schizophreniform disorder, but not due to MS. This male patient showed one isolated white matter (WM) lesion in the globus pallidus on the left side associated with an infectious mononucleosis in his youth. CSF analysis was normal. The two bipolar patients with one positive AI presented with a mixed and a manic episode during the time of lumbar puncture. None of these two patients was finally diagnosed with an organic bipolar disorder.

## Discussion

In this pilot study, we investigated the MRZR in paired CSF and serum samples from 78 patients with bipolar and schizophreniform disorders. We were unable to verify our hypothesis of increased AIs suggestive of an autoimmune-driven intrathecal immune reaction in a relevant subgroup of psychiatric patients. Therefore, our results support the idea that the MRZR is rather specific to MS. Only two schizophreniform patients had a positive MRZR; both patients had schizodepressive disorders without clinical or paraclinical signs of MS [24].

### Earlier findings and clinical relevance of the MRZR

We analyzed the prevalence of a positive MRZR in a relevant psychiatric cohort. Earlier studies focused on patients with demyelinating disorders and OIND [17]. A recent review identified 30 studies that analyzed the MRZR. A positive MRZR was found in 458 of 724 (63.3%) patients with MS and in 19 of 754 control patients (2.5%). Therefore, the MRZR indicates a high cumulative specificity of 97.5% and a cumulative sensitivity of 63.3% for MS [17]. Our findings are in line with these observations, as we found a positive MRZR significantly more frequently in MS patients (48.8%) than in OIND (8.3%), schizophreniform (5.1%), or bipolar (0%) patients (p < 0.001). The prevalence rates in our schizophreniform cohort were comparable with those in the OIND group (5.1 vs. 8.3%; p = 0.557), indicating an association with immunological processes in a small schizophreniform subgroup. Both MRZR-positive schizophreniform patients had schizodepressive disorders without other signs of MS or brain inflammation. Schizodepressive disorders combine aspects of schizophrenia and depression and the distinction between schizophrenia and bipolar disorder is challenging [25]. Patients often show a relapsing–remitting course of the disorder comparable with MS. Male patient 1 had one single WM lesion and a relevant blood–brain barrier dysfunction. In combination with his increased titers of anti-thyroglobulin antibodies, this patient might suffer from Hashimoto encephalopathy [7]. However, no steroid treatment was given because not all clinical criteria were fulfilled (e.g., the patient had normal alpha-EEG and no subacute onset). The other female patient 2 had completely normal paraclinical diagnostics. Earlier research has shown that incipient cases of MS may present as psychosis [26]. Neither of the MRZR-positive patients in our cohort currently fulfill the McDonald diagnostic criteria [24]; however, only the future course can show whether these patients will develop symptoms of MS. In both patients, the AIs were only slightly increased between 1.5 and 1.9. Using a more stringent AI level > 2 as reference value would result in a normal MRZR in both patients, pointing to a

**Table 2 MRZR reaction in the different patient groups**

| MRZR state | Schizophreniform cohort (N = 39) | | | Bipolar cohort (N = 39) | | | Other inflammatory neurological diseases (N = 48) | | | Multiple sclerosis (N = 203) | | |
|---|---|---|---|---|---|---|---|---|---|---|---|---|
| | All AIs negative | MRZR-1 | MRZR positive | All AIs negative | MRZR-1 | MRZR positive | All AIs negative | MRZR-1 | MRZR positive | All AIs negative | MRZR-1 | MRZR positive |
| Number of patients (%) | 33 (84.6) | 4 (10.3) | 2 (5.1) | 37 (94.9) | 2 (5.1) | 0 (0) | 37 (77.1) | 7 (14.6) | 4 (8.3) | 48 (23.6) | 56 (27.6) | 99 (48.8) |

MRZR-1 defined as having only one positive AI, MRZR defined as having 2 or 3 positive AIs

MRZR, MRZ reaction; AI, antibody index

**Table 3 Characteristics of MRZR-positive psychiatric patients**

| | Syndrome | Neurological examination | MRZR | CSF | cMRI | EEG | Other immunological testing |
|---|---|---|---|---|---|---|---|
| Patient 1: 34 year, male | Schizo-depressive syndrome | No neurological signs | M: 1.6 ($\uparrow$) <br> R: $\leftrightarrow$ <br> Z: 1.9 ($\uparrow$) | Cell count: 3 ($\leftrightarrow$) <br> Alb$_Q$: $12 \times 10^{-3}$ ($\uparrow$)[a] <br> OCBs: negative | One unspecific white matter lesion right frontal | Normal | No antineuronal antibodies[b], no rheumatological antibodies[c], C3d slightly increased (9.6, reference < 9 mg/L). Increased anti-TG antibodies (150 IU/mL; reference < 115 IU/mL). Normal anti-TPO antibodies |
| Patient 2: 27 year, female | Schizo-depressive syndrome | No neurological signs | M: 1.7 ($\uparrow$) <br> R: $\leftrightarrow$ <br> Z: 1.5 ($\uparrow$) | Cell count: 3 ($\leftrightarrow$) <br> Alb$_Q$: 3 ($\leftrightarrow$) <br> OCBs: negative | Normal | Normal | No antineuronal antibodies[b], no rheumatological antibodies[c], C3d normal. Normal anti-TPO- and -TG-antibodies |

MRZR, MRZ reaction; M, measles; R, rubella; Z, varicella zoster; CSF, cerebrospinal fluid; cMRI, cerebral magnetic resonance imaging; EEG, electroencephalography; Alb$_Q$, albumin quotient; TG, thyroglobulin; TPO, thyroid peroxidase. $\leftrightarrow$, normal; $\uparrow$, increased

[a] Age dependent reference: $6.5 \times 10^{-3}$

[b] Including antibodies against intracellular onconeural antigens (Yo, Hu, CV2/CRMP5, Ri, Ma1/2, SOX1; measured in serum), against intracellular synaptic antigens (GAD, amphiphysin; in serum) and antibodies against neuronal cell surface antigens [NMDAR, AMPA-R, GABA-B-R, VGKC-complex (LGI1, Caspr2); in CSF]

[c] Antinuclear, anti-neutrophil cytoplasmic, and antiphospholipid antibodies

potential unspecific mechanism. However, a larger study of 99 healthy volunteers found no positive MRZR in all these controls [27]. From our cohort, nine patients were ultimately diagnosed with organic schizophreniform (6 patients) and bipolar (3 patients) disorders. None of these patients had a positive MRZR. One of these patients had only one increased AI; this male patient showed one isolated WM lesion in the globus pallidus associated with a positive history of infectious mononucleosis in his adolescence. The other eight patients with organic psychiatric syndromes had normal AIs. Therefore, a single increased AI to MRZ antigens does not seem to be a strong indicator of an organic psychiatric pathophysiology. Taken together, our data do not support the idea that the MRZR could serve as a biomarker for a potentially autoimmune-driven inflammatory process affecting the CSF in patients with schizophreniform or bipolar disorders. Our findings correspond to the few MRZR-positive patients with OIND or other autoimmune disorders with central nervous involvement, implicating that the MRZR specificity for MS is high, but not 100%. However, the finding of a positive MRZR in a small subgroup of patients with schizophreniform disorders and our earlier reported CSF alterations are compatible with mild neuroinflammation, as proposed in the concept of mild encephalitis [28]. The investigation of further neurotropic agents (e.g., for Borna disease virus, Epstein–barr-virus) and other antineuronal antibodies would have led to the detection of a larger subgroup of patients with mild encephalitis [29].

### Limitations of this study

This study has several limitations. First, we did not assess a healthy control group for comparison. However, this would not have been ethically justified for this type of pilot study which requires CSF sampling. Therefore, we compared our findings with two previously published neurological control cohorts. Second, the study cohort was fairly small, and the gender ratio for bipolar disorder and the OIND group were not representative for the general population. However, our study was a retrospective pilot study of psychiatric patients who were not involved in CSF studies in most psychiatric hospitals. Therefore, in our opinion, the publication of these data from 78 patients, in conjunction with the two earlier published neurological patient cohorts with 251 patients, is still important. Third, the study cohort was inhomogeneous because primary, idiopathic, and secondary organic psychiatric patients were included. We used this approach because we hypothesized that precisely these subgroups of organic psychiatric syndromes would have a positive MRZR in case of a potentially immune-driven inflammatory process underlying the respective disorder. Fourth,

the inclusion of patients was unsystematic, especially for the bipolar patients. However, in light of the negative results in this cohort, this procedure definitely did not lead to false-positive findings. Although the CSF from bipolar patients was investigated to exclude a potential organic cause, none of these patients had a positive MRZR. This implies that the MRZR is not a relevant biomarker for an autoimmune process in the CSF of patients with bipolar disorders. All in all, given the pilot nature of the scientific question explored in this clinical research, we believe that assessing such a question in retrospective analyses is justifiable, if not unavoidable. The alternative would have been to organize a large prospective study, which seems unjustifiable considering the resource input and potential output of such efforts. Nevertheless, we investigated a relevant research question following a logical path of reasoning, and our results are important in terms of planning endeavors for further research in the field.

### Conclusion

In summary, our study supports the high specificity of the MRZR for MS. A positive MRZR was much more frequent in MS than in bipolar and schizophreniform patients, and the difference was highly statistically significant. We detected only two patients with positive MRZR, and both patients suffered from schizodepressive episodes without further evidence of MS. The pathophysiological meaning of this finding remains elusive for the time being but would be compatible with mild encephalitis in these patients [28].

### Abbreviations

AI: antibody index; CSF: cerebrospinal fluid; EEG: electroencephalography; Ig: immunoglobulin; M: measles; MRZR: MRZ reaction; MS: multiple sclerosis; OIND: other inflammatory neurological disorders; R: rubella; WM: white matter; Z: varicella zoster.

### Authors' contributions

DEn, TH, and LTvE initiated the study and performed the data search. DH conducted the lab work. OS, RD, BB, and TH performed the CSF basic analyses. NV performed the rheumatological measurements. DEn performed the statistical analyses and wrote the paper. EP, SH, FS, BF, and DEr critically revised the manuscript. All the authors were crucially involved in theoretical discussions on the study and the performance of the study. All authors read and approved the final manuscript.

### Author details

[1] Section for Experimental Neuropsychiatry, Department of Psychiatry and Psychotherapy, Medical Center-University of Freiburg, Faculty of Medicine, University of Freiburg, Freiburg, Germany. [2] Institute for Virology, Medical Center-University of Freiburg, Faculty of Medicine, University of Freiburg, Freiburg, Germany. [3] Department of Neurology and Neurophysiology, Medical Center-University of Freiburg, Faculty of Medicine, University of Freiburg, Freiburg, Germany. [4] Department of Rheumatology and Clinical Immunology, Medical Center-University of Freiburg, Faculty of Medicine, University of Freiburg, Freiburg, Germany. [5] Institute of Neuropathology, Medical Center-University of Freiburg, Faculty of Medicine, University of Freiburg, Freiburg, Germany. [6] Berta-Ottenstein-Programme, Faculty of Medicine, University of Freiburg, Freiburg, Germany.

## Competing interests

DEn: none. DH: received lecture fees from Serion. RD: none. OS: consulting and lecture fees, grant and research support from Bayer Vital GmbH, Biogen Idec, Genzyme, Merck Serono, Novartis, Sanofi-Aventis and Teva. BB: received travel grants and/or training expenses from Bayer Vital GmbH, Ipsen Pharma GmbH, Novartis, and Genzyme, as well as lecture fees from Ipsen Pharma GmbH. FS: travel support from Bayer healthcare. EP: none. NV: advisory boards, lectures, research or travel grants within the last 3 years: Janssen-Cilag, Roche, Novartis, AbbVie, GSK, Lilly, BMS, Pfizer, Medac. SH: grant and research support from GE Healthcare. BF: grant and research support from Bayer Vital GmbH. DEr: none. TH: travel grants from Bayer Vital GmbH and Novartis. LTVE: advisory boards, lectures, or travel grants within the last 3 years: Eli Lilly, Janssen-Cilag, Novartis, Shire, UCB, GSK, Servier, Janssen, and Cyberonics.

## Funding

The study was financed by the Department for Psychiatry and Psychotherapy of the University Medical Center Freiburg. The article processing charge was funded by the German Research Foundation (DFG) and the University of Freiburg in the funding program Open Access Publishing.

## References

1. Merikangas KR, Jin R, He JP, Kessler R, Lee S, Sampson NA, Viana MC, Andrade LH, Hu C, Karam EG, Ladea M, Medina-Mora ME, Ono Y, Posada-Villa J, Sagar R, Wells JE, Zarkov Z. Prevalence and correlates of bipolar spectrum disorder in the world mental health survey initiative. Arch Gen Psychiatry. 2011;68(3):241–51.

2. Owen M, Sawa A, Mortensen P. Schizophrenia. Lancet. 2016;388(10039):86–97.

3. Tebartz van Elst L. Vom Anfang und Ende der Schizophrenie: Ein Plädoyer für die Abschaffung eines unzeitgemäßen Begriffs und Konzepts. Stuttgart: Kohlhammer; 2017.

4. Lishman A. Lishman's—organic psychiatry—a textbook of neuropsychiatry. 4th ed. Hoboken: Wiley-Blackwell; 2009.

5. Bonnet U, Selle C, Kuhlmann R. Delirious mania associated with autoimmune gastrothyroidal syndrome of a mid-life female: the role of Hashimoto encephalopathy and a 3-year follow-up including serum autoantibody levels. Case Rep Psychiatry. 2016;2016:4168050.

6. Haider A, Alam M, Adetutu E, Thakur R, Gottlich C, DeBacker D, Marks L. Autoimmune schizophrenia? Psychiatric manifestations of Hashimoto's encephalitis. Cureus. 2016;8(7):e672.

7. Endres D, Perlov E, Riering A, Maier V, Stich O, Dersch R, Venhoff N, Erny D, Mader I, Tebartz van Elst L. Steroid-responsive chronic schizophreniform syndrome in the context of mildly increased antithyroid peroxidase antibodies. Front Psychiatry. 2007;8:64.

8. Tebartz van Elst L, Stich O, Endres D. Depressionen und Psychosen bei immunologischen Enzephalopathien. PSYCH up2date. 2015;9(05):265–80.

9. Bechter K, Reiber H, Herzog S, Fuchs D, Tumani H, Maxeiner HG. Cerebrospinal fluid analysis in affective and schizophrenic spectrum disorders: identification of subgroups with immune responses and blood-CSF barrier dysfunction. J Psychiatr Res. 2010;44(5):321–30.

10. Vasic N, Connemann BJ, Wolf RC, Tumani H, Brettschneider J. Cerebrospinal fluid biomarker candidates of schizophrenia: where do we stand? Eur Arch Psychiatry Clin Neurosci. 2012;262(5):375–91.

11. Endres D, Perlov E, Baumgartner A, Hottenrott T, Dersch R, Stich O, Tebartz van Elst L. Immunological findings in psychotic syndromes: a tertiary care hospital's CSF sample of 180 patients. Front Hum Neurosci. 2015;9:476.

12. Endres D, Dersch R, Hottenrott T, Perlov E, Maier S, van Calker D, Hochstuhl B, Venhoff N, Stich O, van Elst LT. Alterations in cerebrospinal fluid in patients with bipolar syndromes. Front Psychiatry. 2016;7:194.

13. Regenold W, Phatak P, Marano C, Sassan A, Conley R, Kling M. Elevated cerebrospinal fluid lactate concentrations in patients with bipolar disorder and schizophrenia: implications for the mitochondrial dysfunction hypothesis. Biol Psychiatry. 2009;65(6):489–94.

14. Stich O, Andres T, Gross C, Gerber S, Rauer S, Langosch J. An observational study of inflammation in the central nervous system in patients with bipolar disorder. Bipolar Disord. 2015;17(3):291–302.

15. Felgenhauer K, Reiber H. The diagnostic significance of antibody specificity indices in multiple sclerosis and herpes virus induced diseases of the nervous system. Clin Investig. 1992;70(1):28–37.

16. Hottenrott T, Dersch R, Berger B, Rauer S, Eckenweiler M, Huzly D, Stich O. The intrathecal, polyspecific antiviral immune response in neurosarcoidosis, acute disseminated encephalomyelitis and autoimmune encephalitis compared to multiple sclerosis in a tertiary hospital cohort. Fluids Barriers CNS. 2015;12:27.

17. Jarius S, Eichhorn P, Franciotta D, Petereit HF, Akman-Demir G, Wick M, Wildemann B. The MRZ reaction as a highly specific marker of multiple sclerosis: re-evaluation and structured review of the literature. J Neurol. 2017;264(3):453–66.

18. Dersch R, Rauer S. Neuroborreliosis—diagnostics, treatment and course. Nervenarzt. 2017;88(4):419–31.

19. Godec MS, Asher DM, Murray RS, Shin ML, Greenham LW, Gibbs CJ Jr, Gajdusek DC. Absence of measles, mumps, and rubella viral genomic sequences from multiple sclerosis brain tissue by polymerase chain reaction. Ann Neurol. 1992;32(3):401–4.

20. Reiber H, Ungefehr S, Jacobi C. The intrathecal, polyspecific and oligoclonal immune response in multiple sclerosis. Mult Scler. 1998;4(3):111–7.

21. Hottenrott T, Dersch R, Berger B, Rauer S, Huzly D, Stich O. The MRZ reaction in primary progressive multiple sclerosis. Fluids Barriers CNS. 2017;14(1):2.

22. Endres D, Dersch R, Hochstuhl B, Fiebich B, Hottenrott T, Perlov E, Maier S, Berger B, Baumgartner A, Venhoff N, Stich O, Tebartz van Elst L. Intrathecal thyroid autoantibody synthesis in a subgroup of patients with schizophreniform syndromes. J Neuropsychiatry Clin Neurosci. 2017;29(4):365–74.

23. Reiber H, Lange P. Quantification of virus-specific antibodies in cerebrospinal fluid and serum: sensitive and specific detection of antibody synthesis in brain. Clin Chem. 1991;37(7):1153–60.

24. Polman CH, Reingold SC, Banwell B, Clanet M, Cohen JA, Filippi M, Fujihara K, Havrdova E, Hutchinson M, Kappos L, Lublin FD, Montalban X, O'Connor P, Sandberg-Wollheim M, Thompson AJ, Waubant E, Weinshenker B, Wolinsky JS. Diagnostic criteria for multiple sclerosis: 2010 revisions to the McDonald criteria. Ann Neurol. 2011;69(2):292–302.

25. Abrams DJ, Rojas DC, Arciniegas DB. Is schizoaffective disorder a distinct categorical diagnosis? A critical review of the literature. Neuropsychiatr Dis Treat. 2008;4(6):1089–109.

26. Bechter K. CSF diagnostics in psychiatry—present status—future projects. Neurol Psychiatry Brain Res. 2016;22(2):69–74.

27. Wurster U, Stachan R, Windhagen A, Petereit H, Leweke F. Reference values for standard cerebrospinal fluid examinations in multiple sclerosis. Results from 99 healthy volunteers. Mult Scler. 2006;12(P248):S62.

28. Bechter K. Updating the mild encephalitis hypothesis of schizophrenia. Prog Neuropsychopharmacol Biol Psychiatry. 2013;42:71–91.

29. Bechter K, Herzog S, Behr W, Schüttler R. Investigations of cerebrospinal fluid in Borna disease virus seropositive psychiatric patients. Eur Psychiatry. 1995;10(5):250–8.

# 18

# Blood–brain and blood–cerebrospinal fluid barrier permeability in spontaneously hypertensive rats

Daphne M. P. Naessens, Judith de Vos, Ed VanBavel and Erik N. T. P. Bakker*

## Abstract

**Background:** Hypertension is an important risk factor for cerebrovascular disease, including stroke and dementia. Both in humans and animal models of hypertension, neuropathological features such as brain atrophy and oedema have been reported. We hypothesised that cerebrovascular damage resulting from chronic hypertension would manifest itself in a more permeable blood–brain barrier and blood–cerebrospinal fluid barrier. In addition, more leaky barriers could potentially contribute to an enhanced interstitial fluid and cerebrospinal fluid formation, which could, in turn, lead to an elevated intracranial pressure.

**Methods:** To study this, we monitored intracranial pressure and estimated the cerebrospinal fluid production rate in spontaneously hypertensive (SHR) and normotensive rats (Wistar Kyoto, WKY) at 10 months of age. Blood–brain barrier and blood–cerebrospinal fluid barrier integrity was determined by measuring the leakage of fluorescein from the circulation into the brain and cerebrospinal fluid compartment. Prior to sacrifice, a fluorescently labelled lectin was injected into the bloodstream to visualise the vasculature and subsequently study a number of specific vascular characteristics in six different brain regions.

**Results:** Blood and brain fluorescein levels were not different between the two strains. However, cerebrospinal fluid fluorescein levels were significantly lower in SHR. This could not be explained by a difference in cerebrospinal fluid turnover, as cerebrospinal fluid production rates were similar in SHR and WKY, but may relate to a larger ventricular volume in the hypertensive strain. Also, intracranial pressure was not different between SHR and WKY. Morphometric analysis of capillary volume fraction, number of branches, capillary diameter, and total length did not reveal differences between SHR and WKY.

**Conclusion:** In conclusion, we found no evidence for blood–brain barrier or blood–cerebrospinal fluid barrier leakage to a small solute, fluorescein, in rats with established hypertension.

**Keywords:** Blood–brain barrier, Blood–cerebrospinal fluid barrier, Cerebrospinal fluid, Hypertension, Interstitial fluid

## Background

Chronic hypertension is a well-established risk factor for cerebrovascular disease, including haemorrhagic stroke, vascular dementia and Alzheimer's disease. It is associated with alterations in the structure and function of cerebral blood vessels, which may contribute to hypoperfusion, microinfarcts, brain atrophy, oedema, and ultimately, cognitive impairment [1, 2]. Although these neuropathological features have been described in many studies, the specific harmful effects of chronic hypertension on these abnormalities remain obscure.

Dysfunction at the blood–brain barrier (BBB) is often regarded as an early and common denominator in cerebrovascular disease. Hypertension could be envisioned to enhance loss of BBB integrity, leading to increased solute permeability of this barrier and leakage of water into the brain parenchyma [1, 2]. The brain extracellular fluids consist of cerebrospinal fluid (CSF), interstitial fluid

*Correspondence: n.t.bakker@amc.uva.nl
Department of Biomedical Engineering and Physics, Academic Medical Center, University of Amsterdam, Meibergdreef 9, 1105 AZ Amsterdam, The Netherlands

(ISF), and blood plasma. Since the experiments of Dandy nearly one century ago [3], it is generally agreed that most of the CSF is formed by the choroid plexuses within the cerebral ventricles. More recent reports described that the remaining CSF stems from an extra-choroidal source [4–7]. This extra-choroidal secretion is believed to derive from the ependymal epithelium and possibly the ISF formation across the BBB of cerebral capillaries that subsequently drains into the CSF compartment [8, 9]. However, the exact contribution of extra-choroidal CSF to the total CSF production is still under debate, and may even play a minimal role under physiological circumstances [10].

Recent work by our group showed that the ISF drainage towards the ventricular system is enhanced in the hippocampus of spontaneously hypertensive rats (SHR) [11]. This animal model recapitulates many of the neuropathological characteristics of chronic hypertension as seen in humans with cerebral small vessel disease. Therefore, these animals are frequently used as a model to study the impact of hypertension on the brain [11, 12]. Whether SHR also develop dysfunction at the BBB remains controversial. A greater permeability of the BBB to large molecular weight solutes has been noted in these animals in certain brain areas, such as the deep cortical layer and nuclei in the brain stem, leading to increased penetration of angiotensin II [12, 13]. However, others have shown that the BBB is intact with respect to large solutes when using labelled albumin, and that SHR are actually protected against acute changes in blood pressure [14]. The enhanced ISF drainage towards the CSF compartment in SHR could be another indication for BBB dysfunction, and may result from leakage of water and electrolytes across this barrier [11]. This same study also demonstrated a tendency for a higher brain parenchyma water content in the hypertensive animals. Lastly, tight junction proteins and ion transporters show and altered expression in SHR, associated with augmented oedema formation after arterial occlusion [13].

In the current study, we determined the effects of hypertension on the BBB and blood–CSF barrier (BCSFB) integrity. We hypothesised that increased leakage across the BBB may lead to enhanced ISF formation, resulting in a greater extra-choroidal contribution to the total CSF production. Apart from this, a more leaky BCSFB may in itself lead to an increased CSF production. Both increased ISF and CSF formation could potentially elevate intracranial pressure (ICP). Therefore, we monitored the ICP and estimated the rate of CSF production in SHR and normotensive controls (Wistar Kyoto, WKY). As a second approach, we assessed the penetration of fluorescein, a relatively small molecule, into the brain parenchyma and CSF compartment as an indicator of subtle BBB and BCSFB dysfunction, in the same animals.

Since all measurements could be affected by vascular parameters such as the total surface of capillaries, we also examined a number of specific vascular characteristics that may be related to the fluid balance in the brain. Lastly, we determined the ionic composition of the CSF, as this may reflect possible alterations in the ISF electrolyte balance associated with dysfunction of the BBB.

## Methods

### Animals

In this study, a total of 20 rats were used. Male spontaneously hypertensive rats (SHR/NCrl) (n = 10) and Wistar Kyoto rats (WKY/NCrl) (n = 10) were purchased from Charles River Laboratories at 12 weeks of age. Animals were kept until $42 \pm 1$ weeks old. All rats were housed in groups and were fed standard laboratory food and water ad libitum. The animals were kept at room temperature on a 12-h light, 12-h dark schedule. All experiments were conducted in accordance with the ARRIVE guidelines and European Union guidelines for the care laboratory animals (Directive 2010/63/EU), and were approved by the Academic Medical Center Animal Ethics Committee.

### Chemicals and reagents

Fluorescein sodium salt (Sigma, 0.4 kDa, $\lambda_{ex}$ 460 nm; $\lambda_{em}$ 515 nm) was used as a tracer to study blood–brain and blood–cerebrospinal fluid barrier leakage. The dye was dissolved in artificial cerebrospinal fluid (aCSF—135 mM NaCl, 5.4 mM KCl, 1 mM $MgCl_2$, 1.8 mM $CaCl_2$, 5 mM HEPES, pH 7.4) to a concentration of 40 mg/ml. DyLight®594 labelled *Lycopersicon Esculentum* (Tomato) Lectin (Vector Laboratories) was used to label the vascular endothelium.

### Blood pressure and heart rate measurements

Blood pressure and heart rate were measured using a non-invasive tail-cuff system (Kent Scientific) prior to the experiments in conscious rats. As blood pressures in SHR are known to increase from 6 weeks of age and are maintained during adulthood [15], the blood pressure and heart rate was only measured once, prior to the experiments. Animals were acclimated to handling and the restrainer for training period of 4 days prior to the measurements. During the procedure, animals were placed in the plastic restrainer on a heating pad to warm up the tail. Four to 13 BP and HR measurements were recorded and were averaged from each individual rat.

### Surgical procedure

Animals were weighed prior to the experimental procedure. All surgical procedures were performed under isoflurane inhalation anaesthesia (2–3.5%). After induction of general anaesthesia, animals were placed on a heating pad to maintain the core body temperature, which was monitored using a rectal thermometer (Greisinger Electronics). Ophthalmic ointment (Duratears®, Alcon) was applied to prevent dryness during the surgical procedure. To study blood–brain and blood–cerebrospinal fluid barrier leakage, fluorescein sodium salt (0.5 kDa) was injected in the dorsal penile vein (40 mg/kg). The animal was turned in the prone position and the head was fixed in a stereotaxic frame (Stoelting). Subsequently, a small longitudinal skin incision was made at the animal's back of the neck and 10% xylocaine (AstraZeneca B.V.) was applied as additional local anaesthesia. The subcutaneous tissues were removed and the neck muscles were separated in order to reach the cisterna magna. To measure the intracranial pressure (ICP), a 29-gauge stainless steel needle was inserted in the cisterna magna, which was connected to a pressure transducer (Edwards) by stiff polythene tubing. After monitoring the physiological baseline ICP, a second 29-gauge needle was inserted that was connected to a polythene catheter and a U-100 insulin syringe (BD Micro-Fine™). 30 min after intravenous injection of fluorescein, the first cerebrospinal fluid (CSF) sample was collected by gentle aspiration until an ICP of 0.5 mmHg was reached. A third 29-gauge needle connected to a polythene catheter and syringe was inserted into the cisterna magna. A second CSF sample was then collected 60 min after the fluorescein injection. After this, all needles were quickly removed from the cisterna magna and the CSF samples were stored at − 80 °C. The animal was turned into the supine position. DyLight®594-labelled *L. esculentum* lectin (1 mg/kg) was injected into the bloodstream via the dorsal penile vein and was allowed to circulate and bind the vascular endothelium for 3 min. Prior to the perfusion fixation, 200 µl of heparin solution (LEO®) was injected intravenously to prevent the formation of blood clots. The chest was opened and a blood sample was taken from the vena cava. The blood samples were centrifuged for 3 min at 3000 rpm and the plasma was stored at − 80 °C. Animals were then transcardially perfused with 60 ml heparinised phosphate buffered saline (PBS) and subsequently with 60 ml 4% paraformaldehyde (PFA). The brains were carefully dissected from the skull, weighed, and cut into three coronal pieces using a rat brain slicer matrix (Zivic Instruments). The front part, containing the olfactory bulb and part of the cortex, and cerebellum were snap frozen in liquid nitrogen and stored at − 80 °C until use. The middle part, containing the cortex and hippocampus, was post-fixed overnight in 4% PFA at 4 °C, and subsequently incubated in 30% sucrose for at least 3 days.

### Blood contamination CSF samples

Blood contamination was assessed in all individual CSF samples from both collection time points. The degree of blood contamination in the CSF samples was quantitatively determined by the detection of haemoglobin. 1 µl of the undiluted individual CSF sample was pipetted onto the window of a TrayCell ultra-micro cell (Hellma Analytics), which was subsequently placed in a LAMBDA Bio + spectrophotometer (PerkinElmer). Samples were considered as blood contaminated when the absorbance spectra of haemoglobin were above the detection limit of the spectrophotometer, and were excluded from further studies.

### Ion and protein concentrations in CSF

Undiluted CSF samples were used to determine concentrations of electrolytes, immunoglobulin G (IgG), glucose, and total protein. Sodium, potassium, and chloride concentrations were analysed using an ion-selective electrode, and glucose levels by hexokinase/glucose-6-phosphate dehydrogenase (c702, Cobas® 8000, Roche Diagnostics). Calcium concentrations were measured by spectrophotometry, IgG levels by immunoturbidimetry, and total protein concentrations by turbidimetry (c502, Cobas® 8000, Roche Diagnostics).

### Intracranial pressure and CSF production rate

After insertion of a 29-gauge needle connected to a pressure transducer into the cisterna magna, the ICP was recorded using a PowerLab acquisition system. Chart™ software (ADInstruments) was used to visualise and analyse the data. To measure the baseline ICP, a stable ICP of at least 40 s was selected and averaged. The CSF production rate was determined by calculating the rate of refilling after withdrawal of the first CSF sample. For this, the following equation was used:

$$\text{CSF production rate } \left(\mu l \, min^{-1}\right) = \left(\frac{V_{CSF}}{\Delta ICP_{Coll}}\right) \times \left(\frac{\Delta ICP_{Refill}}{\Delta t}\right)$$

where $V_{CSF}$ is the total volume of collected CSF, $\Delta ICP_{Coll}$ is the difference in ICP before and after the collection of CSF, and $\Delta ICP_{Refill}$ is the difference in ICP during a certain period ($\Delta t$) in the refill phase.

### Spectrophotometry of plasma, brain and CSF samples

Fluorescence spectrometry was used to quantify the amount of fluorescein in plasma, brain parenchyma and CSF. Plasma and CSF samples were diluted 10,000 and 50 times respectively, in order to be able to measure fluorescence within the range of the spectrophotometer (LS-55, Perkin Elmer). Brain samples comprised the front part of the brain, consisting of the olfactory bulb, cortex and striatum. Care was taken not to include the choroid plexus tissues from the third and lateral ventricle as these tissues may contain high concentrations of fluorescein, thereby interfering with the fluorescein measurements for the brain parenchyma. Brain samples were homogenised in RIPA buffer (150 mM NaCl, 1.0% Triton X100, 0.5% sodium deoxycholate, 0.1% SDS, 50 mM Tris, 1 mM EDTA, pH 8.0) using a Potter–Elvehjem tissue grinder, and an automated homogeniser (Kinematica) to obtain a fully homogenous suspension. Brain homogenates were centrifuged at 7800 rpm for 20 min, the supernatant was removed and used for fluorescence spectrometry.

## Immunohistochemical examination and capillary density quantification

After incubation in 30% sucrose, brains were mounted on a cryostat specimen object disc and subsequently frozen at − 80 °C. Coronal slices of 100 μm were cut on a cryostat (Microm HM 560), transferred to a 48-well plate containing cryoprotectant solution (30% sucrose, 30% ethylene glycol) and stored at − 20 °C until use. Selected sections were collected on SuperFrost glass slides and were allowed to dry for 15 min. Slides were incubated in bisbenzimide (1:100, 3.5 mg/ml, Sigma) for 10 min to visualise the cell nuclei, and coverslipped using fluorescent mounting medium (DAKO). A confocal laser scanning microscope (Leica TCS SP8) was used to acquire brain overview and detailed z-stack images of 70 μm with respectively 10 and 20× objectives. Images were analysed in ImageJ using the automated 'Blood vessel segmentation and network analysis' macro developed by S. Tosi.

## Statistical analysis

All data values were reported as mean ± SEM. Data sets were tested for normality by the Shapiro–Wilk test. The group means of parametric data were compared using an unpaired Student's t-test. The Mann–Whitney U test was applied to test differences between groups in nonparametric data sets. Fluorescein levels were measured in CSF at 30 min and 60 min. Since several samples were contaminated with blood, these data could not be tested with a repeated measurements ANOVA. Therefore, an unpaired Student's t-test was used. Quantifications of a number of vascular parameters were analysed using repeated measurements ANOVA, followed by Bonferroni's post hoc tests. Differences between WKY and SHR were considered significant at $p < 0.05$. All statistical analyses were done using GraphPad Prism software (version 7.03).

## Results

### Physical and biochemical parameters

At 42 ± 1 weeks of age, spontaneously hypertensive rats (SHR) had significantly lower brain wet weights than normotensive Wistar Kyoto rats (WKY) ($p \leq 0.01$). The body weight did not differ between these strains. Both systolic and diastolic blood, as well as the heart rate, were significantly elevated in SHR as compared to WKY ($p \leq 0.0001$) (Table 1).

We measured the concentrations of different solutes in CSF samples that were collected during the experiment. CSF glucose levels were remarkably high in both strains, but were significantly lower in SHR when compared to WKY ($p \leq 0.001$). In addition, we found a small (< 1%), but statistically significant difference in sodium concentrations between SHR and WKY ($p \leq 0.05$), and lower total protein concentrations in SHR ($p \leq 0.05$). IgG levels in both strains were below the detection limit of 0.3 g/l. All other solutes were not different between the two groups (Table 2).

**Table 1  Body and brain weights, blood pressure and heart rate in WKY and SHR rats**

|  | WKY (n = 10) | SHR (n = 10) |
|---|---|---|
| Weight |  |  |
| Body (g) | 401.0 ± 10.1 | 398.4 ± 2.6 |
| Brain (g) | 2.12 ± 0.03 | 2.01 ± 0.01** |
| Blood pressure and heart rate |  |  |
| Systolic (mmHg) | 158.6 ± 2.1 | 190.5 ± 4.0**** |
| Diastolic (mmHg) | 103.9 ± 2.3 | 145.7 ± 4.5**** |
| Heart rate (bpm) | 386.1 ± 8.6 | 460.9 ± 7.0**** |

Body weight did not differ between WKY and SHR, while brain wet weights were significantly lower in SHR. Both systolic and diastolic blood pressure, and heart rate were significantly elevated in SHR as compared to WKY. Values are mean ± SEM

*WKY* Wistar Kyoto rat, *SHR* spontaneously hypertensive rat

** $p \leq 0.01$ and **** $p \leq 0.0001$ vs. WKY (unpaired Student's t-test or Mann–Whitney U test)

**Table 2  Ionic composition and concentrations of various other solutes in the CSF of WKY and SHR rats**

|  | WKY | SHR |
|---|---|---|
| Na$^+$ | 156.3 ± 0.31 (n = 4) | 157.5 ± 0.25 (n = 4)* |
| K$^+$ | 2.76 ± 0.02 (n = 4) | 2.77 ± 0.01 (n = 4) |
| Cl$^-$ | 130.1 ± 0.31 (n = 4) | 131.3 ± 0.54 (n = 4) |
| Ca$^{2+}$ | 1.29 ± 0.01 (n = 3) | 1.27 ± 0.01 (n = 4) |
| Glucose | 8.11 ± 0.30 (n = 4) | 5.26 ± 0.20 (n = 4)*** |
| IgG | < 0.30 (n = 3) | < 0.30 (n = 8) |
| Total protein | 0.15 ± 0.002 (n = 5) | 0.11 ± 0.01 (n = 7)* |

Glucose levels were significantly lower in SHR as compared to WKY, but were remarkably high in both groups

*WKY* Wistar Kyoto rat, *SHR* spontaneously hypertensive rat; IgG, Immunoglobulin G

Na$^+$ concentrations were significantly higher in SHR, whereas none of the other ion concentrations were different. Total protein concentrations were significantly lower in SHR. Na$^+$, K$^+$, Cl$^-$, Ca$^{2+}$, and glucose levels are in mmol/L, whereas IgG and total protein are in g/L. Values are mean ± SEM. * $p \leq 0.05$, *** $p \leq 0.001$ vs. WKY (unpaired Student's t-test)

### Intracranial pressure and CSF production rate

Increased fluid leakage from parenchymal and choroidal capillaries as a consequence of hypertension could potentially elevate intracranial pressure (ICP) and CSF formation. Therefore, we recorded the ICP prior to and during withdrawal of CSF from the cisterna magna. Figure 1a shows an example of the ICP recording during the experiment, showing a pulsatile ICP and a clear drop in pressure upon CSF withdrawal. This drop in pressure was followed by a 'refill-phase' in which the animal was allowed to restore CSF volume for another 30 min. The inset shows a zoom in on the oscillatory patterns observed in the ICP recordings, which were attributable to the respiration and heart rate of approximately

1 breath and 4 to 5 heart beats per second. Prior to the first CSF collection, we measured the baseline ICP over a stable period of at least 40 s. In the example shown in Fig. 1a, the mean baseline ICP was 4.0 mmHg and was averaged over a period of approximately 5 min. Figure 1b shows the mean baseline ICP in WKY and SHR, with $5.19 \pm 0.52$ mmHg and $4.75 \pm 0.28$ mmHg respectively.

The CSF production rate was estimated from the rate of refilling after withdrawal of CSF. Since the CSF is formed by the choroid plexus, together with a possible contribution from ISF formed across the BBB, both an increased BBB and BCSFB permeability could lead to an enhanced CSF formation. However, CSF production rates did not significantly differ between WKY and SHR, with values

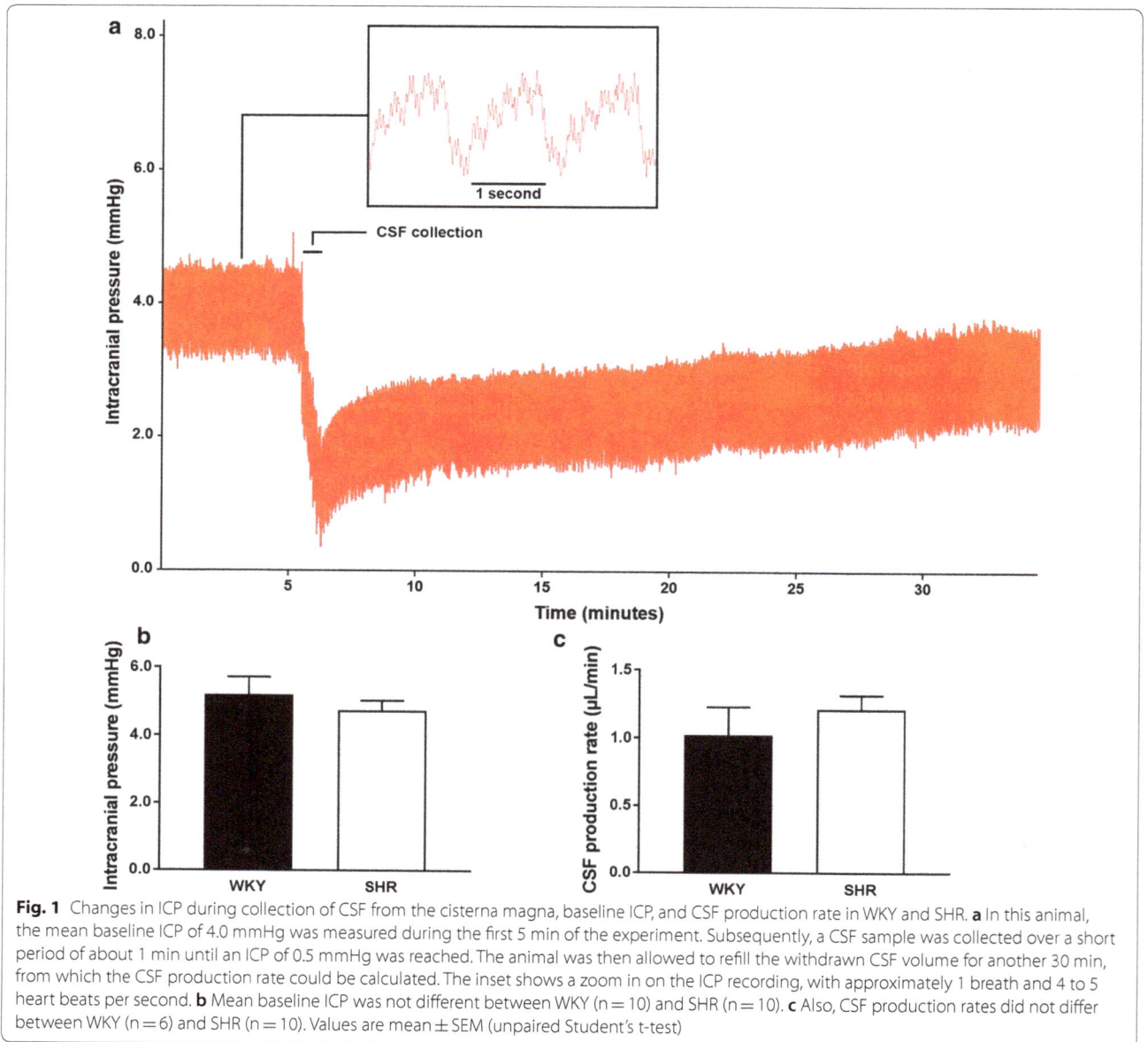

**Fig. 1** Changes in ICP during collection of CSF from the cisterna magna, baseline ICP, and CSF production rate in WKY and SHR. **a** In this animal, the mean baseline ICP of 4.0 mmHg was measured during the first 5 min of the experiment. Subsequently, a CSF sample was collected over a short period of about 1 min until an ICP of 0.5 mmHg was reached. The animal was then allowed to refill the withdrawn CSF volume for another 30 min, from which the CSF production rate could be calculated. The inset shows a zoom in on the ICP recording, with approximately 1 breath and 4 to 5 heart beats per second. **b** Mean baseline ICP was not different between WKY (n = 10) and SHR (n = 10). **c** Also, CSF production rates did not differ between WKY (n = 6) and SHR (n = 10). Values are mean ± SEM (unpaired Student's t-test)

of $1.02 \pm 0.21$ µl/min for WKY and $1.21 \pm 0.10$ µl/min for SHR (Fig. 1c).

## Fluorescein levels as a marker for BBB and BCSFB permeability

BBB and BCSFB permeability to small molecules was assessed by intravenous injection of a relatively small fluorescent tracer (sodium fluorescein, 0.4 kDa) into the bloodstream. The tracer was allowed to circulate for 60 min. After 30 and 60 min, CSF samples were collected from the cisterna magna, while plasma and brain samples were only obtained 60 min after infusion of fluorescein. Spectrophotometric analysis revealed that there were no significant differences in the fluorescein concentrations in both plasma ($10.56 \pm 0.34$ mg/l in WKY vs. $9.80 \pm 0.74$ mg/l in SHR) and brain ($0.11 \pm 0.012$ mg/l in WKY vs. $0.090 \pm 0.013$ mg/l in SHR) samples (Fig. 2a and b). In contrast, fluorescein concentration in CSF samples at both collection time points was significantly lower in SHR as compared to WKY. CSF fluorescein concentrations 30 min after fluorescein injection were about twice as high in WKY ($0.040 \pm 0.0047$ mg/l) than SHR ($0.022 \pm 0.0011$ mg/l) ($p \leq 0.001$). At the second CSF collection time point, fluorescein concentrations were $0.027 \pm 0.0012$ in WKY and $0.021 \pm 0.0023$ mg/l in SHR ($p \leq 0.05$) (Fig. 2c).

## Quantification of vascular anatomy

To further study the impact of hypertension on the cerebral microcirculation, we quantified the mean vessel diameter, number of branches, and volume fraction occupied by vessels. Fluorescently labelled *L. esculentum* lectin was injected into the bloodstream prior to sacrifice and perfusion fixation. This compound rapidly binds the vascular endothelium, which makes it an effective marker of perfused blood vessels. Six different brain regions were imaged to assess whether there were differences in the microvascular density or mean vessel diameter between SHR and WKY. Figure 3a shows an overview of a rat brain section in which these different brain regions are indicated. The images in Fig. 3b and c represent higher magnifications of the lectin staining in the field CA3 of the hippocampus and ventromedial thalamic nucleus respectively. These detail images were subsequently used for the quantification of several vascular parameters in ImageJ. As shown in Fig. 3d, no significant differences

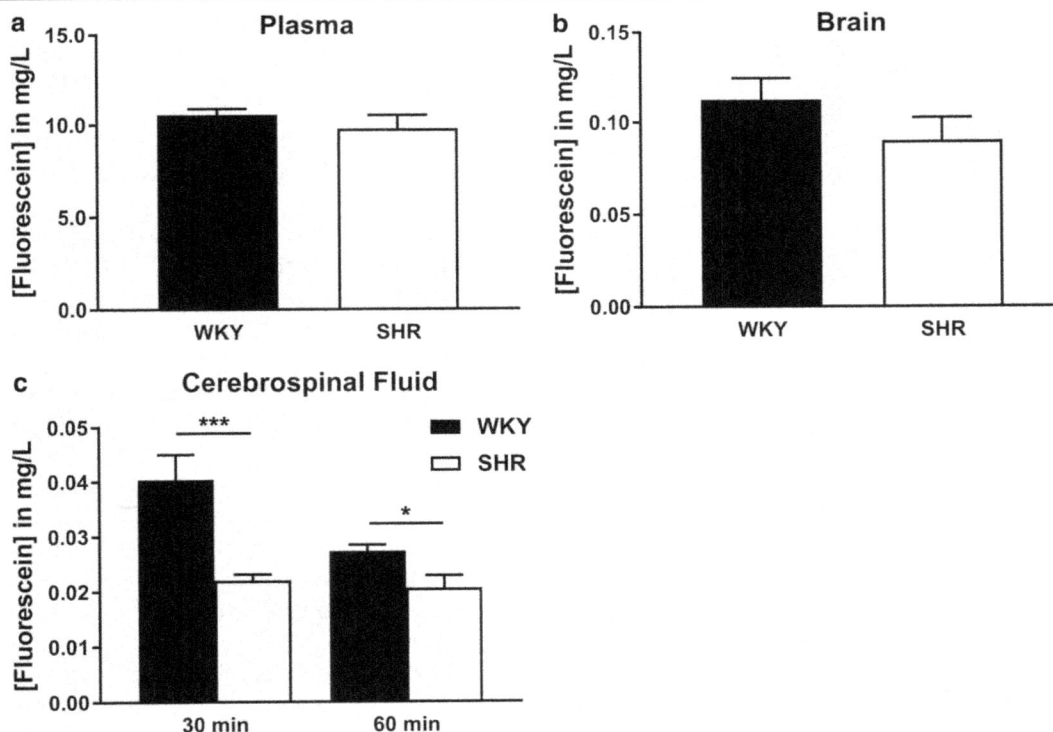

**Fig. 2** Fluorescein concentrations in plasma, brain and CSF. Fluorescein concentrations were quantified by spectrophotometric analysis in plasma (**a**), brain (**b**), and CSF (**c**) samples of WKY (n = 10 for plasma and brain, n = 7 at CSF 30 min, and n = 5 at CSF 60 min) and SHR (n = 10 for plasma and brain, n = 9 at CSF 30 min, and n = 6 at CSF 60 min). Values are mean ± SEM. *p ≤ 0.05, ***p ≤ 0.001. (unpaired Student's t-test or Mann–Whitney U test)

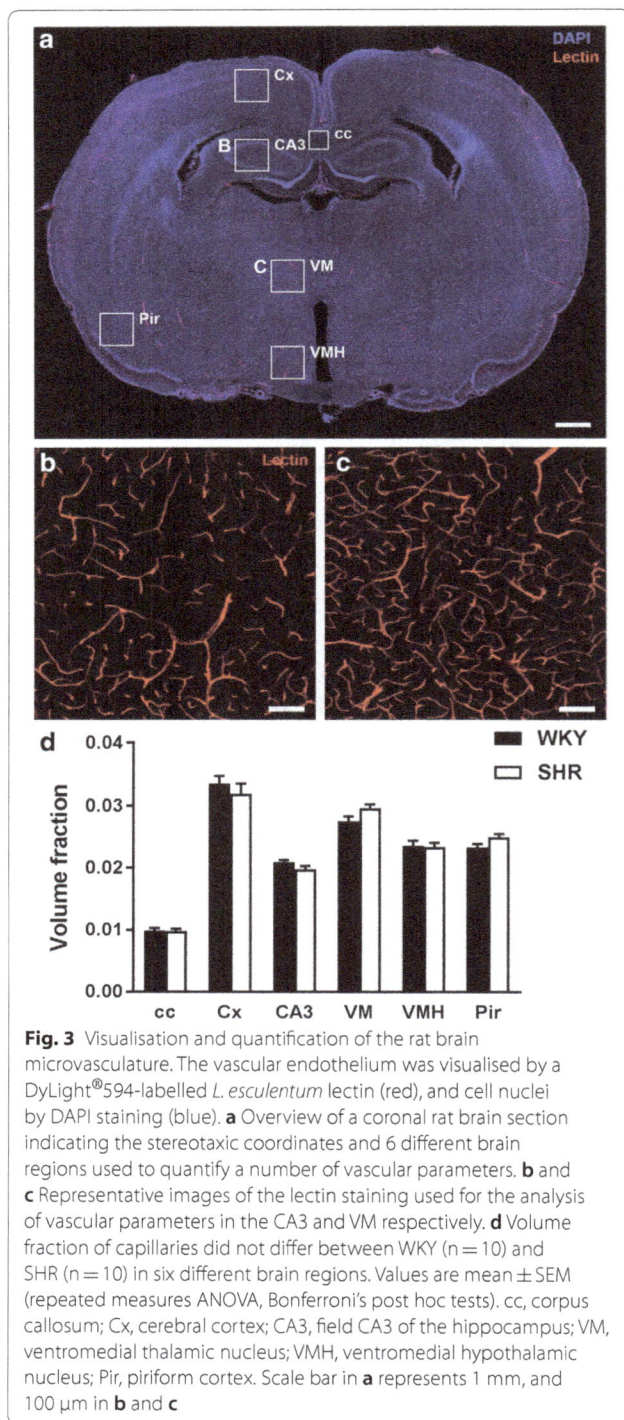

**Fig. 3** Visualisation and quantification of the rat brain microvasculature. The vascular endothelium was visualised by a DyLight®594-labelled *L. esculentum* lectin (red), and cell nuclei by DAPI staining (blue). **a** Overview of a coronal rat brain section indicating the stereotaxic coordinates and 6 different brain regions used to quantify a number of vascular parameters. **b** and **c** Representative images of the lectin staining used for the analysis of vascular parameters in the CA3 and VM respectively. **d** Volume fraction of capillaries did not differ between WKY (n = 10) and SHR (n = 10) in six different brain regions. Values are mean ± SEM (repeated measures ANOVA, Bonferroni's post hoc tests). cc, corpus callosum; Cx, cerebral cortex; CA3, field CA3 of the hippocampus; VM, ventromedial thalamic nucleus; VMH, ventromedial hypothalamic nucleus; Pir, piriform cortex. Scale bar in **a** represents 1 mm, and 100 μm in **b** and **c**

between WKY and SHR were found for the vascular volume fraction. Also mean vessel diameter, the number of branches, and total vessel length did not differ between the two strains (Additional file 1).

## Discussion

In the present study, we examined the effects of chronic hypertension on fluid management in the brains of rats at 10 months of age. No differences in either ICP values or CSF production rates were found between SHR and WKY. BBB and BCSFB integrity was subsequently determined by measuring the penetration of sodium fluorescein from the circulation into the brain parenchyma and CSF. Brain fluorescein concentrations in SHR were similar to those found in WKY rats, whereas the levels of this marker were higher in the CSF of the normotensive control animals. Ultimately, we quantified various vascular parameters in different brain regions, which did not reveal any differences between the two strains.

A general characterisation of SHR rats in this study confirmed an elevated systolic and diastolic blood pressure, higher heart rate, and a significant loss of brain mass, when compared to WKY rats. Electrolyte concentrations in the CSF did not reveal substantial differences between SHR and WKY. However, CSF glucose concentrations were significantly lower in SHR. The reason for this difference is unclear, but could hint towards altered metabolic activity between strains. Total CSF protein concentrations were significantly lower in SHR, while IgG levels were below the detection limit in both strains. These observations suggest an intact BBB and BCSFB in SHR, as concentrations of these plasma proteins would expectedly be higher in case of a leaky barrier. Others did find differences in the protein composition of CSF between SHR and WKY, which includes a relatively low level of transthyretin [16]. This could reflect dysfunction of the choroid plexus in SHR, other than increased permeability.

The significantly lower brain weights in SHR suggest cerebral atrophy in these animals. This was also previously reported by Gesztelyi et al. [17] and interpreted as a loss in microvascular tissue and neurons. Consequently, this brain tissue atrophy may result in ventricular enlargement as observed in SHR, a feature that is also observed in hypertensive patients [18–20]. Another possibility is that ventricular enlargement could result from altered fluid production due to hypertension. Thus, hypertension might lead to increased formation of ISF and CSF due to elevated fluid leakage from parenchymal and choroidal blood vessels, which could result in an elevated ICP [20]. To study this, we monitored the ICP via the cisterna magna prior to and during collection of CSF. This showed a highly oscillatory pressure profile generated by the heartbeat and respiration. However, mean ICPs did not differ significantly between SHR and WKY, and correspond well to values reported in the study by Ritter et al. [21]. It may be possible that SHR experience episodic variations in ICP which could not be detected during our experiments.

Determining the CSF production rate is still technically challenging and a number of different techniques have been tested [5], yielding varying production rates. In this study, we estimated CSF production rates from the refill rate after collection of a known volume of CSF according to the procedure described by Masserman [22]. The values we found were similar to those found in rats using the ventriculo-cisternal perfusion method [23, 24], but might be slightly underestimated since the animals were not artificially ventilated. In mice, artificial ventilation was recently found to increase CSF production [25]. The CSF production rates tended to be slightly higher in SHR, but were not statistically different from the normotensive control animals. This suggests that there is no markedly enhanced BBB or BCSFB permeability in SHR, as this would result a more rapid recovery to the ICP after CSF collection, and therefore a higher CSF production rate. However, another possibility may be that the contribution of the extra-choroidal CSF formation across the BBB is too small to detect differences in the presence of a large background of choroidal CSF formation.

We do not expect that differences in ventricular volume affect the calculated CSF production. In the current procedure, we obtained a sample of CSF. From the volume of the sample and the accompanying decrease in pressure we could derive the compliance (delta V/delta P). In case differences in ventricular volume play a role, this is reflected herein. Yet, the compliance was the same in WKY and SHR (data not shown). Thus, refilling of the CSF induces the same gradual increase in pressure in both rat strains, irrespective of the ventricle volume. Another potential limitation is that withdrawal of a CSF sample might lead to a redistribution between ISF and CSF that affects the estimation of CSF production. Thus, the refilling of the CSF compartment after fluid withdrawal might to some extent have originated from the ISF compartment rather than the choroid plexus. Estimation of this contribution would require data on interstitial compliance and resistance for ISF-CSF fluid flow. There are two extreme cases: first, the ISF volume might not change at all in the time course of the experiment, because of low compliance or high resistance. Second, resistance is low enough to allow a rapid equilibrium between these compartments. In either case the presence of the ISF compartment would not affect the estimation of CSF production, although the interpretation of compliance differs. Yet, in intermediate cases of ISF-CSF convection dynamics, a two-compartment model would be needed to more carefully interpret these findings.

BBB and BCSFB integrity was further studied by measuring sodium fluorescein passage across these barriers using spectrophotometry. For the brain tissue samples, care was taken not to include choroid plexus tissue, as preliminary experiments showed that the choroid vascular and stromal tissue contained high concentrations of fluorescein. We used sodium fluorescein as it is described as the most suitable marker to detect more subtle changes in BBB and BCSF integrity because of its low molecular weight of 0.4 kDa. Fluorescein is also less toxic and only weakly binds to plasma proteins such as albumin when compared to Evans blue, which is still the most commonly used dye in BBB permeability studies [26]. One hour after injection of fluorescein, we measured the levels of this dye in plasma, brain parenchyma, and CSF. Measurement of fluorescein in plasma is of importance, as differences in clearance from the blood between SHR and WKY would obscure brain and CSF permeability measurements. However, no differences in plasma fluorescein concentrations were found between SHR and WKY, indicating that the clearance rate from the blood is similar in these strains. Brain fluorescein concentrations were also nearly identical between hypertensive and normotensive rats, and were around 1% of those present in plasma. This finding suggests that the BBB in these rats is still intact, which seems to be in contrast to one study showing decreased BBB permeability [27]. This may relate to a large difference in the time point of the measurements (15 s after tracer infusion versus 30 and 60 min in the current study). Alternatively, the type of anesthesia, the age of the rats, or the use of a different marker for the assessment of BBB integrity, radiolabelled [14]C-sucrose, which has been criticised [28], may play a role [27]. In a study by Kaiser et al. [12], whole brain permeability to Evans blue was not statistically different between SHR and WKY, whereas the deep cortical region was found to be more permeable in SHR.

Cerebrospinal fluid fluorescein concentrations were significantly lower in SHR as compared to WKY, with roughly a twofold difference at the first collection point. As CSF production rates were similar in the two strains, the latter finding could not be explained by an elevated CSF turnover. While the data might seem to suggest actually a higher leakage of fluorescein in the WKY, a more likely explanation is the increased ventricle volume by about a factor of two in SHR in which the fluorescein dilutes [12, 19, 20, 29]. Taken together, these findings indicate an intact BBB and BCSFB in the hypertensive rats. This is in agreement with a study by Calcinaghi et al. [29], which showed that there is no leakage of the body's own macromolecules from the circulation across the BBB. Another study by Mueller and Heistad [14] demonstrated an even less permeable BBB in SHR when compared to WKY. The lack of BBB damage might be explained by protective mechanisms, such as inward remodelling of the arteries and autoregulatory responses, which limit increases in pressure at the level of the capillaries.

Chronic hypertension is associated with changes in the structure of the cerebral arteries both in humans and animal models such as the inward remodelling mentioned above [1], but data regarding the capillary network are less clear. A detailed analysis of the microvascular network, including average vessel diameter, number of branches, and volume fraction was done in an automated manner using ImageJ software. This unbiased approach revealed no differences between SHR and WKY in six different brain areas, and is consistent with other studies showing similar findings in the same brain regions [17, 29, 30]. In contrast, Kaiser et al. [12] demonstrated an augmented vessel volume in SHR. This total vessel volume was quantified in the deep cortical region only, which may be one brain area specifically affected by hypertension and might therefore not be considered as a general feature of the hypertensive brain. In addition, the study by Ritz et al. [31] showed higher cerebral small vessel densities in the cortex and putamen of younger SHR, but similar densities in these brain regions in hypertensive and normotensive animals of 9 months of age.

## Conclusions

In summary, we found no evidence for increased BBB and BCSFB permeability to a small compound in hypertensive rats. This was based on quantification of fluorescein leakage from blood into brain parenchyma and CSF. Also indirect consequences of increased fluid leakage, such as elevated ICP or CSF formation, were not evident. However, it remains to be established whether these barriers show differences in permeability to even smaller molecules, such as water, in hypertension. Finally, the brain microvasculature of SHR was not affected in terms of vessel volume, vessel diameter, and the number of branches. From this we conclude that several established features of mature SHR, including the lower brain weight, larger ventricular volume [19, 20], small artery remodelling [12], and increased sensitivity to stroke [32] are not paralleled by a physical loss of BBB and BCSFB integrity.

## Abbreviations
BBB: blood–brain barrier; BCSFB: blood–cerebrospinal fluid barrier; CSF: cerebrospinal fluid; ICP: intracranial pressure; IgG: immunoglobulin G; ISF: interstitial fluid; SHR: spontaneously hypertensive rat; WKY: Wistar Kyoto rat.

## Authors' contributions
DN, EvB, and EB designed the study and wrote the manuscript. DN, EB, and JdeV performed the animal experiments. All authors read and approved the final manuscript.

## Acknowledgements
We would like to thank J.J. de Groot for his help with the electrolyte and protein measurements.

## Competing interests
The authors declare that they have no competing interests.

## Funding
This project was funded by Alzheimer Nederland and is part of the Deltaplan Dementie.

## References
1. Iadecola C, Yaffe K, Biller J, Bratzke LC, Faraci FM, Gorelick PB, et al. Impact of hypertension on cognitive function: a scientific statement from the American Heart Association. Hypertension. 2016;68(6):e67–94.
2. Ishida H, Takemori K, Dote K, Ito H. Expression of glucose transporter-1 and aquaporin-4 in the cerebral cortex of stroke-prone spontaneously hypertensive rats in relation to the blood-brain barrier function. Am J Hypertens. 2006;19(1):33–9.
3. Dandy WE. Experimental hydrocephalus. Ann Surg. 1919;70(2):129–42.
4. Hladky SB, Barrand MA. Mechanisms of fluid movement into, through and out of the brain: evaluation of the evidence. Fluids Barriers CNS. 2014;11(1):26.
5. Segal MB, Pollay M. The secretion of cerebrospinal fluid. Exp Eye Res. 1977;25(Suppl):127–48.
6. Spector R, Robert Snodgrass S, Johanson CE. A balanced view of the cerebrospinal fluid composition and functions: focus on adult humans. Exp Neurol. 2015;273:57–68.
7. Milhorat TH. Choroid plexus and cerebrospinal fluid production. Science (New York, NY). 1969;166(3912):1514–6.
8. Hladky SB, Barrand MA. Fluid and ion transfer across the blood-brain and blood–cerebrospinal fluid barriers; a comparative account of mechanisms and roles. Fluids Barriers CNS. 2016;13(1):19.
9. Pollay M, Curl F. Secretion of cerebrospinal fluid by the ventricular ependyma of the rabbit. Am J Physiol. 1967;213(4):1031–8.
10. Sakka L, Coll G, Chazal J. Anatomy and physiology of cerebrospinal fluid. Eur Ann Otorhinolaryngol Head Neck Dis. 2011;128(6):309–16.
11. Bedussi B, Naessens DM, de Vos J, Olde Engberink R, Wilhelmus MM, Richard E, et al. Enhanced interstitial fluid drainage in the hippocampus of spontaneously hypertensive rats. Sci Rep. 2017;7(1):744.
12. Kaiser D, Weise G, Moller K, Scheibe J, Posel C, Baasch S, et al. Spontaneous white matter damage, cognitive decline and neuroinflammation in middle-aged hypertensive rats: an animal model of early-stage cerebral small vessel disease. Acta Neuropathol Commun. 2014;2:169.
13. Hom S, Fleegal MA, Egleton RD, Campos CR, Hawkins BT, Davis TP. Comparative changes in the blood-brain barrier and cerebral infarction of SHR and WKY rats. Am J Physiol Regul Integr Comp Physiol. 2007;292(5):R1881–92.
14. Mueller SM, Heistad DD. Effect of chronic hypertension on the blood-brain barrier. Hypertension. 1980;2(6):809–12.
15. Bakker EN, Groma G, Spijkers LJ, de Vos J, van Weert A, van Veen H, et al. Heterogeneity in arterial remodeling among sublines of spontaneously hypertensive rats. PLoS ONE. 2014;9(9):e107998.
16. Gonzalez-Marrero I, Castaneyra-Ruiz L, Gonzalez-Toledo JM, Castaneyra-Ruiz A, de Paz-Carmona H, Castro R, et al. High blood pressure effects on the blood to cerebrospinal fluid barrier and cerebrospinal fluid protein composition: a two-dimensional electrophoresis study in spontaneously hypertensive rats. Int J Hypertens. 2013;2013:164653.
17. Gesztelyi G, Finnegan W, DeMaro JA, Wang JY, Chen JL, Fenstermacher J. Parenchymal microvascular systems and cerebral atrophy in spontaneously hypertensive rats. Brain Res. 1993;611(2):249–57.

18. Salerno JA, Murphy DG, Horwitz B, DeCarli C, Haxby JV, Rapoport SI, et al. Brain atrophy in hypertension. A volumetric magnetic resonance imaging study. Hypertension. 1992;20(3):340–8.

19. Bendel P, Eilam R. Quantitation of ventricular size in normal and spontaneously hypertensive rats by magnetic resonance imaging. Brain Res. 1992;574(1–2):224–8.

20. Ritter S, Dinh TT. Progressive postnatal dilation of brain ventricles in spontaneously hypertensive rats. Brain Res. 1986;370(2):327–32.

21. Ritter S, Dinh TT, Stone S, Ross N. Cerebroventricular dilation in spontaneously hypertensive rats (SHRs) is not attenuated by reduction of blood pressure. Brain Res. 1988;450(1–2):354–9.

22. Masserman JH. Cerebrospinal hydrodynamics: Iv. clinical experimental studies. Arch Neurol Psychiatry. 1934;32(3):523–53.

23. Preston JE. Ageing choroid plexus-cerebrospinal fluid system. Microsc Res Tech. 2001;52(1):31–7.

24. Cserr H. Potassium exchange between cerebrospinal fluid, plasma, and brain. Am J Physiol. 1965;209(6):1219–26.

25. Steffensen AB, Oernbo EK, Stoica A, Gerkau NJ, Barbuskaite D, Tritsaris K, et al. Cotransporter-mediated water transport underlying cerebrospinal fluid formation. Nat Commun. 2018;9(1):2167.

26. Saunders NR, Dziegielewska KM, Mollgard K, Habgood MD. Markers for blood-brain barrier integrity: how appropriate is Evans blue in the twenty-first century and what are the alternatives? Front Neurosci. 2015;9:385.

27. Al-Sarraf H, Philip L. Effect of hypertension on the integrity of blood brain and blood CSF barriers, cerebral blood flow and CSF secretion in the rat. Brain Res. 2003;975(1–2):179–88.

28. Miah MK, Chowdhury EA, Bickel U, Mehvar R. Evaluation of [(14)C] and [(13)C]Sucrose as blood–brain barrier permeability markers. J Pharm Sci. 2017;106(6):1659–69.

29. Calcinaghi N, Wyss MT, Jolivet R, Singh A, Keller AL, Winnik S, et al. Multimodal imaging in rats reveals impaired neurovascular coupling in sustained hypertension. Stroke. 2013;44(7):1957–64.

30. Lin SZ, Sposito N, Pettersen S, Rybacki L, McKenna E, Pettigrew K, et al. Cerebral capillary bed structure of normotensive and chronically hypertensive rats. Microvasc Res. 1990;40(3):341–57.

31. Ritz MF, Fluri F, Engelter ST, Schaeren-Wiemers N, Lyrer PA. Cortical and putamen age-related changes in the microvessel density and astrocyte deficiency in spontaneously hypertensive and stroke-prone spontaneously hypertensive rats. Curr Neurovasc Res. 2009;6(4):279–87.

32. Kang BT, Leoni RF, Silva AC. Impaired CBF regulation and high CBF threshold contribute to the increased sensitivity of spontaneously hypertensive rats to cerebral ischemia. Neuroscience. 2014;269:223–31.

# 19

# Pulsatile flow drivers in brain parenchyma and perivascular spaces: a resistance network model study

Julian Rey and Malisa Sarntinoranont[*]

## Abstract

**Background:** In animal models, dissolved compounds in the subarachnoid space and parenchyma have been found to preferentially transport through the cortex perivascular spaces (PVS) but the transport phenomena involved are unclear.

**Methods:** In this study two hydraulic network models were used to predict fluid motion produced by blood vessel pulsations and estimate the contribution made to solute transport in PVS and parenchyma. The effect of varying pulse amplitude and timing, PVS dimensions, and tissue hydraulic conductivity on fluid motion was investigated.

**Results:** Periodic vessel pulses resulted in oscillatory fluid motion in PVS and parenchyma but no net flow over time. For baseline parameters, PVS and parenchyma peak fluid velocity was on the order of 10 µm/s and 1 nm/s, with corresponding Peclet numbers below $10^3$ and $10^{-1}$ respectively. Peak fluid velocity in the PVS and parenchyma tended to increase with increasing pulse amplitude and vessel size, and exhibited asymptotic relationships with hydraulic conductivity.

**Conclusions:** Solute transport in parenchyma was predicted to be diffusion dominated, with a negligible contribution from convection. In the PVS, dispersion due to oscillating flow likely plays a significant role in PVS rapid transport observed in previous in vivo experiments. This dispersive effect could be more significant than convective solute transport from net flow that may exist in PVS and should be studied further.

**Keywords:** Rat cerebral cortex, Biotransport, Glymphatic theory, Extracellular flow, Bulk flow, Interstitial flow, Lumped parameter, Porous media, Cerebrospinal fluid, Fluid mechanics, Diffusion

## Background

Since the 1970s the perivascular spaces (PVS) surrounding blood vessels have been thought to play a role in solute transport through brain tissue, specifically as conduits for rapid transport [1, 2]. The PVS are extracellular spaces formed by cylindrical arrangements of glial cells that surround intracortical arterioles and veins [3]. Rennels et al. [2] and more recently Iliff et al. [4] found that tracers injected into the subarachnoid space (SAS) of animal models were preferentially transported through the PVS of intracortical arteries at rates faster than would

be expected from diffusion alone. In these studies, tracer moved in the direction of blood flow. Ichimura et al. [5] injected fluorescently labeled albumin into cortical perivascular spaces of rats with an open cranial window preparation and using video-densitometric measurements described slow oscillatory tracer motion within the PVS that was not biased in either direction. Carare et al. [6] and more recently Morris et al. [7] observed tracers injected into the parenchyma quickly located in the basal lamina of capillaries and moved through the basal lamina of arterioles opposite the direction of blood flow. Other recent experiments have confirmed observations of rapid tracer transport via PVS [8, 9]. In humans, cerebrospinal fluid (CSF) tracers have been found along the large leptomeningeal arterial trunks with MRI [10].

*Correspondence: msarnt@ufl.edu
Department of Mechanical and Aerospace Engineering, University of Florida, PO Box 116250, Gainesville, FL 32611, USA

Together, these findings suggest that a network of intra-mural and extravascular channels may serve as a means for facilitated transport of dissolved compounds and exchange between interstitial fluid (ISF) and CSF. As such, it may substitute for an absent lymphatic vessel network in the parenchyma by collecting excess ISF and metabolic wastes [11]. Insights into Alzheimer's disease, Parkinson's disease, hydrocephalus, and other neurologi-cal diseases may be predicated on a precise understand-ing of how these solute and fluid transport pathways malfunction.

Despite discrepancies in the literature with regard to the direction of solute transport and the anatomical structures involved, strong correlation with vascular pul-satility is a point of agreement [12]. Pulsatility refers to the periodic changes in blood vessel volume caused by heart contractions. The rate of imaging tracer transport from the SAS into the PVS of penetrating arterioles has been positively correlated with arterial pulsatility in ani-mal models [2, 13]. Clearance of beta-amyloid from the parenchyma of mice [13] and of liposomes introduced by intraparenchymal convection enhanced delivery [14] both decreased with decreased pulsatility. Rapid tracer localization within the capillary basal lamina ceased shortly after animal sacrifice [6]. The rate of transport in PVS and its apparent relationship with pulsatility sug-gests convective transport generated by pulsatility is involved. Convection is here defined as solute transport along with the net flow of its solvent fluid. A number of investigators have developed pulsatility models for fluid flow in the PVS. Coloma et al. [15] and Sharp et al. [16] have examined vascular reflection waves and unsteady PVS hydraulic resistance as drivers of net fluid flow within the PVS, specifically the arterial basement mem-branes. However, Asgari et al. [17] simulated flow in the PVS due to vascular pulse wave propagation using com-putational fluid dynamics (CFD) and observed oscillating flow was $10^3$ times greater that net axial flow, evidence against net convective solute transport by peristalsis.

Iliff et al. [4] proposed the glymphatic theory in which CSF enters the PVS surrounding cortical arteries and flows through parenchyma while convectively transport-ing metabolic wastes to the PVS surrounding veins from which they are ultimately cleared. Astrocytic endfeet expressing AQP4 at the PVS boundary were proposed to play an essential role in this process. Subsequent compu-tational models and experiments have sought to test the glymphatic theory and have challenged many of its ten-ets, particularly that solutes are transported via convec-tion in the parenchyma [8, 9, 17–19].

Asgari et al. [20] modeled fluid motion through and around astrocytes in the parenchyma with a hydraulic resistance network. Fluid was driven by a constant pres-sure difference between arterial and venous perivas-cular spaces and resistances were varied to simulate the effect of AQP4 knockout and increased extracel-lular volume. More recently, this group has addressed whether arterial pulsatility modeled with CFD pro-duced bulk flow in parenchyma and argued diffusion dominates solute transport there [17]. Jin et al. [18] and Holter et al. [19] imposed pressure differences between arterial and venous PVS in porous media CFD models and concluded solute transport in parenchyma can be explained by diffusion alone.

In this study, a one vessel and two vessel hydraulic network model was developed to explore how pulsa-tility may drive fluid motion within cortical PVS and parenchyma of the rat. The one vessel model parameters such as pulse amplitude, PVS size, and tissue hydrau-lic conductivity were varied to predict their effect on fluid motion and solute transport. A two vessel model was also developed to study the effect of pulse ampli-tude and timing differences between arteries and veins in proximity. A 2D resistance network is a simple tool that captures the essential physics involved, reveals the effect of varying tissue properties, and can help validate future CFD models. Unlike previous resistance network and CFD models [17–20], the present model predicts fluid motion in the PVS and parenchyma together and does not assume a pressure gradient between the arte-rial and venous PVS, but is instead based on observed changes in vessel diameter during the cardiac cycle. How the predicted fluid motion may result in previ-ously reported tracer transport patterns is discussed.

## Methods
Two hydraulic network models of the PVS and sur-rounding parenchyma in rat cortex were developed to simulate the fluid motion produced by vascular pulsa-tions: a one vessel model of an arteriole segment, and a two vessel model of arteriole and vein segments (Fig. 1). The vessel segment length and separation were 300 and 200 μm, respectively, which are comparable to mean values found in the literature [19, 21]. Fluid motion through the resistors in the network was governed by the hydraulic equivalent of Ohm's law.

$$\Delta p = Rq \qquad (1)$$

where $\Delta p$ is the pressure difference across the resistor, $q$ is the volumetric flow rate through the resistor, and $R$ is the reciprocal of the hydraulic conductivity, or the hydraulic resistance. The one and two vessel models were imple-mented and run in MATLAB R2018a (MathWorks®, Natick, MA).

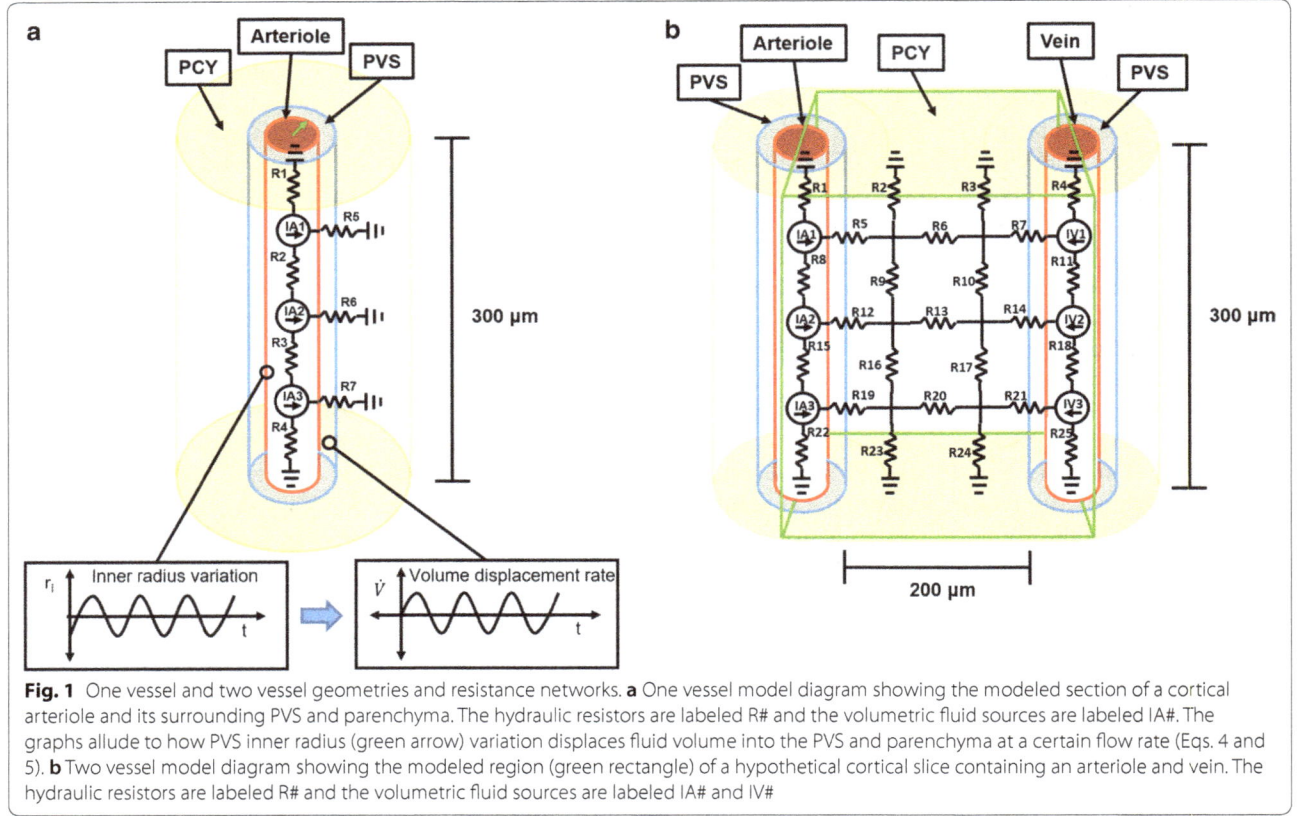

**Fig. 1** One vessel and two vessel geometries and resistance networks. **a** One vessel model diagram showing the modeled section of a cortical arteriole and its surrounding PVS and parenchyma. The hydraulic resistors are labeled R# and the volumetric fluid sources are labeled IA#. The graphs allude to how PVS inner radius (green arrow) variation displaces fluid volume into the PVS and parenchyma at a certain flow rate (Eqs. 4 and 5). **b** Two vessel model diagram showing the modeled region (green rectangle) of a hypothetical cortical slice containing an arteriole and vein. The hydraulic resistors are labeled R# and the volumetric fluid sources are labeled IA# and IV#

## One vessel model

A cylindrical segment of a penetrating arteriole with a baseline radius of 10 µm [4] and its surrounding PVS and parenchyma were modeled as a network with seven resistors (Fig. 1a). Fluid could enter or leave the network axially through the modeled PVS or radially through the parenchyma. Here the PVS was simply considered a low resistance pathway around the vessel that included the basement membrane of smooth muscle cells [7], the space between the vessel and pial sheath, and the space between the pial sheath and the glia limitans. The existence of true spaces between these membranes is debated [7, 22], but a broad description of PVS as is adopted here was provided in a review by Abbott et al. [3] and reflects uncertainty about what spaces are involved in rapid tracer transport and communication between these spaces. This model did not explicitly model aquaporins on the astrocytic endfeet surrounding the PVS but accounts for their effect as a change in parenchyma hydraulic conductivity.

The PVS hydraulic resistance was derived from the Navier–Stokes solution for steady pressure-driven flow through a straight annulus [23].

$$R_{PVS} = \frac{8\mu l}{\pi R_o^4 \left[1 - E^4 + \frac{(E^2 - 1)^2}{lnE}\right]} \qquad (2)$$

Here $\mu$, $l$, $R_o$, and $E$ are the fluid dynamic viscosity, the PVS length modeled by the resistor, the PVS outer radius, and the ratio of PVS inner to outer radius, respectively. Parameters and their values are listed in Table 1. Because the PVS is a complex physiological space occupied by proteins and other molecules, this hydraulic resistance was considered a lower bound for hydraulic resistance in vivo.

The parenchyma hydraulic resistance was derived by simplifying Darcy's law for flow through rigid porous media to one-dimensional radial flow through a cylindrical shell.

$$R_{PCY} = \frac{\ln\left(R_o^{PCY}/R_i^{PCY}\right)}{2\pi h K_{PCY}} \qquad (3)$$

Here $R_o^{PCY}$, $R_i^{PCY}$, $h$, $K_{PCY}$, are the outer and inner radii of the parenchymal cylindrical shell, the shell height, and the parenchyma hydraulic conductivity, respectively [33].

**Table 1  One vessel and two vessel model parameters**

| Symbol | Description | Baseline value | Simulated range | Source |
|---|---|---|---|---|
| $R_i$ | PVS inner radius | 10 μm | 1–29 μm | [4, 13, 21] |
| $R_o$ | PVS outer radius | 30 μm | 2–30 μm | [4] |
| $L_{PVS}$ | PVS segment length | 300 μm | – | [17, 21] |
| $L_{PCY}$ | Distance between vessels | 200 μm | – | [19] |
| $b$ | Wave amplitude | 0.25 μm | 0–0.37 μm | [13] |
| $f$ | Pulse frequency | 5 Hz | – | [14] |
| – | Wave speed | 1 m/s | | [24–26] |
| $K$ | Hydraulic conductivity | $5.63 \times 10^{-12}$ m²/(Pa s) | $10^2$–$10^{11}$ μm³ s/kg | [27] |
| $\mu$ | Dynamic viscosity | $0.9 \times 10^{-3}$ Pa s | – | [28, 29] |
| $\rho$ | Interstitial fluid density | 993.2 kg/m³ | – | [30] |
| $\varphi$ | Porosity | 0.2 | | [31] |
| $D*^b$ | Solute diffusivity | – | $10^1$–$10^3$ μm²/s | [31, 19] |
| $l^a$ | Resistance length | 50; 100 μm | | Model dependent |
| $h$ | Resistance height | 100 μm | | Model dependent |
| $d$ | Resistance depth | 200 μm | | Model dependent |
| $R_i^{PCY}$ | Parenchyma inner radius | 10 μm | | [4] |
| $R_o^{PCY}$ | Parenchyma outer radius | 300 μm | | Model dependent |
| $\eta$ | Pore size | 60 nm | | [32] |
| $\theta$ | Phase shift | 0 | 0–2π | Model dependent |
| $\xi$ | Pulsatility ratio | 0.80 | 0–1 | [13] |

a  R2, R3 in the one vessel model and R6, R8, R9, R10, R11, R13, R15, R16, R17, R18, and R20 in the two vessel model had lengths of 100 μm. All others resistors had lengths of 50 μm except R5, R6, and R7 in the one vessel model which were defined as in Eq. 3

b  D* refers to the effective solute diffusion coefficient in brain tissue

The outer radius of the parenchymal shell was taken as much larger than the inner radius to reflect the scale of the parenchyma theoretically available for flow.

Volumetric fluid sources were introduced into the network to account for fluid displaced by the arterial pulses in the cardiac cycle (Fig. 1a). No pressure gradients were imposed anywhere in the model and these volumetric fluid sources were the only drivers of fluid motion present. In-vivo measurements indicate that cortical vessel diameter variation in time is roughly sinusoidal [4]. An arterial wave speed of order 1 m/s [26] and pulse frequency of 5 Hz [14] correspond to a wavelength of 20 cm, much longer than the modeled 300 μm arteriole segment. It was therefore fair to assume a PVS inner radius that varies uniformly along its length [17] and sinusoidally in time. An expression for the rate of volume displacement due to uniform motion of the PVS inner boundary was found by differentiating the volume contained by the inner boundary with respect to time. Fluid volume displaced by the inner boundary moved into the PVS and parenchyma and appeared as a volumetric fluid source in the network model.

$$q = \dot{V} = 2\pi l r_i \dot{r}_i \tag{4}$$

Here $q$, $V$, $l$, and $r_i$ are the volumetric flow rate, volume contained by the PVS inner boundary, the segment length modeled by the fluid source, and the PVS inner radius as a function of time, respectively.

The inner radius varied in time according to

$$r_i = -b\cos(2\pi f) + R_i \tag{5}$$

Here $f$ and $b$ are the frequency and amplitude of inner wall motion, or the pulse frequency and amplitude. $R_i$ is the time-averaged PVS inner radius value. Substituting Eq. 5 into Eq. 4 the flow rate became

$$q = 4\pi^2 lfb\big(R_i \sin(2\pi ft) - b\sin(2\pi ft)\cos(2\pi ft)\big) \tag{6}$$

Because the ratio of coefficients for the second and first term is $b/R_i$, the first term dominates when $b$ is much smaller than $R_i$ and the flow rate is approximately

$$q \approx 4\pi^2 lfbR_i \sin(2\pi ft) \tag{7}$$

Although the expression for PVS hydraulic resistance was derived for steady, axial pressure-driven flow, it serves as a reasonable approximation because the PVS thickness is much smaller than the pulse wavelength and the Womersley number, $\alpha = 2(R_o - R_i)\sqrt{2\pi f \rho/\mu}$, is small [34]. Twice the value of PVS thickness is the hydrodynamic radius [23] and $\rho$ is the fluid density, approximately that of water at body temperature [30]. When PVS thickness is much smaller than wavelength, lubrication theory says radial velocity and pressure gradients can be assumed negligible, and axial velocity and pressure gradients dominate. When $\alpha$ is small, oscillatory flow can be approximated by the steady-state profile corresponding to the instantaneous axial pressure gradient in the segment [34]. The pulse amplitude was selected so that the free fluid hydraulic resistance of the PVS never varied by more than 5% and could be assumed constant when solving for pressure and velocity in the network.

To account for the presence of solid components in the PVS, an alternative resistance was derived by simplifying Darcy's law for axial flow through an annulus of rigid porous media.

$$R_{PVS} = \frac{l}{\pi(R_o^2 - R_i^2)K_{PVS}} \qquad (8)$$

Here $l$, $R_o$, $R_i$, $K_{PVS}$, are the PVS length modeled by the resistor, the PVS outer radius, the PVS inner radius, and the PVS hydraulic conductivity, respectively.

**Two vessel model**

A planar portion of tissue which included segments of a cortical arteriole and vein, surrounding PVS and parenchyma were modeled as a network with 25 resistors (Fig. 1b). Vessels had a baseline radii of 10 µm [4] and were separated by 200 µm [19]. Fluid could enter or leave the network at the upper and lower boundaries of the modeled parenchyma and PVS. Because the flow produced by vessel pulsation was assumed to be radially symmetric, half of the radial flow produced by each vessel entered the modeled parenchyma and the flow rate for each arterial volumetric fluid source became.

$$q \approx 2\pi^2 lfbR_i \sin(2\pi ft) \qquad (9)$$

Accordingly, axial flow along half the PVS was modeled for the arteriole and the vein. The PVS resistances were therefore double those derived in the one vessel model because only half the annulus was available for flow.

The flow rate for each venous volumetric fluid source was determined by considering the pulsatility ratio between cortex arterioles and veins where pulsatility is defined as.

$$\Pi = 2\int_0^T |r_i - R_i| dt \qquad (10)$$

This formulation for pulsatility is based on Iliff et al. [13] where $T$ is the measurement interval. Substituting Eq. 5 for inner radius variation over time into Eq. 10 revealed that pulsatility was proportional to pulse amplitude and inversely proportional to pulse frequency, $\Pi = b/\pi f$. The ratio of venous to arterial pulsatility, $\xi$, was used to determine the venous pulse amplitude for a given arterial pulse amplitude. Substituting the venous pulse amplitude into Eq. 9 produced the flow rate for each venous fluid source.

To assess the mode of solute transport in both the models, the Peclet number was computed for the PVS and parenchyma.

$$Pe = L_{PVS}v/D^* \qquad (11)$$

$$Pe = L_{PCY}v/\phi D^* \qquad (12)$$

$$Pe = \eta v/\phi D^* \qquad (13)$$

Here $\phi$ and $D^*$ are the parenchyma porosity and solute diffusivity, respectively. The Peclet number formulation for the PVS, Eq. 11, includes $L_{PVS}$, the full vessel segment length, and $v$, the average axial velocity. Two Peclet number formulations, Eqs. 12 and 13, were used for the parenchyma, differing in their characteristic length scale. The former includes $L_{PCY}$, the distance between the arteriole and vein [19], and the latter includes $\eta$, an estimate of the parenchyma pore size [35].

Parameter sweeps were conducted to explore their effect on fluid motion in PVS and parenchyma. Parameters such as pulse amplitude, PVS inner and outer radius, and PVS and parenchyma hydraulic conductivity were varied for both the one vessel and two vessel models. In addition, the pulsatility ratio and pulse timing between arterial and venous pulses were varied in the two vessel model. Pulse timing was varied by adding a phase shift, $\theta$, to the venous fluid production function.

$$q \approx 2\pi^2 lfbR_i \sin(2\pi ft - \theta) \qquad (14)$$

When a particular parameter(s) was varied the others remained at baseline values (Table 1) except in the PVS radii sweep where the pulse amplitude was reduced to 16.2 nm to account for PVS gap thicknesses as small as 1 µm without varying the PVS free-fluid hydraulic resistance by more than 5%

The authors use the term "oscillatory fluid motion", "net fluid motion", and "net flow" to refer to movement of fluid and reserve "solute transport", "diffusion", "dispersion", and "convection" for the transport of solutes in the fluid medium. Oscillatory fluid motion is fluid motion that does not displace the mean position of the fluid over time unlike net fluid motion and net flow. Diffusion is the solute transport due to random molecular motion.

Dispersion in this context is enhanced diffusion due to oscillatory fluid motion, and convection is solute transport along with a fluid undergoing net flow.

## Results

### One vessel model

Cyclic variation in arteriole diameter in the one vessel model produced oscillatory fluid motion in both the PVS and parenchyma, but no net fluid motion (net flow) in any direction. Peak fluid velocity and pressure in the PVS were about 30 μm/s and 60 mPa, respectively (Fig. 2 a, b). Peak fluid velocity in the parenchyma close to the PVS was below 6 nm/s, and at a distance 50 μm from the PVS outer boundary decreased to less than 3 nm/s (Fig. 2 c). Peclet numbers for hypothetical solutes with diffusivities spanning $10–10^3$ μm$^2$/s were mostly below $10^{-1}$ in the parenchyma indicating transport of physiological solutes there was diffusion dominated (Fig. 2e). In contrast, PVS Peclet numbers varied between $10^3$ and $10^1$ for the same span of diffusivities, suggesting physiological solute transport there had a convective component (Fig. 2d).

### Two vessel model

Cyclic diameter variation in the arteriole and vein also produced oscillatory fluid motion in both the PVS and parenchyma, but no net fluid motion. For the baseline case, peak fluid velocity in the arterial PVS was approximately 15 μm/s, about half the peak velocity in the one vessel model, and peak pressure was 60 mPa which was similar to the one vessel model value (Fig. 3 a, b). Peak fluid velocity within the parenchyma was determined between 50 and 150 μm from the arterial PVS outer boundary, and it was found to be below 3 nm/s in both perpendicular and parallel directions to the vessels (Fig. 3c). Peak fluid velocity increased with proximity to the vessel which was in agreement with the one vessel model results (compare R12 and R13 in Fig. 3c). As in the one vessel model, Peclet numbers for hypothetical solutes with diffusivities spanning $10–10^3$ μm$^2$/s were above 1 in the PVS (Fig. 3d) and below $10^{-1}$ in the parenchyma (Fig. 3e).

### Parameter sweeps

In the one vessel model, peak fluid velocity in parenchyma increased linearly with pulse amplitude and decayed with distance from the PVS outer boundary

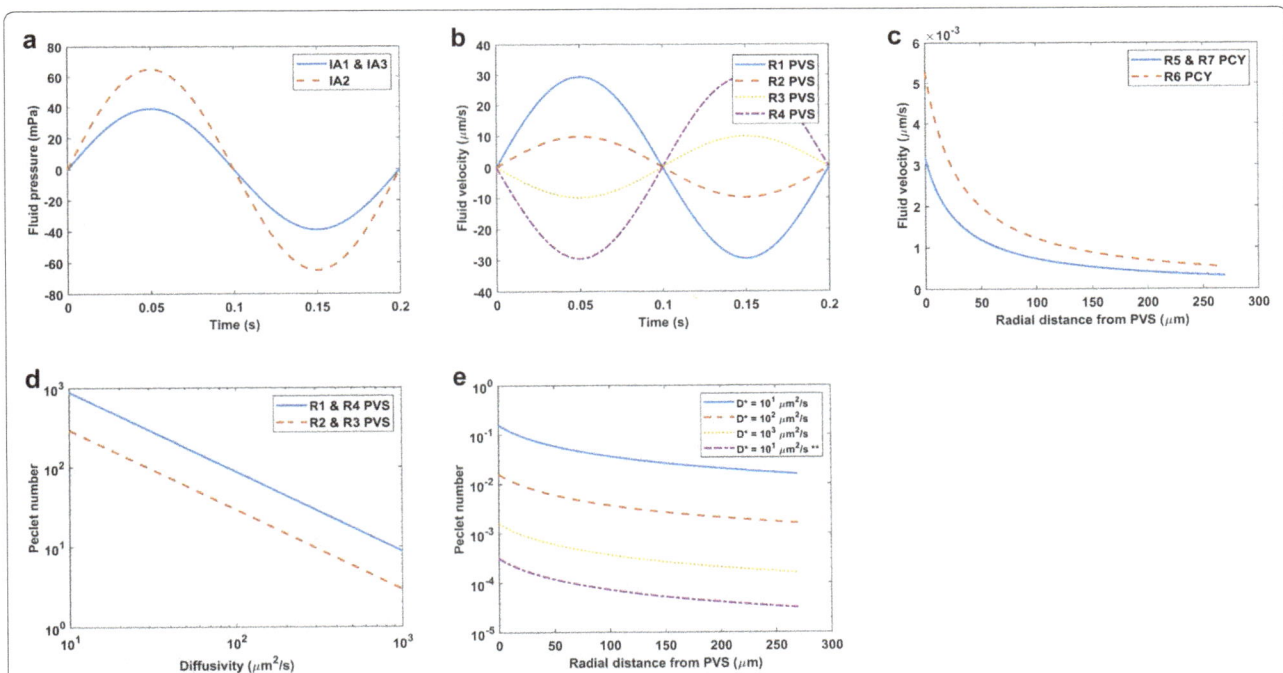

**Fig. 2** One vessel model baseline results. **a** Fluid pressure produced by volumetric fluid sources IA1, IA2, and IA3 over the course of one period. See Fig. 1 for source labels. **b** PVS fluid velocity over the course of one period for each PVS resistor. See Fig. 1 for resistor labels. **c** Parenchyma peak fluid velocity with distance from the PVS outer radius. **d** PVS Peclet numbers for a range of physiologically relevant diffusivities. **e** Parenchyma Peclet numbers with radial distance from the PVS outer radius for a range of physiologically relevant diffusivities. Peclet numbers were computed with the distance between vessels as the characteristic length (Eq. 12) for all diffusivities except that marked (**) for which pore size was the characteristic length (Eq. 13)

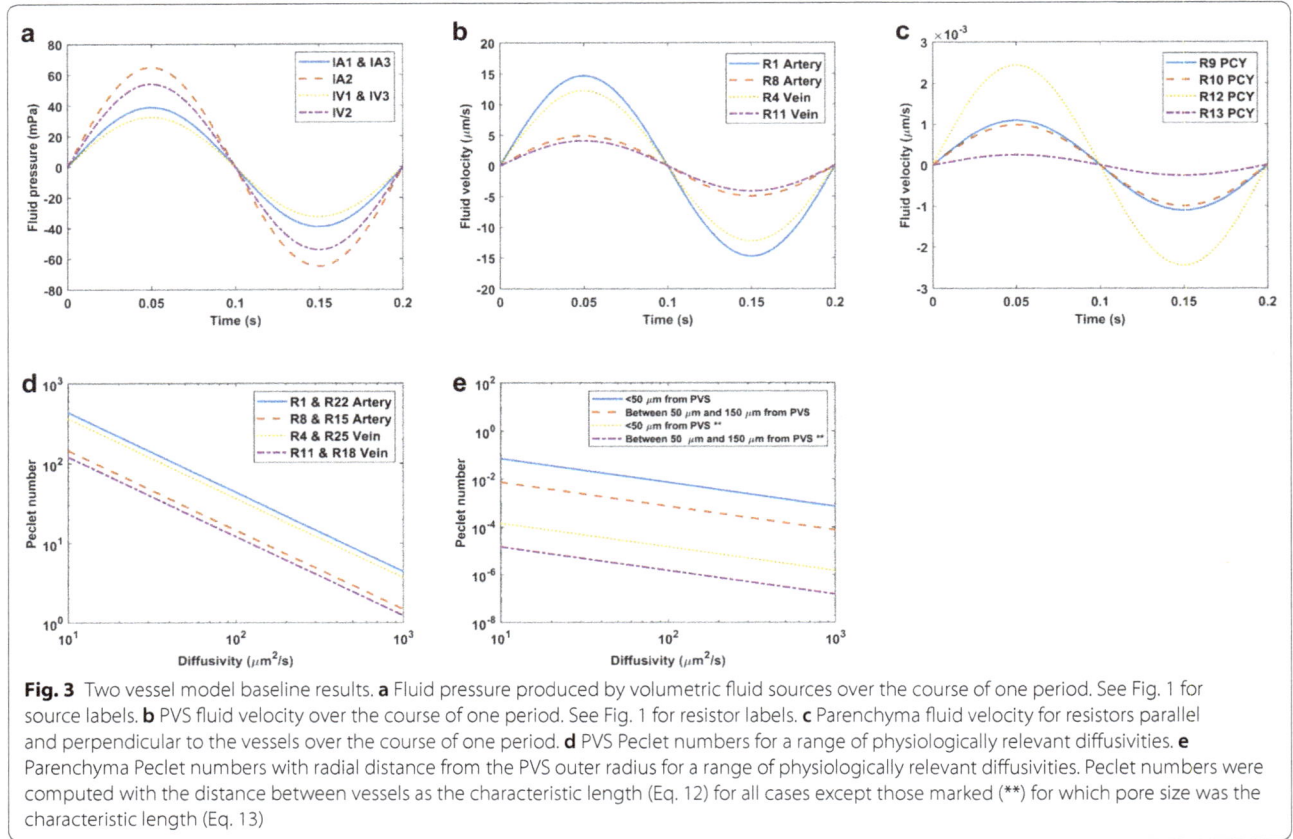

**Fig. 3** Two vessel model baseline results. **a** Fluid pressure produced by volumetric fluid sources over the course of one period. See Fig. 1 for source labels. **b** PVS fluid velocity over the course of one period. See Fig. 1 for resistor labels. **c** Parenchyma fluid velocity for resistors parallel and perpendicular to the vessels over the course of one period. **d** PVS Peclet numbers for a range of physiologically relevant diffusivities. **e** Parenchyma Peclet numbers with radial distance from the PVS outer radius for a range of physiologically relevant diffusivities. Peclet numbers were computed with the distance between vessels as the characteristic length (Eq. 12) for all cases except those marked (**) for which pore size was the characteristic length (Eq. 13)

(Fig. 4a). This velocity never exceeded 3 nm/s for the range of pulse amplitudes examined. Peak fluid velocity in the PVS also increased linearly with pulse amplitude and was greater near the ends of the PVS segment (Fig. 5a). For a given PVS outer radius, increasing the inner radius (without varying the pulse amplitude), increased peak fluid velocity in the PVS and parenchyma by several orders of magnitude (Fig. 4b, 5b). As the PVS became narrower, PVS resistance to flow increased, thus promoting flow into the parenchyma while restricting flow in the PVS. Peak fluid velocity in PVS and parenchyma varied non-linearly with changes in PVS inner and outer radii. Modeling the PVS as porous media revealed that as PVS hydraulic conductivity became unnaturally low the peak fluid velocity in parenchyma remained of order 1 µm/s. Alternatively, as PVS hydraulic conductivity approached that corresponding to a free fluid cavity ($\sim 10^{10}$ µm$^3$ s/kg), peak fluid velocity in the parenchyma dropped three orders of magnitude and fluid velocity in the PVS remained of order 10 µm/s (Fig. 4c) for R2 in the one vessel model. A similar pattern was also evident when parenchyma hydraulic conductivity was varied and the PVS was considered a free fluid cavity (Fig. 4d).

The two vessel model demonstrated a linear increase in parenchyma peak fluid velocity as pulse amplitude increased as in the one vessel model, but also showed that increasing the pulse amplitude difference between the arteriole and vein by decreasing venous pulsatility increased the peak fluid velocity in parenchyma perpendicular to the vessels (Fig. 4e). This decrease in venous pulsatility also decreased venous PVS peak fluid velocity but did not affect arterial PVS peak fluid velocity (Fig. 5c). Delaying the cyclic diameter variation of the vein with respect to the arteriole produced changes in parenchyma fluid velocity parallel and perpendicular to the vessels, but both velocities remained of order $10^{-3}$ µm/s at a distance of 50 µm from the arterial PVS outer boundary (Fig. 4f). Fluid velocity was measured a fourth period into the arterial fluid production waveform (Eq. 9). Arterial PVS fluid velocity was unaffected by this delay, but venous fluid velocity varied such that for some phase shifts arterial and venous PVS velocities were in opposite directions (Fig. 5d). The two vessel model followed similar trends as the one vessel model for variation in PVS radii and hydraulic conductivities (not shown).

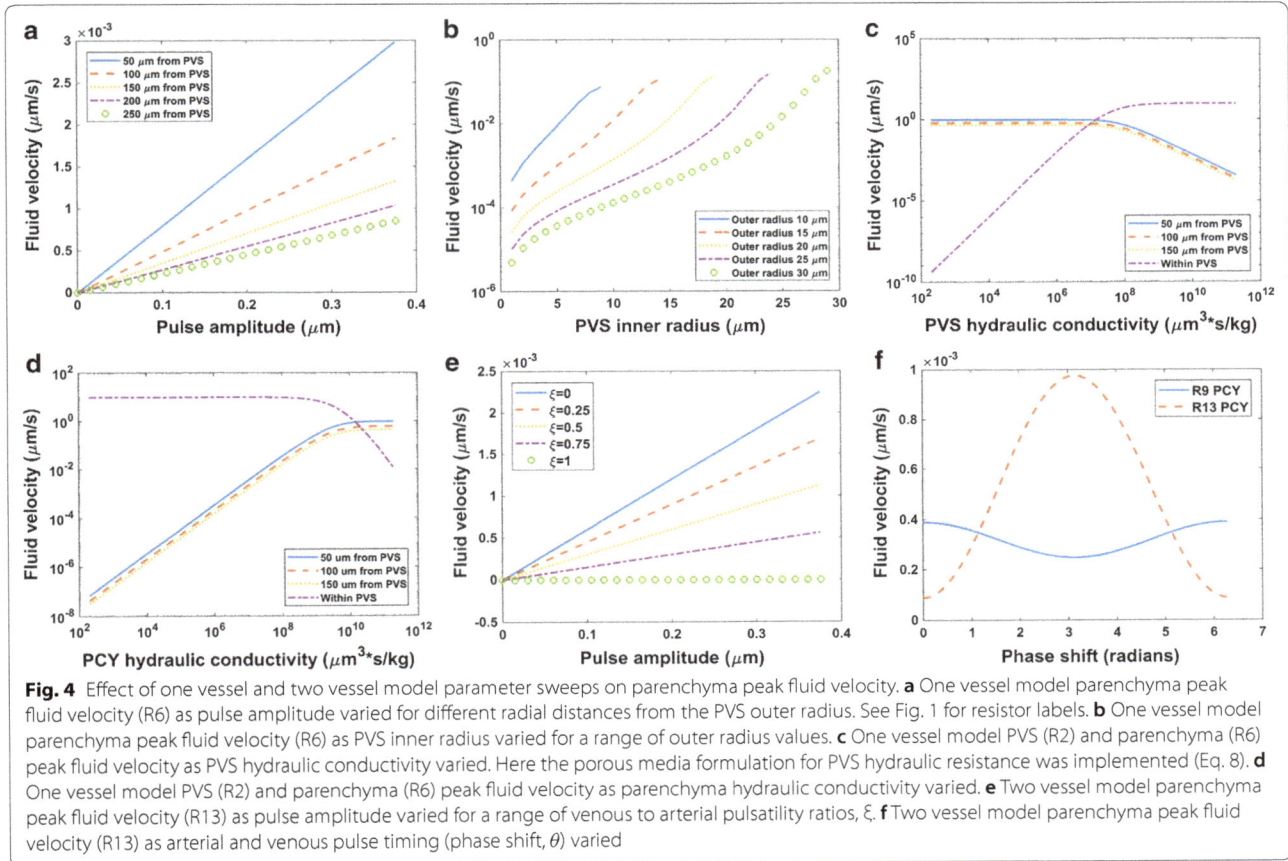

**Fig. 4** Effect of one vessel and two vessel model parameter sweeps on parenchyma peak fluid velocity. **a** One vessel model parenchyma peak fluid velocity (R6) as pulse amplitude varied for different radial distances from the PVS outer radius. See Fig. 1 for resistor labels. **b** One vessel model parenchyma peak fluid velocity (R6) as PVS inner radius varied for a range of outer radius values. **c** One vessel model PVS (R2) and parenchyma (R6) peak fluid velocity as PVS hydraulic conductivity varied. Here the porous media formulation for PVS hydraulic resistance was implemented (Eq. 8). **d** One vessel model PVS (R2) and parenchyma (R6) peak fluid velocity as parenchyma hydraulic conductivity varied. **e** Two vessel model parenchyma peak fluid velocity (R13) as pulse amplitude varied for a range of venous to arterial pulsatility ratios, $\xi$. **f** Two vessel model parenchyma peak fluid velocity (R13) as arterial and venous pulse timing (phase shift, $\theta$) varied

## Discussion

Evidence has shown that transport of dissolved compounds in PVS cannot be explained by diffusion alone [3]. Consequently, convective solute transport by net flow through the PVS driven by vascular pulsatility has been forwarded as a rationale for rapid transport rates. This viewpoint is supported by evidence of reduced PVS uptake and clearance of compounds injected into CSF and parenchyma when vascular pulsatility is dampened [2, 13].

In the one vessel and two vessel models developed here, vascular pulsatility produced oscillating fluid motion in the PVS but did not produce net flow which is needed for convection to occur. As a result, it is more difficult to explain net solute uptake or clearance by convection. During vessel expansion, fluid moved out of the PVS segment through both ends. During vessel retraction, the flow direction was reversed such that no net flow was observed. This prediction aligns with previous observations of oscillatory tracer movement within PVS and computational predictions [5, 17]. Though no net flow was observed, the PVS Peclet numbers ranged between 1 and $10^3$ in the PVS (Fig. 2d; Fig. 3d) such that the fluid

motion could promote solute transport by dispersion, as has been discussed previously [12, 17, 36]. Spatial variation in fluid velocity within the PVS may create temporary concentration gradients that enhance axial diffusion without net fluid flow. Dispersion could help explain discrepancies in transport direction through PVS seen in previous tracer uptake studies (influx into versus efflux from parenchyma) and the preference of solutes for arterial rather than venous PVS because of greater dispersion in the former [36].

The degree to which dispersion enhances axial diffusion for oscillating flow in a fluid filled annulus is proportional to the square of the volume displaced in each oscillation, also known as the tidal or stroke volume [37]. The tidal volume was greater in the arterial PVS than in venous PVS for the baseline case (Fig. 3b) and this difference grew with decreasing venous pulsatility (Fig. 5c). An increase in effective diffusion coefficient by up to a factor of two was previously predicted for solutes with diffusivities of 2 $\mu m^2/s$ for oscillating flow in a 250 $\mu m$ PVS segment [17]. Given the average fluid velocity computed from their maximum flow rate (1590 $\mu m/s$) and cross-sectional area was less than the peak outlet velocity for

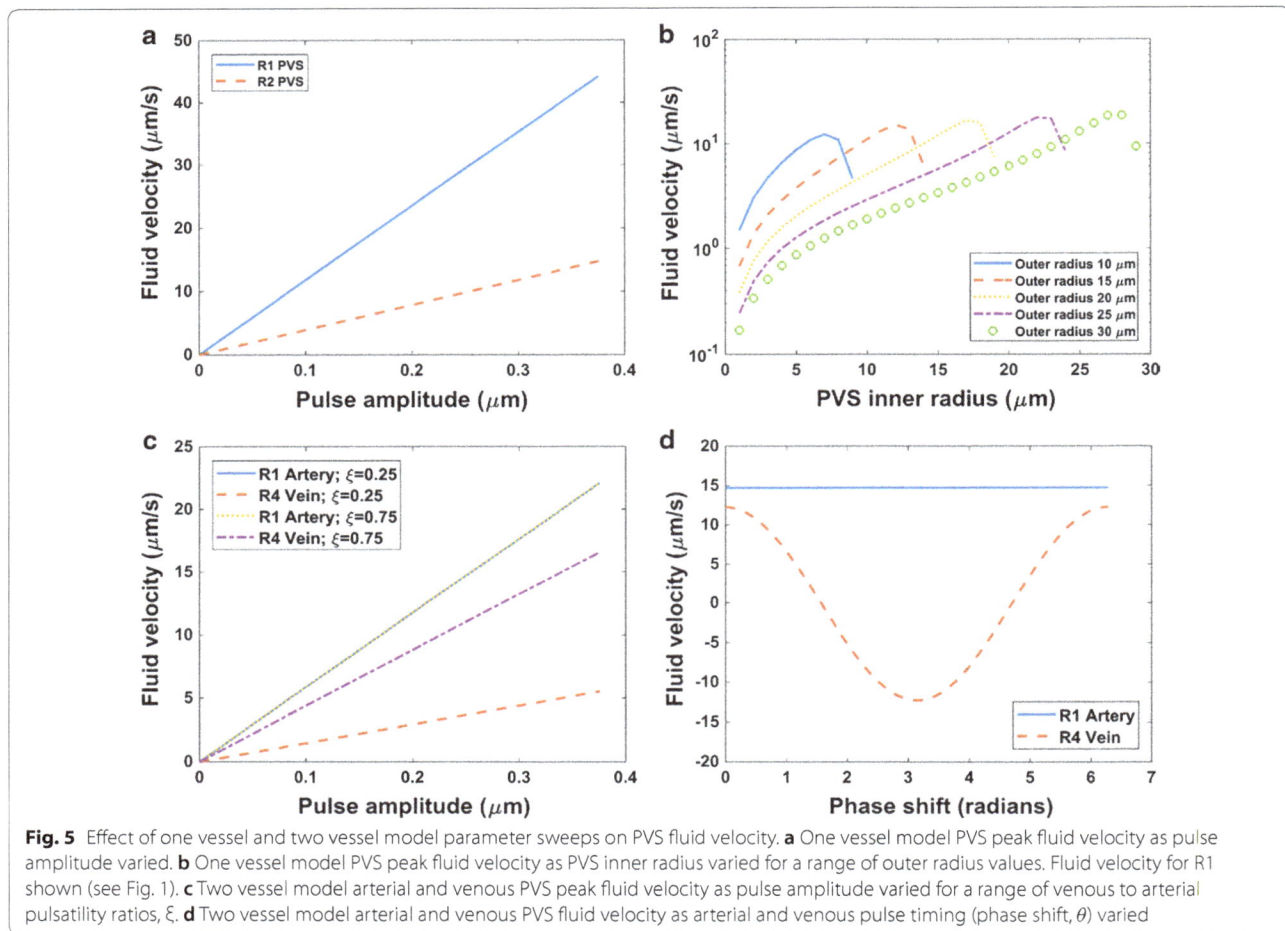

**Fig. 5** Effect of one vessel and two vessel model parameter sweeps on PVS fluid velocity. **a** One vessel model PVS peak fluid velocity as pulse amplitude varied. **b** One vessel model PVS peak fluid velocity as PVS inner radius varied for a range of outer radius values. Fluid velocity for R1 shown (see Fig. 1). **c** Two vessel model arterial and venous PVS peak fluid velocity as pulse amplitude varied for a range of venous to arterial pulsatility ratios, ξ. **d** Two vessel model arterial and venous PVS fluid velocity as arterial and venous pulse timing (phase shift, θ) varied

arterial PVS reported here (30 μm/s) and that these predictions are likely underestimations that do not account for fluid volume displaced by vessel expansion downstream from the modeled segment, the dispersive effect could be greater still. PVS tapering likely influences PVS fluid motion and solute dispersion as well. As inner radius increased for a given outer radius, the volume displaced by the same pulse amplitude increased, and as outer radius decreased for a given inner radius, the PVS cross sectional area decreased both of which lead to an increase in fluid velocity except when the PVS gap thickness was small (Fig. 5b). Additional analysis of PVS branching networks is needed to determine the effect of downstream pulsatility and PVS tapering on flow velocity and dispersion within the PVS, especially when modeled as a porous media.

Both the one vessel and two vessel models predicted oscillatory fluid motion in the parenchyma but the peak fluid velocity was so small ($\leq 6$ nm/s) that the main solute transport mode was diffusion (Pe $< 10^{-1}$) as in many other experiments and models [8, 9, 17–19]. Parenchyma fluid

velocity of up to 16 nm/s and Peclet number of order $10^{-1}$ for a pressure difference of 1 mmHg/mm between arterial and venous PVS was recently predicted in a porous media computational model [19]. This fluid velocity is likely higher than that reported here because the pressure drop for the present baseline case is of order $10^{-3}$ mmHg/mm (Fig. 3a). Fluid velocity in the parenchyma increased with pulse amplitude (Fig. 4a), increasing pulse amplitude difference between the arteriole and vein (Fig. 4e), increasing PVS inner radius for a given outer radius, and decreasing PVS outer radius for a given inner radius (Fig. 4b) because of corresponding changes in volume displacement and PVS hydraulic conductivity. However, the parenchyma fluid velocity remained less than order $10^{-1}$ μm/s even for narrow PVS gap thicknesses. Variation in PVS and parenchyma hydraulic conductivity when PVS was considered a porous media indicated that even when PVS hydraulic conductivity was made to be unnaturally low, fluid velocity in the parenchyma was at most order 1 μm/s and decreased rapidly at high PVS hydraulic conductivity ranges (Fig. 4c). Computing

Peclet number with pore size taken as the characteristic length as is often done in porous media [35] instead of the distance between the arteriole and vein suggests that even in these limiting cases, transport in parenchyma is expected to be diffusion dominated (Fig. 2e for baseline case). Parenchyma fluid velocity increased with increasing hydraulic conductivity as may be found along white matter tracts (Fig. 4d). Delaying the venous pulse relative to the arterial pulse did not produce changes in parenchyma fluid velocity large enough to affect this conclusion (Fig. 4f).

While the results show no net flow over time in the PVS (Fig. 2b; Fig. 3b), they do not rule out net flow produced by other phenomena not explicitly modeled such as time-varying PVS hydraulic conductivity [16, 38] and transient pressure differences between CSF and PVS spaces [38]. For example, a pressure gradient driving fluid into the PVS could be established when PVS hydraulic conductivity is high and a reversed gradient could be present when conductivity is low thus producing a net flow through PVS. This relies on timing differences between vascular and CSF pressure pulses [38]. Other drivers of net flow may include fluid exudation through the blood brain barrier at the capillary level [3, 12] and global pressure gradients responsible for CSF circulation. Capillary fluid production has been included as a global fluid source in previous convection enhanced drug delivery models [39, 40]. Net fluid movement could be established in an unverified, continuous arterial PVS to peri-capillary space to venous PVS path [2, 9], or an arterial PVS to parenchyma to venous PVS path [4]. The latter does not necessarily imply convective solute transport through parenchyma as proposed in glymphatic theory [4] because fluid velocity could be very low there (as expected) while maintaining net flow from arterial to venous PVS. However the magnitude, direction, and mechanical drivers of such net flows within PVS remain unclear. It is therefore important to quantify the degree to which dispersion via oscillatory flow due to vascular expansion can explain experimental solute transport in PVS, or if net flow caused by other factors must be present. It is even possible to imagine solute transport occurring down a concentration gradient opposite to the direction of net flow in the PVS if net flow is small relative to oscillatory flow. A distinguishing feature of solute transport by dispersion versus convection due to net flow is that the rate of the former varies with solute diffusivity [37] whereas the latter is independent of diffusivity. However, other complications to consider are tracer size-exclusion and the possibility of opposing flow directions within different regions of the PVS [7].

While the one and two vessel hydraulic resistance networks developed here are a coarse discretization of the flow domain they can nonetheless capture the effects of vessel diameter variation and tissue property changes on fluid motion within the PVS and parenchyma simultaneously. Because the parenchyma was modeled as rigid porous media, these models did not capture parenchyma deformation expected to accompany vessel volume change in vivo which might result in unsteady variation in PVS hydraulic conductivity. Non-linear, viscoelastic tissue properties might play a role in producing net fluid motion as hydraulic conductivity could vary with unsteady deformation rates during the cardiac cycle. CFD models that account for interaction between fluid–solid interfaces and viscoelastic tissue properties would provide further insight into fluid motion and solute transport.

## Conclusions

Two hydraulic network models were developed to predict the fluid motion produced by blood vessel pulsations in PVS and parenchyma. Periodic changes in vessel volume resulted in oscillatory fluid motion in PVS and parenchyma but no net flow over time. Peclet numbers indicated solute transport is diffusion dominated in parenchyma but might be enhanced by dispersion in PVS. Peak fluid velocity in the PVS tended to increase with increasing pulse amplitude and vessel size. While these results to do not rule out possible net flow in the PVS due to unsteady PVS hydraulic resistance and non-linear tissue properties, they do encourage further investigation into dispersion as an alternative mechanism for rapid solute transport in PVS.

**Abbreviations**
PVS: perivascular space(s); SAS: subarachnoid space(s); ISF: interstitial fluid; CSF: cerebrospinal fluid; CFD: computational fluid dynamics; PCY: parenchyma; R#: resistance number; IA#: arterial source number; IV#: venous source number; Pe: Peclet number.

**Author's contributions**
JR contributed to model design, implemented the model, performed simulations, and was a major contributor to writing the manuscript. MS established the project's focus, contributed to model design, data analysis, and manuscript revision. Both authors read and approved the final manuscript.

**Acknowledgements**
We thank Charles Nicholson (NYU School of Medicine) for helpful discussions that led to the development of this model. We also thank Magdoom Kulam for comments and editorial assistance.

**Competing interests**
The authors declare that they have no competing interests.

**Funding**

The Chiari & Syringomyelia Foundation provided seed funding for this project.

**References**

1.  Cserr HF, Cooper DN, Milhorat TH. Flow of cerebral interstitial fluid as indicated by removal of extracellular markers from rat caudate-nucleus. Exp Eye Res. 1977;25:461–73.

2.  Rennels ML, Gregory TF, Blaumanis OR, Fujimoto K, Grady PA. Evidence for a paravascular fluid circulation in the mammalian central nervous-system, provided by the rapid distribution of tracer protein throughout the brain from the subarachnoid space. Brain Res. 1985;326:47–63.

3.  Abbott NJ, Pizzo ME, Preston JE, Janigro D, Thorne RG. The role of brain barriers in fluid movement in the cns: is there a 'glymphatic' system? Acta Neuropathol. 2018;135:387–407.

4.  Iliff JJ, Wang MH, Liao YH, Plogg BA, Peng WG, Gundersen GA, Benveniste H, Vates GE, Deane R, Goldman SA, Nagelhus EA, Nedergaard M. A paravascular pathway facilitates csf flow through the brain parenchyma and the clearance of interstitial solutes, including amyloid beta. Sci Transl Med. 2012;4:11.

5.  Ichimura T, Fraser PA, Cserr HF. Distribution of extracellular tracers in perivascular spaces of the rat-brain. Brain Res. 1991;545:103–13.

6.  Carare RO, Bernardes-Silva M, Newman TA, Page AM, Nicoll JAR, Perry VH, Weller RO. Solutes, but not cells, drain from the brain parenchyma along basement membranes of capillaries and arteries: significance for cerebral amyloid angiopathy and neuroimmunology. Neuropathol Appl Neurobiol. 2008;34:131–44.

7.  Morris AWJ, Sharp MM, Albargothy NJ, Fernandes R, Hawkes CA, Verma A, Weller RO, Carare RO. Vascular basement membranes as pathways for the passage of fluid into and out of the brain. Acta Neuropathol. 2016;131:725–36.

8.  Smith AJ, Yao XM, Dix JA, Jin BJ, Verkman AS. Test of the 'glymphatic' hypothesis demonstrates diffusive and aquaporin-4-independent solute transport in rodent brain parenchyma. eLife. 2017;6:16.

9.  Pizzo ME, Wolak DJ, Kumar NN, Brunette E, Brunnquell CL, Hannocks MJ, Abbott NJ, Meyerand ME, Sorokin L, Stanimirovic DB, Thorne RG. Intrathecal antibody distribution in the rat brain: surface diffusion, perivascular transport and osmotic enhancement of delivery. J Physiol. 2018;596:445–75.

10. Ringstad G, Vatnehol SAS, Eide PK. Glymphatic mri in idiopathic normal pressure hydrocephalus. Brain. 2017;140:2691–705.

11. Hall JE, Guyton AC. Guyton and hall textbook of medical physiology. 12th ed. Philadelphia: Saunders/Elsevier; 2011.

12. Bakker E, Bacskai BJ, Arbel-Ornath M, Aldea R, Bedussi B, Morris AWJ, Weller RO, Carare RO. Lymphatic clearance of the brain: perivascular, paravascular and significance for neurodegenerative diseases. Cell Mol Neurobiol. 2016;36:181–94.

13. Iliff JJ, Wang MH, Zeppenfeld DM, Venkataraman A, Plog BA, Liao YH, Deane R, Nedergaard M. Cerebral arterial pulsation drives paravascular csf-interstitial fluid exchange in the murine brain. J Neurosci. 2013;33:18190–9.

14. Hadaczek P, Yamashita Y, Mirek H, Tamas L, Bohn MC, Noble C, Park JW, Bankiewicz K. The, "perivascular pump" driven by arterial pulsation is a powerful mechanism for the distribution of therapeutic molecules within the brain. Mol Ther. 2006;14:69–78.

15. Coloma M, Schaffer JD, Carare RO, Chiarot PR, Huang P. Pulsations with reflected boundary waves: a hydrodynamic reverse transport mechanism for perivascular drainage in the brain. J Math Biol. 2016;73:469–90.

16. Sharp MK, Diem AK, Weller RO, Carare RO. Peristalsis with oscillating flow resistance: a mechanism for periarterial clearance of amyloid beta from the brain. Ann Biomed Eng. 2016;44:1553–65.

17. Asgari M, de Zelicourt D, Kurtcuoglu V. Glymphatic solute transport does not require bulk flow. Sci Rep. 2016;6:11.

18. Jin BJ, Smith AJ, Verkman AS. Spatial model of convective solute transport in brain extracellular space does not support a "glymphatic" mechanism. J Gen Physiol. 2016;148:489–501.

19. Holter KE, Kehlet B, Devor A, Sejnowski TJ, Dale AM, Omholt SW, Ottersen OP, Nagelhus EA, Mardal KA, Pettersen KH. Interstitial solute transport in 3d reconstructed neuropil occurs by diffusion rather than bulk flow. Proc Natl Acad Sci USA. 2017;114:9894–9.

20. Asgari M, de Zelicourt D, Kurtcuoglu V. How astrocyte networks may contribute to cerebral metabolite clearance. Sci Rep. 2015;5:13.

21. Yoshihara K, Takuwa H, Kanno I, Okawa S, Yamada Y, Masamoto K. 3d analysis of intracortical microvasculature during chronic hypoxia in mouse brains. Adv Exp Med Biol. 2013;765:357–63.

22. Weller RO, Sharp MM, Christodoulides M, Carare RO, Mollgard K. The meninges as barriers and facilitators for the movement of fluid, cells and pathogens related to the rodent and human cns. Acta Neuropathol. 2018;135:363–85.

23. Bird RB, Stewart WE, Lightfoot EN. Transport phenomena. 2nd ed. New York: Wiley; 2007.

24. Gladdish S, Manawadu D, Banya W, Cameron J, Bulpitt CJ, Rajkumar C. Repeatability of non-invasive measurement of intracerebral pulse wave velocity using transcranial doppler. Clin Sci. 2005;108:433–9.

25. Hoeks APG, Brands PJ, Willigers JM, Reneman RS. Non-invasive measurement of mechanical properties of arteries in health and disease. Proc Inst Mech Eng. 1999;213:195–202.

26. Lightfoot EN. Transport phenomena and living systems; biomedical aspects of momentum and mass transport. New York: Wiley; 1973.

27. Neeves KB, Lo CT, Foley CP, Saltzman WM, Olbricht WL. Fabrication and characterization of microfluidic probes for convection enhanced drug delivery. J Control Release. 2006;111:252–62.

28. Bloomfield IG, Johnston IH, Bilston LE. Effects of proteins, blood cells and glucose on the viscosity of cerebrospinal fluid. Pediatr Neurosurg. 1998;28:246–51.

29. Wang P, Olbricht WL. Fluid mechanics in the perivascular space. J Theor Biol. 2011;274:52–7.

30. Kundu PK, Cohen IM, Dowling DR, Tryggvason GT. Fluid mechanics. 6th ed. Boston: Elsevier/AP; 2016.

31. Sykova E, Nicholson C. Diffusion in brain extracellular space. Physiol Rev. 2008;88:1277–340.

32. Thorne RG, Nicholson C. In vivo diffusion analysis with quantum dots and dextrans predicts the width of brain extracellular space. Proc Natl Acad Sci USA. 2006;103:5567–72.

33. Berger SA, Goldsmith W, Lewis ER. Introduction to bioengineering. New York: Oxford University Press; 2000.

34. Truskey GA, Yuan F, Katz DF. Transport phenomena in biological systems. 2nd ed. Upper Saddle River: Pearson Prentice Hall; 2009.

35. Bear J. Dynamics of fluids in porous media. New York: Dover Publications; 1972.

36. Hladky SB, Barrand MA. Mechanisms of fluid movement into, through and out of the brain: evaluation of the evidence. Fluids Barriers CNS. 2014;11:26.

37. Tsangaris S, Athanassiadis N. Diffusion in oscillatory flow in an annular pipe. Z Angew Math Mech. 1985;65:T252–4.

38. Bilston LE, Stoodley MA, Fletcher DF. The influence of the relative timing of arterial and subarachnoid space pulse waves on spinal perivascular cerebrospinal fluid flow as a possible factor in syrinx development laboratory investigation. J Neurosurg. 2010;112:808–13.

39. Kim JH, Astary GW, Kantorovich S, Mareci TH, Carney PR, Sarntinoranont M. Voxelized computational model for convection-enhanced delivery in the rat ventral hippocampus: comparison with in vivo mr experimental studies. Ann Biomed Eng. 2012;40:2043–58.

40. Dai W, Astary GW, Kasinadhuni AK, Carney PR, Mareci TH, Sarntinoranont M. Voxelized model of brain infusion that accounts for small feature fissures: comparison with magnetic resonance tracer studies. J Biomech Eng. 2016;138:13.

# 20

# Accurate, strong, and stable reporting of choroid plexus epithelial cells in transgenic mice using a human transthyretin BAC

Brett A. Johnson[1,2], Margaret Coutts[1,2], Hillary M. Vo[1,2], Xinya Hao[1,2], Nida Fatima[1,2], Maria J. Rivera[4], Robert J. Sims[4], Michael J. Neel[1,2], Young-Jin Kang[1,2] and Edwin S. Monuki[1,2,3*]

## Abstract

**Background:** Choroid plexus epithelial cells express high levels of transthyretin, produce cerebrospinal fluid and many of its proteins, and make up the blood-cerebrospinal fluid barrier. Choroid plexus epithelial cells are vital to brain health and may be involved in neurological diseases. Transgenic mice containing fluorescent and luminescent reporters of these cells would facilitate their study in health and disease, but prior transgenic reporters lost expression over the early postnatal period.

**Methods:** Human bacterial artificial chromosomes in which the transthyretin coding sequence was replaced with DNA for tdTomato or luciferase 2 were used in pronuclear injections to produce transgenic mice. These mice were characterized by visualizing red fluorescence, immunostaining, real-time reverse transcription polymerase chain reaction, and luciferase enzyme assay.

**Results:** Reporters were faithfully expressed in cells that express transthyretin constitutively, including choroid plexus epithelial cells, retinal pigment epithelium, pancreatic islets, and liver. Expression of tdTomato in choroid plexus began at the appropriate embryonic age, being detectable by E11.5. Relative levels of tdTomato transcript in the liver and choroid plexus paralleled relative levels of transcripts for transthyretin. Expression remained robust over the first postnatal year, although choroid plexus transcripts of tdTomato declined slightly with age whereas transthyretin remained constant. TdTomato expression patterns were consistent across three founder lines, displayed no sex differences, and were stable across several generations. Two of the tdTomato lines were bred to homozygosity, and homozygous mice are healthy and fertile. The usefulness of tdTomato reporters in visualizing and analyzing live Transwell cultures was demonstrated. Luciferase activity was very high in homogenates of choroid plexus and continued to be expressed through adulthood. Luciferase also was detectable in eye and pancreas.

**Conclusions:** Transgenic mice bearing fluorescent and luminescent reporters of transthyretin should prove useful for tracking transplanted choroid plexus epithelial cells, for purifying the cells, and for reporting their derivation from stem cells. They also should prove useful for studying transthyretin synthesis by other cell types, as transthyretin has been implicated in many functions and conditions, including clearance of β-amyloid peptides associated with Alzheimer's disease, heat shock in neurons, processing of neuropeptides, nerve regeneration, astrocyte metabolism, and transthyretin amyloidosis.

**Keywords:** Transthyretin, Choroid plexus, Cerebrospinal fluid, Retinal pigment epithelium, Hepatocytes, Islets

*Correspondence: emonuki@uci.edu
[1] Department of Pathology and Laboratory Medicine, UC Irvine, Irvine, USA
Full list of author information is available at the end of the article

## Background

Choroid plexus epithelial cells (CPECS) represent an under-studied cell type that contributes vitally to the health of the brain. CPECs, which reside in all four brain ventricles, produce cerebrospinal fluid (CSF), pumping water from the blood into the ventricles and manufacturing and secreting a variety of important CSF proteins such as growth factors and the thyroxine-carrier transthyretin (TTR) [1, 2]. The CSF in turn mechanically cushions the brain and provides a circulatory system communicating with brain interstitial fluid, both delivering beneficial substances and removing metabolic waste [2, 3]. Tight junctions between the CPECs are responsible for establishing the blood-CSF barrier [4], and yet CPECs also possess various transport systems that actively insure the delivery of certain substances from the blood into the CPECs as well as into the CSF [5, 6].

Choroid plexus epithelial cells decline in number and health with age and in association with several neurological diseases [1, 7, 8]. Indeed, deterioration of CPECs has been hypothesized to contribute to the progression of these diseases, with a particular emphasis on the potential role of TTR in the removal of β-amyloid in Alzheimer's disease [7–9]. CPECs may also be critically involved in immune cell activation and entry into the CNS in the development of multiple sclerosis and other inflammatory conditions [10, 11]. On the other hand, the discovery both that CPECs can be derived from human stem cells and that they can become integrated into the recipient choroid plexus (ChP) after transplantation suggests a potential use of engineered CPECs in cell-based therapies for neurological disorders [12].

To better explore the basic biology of CPECs, track them in disease models, monitor their differentiation from stem cells, purify them, and assess their integration, survival, and health after transplantation, it would be useful to have transgenic mice in which these cells express fluorescent and/or luminescent reporters. The most abundant and selective mRNA in the CPEC transcriptome is TTR [13, 14], which is produced in a limited set of other tissues including the liver, pancreas, and retinal pigment epithelium [15], as well as in neurons as a heat shock protein under conditions of stress and disease [16]. TTR's abundance in CPECs, its tissue selectivity, and its long-term expression suggest that its gene regulatory sequences would be effective for directing the expression of CPEC reporter proteins.

To study the development of the visceral endoderm, Kwon and Hadjantonakis previously created transgenic mice using a plasmid vector in which a red fluorescent protein (mRFP1) was expressed under the direction of 3 kb upstream regulatory sequence of the mouse TTR gene [17]. Expression of RFP in these mice did occur in CPECs of embryonic and neonatal mice and were useful for monitoring initial CPEC derivation from stem cells [12] and fluorescence activated cell sorting of CPECs from young mice [14]; however, the expression in embryonic choroid plexus was found to be mosaic and to decline markedly with age [14].

In the present paper, we describe the generation of transgenic CPEC reporter mice using a human bacterial artificial chromosome (BAC). The large expanse of DNA in a BAC transgene not only holds the promise of including more extensive TTR regulatory sequences, but also should preclude the type of positional effects that plague the use of smaller transgenic constructs, such as ectopic and mosaic expression as well as extinction [18]. We characterize these mice with special attention to CPECs to establish that the reporters accurately reflect the tissue distribution of TTR, that they display an appropriate embryonic developmental profile, and that they continue to be expressed well into adulthood. We conclude that these mice will be useful tools for the investigation of not only CPECs but also other cell types expressing TTR.

## Methods

### Recombineering of a human TTR BAC

The RP11-571I2 BAC, which contains the human TTR gene and flanking 5'- and 3'-proximal genomic sequences of 126 and 41 kb, respectively, was obtained from CHORI BAC PAC Resources Center (https://bacpacresources.org/) and recombineered by the UC Davis Mouse Biology Program to replace the coding sequence of the human TTR gene (from start codon to stop codon, including introns) with either tdTomato or luciferase2 (luc2) cDNA. The clones were constructed using BAC recombineering methods adapted from Chan et al. [19], using the pSIM18 plasmid and Wang et al. [20], using the RspL counter selection method.

The TTR coding sequence in RP11-571I2 was first replaced with the RspL counter selection cassette in opposite orientation from TTR. (Previous attempts in the same orientation failed to yield stable intermediate clones.) E. coli clones in 96 well plates were PCR screened using primers spanning recombination junctions, with twelve subsequently verified by pulse field gel electrophoresis (PFGE) of SbfI digested BAC DNA. Two were then electroporated into E. coli DH10 cells and grown with kanamycin and chloramphenicol to separate the hTTR-RspKan-RC clone from unmodified BAC DNA, with all clones tested (four each for the two separation transformations) showing the expected SbfI restriction pattern by PFGE. To replace the RspL counter selection cassette with luc2 or tdTomato, the selected intermediate clone was made "recombineering-ready" by transformation with the pSIM18 plasmid, then luc2 or tdTomato cassettes were introduced and grown in chloramphenicol and streptomycin.

For luc2, PCR screening identified 14 putative clones, then pooled BAC DNA from these clones were transformed into DH10 cells to separate hTTR-luc2 and intermediate clones. Seven clones were selected based on PCR screening, and all seven were verified to be hTTR-luc2 clones by PFGE of SalI-digested DNA. The luc2 insert was also PCR amplified from all seven clones, and five were verified by sequencing for luc2 coding sequence integrity and TTR replacement. For tdTomato, BAC DNA from 6 PCR-verified clones were pooled for separation transformation into DH10 cells, with six hTTR-tdTomato clones verified by PFGE of SalI-digested BAC DNA and sequencing of tdTomato inserts. Subsequent restriction analysis of the tdTomato BAC by the UC Irvine Transgenic Mouse Facility indicated loss of an expected Sbf1 restriction site, which ultimately did not impact the generation of useful transgenic reporter lines.

## Generation of transgenic mice

Transgenic mice were produced by the UC Irvine Transgenic Mouse Facility by pronuclear injection of intact circular (tdTomato) or Sbf1-linearized (luc2) DNA. B6SJLF1/J mice were used as egg donors. Subsequent breeding used CD1 mice. Successful BAC insertion was judged by PCR of F1 genomic DNA employing primer pairs distributed throughout the BAC (Fig. 2, Table 1). Results reported here involve progeny of the original founders through four generations of CD1 breeding. Routine genotyping involved PCR of reporter coding sequences (Table 1). Both male and female mice were studied. Euthanasia involved either $CO_2$ inhalation or intraperitoneal injection of Euthasol (Virbac AH, Inc., Fort Worth, TX).

## Analysis of mRNA levels by real-time reverse transcription quantitative PCR (RT-qPCR)

Choroid plexus was rapidly collected from lateral and fourth ventricles while brains were submerged in cold PBS, frozen together on the walls of microcentrifuge tubes sitting on dry ice, then stored at −80 °C or lysed with 50–100 μL of HLY lysis buffer (Biomiga, San Diego, CA) added to tubes on dry ice followed by homogenization using plastic pestles. Additional HLY was added to a final volume of 350 μL, with further homogenization, and homogenates were stored at −80 °C. Pieces of liver (20–40 mg) were also rapidly dissected and minced immediately after collection, followed by homogenization in 200 μL of cold HLY buffer. Additional HLY buffer was added to a final volume of 500–700 μL, with

**Table 1 PCR primers used in the study**

| Category | Primer pair | Direction | Sequence (5′ to 3′) | Amplicon (bp) |
|---|---|---|---|---|
| genotyping | tdTom internal | Forward | CACCATCGTGGAACAGTACG | 142 |
| | | Reverse | GCGCATGAACTCTTTGATGA | |
| | BAC 100 kb 5′ #1 | Forward | TTAGGATTCAGGTGGCCTTG | 148 |
| | | Reverse | TGCACATCCTTGGCAATAAA | |
| | BAC 100 kb 5′ #2 | Forward | AATGAAGAGGCTGCCAAAGA | 192 |
| | | Reverse | AGTGGATCCCACGACAGTTC | |
| | BAC 60 kb 5′ | Forward | AAGCCCAAGATCAAAGCAGA | 202 |
| | | Reverse | CTCACGTGCTGAAATCCTGA | |
| | BAC 40 kb 3′ | Forward | TCAGCAGCTTCCTGCTACAC | 500 |
| | | Reverse | GCTAGACAGGTACCCAGGGA | |
| | luc2 internal | Forward | ACAGAAACAACCAGCGCCATTCTG | 590 |
| | | Reverse | TCCAACTTGCCGGTCAGTCCTTTA | |
| | JAX control | Forward | CTAGGCCACAGAATTGAAAGATCT | 324 |
| | | Reverse | GTAGGTGGAAATTCTAGCATCATCC | |
| RT-qPCR | tdTomato | Forward | ATCGTGGAACAGTACGAGCG | 133 |
| | | Reverse | TGAACTCTTTGATGACGGCCA | |
| | transthyretin | Forward | ATCGTACTGGAAGACACTTGGC | 131 |
| | | Reverse | CCGTGGTGCTGTAGGAGTAT | |
| | 18S ribosomal | Forward | CGGCTACCACATCCAAGGAA | 187 |
| | | Reverse | GCTGGAATTACCGCGGCT | |
| | cyclophilin A | Forward | GAGCTGTTTGCAGACAAAGTTC | 125 |
| | | Reverse | CCCTGGCACATGAATCCTGG | |

further homogenization, and homogenates were stored at $-80\,^\circ$C.

Total RNA was isolated from homogenates of liver or ChP using Biomiga EZgene tissue RNA kits. Yield and purity were judged by absorbance at 230, 260 and 280 nm (NanoDrop 2000c spectrophotometer, ThermoFisher, Waltham, MA). cDNA was synthesized using random hexamers, dNTPs, RNAsin (Promega, Madison, WI), and Moloney Murine Leukemia Virus reverse transcriptase (Promega). For every sample, minus-RT control incubations were performed using DEPC-treated water in place of reverse transcriptase. RT-qPCR reactions used iTaq Universal SYBR Green Supermix (Bio-Rad, Hercules, CA) on a Roche LightCycler 480II in 96-well plate format, and primer pairs for tdTomato, TTR, cyclophilin A, or 18S ribosomal RNA (see Table 1) on samples and water-only controls. Primers were validated for log-linearity of Ct values using serially-diluted ChP and liver RNA samples, >90% doubling efficiencies, homogeneous melt curves, and single amplicons of appropriate size by gel electrophoresis. Results were excluded if amplification was detected in water-only controls or if +RT and $-$RT samples displayed a Ct value difference of less than 10 cycles with the 18S primer set.

RT-qPCR results were reported as $\Delta\Delta$Ct, subtracting target Ct values (tdTomato and TTR) from the average of two reference Ct values (18S and cyclophilin A) for the same experimental sample [21], and then subtracting experimental sample values from the average value obtained across all samples of wild type mice (22 total). More positive values indicate more mRNA.

### Immunostaining and imaging

Brains or dissected tissues were fixed by submersion in 4% paraformaldehyde in phosphate-buffered saline (PBS) (4–48 h), followed by overnight cryoprotection in PBS containing 30% sucrose, both at 4 °C. Tissues then were embedded in O.C.T. compound (TissueTek, Sakura Finetek, Torrance, CA) in specimen molds, frozen on dry ice, and stored at $-80\,^\circ$C until sectioning. Tissue blocks were sectioned at 20-μm thickness in a Leica CM3050 S cryostat, and slices were collected on Superfrost plus slides.

Sections were washed thrice with PBS (5 min/wash at room temperature), followed by blocking with 5% serum in PBS containing 0.3% Triton X-100 and overnight incubation in primary antibody at 4 °C. After three additional washes, incubations with secondary antibodies (1:500) were carried out for 1 h at room temperature, followed by three additional washes and mounting with Fluoromount-G containing DAPI fluorescent counterstain (SouthernBiotech, Birmingham, AL). Antibodies were diluted in 1% serum in PBS containing 0.3% Triton X-100. Primary antibodies were rabbit anti-RFP (1:1000,

600-401-379, Rockland, Limerick, PA), goat anti-anion exchange protein 2 (AE2, 1:250, sc46710, Santa Cruz Biotechnology, Dallas, TX), rabbit anti-glucagon (1:200, 2760S, Cell Signaling Technology, Danvers, MA), sheep anti-TTR (1:500, Abcam, ab9015), and guinea pig anti-insulin (1:500, Dako A0564, Agilent Technologies, Santa Clara, CA). Secondary antibodies (1:500, Life Technologies, ThermoFisher) included Alexa 488-conjugated donkey anti-rabbit (to detect anti-glucagon antibodies), donkey anti-goat, donkey anti-sheep, and goat anti-guinea pig IgG, as well as Alexa 555-conjugated donkey anti-rabbit IgG (to detect tdTomato).

Fluorescent (RFP filters) and brightfield imaging of fresh tissues used either an AMG EVOS fl microscope or a Nikon SMZ1500 dissecting fluorescent microscope and an SD-Ri1 digital camera. Immunofluorescence on slides was evaluated using a Nikon Eclipse E400 microscope fitted with DAPI, FITC, and TRITC filters and imaged using a Nuance FX camera (Perkin Elmer). Image contrasts were adjusted automatically by the Nuance software using the "Clip/Stretch" display function. Channels were blended in Adobe Photoshop, and further adjustments to contrast were made in Photoshop to give a more balanced representation of the channels. For comparative panels in figures, image adjustments were made in parallel.

### Primary transwell cultures of CPECs

Choroid plexus was rapidly dissected from the lateral and fourth ventricles of four P2 mice and collected in 500 μL ice-cold HBSS containing 0.6% sucrose. Enzymatic dissociation of CPECs was performed with 500 μL of 1000 U/mL collagenase II (Sigma 234155) in 3 mM $CaCl_2$. The mixture was incubated at 37 °C for 40 min, with vigorous agitation every 5 min, at the end of which no large aggregates of tissue could be visualized by eye. After trituration, the suspension was then centrifuged at 805$g$ for 3 min, the supernatant was discarded, and the pellet containing cells and small cell aggregates was resuspended in 500 μL TrypLE Express (Gibco 12605028) and incubated at 37 °C for 5 min. After trituration, this suspension was centrifuged at 805$g$ for 3 min, the supernatant was discarded, the cell pellet was resuspended in 510 μL of CPEC media (DMEM/F12 (Gibco 11320033), 10% fetal bovine serum (Hyclone SH 300703), antimicrobial-antimycotic supplement ("anti-anti", Gibco 15240062), and the cell suspension was plated in 0.33 cm$^2$ Transwell chambers (Corning 3470) previously coated with poly-D-lysine and laminin and cultured for various durations, with media replacements every other day. Nutrient media was supplemented with 20 μM cytosine β-D arabinofuranoside (AraC, Sigma C6645) during days 0–4 of culture, and serum was withdrawn on day 4.

The EVOM2 apparatus equipped with the Endohm 6 attachment, specifically designed for use with 0.33 cm$^2$ transwell inserts (World Precision Instruments) was used to measure trans-epithelial electrical resistance. Values of >65 $\Omega$ cm$^2$ have been reported as indicative of monolayer confluency for primary mouse CPEC culture [22]. Fluorescence (RFP filter) and phase contrast images were obtained using an AMG EVOS fl microscope.

### Luciferase assays

Lateral and fourth ventricle ChP from each single mouse were combined and homogenized in 100 µL of passive lysis buffer (PLB, Promega), using a plastic pestle in a microcentrifuge tube. Other tissues were homogenized in 1–2 mL of PLB using a PowerGen 125 tissue homogenizer (Fisher Scientific) typically set at medium speed, twice for 15 s each. Harder tissues such as heart, kidney, and eye were minced with scissors prior to homogenization. Homogenates were frozen at −80 °C. Upon thawing, homogenates were centrifuged for 10 min at 10,000g, 4 °C, and the supernatants were taken for determination of protein concentration and luciferase activity. Protein was assayed using BioRad Bradford dye reagent and bovine serum albumin standards. Luciferase activity was measured using an E1500 assay kit (Promega). A BioTek Synergy HT microplate reader was used to measure absorbance in protein assays and luminescence in luciferase assays. Results were expressed as plate reader light units per mg of protein. The luciferase assay was

determined to be linear across six tenfold serial dilutions of a sample yielding the maximum detected activity level.

## Results

### Loss of fluorescence in postnatal Ttr::RFP mice

Although we confirmed the robust fluorescence of CPECs in embryonic and neonatal Ttr::RFP transgenic mice produced by integration of a plasmid vector [17], we found that RFP expression was mosaic in embryonic mouse ChP [14], and the number of cells expressing fluorescence declined precipitously after birth. Figure 1 shows ChP from a 3-week old Ttr::RFP mouse. Only a few sporadic, brightly labeled cells were still detectable in the lateral ventricle ChP (arrows) at this age, and the third ventricle ChP was devoid of fluorescence. Fewer than half of the CPECs in the fourth ventricle ChP were fluorescent. The loss of fluorescence indicated that the reporter was not tightly linked to TTR expression over the lifetime of the mice, making it incompatible with many of our intended uses. Thus, we were motivated to generate transgenic mice with more stable reporter expression that better matched TTR.

### Generation of human TTR BAC-tdTomato mice

To confer more faithful regulation of expression, we decided to use as a starting point bacterial artificial chromosome (BAC) RP11-571I2, which contains the human TTR gene (Fig. 2A). A human BAC was chosen over mouse to enable interpretations of expression studies that more likely extend to human TTR, a

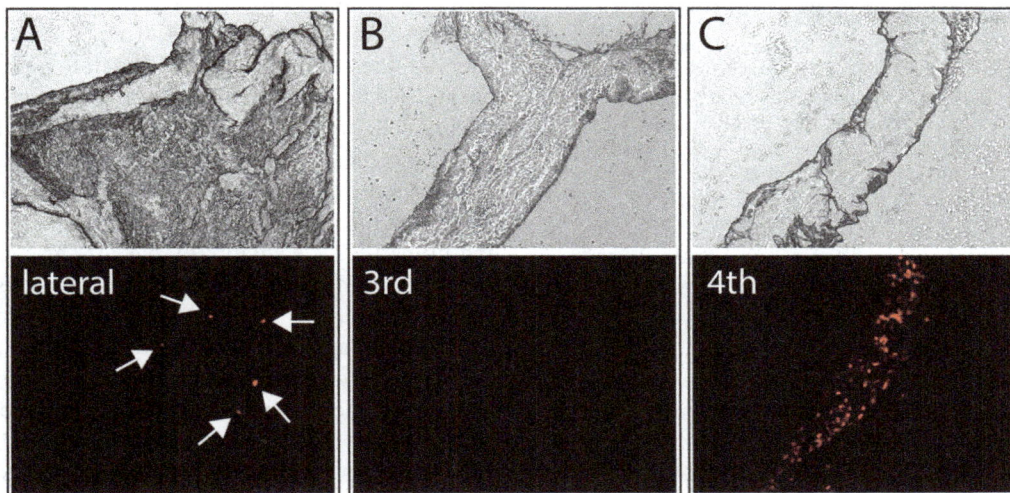

**Fig. 1** Choroid plexus fluorescence is diminished in weanling Ttr::RFP transgenic mice. Upper panels show images of transmitted light and bottom panels show corresponding images of red fluorescence taken for choroid plexus dissected from a 21-day old Ttr::RFP transgenic mouse. A few scattered fluorescent CPECs were visible in the lateral ventricle ChP (**A**, arrows), but none were found in the third ventricle ChP (**B**). A larger number of fluorescent CPECs were detected in the fourth ventricle ChP, although expression was clearly mosaic (**C**)

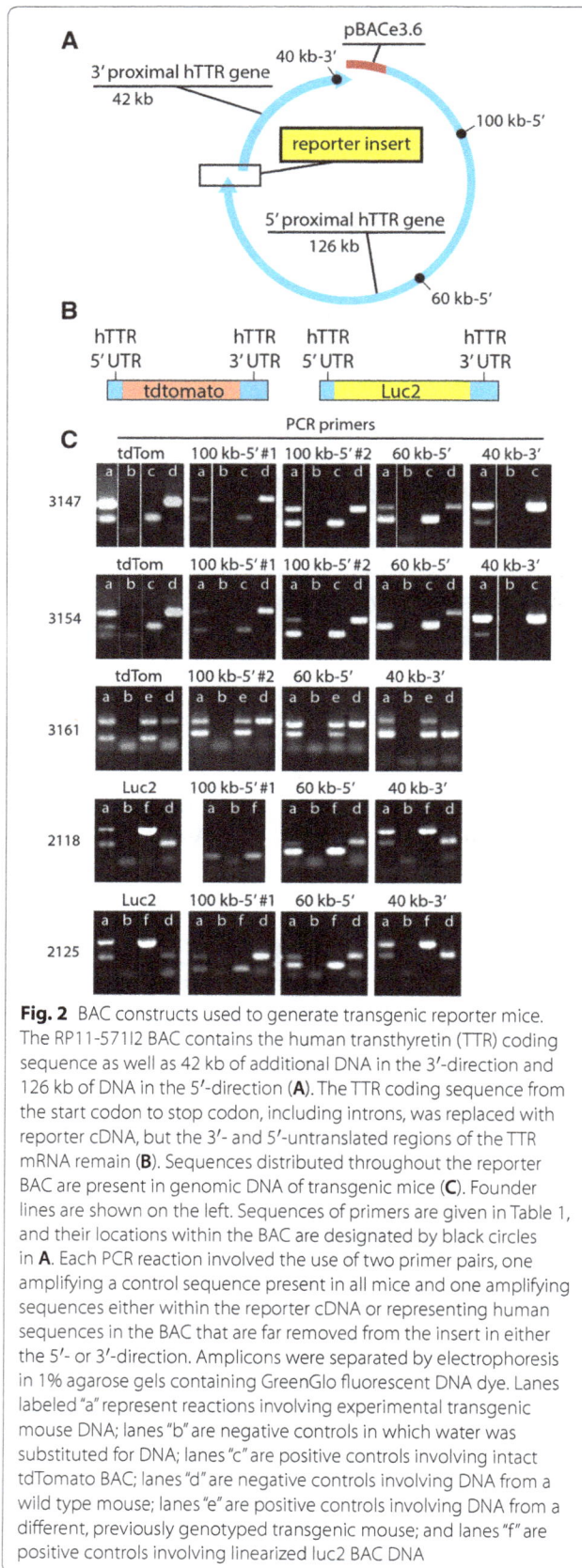

**Fig. 2** BAC constructs used to generate transgenic reporter mice. The RP11-571I2 BAC contains the human transthyretin (TTR) coding sequence as well as 42 kb of additional DNA in the 3′-direction and 126 kb of DNA in the 5′-direction (**A**). The TTR coding sequence from the start codon to stop codon, including introns, was replaced with reporter cDNA, but the 3′- and 5′-untranslated regions of the TTR mRNA remain (**B**). Sequences distributed throughout the reporter BAC are present in genomic DNA of transgenic mice (**C**). Founder lines are shown on the left. Sequences of primers are given in Table 1, and their locations within the BAC are designated by black circles in **A**. Each PCR reaction involved the use of two primer pairs, one amplifying a control sequence present in all mice and one amplifying sequences either within the reporter cDNA or representing human sequences in the BAC that are far removed from the insert in either the 5′- or 3′-direction. Amplicons were separated by electrophoresis in 1% agarose gels containing GreenGlo fluorescent DNA dye. Lanes labeled "a" represent reactions involving experimental transgenic mouse DNA; lanes "b" are negative controls in which water was substituted for DNA; lanes "c" are positive controls involving intact tdTomato BAC; lanes "d" are negative controls involving DNA from a wild type mouse; lanes "e" are positive controls involving DNA from a different, previously genotyped transgenic mouse; and lanes "f" are positive controls involving linearized luc2 BAC DNA

protective and clinically relevant protein [23–26]. The contiguous TTR coding region (start codon to stop codon, including introns) was replaced with cDNA for either tdTomato or luc2, and transgenic mice were generated via random BAC integration following pronuclear injection into fertilized eggs (Fig. 2B; see "Methods" for details). 5′ and 3′ untranslated TTR regions, which contain likely transcriptional and mRNA stability elements, were retained. Tdtomato was chosen for its bright, red-shifted fluorescence [27], and luc2 was chosen to confer the possibility of repeated, highly sensitive in vivo imaging (and highly quantitative in vitro measurement) of emitted light in the presence of luciferin substrate and ATP [28].

A total of 63 mice were born from eggs injected with the tdTomato reporter BAC. Of these, 25 possessed tdTomato reporter sequences by PCR, and 21 were also PCR-positive for human TTR regulatory elements (100 kb upstream, 60 kb upstream, and 40 kb downstream of coding sequence; Fig. 2A, C, Table 1). Nine founder mice were then bred. All nine displayed germline transmission and showed red fluorescence in dissected, unfixed ChP (evaluated at P21–28). Of these, two founder lines yielded offspring with only weakly fluorescent ChP (RFP fluorescence barely detectable using an EVOS microscope at 10X, 100% lamp intensity, 1 s exposure), two yielded moderately fluorescent ChP (fluorescence clear at 10X, but not at 4X), and five yielded strongly fluorescent ChP (fluorescence clear at 4X). Three of these strongly fluorescent founder lines were bred further, and hemizygous mice from these lines were characterized in greater detail in this paper (founder lines 3147, 3154, and 3161). All three lines have been archived by cryopreservation of sperm that have been verified for fertility after thawing.

Pairs of hemizygous mice from each of the three founder lines were also bred to generate homozygous offspring. We first identified putative homozygotes by quantifying PCR amplicons that spanned the hTTR-tdTomato BAC. Specifically, we performed multiplex PCR reactions (two primer pairs per reaction) for JAX control mouse DNA and for either tdTomato coding sequence or flanking human TTR elements (Table 1). Three or four multiplex reactions were performed per mouse, subjected to gel electrophoresis (Fig. 3a), and analyzed by densitometry using ImageJ (Fig. 3b). The relative areas of the peaks corresponding to the BAC and control bands were calculated for each lane, and the ratios were plotted against those obtained for other sets of primer pairs (Fig. 3c). In these plots, individual mice typically clustered based on amplicon abundance (e.g. see mice 891 and 892 in red in Fig. 3). Mice with the most abundant BAC amplicons (i.e. putative homozygotes) were then bred with wild-type mice to test for homozygosity. Of the ten

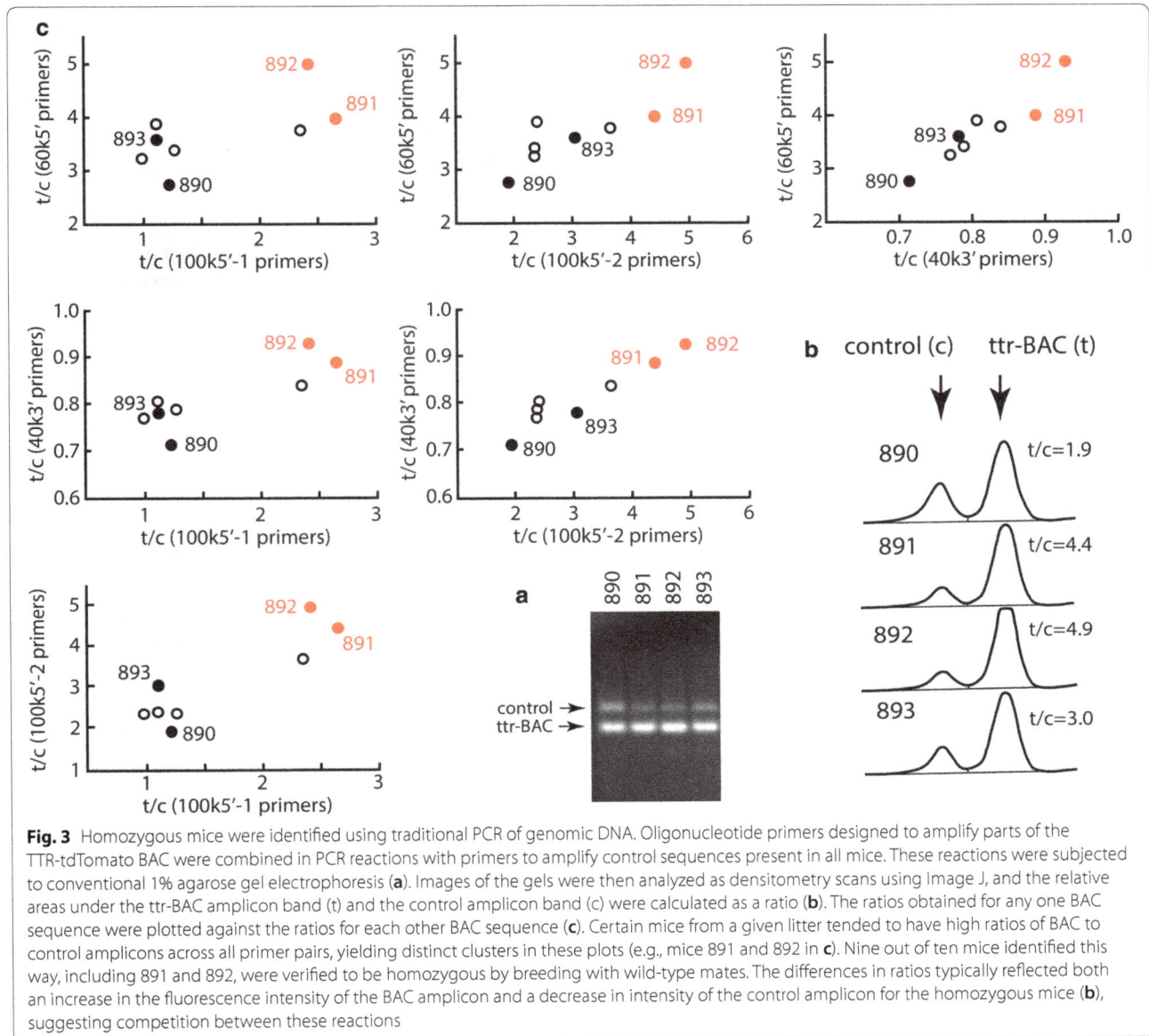

**Fig. 3** Homozygous mice were identified using traditional PCR of genomic DNA. Oligonucleotide primers designed to amplify parts of the TTR-tdTomato BAC were combined in PCR reactions with primers to amplify control sequences present in all mice. These reactions were subjected to conventional 1% agarose gel electrophoresis (a). Images of the gels were then analyzed as densitometry scans using Image J, and the relative areas under the ttr-BAC amplicon band (t) and the control amplicon band (c) were calculated as a ratio (b). The ratios obtained for any one BAC sequence were plotted against the ratios for each other BAC sequence (c). Certain mice from a given litter tended to have high ratios of BAC to control amplicons across all primer pairs, yielding distinct clusters in these plots (e.g., mice 891 and 892 in c). Nine out of ten mice identified this way, including 891 and 892, were verified to be homozygous by breeding with wild-type mates. The differences in ratios typically reflected both an increase in the fluorescence intensity of the BAC amplicon and a decrease in intensity of the control amplicon for the homozygous mice (b), suggesting competition between these reactions

mice successfully bred, nine produced solely transgenic offspring (17–36 pups genotyped) and were deemed homozygous.

For founder line 3147, four homozygous males and two homozygous females were identified, and for founder line 3154, two homozygous females and one homozygous male were identified. All homozygous mice appeared normal, grew at indistinguishable rates from wild-type siblings, and successfully interbred to generate homozygous 3147 and 3154 lines, all offspring of which appear normal. For founder line 3161, 20 pups (three litters) from two hemizygous pairs were screened, but no putative homozygotes were identified; thus, no further

attempts were made at achieving homozygosis of this line.

### Embryonic onset of tdTomato fluorescence in choroid plexus

Red fluorescence could be detected in heads of whole, unfixed embryos as early as E11.5. At E11.5 and E12.5, the greatest signal was detected in the hindbrain region (Fig. 4A, open arrowhead), which is consistent with the first appearance of the ChP [29, 30]. By E14.5, fluorescence in the forebrain had clearly taken on the bicornuate form of the two lateral ventricles (Fig. 4B, solid

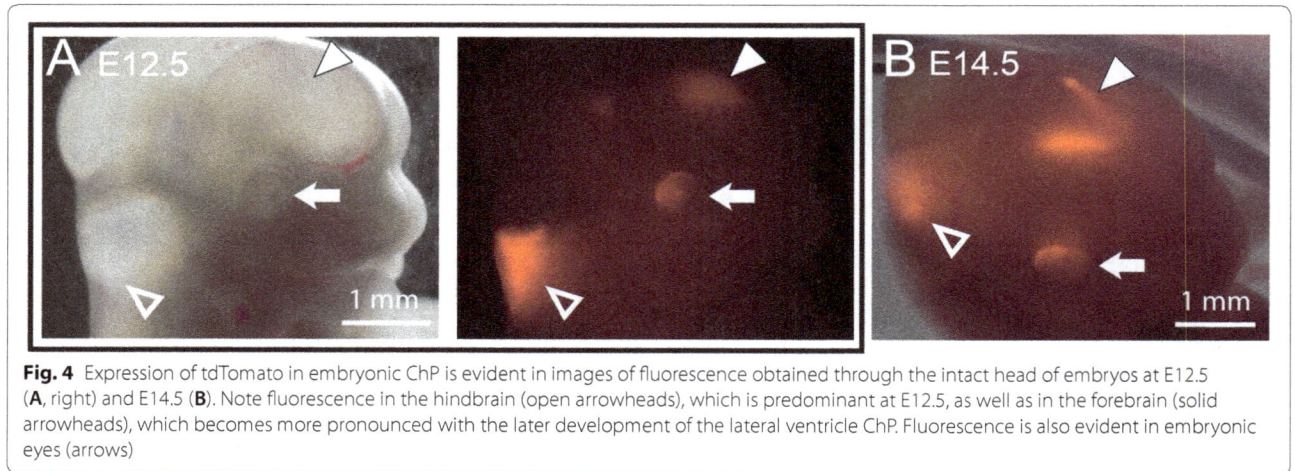

**Fig. 4** Expression of tdTomato in embryonic ChP is evident in images of fluorescence obtained through the intact head of embryos at E12.5 (**A**, right) and E14.5 (**B**). Note fluorescence in the hindbrain (open arrowheads), which is predominant at E12.5, as well as in the forebrain (solid arrowheads), which becomes more pronounced with the later development of the lateral ventricle ChP. Fluorescence is also evident in embryonic eyes (arrows)

arrowhead), reflecting the development of the telencephalic choroid plexus.

We also detected tdTomato fluorescence in the eyes of whole, unfixed embryos as early as E12.5 (Fig. 4A, B, arrows). This fluorescence reflects transthyretin expression in retinal pigment epithelium, which will be discussed in more detail below.

### tdTomato is strongly expressed in choroid plexus throughout the postnatal period

We successfully imaged tdTomato in both unfixed and fixed ChP, with or without immunostaining, across a wide range of ages. Figure 5A shows images taken through a dissecting scope of whole mounts of unfixed lateral ventricle ChP dissected from weanling mice of three founder lines. The ChP of hemizygous mice (+) were bright from native tdTomato fluorescence, whereas the ChP from wild-type siblings that were imaged alongside (−) showed no fluorescence. All regions of the lateral and fourth ventricle ChP appeared to fluoresce, a strong contrast to the results with the previous mRFP1 reporter (Fig. 1).

We found that native tdTomato fluorescence photobleached rapidly, so we frequently chose to perform indirect immunofluorescence staining using an anti-RFP antibody (Rockland, 600-401-379) that reacts with

tdTomato. TdTomato immunofluorescence was detected in all four ventricles of a P3 mouse (Fig. 5B) and was clearly present in the ChP and CPECs based on double-labeling with the CPEC marker AE2 (Fig. 5B, right panel). TdTomato expression remained robust in ChP from all ventricles at P314 (10.5 months of age; Fig. 5C–E), attesting to the longevity of tdTomato expression. Moreover, essentially every CPEC bearing TTR (green fluorescence) appeared also to express tdTomato (red fluorescence) in these images.

### TdTomato is expressed in a subset of cells in pancreatic islets

TdTomato fluorescence was detected in pancreatic tissue from every transgenic mouse investigated, which included animals from P3 to 10.5 months of age. Figure 6A shows fluorescence in a wet mount of pancreas from a 6-month old transgenic mouse (+) alongside pancreas from a wild-type mouse (−). The observed patchy distribution of red fluorescence was consistent with the known expression of transthyretin in pancreatic islets [31]. In cryosections, some weak immunostaining for tdTomato more centrally within islets co-localized with insulin immunostains (arrows in Fig. 6B), suggesting low-level tdTomato expression in β-cells [31, 32], but more intense tdTomato staining occurred in the largely

(See figure on next page.)
**Fig. 5** TdTomato continues to be expressed in postnatal choroid plexus of BAC transgenic mice. **A** Show paired images of transmitted light and tdTomato fluorescence in wet mounts of dissected lateral ventricle ChP from post-weanling mice from three founder lines. Whereas transgenic ChP (+) fluoresce brightly, ChP from wild-type siblings (−) do not. **B** Show immunofluorescence in cryostat sections from a P3 brain. TdTomato was detected in all four ventricles and was co-localized with anion exchanger 2 (AE2, right). **C–E** Shows immunofluorescence in microtome sections of brains from 314-day-old mice, verifying the long-term expression of the reporter in CPECs of the lateral (**C**), third (**D**), and fourth (**E**) ventricle. The selective localization of tdTomato in CPECs is confirmed by associated staining with antibodies to TTR. The location of nuclei is indicated by DAPI staining

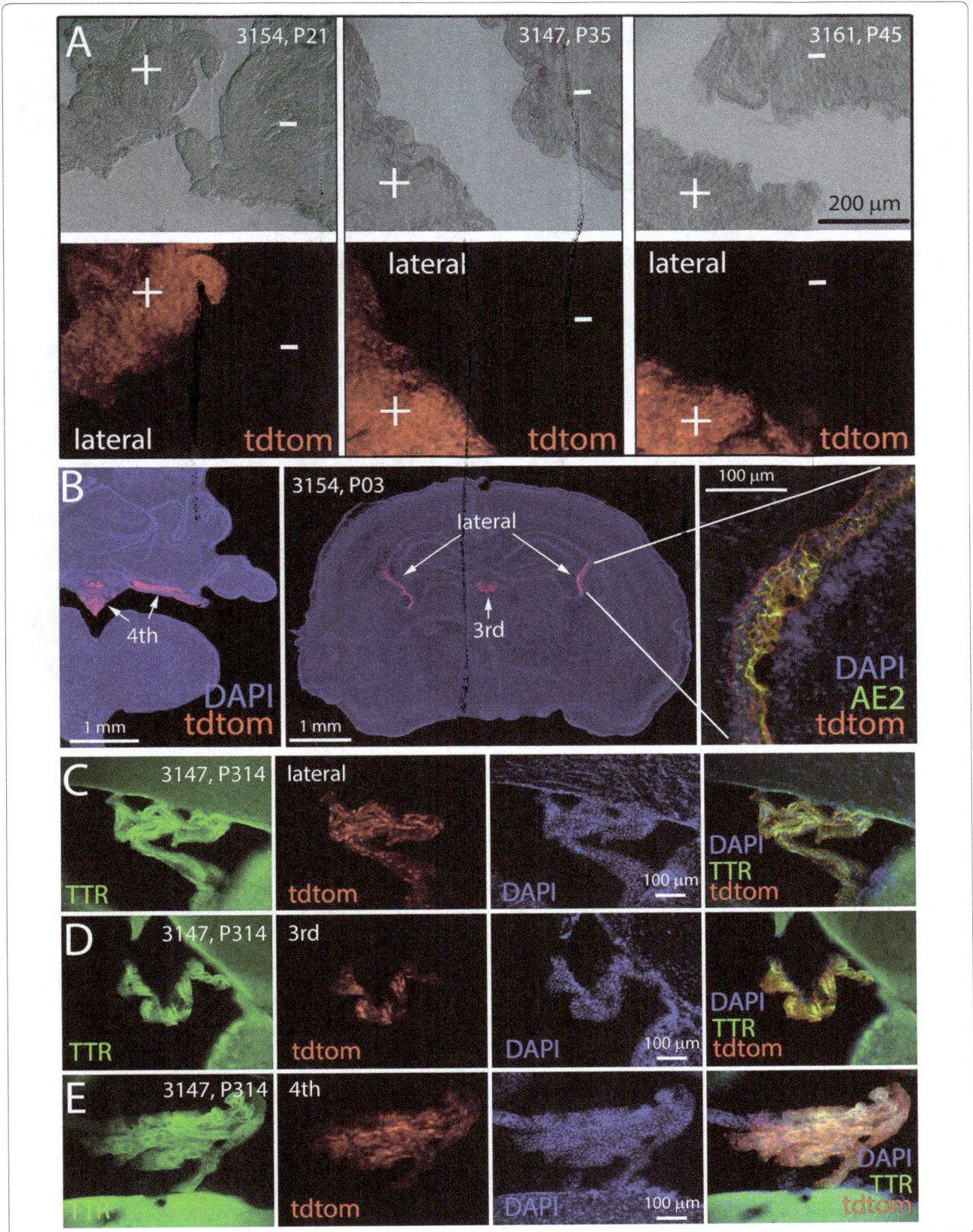

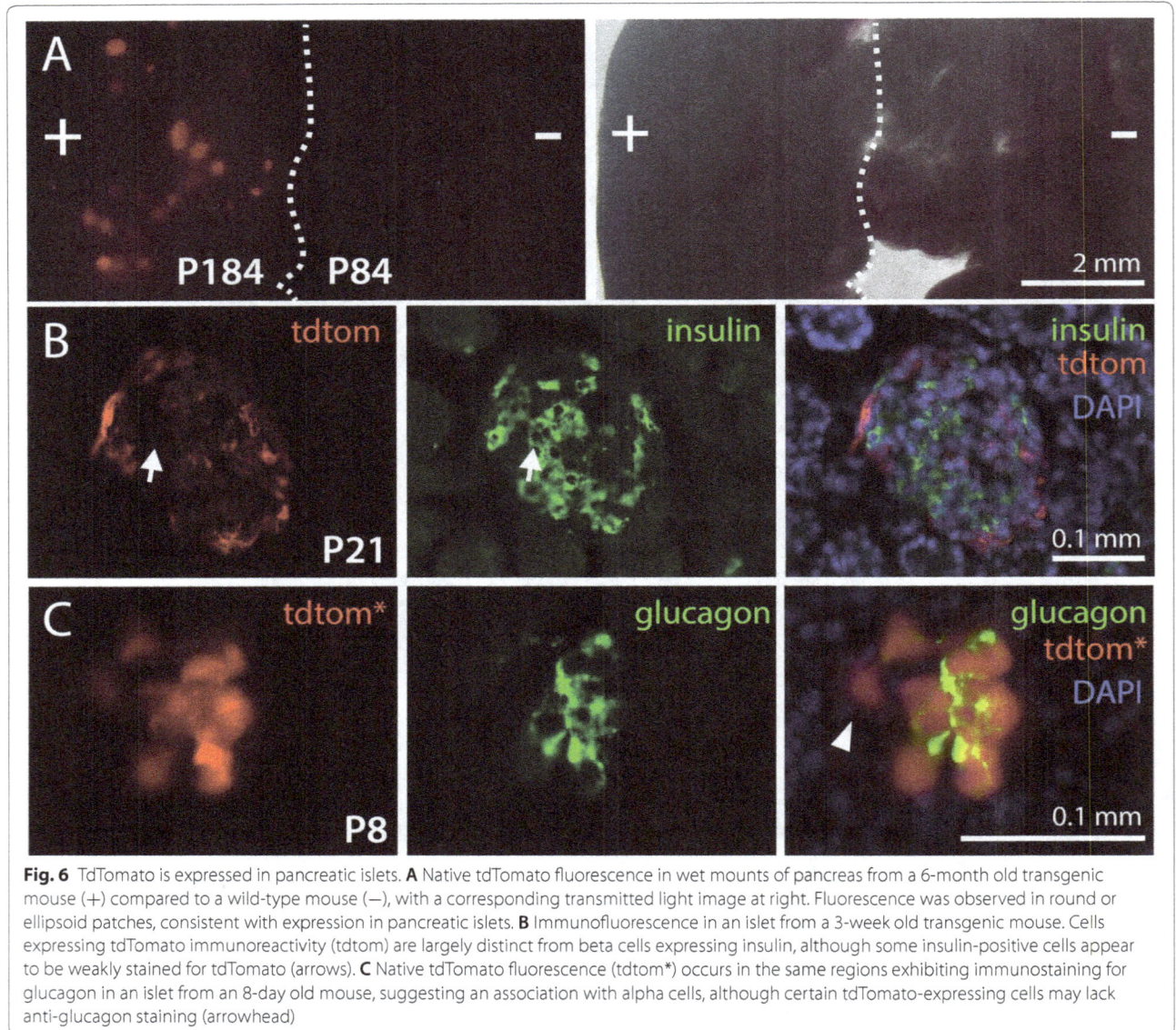

**Fig. 6** TdTomato is expressed in pancreatic islets. **A** Native tdTomato fluorescence in wet mounts of pancreas from a 6-month old transgenic mouse (+) compared to a wild-type mouse (−), with a corresponding transmitted light image at right. Fluorescence was observed in round or ellipsoid patches, consistent with expression in pancreatic islets. **B** Immunofluorescence in an islet from a 3-week old transgenic mouse. Cells expressing tdTomato immunoreactivity (tdtom) are largely distinct from beta cells expressing insulin, although some insulin-positive cells appear to be weakly stained for tdTomato (arrows). **C** Native tdTomato fluorescence (tdtom*) occurs in the same regions exhibiting immunostaining for glucagon in an islet from an 8-day old mouse, suggesting an association with alpha cells, although certain tdTomato-expressing cells may lack anti-glucagon staining (arrowhead)

insulin-negative periphery of islets (Fig. 6B). At the periphery, bright native tdTomato fluorescence partially co-localized with immunostains for glucagon (Fig. 6C), consistent with TTR expression in α-cells [31–34]. However, peripheral tdTomato native fluorescence was also seen in glucagon-negative cells, suggesting the possibility of reporter expression in other non-α or -β islet cell types.

### TdTomato is highly expressed in retinal pigment epithelium (RPE)

TdTomato fluorescence was also detected in eyes from every transgenic mouse investigated from E12.5 (Fig. 4) to 10 months of age and from all three transgenic lines.

Figure 7A shows an image looking down through the lens of an intact, unfixed E18.5 transgenic eye (+) alongside an eye from a wild-type sibling (−). Most of the transgenic retina fluoresced, with the exception of the optic disk where retina is normally absent (arrow). Figure 7B shows a side view of eyes from P45 transgenic (+) and wild-type siblings (−), illustrating the persistence of fluorescence into the second postnatal month. In cryosections, immunostaining for tdTomato was most intense in the RPE (Fig. 7C), consistent with the known TTR expression in that layer [35, 36]. Apparent staining of sparsely distributed cells in the retina was also observed (arrowheads), which may represent horizontal or amacrine cells, although TTR mRNA detected by in situ

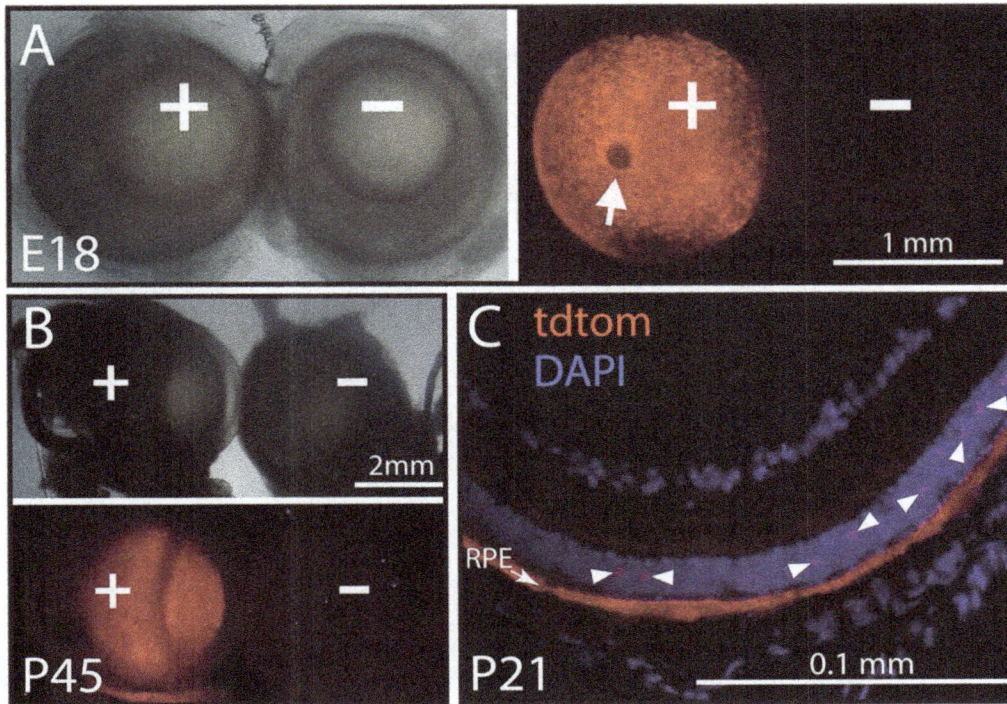

**Fig. 7** TdTomato is expressed in retinal pigment epithelium. **A** Shows corresponding brightfield (left) and red fluorescence (right) images of intact eyes dissected from a transgenic tdTomato E18 embryo (+) and a wild-type sibling (−). The back of the transgenic eye is fluorescent, except for the circular optic disk (arrow), where the retina is interrupted by outgoing axons of the optic nerve. **B** Shows similar images of eyes from a 1.5-month old pair of transgenic (+) and wild-type (−) siblings. **C** Shows immunofluorescence for tdTomato in a cryostat section taken transverse to the plane of the retina from a 3-week old transgenic mouse. The immunoreactive arc corresponds in location to the retinal pigment epithelium (RPE), known to express TTR. Intermittent immunostained large cells in the retinal layer were also observed (arrowheads)

hybridization has been reported to be absent outside of the RPE in the rat eye [34].

### TdTomato fluorescence is detectable in the liver

Transthyretin is well known to be synthesized by hepatocytes, the main source of TTR in plasma [37]. Accordingly, tdTomato fluorescence was detected in wet mounts of thin liver slices taken from transgenic mice ranging in age from E18 through P22 (Fig. 8). However, longer exposures were invariably required to detect fluorescence compared to the previously described tissues, and comparisons to wild-type liver slices were essential to distinguish signal definitively from autofluorescence.

### Real time RT-qPCR confirms long-term expression of tdTomato

To evaluate whether tdTomato expression accurately reports TTR expression, we used real-time RT-qPCR to quantify relative levels of tdTomato and TTR mRNA in ChP and liver in hemizygous mice. Average Ct values for 18S rRNA and cyclophilin mRNA together were used as reference standards to calculate $\Delta Ct$ values.

The RT-qPCR assay clearly detected tdTomato mRNA, as $\Delta Ct$ values for hemizygous mice (n=56) differed significantly from values for wild-type mice (n=24) in both tissues (ChP: hemizygous $\Delta Ct=-11.1\pm1.5$ (s.d.), wild type $\Delta Ct=-20.5\pm3.8$, two-tailed t=15.7, p=$8.5\times10^{-26}$; liver: hemizygous $\Delta Ct=-14.8\pm1.7$, wild type-$21.9\pm2.7$, t=14.2, p=$2.2\times10^{-23}$). We also measured levels of TTR, which did not differ between hemizygous and wild-type mice (ChP: hemizygous $\Delta Ct=-0.2\pm0.8$, wild type $\Delta Ct=-0.2\pm1.1$, t=0.05, p=0.96; liver: hemizygous $\Delta Ct=-4.2\pm0.9$, wild type $\Delta Ct=-4.0\pm1.0$, t=−0.99, p=0.32). The fact that levels of TTR mRNA did not differ between transgenic and wild-type mice indicates that the reporter sequence did not interfere significantly with transcription of the endogenous TTR gene.

Figure 9a shows the $\Delta\Delta Ct$ values obtained for ChP and liver from all mice we investigated from the 3154 founder line (n=32 hemizygotes). Consistent with the brighter native tdTomato fluorescence of the ChP compared to the liver, RT-qPCR showed that ChP expressed greater levels of both tdTomato and TTR transcripts than did

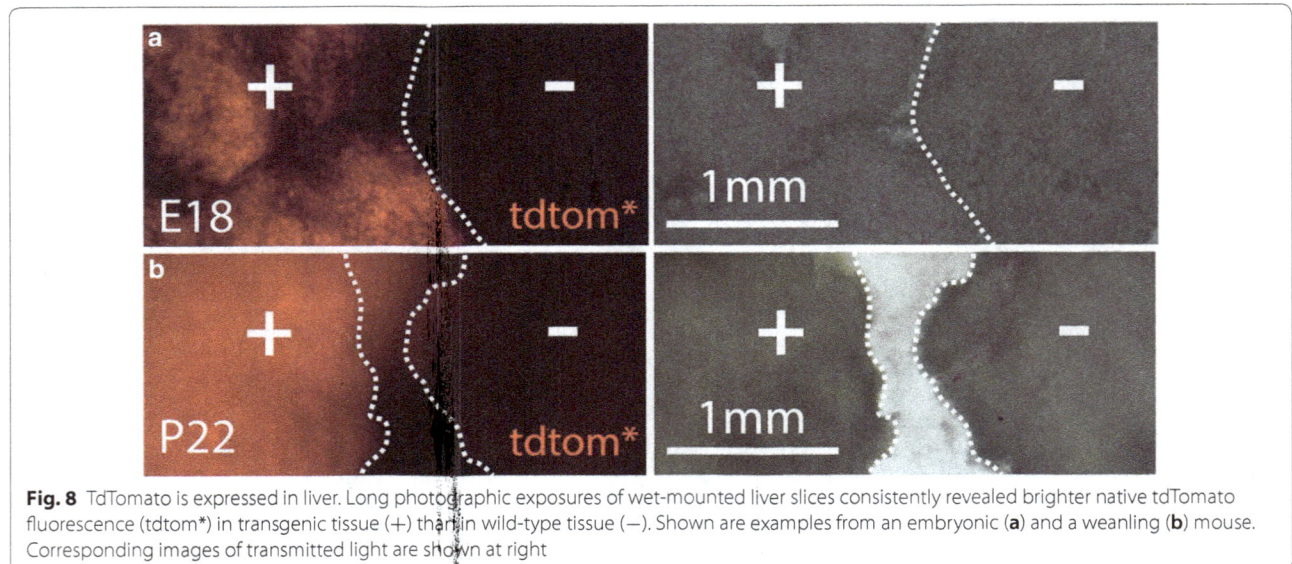

**Fig. 8** TdTomato is expressed in liver. Long photographic exposures of wet-mounted liver slices consistently revealed brighter native tdTomato fluorescence (tdtom*) in transgenic tissue (+) than in wild-type tissue (−). Shown are examples from an embryonic (**a**) and a weanling (**b**) mouse. Corresponding images of transmitted light are shown at right

liver. The ChP-liver difference was also similar for the two transcripts [$2.8 \pm 1.9$ (s.d.) Ct values for tdTomato and $3.2 \pm 0.9$ Ct values for TTR, paired $t$ test: $t = -0.94$, $p = 0.35$], corresponding to ~8-fold higher transcript levels in ChP than in liver. The fact that ChP and liver displayed similar differences in transcription of tdTomato and TTR implies that the human TTR regulatory sequences in the BAC are similarly interpreted by the mouse transcription factors that specify tissue dependence and levels.

Figure 9b shows the $\Delta\Delta$Ct values from the 3154 founder line as a function of mouse age. Whereas TTR displayed no significant differences with age in either the ChP or the liver, regression analysis indicated a small, but statistically significant, age-related decline in tdTomato transcripts in the ChP ($-0.0036$ Ct value/day, $r = 0.40$, $F = 5.78$, $p = 0.022$) and a significant but small age-related increase in the liver ($0.0055$ Ct value/day, $r = 0.37$, $F = 4.66$, $p = 0.039$).

There were no significant differences in ChP tdTomato $\Delta\Delta$Ct values across the three founder lines that were chosen for detailed analysis (single-factor analysis of variance (ANOVA) $F_{(2,53)} = 0.34$, $p = 0.72$); however, tdTomato $\Delta\Delta$Ct values in liver did show significant differences (one-way ANOVA $F_{(2,53)} = 4.59$, $p = 0.016$). Post-hoc t-tests revealed a significant difference between the 3154 line and the 3147 line ($t = 2.49$, $p = 0.016$), while the difference between 3154 and 3161 lines did not reach the significance threshold ($p = 0.059$). The slight age-dependent decline in tdTomato $\Delta\Delta$Ct values in the ChP in the 3154 line (Fig. 9b) was also significant for the 3147 line, despite being assessed with fewer data points ($-0.0030$

Ct value/day, $r = 0.72$, $F = 11.0$, $p = 0.0077$) (Fig. 9c). A similar trend towards age-related decline was apparent for the 3161 line (Fig. 9d), but was not found to be significant ($r = 0.49$, $F = 2.80$, $p = 0.13$). Unlike the 3154 line, however, the 3147 and 3161 founder lines did not show any age-dependent increase in liver tdTomato transcripts (Fig. 9c, d). Similar to the 3154 line, TTR transcripts did not change significantly with age in either 3147 or 3161 founder lines (Fig. 9c, d). The fact that all three founder lines showed a slight age-related tdTomato decline in the ChP, while TTR transcripts remained unchanged, suggests the possibility of a human-mouse difference in TTR regulation that is independent of integration site.

Real-time RT-qPCR further indicated that mRNA levels for tdTomato and TTR did not differ between sexes in either tissue of the 3154 founder line (Fig. 9e, $n = 15$ males and 9 females), consistent with prior experiments showing no sex difference in TTR transcripts in the mouse liver [38]. Figure 9f shows that there was no consistent decline in tdTomato $\Delta\Delta$Ct values over four successive generations in the 3154 founder line, suggesting stability of the BAC transgene and its expression in the ChP and liver. (The liver values were not statistically different: single-factor ANOVA $F_{(3,28)} = 1.29$, $p = 0.30$).

Thus, the real-time RT-qPCR data indicates that the human TTR BAC tdTomato reporter largely parallels the expression of the endogenous mouse TTR gene in terms of ChP and liver expression profiles in a fashion that is gender-independent, integration site-independent, and stable across generations, with consistently higher levels of TTR and tdTomato in ChP compared to liver. There were, however, small but significant age-related declines

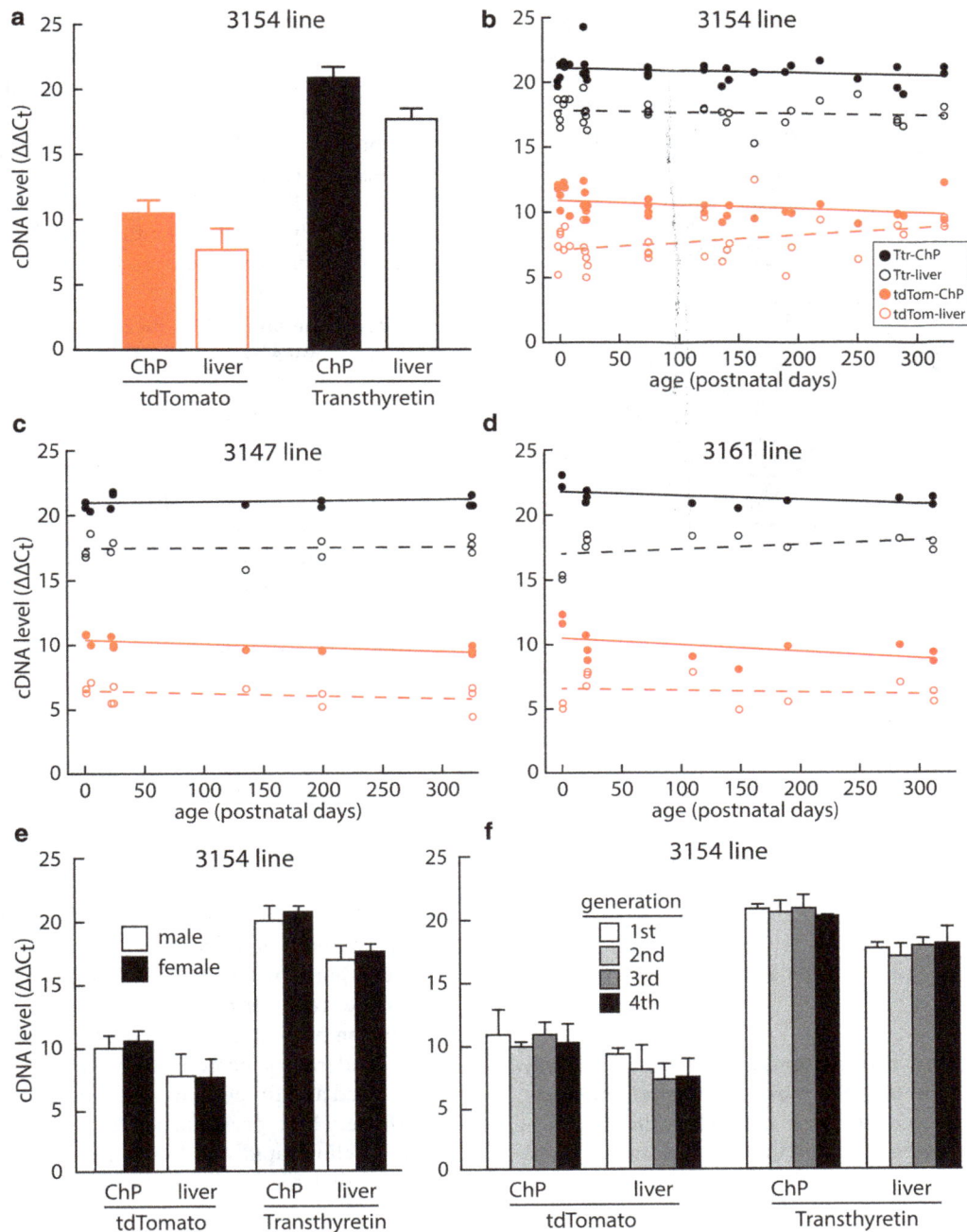

**Fig. 9** Real-time rt-qPCR revealed long-term expression of TTR and tdTomato mRNA. **a** Values across all animals from the 3154 founder line indicated a greater abundance of tdTomato transcript in the ChP than in the liver, and the difference was similar to that detected for transthyretin. **b** When expressed as a function of age, tdTomato transcripts in the ChP declined slightly but significantly in the 3154 founder line, whereas tdTomato transcripts in the liver increased significantly. In contrast, transthyretin transcripts remained steady with age in both ChP and liver. The small decline in tdTomato expression across age in the 3154 line was recapitulated in both the 3147 (**c**) and 3161 (**d**) founder lines, but the increase in tdTomato transcript in the liver was not observed for the 3147 and 3161 lines. Levels of transthyretin transcripts did not change significantly with age in either the ChP or liver in either the 3147 or 3161 founder line. TdTomato and transthyretin in the 3154 founder line did not differ between the sexes (**e**) or across generations (**f**). Heights of bars indicate mean values, error bars denote standard deviations, and trendlines are the results of linear regression

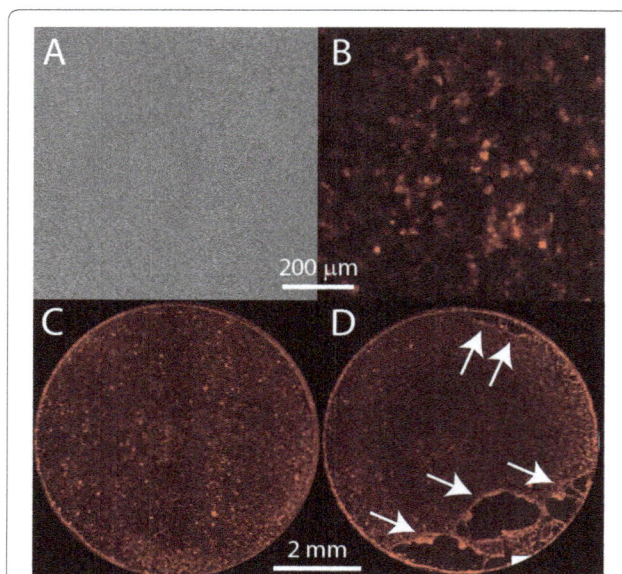

**Fig. 10** The tdTomato reporter facilitates visualization of cultured CPECs on Transwell membranes. **A** CPECs growing on Transwell membranes are not easily visible using phase contrast microscopy. **B** When visualized using red epifluorescence, the same field as in **A** could be seen to possess a confluent monolayer of primary CPECs originally dissociated from the ChP of homozygous TTR BAC-tdTomato transgenic mice (3147 founder line). **C** Stitched images of tdTomato fluorescence revealed nearly 100% coverage of the Transwell membrane after 4 days of undisturbed culture. The monolayer displayed a respectable trans-epithelial electrical resistance of 110 $\Omega$ cm$^2$. **D** The same membrane as in **C** was imaged after 3 days of experimental manipulation. Holes in the coverage were clearly evident (arrows), explaining a measure decrease of resistance to 44 $\Omega$ cm$^2$

in ChP transcription of tdTomato across lines that were not observed for TTR.

### The TTR BAC-tdTomato reporter is useful in characterizing monolayer cultures of CPECs grown in transwell chambers

Primary monolayer cultures of CPECs in Transwell chambers are useful for studying the barrier and transport functions of the ChP [22, 39–41]. It would be beneficial to monitor the coverage of the Transwell membrane by these live cells over time and across different experimental conditions, but the cells can be difficult to visualize by phase contrast microscopy because of the strong pattern from the porous membrane upon which they are grown (Fig. 10A). Fortunately, primary Transwell cultures derived from homozygous TTR BAC-tdTomato mice could be easily visualized by way of their red fluorescence (Fig. 10B). Furthermore, the presence of fluorescence throughout the cytoplasm of these cells supports an evaluation of the confluence of cells when the entire membrane is imaged by way of stitching together

spatially-ordered snapshots of a culture (Fig. 10C). The ability to evaluate confluence non-invasively has aided in the interpretation of the loss of barrier function sometimes observed after having performed multiple experiments on the same culture over time. For example, the culture shown in Fig. 10C displayed a healthy trans-epithelial electrical resistance of 110 $\Omega$ cm$^2$, whereas a drop in the value to 44 $\Omega$ cm$^2$ observed after 2 days of experiments was clearly associated with a detached monolayer when tdTomato fluorescence was evaluated (Fig. 10D).

### Generation of human TTR BAC-luc2 reporter mice

A total of 11 mice were born from eggs injected with the luc2 reporter BAC. (See "Methods" for details.) PCR showed that five of these mice possessed both internal sequences of luc2 cDNA and human BAC sequences flanking the reporter (Fig. 2). Two of the positive mice were bred to test for expression of luciferase activity in various tissues of their progeny. Both of these strains have been archived by sperm cryopreservation, and the sperm has been verified for fertility after thawing.

### Long-term persistence of luciferase activity in TTR-expressing tissues of transgenic mice

The tissue distribution of specific luciferase activity was very similar between the two founder lines, although line 2118 had twice the activity of line 2125 (Fig. 11a). Of the tissues examined, ChP had by far the greatest specific activity, 100 times that of the eye, the second most active tissue. Activity was low, but detectable in the pancreas, but was not detected in the liver. The presence of luc2 activity in ChP, eye, and pancreas is consistent with the tdTomato reporter and the known expression of TTR, while the absence of activity in liver was surprising given the tdTomato reporter data (Figs. 8 and 9), but was consistent for the two independent luc2 founder lines.

When luciferase specific activity in the ChP and eye were followed as a function of age in tissue from founder line 2118, very high perinatal activity in both tissues was found to decline rapidly to lower, but still easily detectable, levels that then remained stable from 2 weeks to 6 months of age (Fig. 11b). Thus, the sustained expression of the luciferase reporter and the rank order of tissue expression were similar to those of the tdTomato reporter, and the consistency across the two luc2 lines recalls the similarity in expression across the three tdTomato founder lines that we studied.

### Discussion

We have demonstrated accurate reporting of transthyretin expression in transgenic mice expressing tdTomato fluorescent protein by way of randomly integrated human TTR BACs. The major tissues in which TTR is

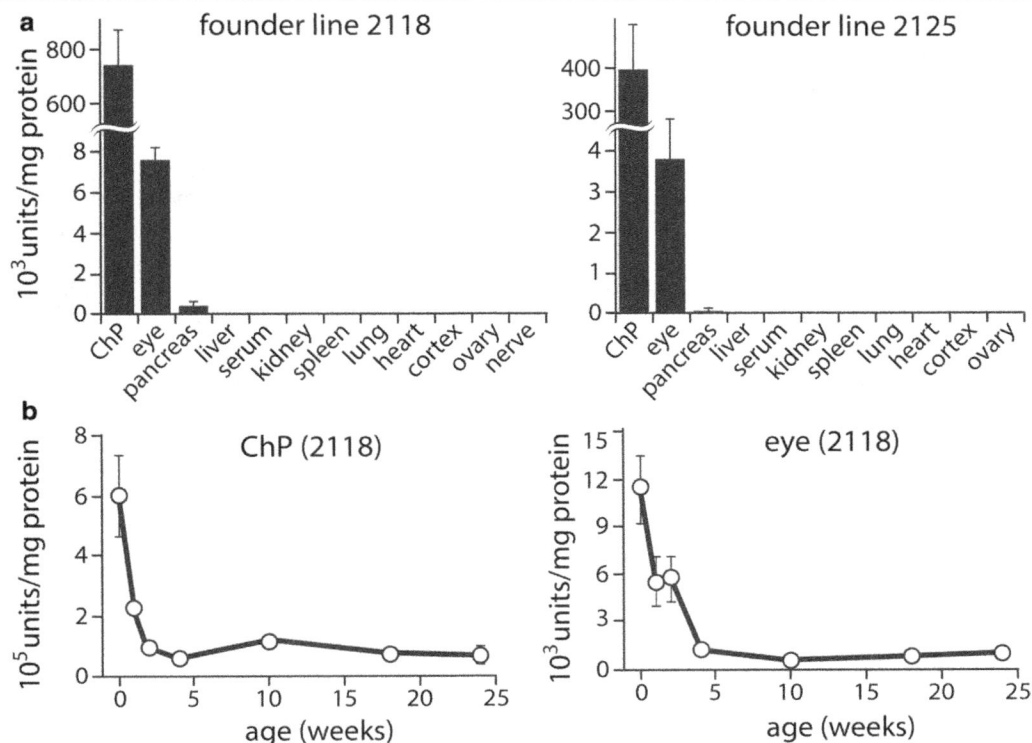

**Fig. 11** Luciferase activity is high in the ChP of transgenic mice. Luciferase activity measured in lysates of various tissues in two different founder lines showed a rank order largely consistent with the intensity of tdTomato native fluorescence, with no detection of luciferase in tissues that do not express TTR (**a**). The specific activity of luciferase in both the ChP and the eye declined rapidly from high perinatal values to steadily detectable levels that persisted well into adulthood (**b**). Error bars denote standard deviations

expressed postnatally and constitutively (choroid plexus, liver, retinal pigment epithelium, and pancreatic islets) all displayed endogenous red fluorescence when compared to wild type controls, and no ectopic expression was detected. Quantitative evaluation of transcription by rt-qPCR showed that relative expression of tdTomato in the liver and ChP paralleled relative expression of TTR in those two tissues. No sex differences were detected, and expression was maintained over successive generations. Appropriate cellular specificity was documented by immunostaining using antibodies that recognize the tdTomato protein. Expression of tdTomato in the embryonic choroid plexus coincided with the known onset of TTR expression [29, 30, 42], and ChP tdTomato expression persisted far into adulthood. Similarity across three independent founder lines indicated that the characteristics of expression were independent of integration site, a typical advantage of BAC transgenes [18]. Activity of luc2 was also similar in two independent reporter lines generated from the human TTR BACs.

A prior TTR::RFP reporter transgenic mouse [17] was based on a TTR minigene involving 3kbp of DNA upstream of the mouse TTR coding sequence, a region that had been shown in prior studies to contain the positive elements required for ChP expression [43, 44]. Despite expression of this minigene in the ChP, ectopic expression in brain regions other than the ChP was also observed [17, 43], and embryonic expression of RFP and Cre were detected in regions of the limb that have not previously been associated with TTR expression [17]. As previously mentioned, expression of the RFP reporter was mosaic in the ChP and disappeared from the lateral and third ventricle in the first few postnatal weeks. These anomalies could reflect the absence of important regulatory elements from the 3-kbp portion of the mouse gene, or they could reflect positional effects on expression caused by the site of integration in the mouse chromosome [18].

Positive elements in the human TTR gene that are required for expression of a mutant TTR in transgenic mouse ChP were found to be within 6 kbp upstream of the TTR coding sequence [45]. The presence of these regulatory sequences in the human TTR BAC, as well as the very large expanse of DNA from the BAC that would tend to obviate positional effects, may explain the more faithful expression of tdTomato in the human TTR BAC transgenic mice.

In the 6 kbp mutant human TTR transgenic mouse, it was noted that levels of liver transcripts for the mutant TTR increased with age following birth, while postnatal levels of the native mouse TTR transcript remained constant following an embryonic increase, and it was suggested that the postnatal increase in human TTR may reflect a difference in the regulation of the human TTR gene in the mouse liver [45]. In one of our founder lines (3154), we also observed a postnatal increase in transcription of tdTomato in the liver; however, this increase was not observed in the other two founder lines. On the other hand, all three founder lines we investigated displayed a small postnatal decrease in transcription of the tdTomato reporter in the ChP over the course of the first postnatal year, while levels of the native mouse TTR transcript in ChP remained constant, which may be evidence of a difference in regulation of the human and mouse genes in the ChP of transgenic mice. Although we found no changes in the level of the native mouse TTR transcript over the course of the first postnatal year, there has been one report of a decrease in CSF TTR protein levels in 18-month-old mice [46]. We cannot rule out the possibility that we would have detected declines in ChP TTR transcripts had we investigated such older mice.

The TTR reporters developed here should facilitate future studies of CPEC biology. In addition to the enhanced ability to visualize and analyze CPECs in Transwell cultures that we have demonstrated in the current paper, the reporters should provide tools to track CPECs following transplantation, to purify CPECs for detailed study and manipulation, and to report on CPEC derivation from stem cells. TTR reporters may be similarly useful in studying retinal pigment epithelial cells, pancreatic islet cells, and hepatocytes. In addition to these important uses, the myriad functions being revealed for TTR [9, 47] suggest that these reporters may enjoy a broader set of applications. Originally known as prealbumin, transthyretin was renamed for its ability to transport thyroxine and retinol binding protein; now, TTR is known to bind to numerous other proteins and to function as a protease, cleaving such important substrates as beta-amyloid peptide [48], apolipoprotein AI [49], and neuropeptide Y [50]. The ability of TTR to fragment the Alzheimer's disease-related beta-amyloid peptide recently has been reported to be central to its ability to decrease the toxicity of this peptide [51], and TTR also participates in the transport of beta-amyloid out of the brain to the liver [52]. TTR is expressed in neurons during heat shock and during the progression of mouse models of familial Alzheimer's disease [16, 24]. TTR also binds to cell surface receptors directly and independently

of binding thyroxine or retinol binding protein to promote nerve regeneration [53] and to affect synthesis of metabolic enzymes in astrocytes [54]. Aggregates of mutated and wild type TTR are responsible for various TTR amyloidoses, and treatment options currently being tested include genetic strategies to knock down synthesis of the protein [25]. Transgenic mice bearing reporters of TTR synthesis should be particularly useful for studying responses of the cell types involved in these myriad functions as well as to screen drugs to enhance or interfere with synthesis of TTR. The presence of human regulatory sequences in the BAC transgenes should increase the biomedical relevance of such studies.

The consistency of reporter expression across multiple founder lines suggests that TTR BACs may prove to be a reliable means to overexpress, knock down (via regulatory RNA expression), or knockout (via Cre recombinase expression and matings with floxed null mice) expression of other proteins in CPECs and other TTR-expressing cells.

## Conclusions

Transgenic mice bearing fluorescent and luminescent reporters of transthyretin have been developed and characterized. We have found that reporter expression profiles match those expected for transthyretin, and they remain expressed into adulthood. These reporter mice should prove useful for tracking transplanted choroid plexus epithelial cells, for purifying the cells for further study, and for reporting their derivation from stem cells. They also should prove useful for studying transthyretin synthesis by other cell types, as transthyretin has been implicated in many functions and conditions, including clearance of β-amyloid peptides associated with Alzheimer's disease, heat shock in neurons, processing of neuropeptides, nerve regeneration, astrocyte metabolism, and transthyretin amyloidosis.

**Abbreviations**
AE2: anion-exchange protein 2; ANOVA: analysis of variance; BAC: bacterial artificial chromosome; ChP: choroid plexus; CPEC: choroid plexus epithelial cell; CSF: cerebrospinal fluid; PBS: phosphate-buffered saline; RFP: red fluorescent protein; RPE: retinal pigment epithelium; RT-qPCR: reverse transcription quantitative polymerase chain reaction; TTR: transthyretin.

**Authors' contributions**
BAJ designed portions of the study involving tdTomato, drafted the manuscript, supervised student researchers, and conducted experiments involving immunostaining, microscopy, and PCR. MC characterized founder lines and designed and performed portions of the study involving luciferase2. HMV performed and analyzed experiments involving rt-qPCR. XH analyzed homozygosity of mice and performed experiments involving immunostaining and microscopy. NF characterized embryonic expression of tdTomato. MJR designed, performed, and analyzed experiments involving rt-qPCR. RJS designed, performed, and analyzed experiments involving primary culture of CPECs in Transwell chambers. MJN performed experiments involving immunostaining and microscopy. YJK characterized postnatal RFP expression. ESM

conceived the study and guided both the experiments and the writing of the manuscript. All authors read and approved the final manuscript.

## Author details
[1] Department of Pathology and Laboratory Medicine, UC Irvine, Irvine, USA. [2] Sue and Bill Gross Stem Cell Research Center, UC Irvine, Irvine, USA. [3] Department of Developmental and Cell Biology, UC Irvine, Irvine, USA. [4] Department of Biological Sciences, California State University, Long Beach, USA.

## Acknowledgements
We are grateful for the technical support, products, and services provided to our research by the Mouse Biology Program (MBP) at the University of California Davis. We also are grateful to Jon Neumann at the UCI Transgenic Mouse Facility for pronuclear injections and advice in characterizing the transgenic mice. We thank Cecilia Urbina, Fangzhou Bian, Priscilla Encinas, Midori Thomas, Chi V.T. Pham, and Dylan Jamner for their excellent technical assistance, Dr. Steven Chessler for his gift of antibodies to insulin and glucagon, and Dr. Anna-Katerina Hadjantonakis for her gift of Ttr::RFP transgenic mice.

## Competing interests
The authors declare that they have no competing interests.

## Funding
Portions of this work were supported by CIRM EDUC2-08383.

## References
1. Lehtinen MK, Bjornsson CS, Dymecki SM, Gilbertson RJ, Holtzman DM, Monuki ES. The choroid plexus and cerebrospinal fluid: emerging roles in development, disease, and therapy. J Neurosci. 2013;33:17553–9.
2. Spector R, Keep RF, Robert Snodgrass S, Smith QR, Johanson CE. A balanced view of choroid plexus structure and function: focus on adult humans. Exp Neurol. 2015;267:78–86.
3. Wright BL, Lai JT, Sinclair AJ. Cerebrospinal fluid and lumbar puncture: a practical review. J Neurol. 2012;259:1530–45.
4. Angelow S, Galla HJ. Junctional proteins of the blood-CSF barrier. In: Zheng W, Chodobski, editors. The blood-cerebrospinal fluid barrier. Boca Raton: Chapman & Hall/CRC; 2005. p. 53–80.
5. Brown PD, Speake T, Davies SL, Millar ID. Ion transporters and channels involved in CSF formation. In: Zheng W, Chodobski, editors. The blood-cerebrospinal fluid barrier. Boca Raton: Chapman & Hall/CRC; 2005. p. 119–45.
6. Miller DS, Lowes S, Pritchard JB. The molecular basis of xenobiotic transport and metabolism. In: Zheng W, Chodobski, editors. The blood-cerebrospinal fluid barrier. Boca Raton: Chapman & Hall/CRC; 2005. p. 147–73.
7. Serot JM, Béné MC, Faure GC. Choroid plexus, aging of the brain, and Alzheimer's disease. Front Biosci. 2003;8:s515–21.
8. Emerich DF, Skinner SJ, Borlongan CV, Vasconcellos AV, Thanos CG. The choroid plexus in the rise, fall and repair of the brain. BioEssays. 2005;27:262–74.
9. Fleming CE, Nunes AF, Sousa MM. Transthyretin: more than meets the eye. Prog Neurobiol. 2009;89:266–76.
10. Reboldi A, Coisne C, Baumjohann D, Benvenuto F, Bottinelli D, Lira S, Uccelli A, Lanzavecchia A, Engelhardt B, Sallusto F. C-C chemokine receptor 6-regulated entry of TH-17 cells into the CNS through the choroid plexus is required for the initiation of EAE. Nat Immunol. 2009;10:514–23.
11. Zhang X, Wu C, Song J, Götte M, Sorokin L. Syndecan-1, a cell surface proteoglycan, negatively regulates initial leukocyte recruitment to the brain across the choroid plexus in murine experimental autoimmune encephalomyelitis. J Immunol. 2013;191:4551–61.
12. Watanabe M, Kang YJ, Davies LM, Meghpara S, Lau K, Chung CY, Kathiriya J, Hadjantonakis AK, Monuki ES. BMP4 sufficiency to induce choroid plexus epithelial fate from embryonic stem cell-derived neuroepithelial progenitors. J Neurosci. 2012;32:15934–45.

13. Marques F, Sousa JC, Coppola G, Gao F, Puga R, Brentani H, Geschwind DH, Sousa N, Correia-Neves M, Palha JA. Transcriptome signature of the adult mouse choroid plexus. Fluids Barriers CNS. 2011;8:10.
14. Lun MP, Johnson MB, Broadbelt KG, Watanabe M, Kang YJ, Chau KF, Springel MW, Malesz A, Sousa AM, Pletikos M, Adelita T, Calicchio ML, Zhang Y, Holtzman MJ, Lidov HG, Sestan N, Steen H, Monuki ES, Lehtinen MK. Spatially heterogeneous choroid plexus transcriptomes encode positional identity and contribute to regional CSF production. J Neurosci. 2015;35:4903–16.
15. Richardson SJ. Cell and molecular biology of transthyretin and thyroid hormones. Int Rev Cytol. 2007;258:137–93.
16. Wang X, Cattaneo F, Ryno L, Hulleman J, Reixach N, Buxbaum JN. The systemic amyloid precursor transthyretin (TTR) behaves as a neuronal stress protein regulated by HSF1 in SH-SY5Y human neuroblastoma cells and APP23 Alzheimer's disease model mice. J Neurosci. 2014;34:7253–65.
17. Kwon GS, Hadjantonakis AK. Transthyretin mouse transgenes direct RFP expression or Cre-mediated recombination throughout the visceral endoderm. Genesis. 2009;47:447–55.
18. Yang XW, Gong S. An overview on the generation of BAC transgenic mice for neuroscience research. Curr Protoc Neurosci. 2005;31:5.20.1–20.11.
19. Chan W, Costantino N, Li R, Lee SC, Su Q, Melvin D, Court DL, Liu P. A recombineering based approach for high-throughput conditional knockout targeting vector construction. Nucleic Acids Res. 2007;35:e64.
20. Wang S, Zhao Y, Leiby M, Zhu J. A new positive/negative selection scheme for precise BAC recombineering. Mol Biotechnol. 2009;42:110–6.
21. Vandesompele J, De Preter K, Pattyn F, Poppe B, Van Roy N, De Paepe A, Speleman F. Accurate normalization of real-time quantitative RT-PCR data by geometric averaging of multiple internal control genes. Genome Biol. 2002;3:RESEARCH0034.
22. Monnot AD, Zheng W. Culture of choroid plexus epithelial cells and in vitro model of blood-CSF barrier. Methods Mol Biol. 2013;945:13–29.
23. Costa R, Gonçalves A, Saraiva MJ, Cardoso I. Transthyretin binding to A-Beta peptide–impact on A-Beta fibrillogenesis and toxicity. FEBS Lett. 2008;582:936–42.
24. Li X, Buxbaum JN. Transthyretin and the brain re-visited: is neuronal synthesis of transthyretin protective in Alzheimer's disease? Mol Neurodegener. 2011;6:79.
25. Sekijima Y. Transthyretin (ATTR) amyloidosis: clinical spectrum, molecular pathogenesis and disease-modifying treatments. J Neurol Neurosurg Psychiatry. 2015;86:1036–43.
26. Alemi M, Silva SC, Santana I, Cardoso I. Transthyretin stability is critical in assisting beta amyloid clearance—relevance of transthyretin stabilization in Alzheimer's disease. CNS Neurosci Ther. 2017;23:605–19.
27. Shaner NC, Campbell RE, Steinbach PA, Giepmans BN, Palmer AE, Tsien RY. Improved monomeric red, orange and yellow fluorescent proteins derived from Discosoma sp. red fluorescent protein. Nat Biotechnol. 2004;22:1567–72.
28. Paguio A, Almond B, Fan F, Stecha P, Garvin D, Wood M, Wood K. pGL4 vectors: a new generation of luciferase reporter vectors. Promega Notes. 2005;89:7–10.
29. Dziegielewska KM, Ek J, Habgood MD, Saunders NR. Development of the choroid plexus. Microsc Res Tech. 2001;52:5–20.
30. Currle DS, Cheng X, Hsu CM, Monuki ES. Direct and indirect roles of CNS dorsal midline cells in choroid plexus epithelia formation. Development. 2005;132:3549–59.
31. Jacobsson B, Collins VP, Grimelius L, Pettersson T, Sandstedt B, Carlström A. Transthyretin immunoreactivity in human and porcine liver, choroid plexus, and pancreatic islets. J Histochem Cytochem. 1989;37:31–7.
32. Dorrell C, Grompe MT, Pan FC, Zhong Y, Canaday PS, Shultz LD, Greiner DL, Wright CV, Streeter PR, Grompe M. Isolation of mouse pancreatic alpha, beta, duct and acinar populations with cell surface markers. Mol Cell Endocrinol. 2011;339:144–50.
33. Westermark GT, Westermark P. Transthyretin and amyloid in the islets of Langerhans in type-2 diabetes. Exp Diabetes Res. 2008;2008:429274.
34. Su Y, Jono H, Misumi Y, Senokuchi T, Guo J, Ueda M, Shinriki S, Tasaki M, Shono M, Obayashi K, Yamagata K, Araki E, Ando Y. Novel function of transthyretin in pancreatic alpha cells. FEBS Lett. 2012;586:4215–22.
35. Cavallaro T, Martone RL, Dwork AJ, Schon EA, Herbert J. The retinal pigment epithelium is the unique site of transthyretin synthesis in the rat eye. Invest Ophthalmol Vis Sci. 1990;31:497–501.

36. Dwork AJ, Cavallaro T, Martone RL, Goodman DS, Schon EA, Herbert J. Distribution of transthyretin in the rat eye. Invest Ophthalmol Vis Sci. 1990;31(489–96):34.

37. Felding P, Fex G. Cellular origin of prealbumin in the rat. Biochim Biophys Acta. 1982;716:446–9.

38. Gonçalves I, Alves CH, Quintela T, Baltazar G, Socorro S, Saraiva MJ, Abreu R, Santos CR. Transthyretin is up-regulated by sex hormones in mice liver. Mol Cell Biochem. 2008;317:137–42.

39. Lazarevic I, Engelhardt B. Modeling immune functions of the mouse blood-cerebrospinal fluid barrier in vitro: primary rather than immortalized mouse choroid plexus epithelial cells are suited to study immune cell migration across this brain barrier. Fluids Barriers CNS. 2016;13:2.

40. Baehr C, Reichel V, Fricker G. Choroid plexus epithelial monolayers—a cell culture model from porcine brain. Cerebrospinal Fluid Res. 2006;3:13.

41. Hakvoort A, Haselbach M, Galla HJ. Active transport properties of porcine choroid plexus cells in culture. Brain Res. 1998;795:247–56.

42. Murakami T, Yasuda Y, Mita S, Maeda S, Shimada K, Fujimoto T, Araki S. Prealbumin gene expression during mouse development studied by in situ hybridization. Cell Differ. 1987;22:1–9.

43. Yan C, Costa RH, Darnell JE Jr, Chen JD, Van Dyke TA. Distinct positive and negative elements control the limited hepatocyte and choroid plexus expression of transthyretin in transgenic mice. EMBO J. 1990;9:869–78.

44. Costa RH, Van Dyke TA, Yan C, Kuo F, Darnell JE Jr. Similarities in transthyretin gene expression and differences in transcription factors: liver and yolk sac compared to choroid plexus. Proc Natl Acad Sci USA. 1990;87:6589–93.

45. Nagata Y, Tashiro F, Yi S, Murakami T, Maeda S, Takahashi K, Shimada K, Okamura H, Yamamura K. A 6-kb upstream region of the human transthyretin gene can direct developmental, tissue-specific, and quantitatively normal expression in transgenic mouse. J Biochem. 1995;117:169–75.

46. Sousa JC, Marques F, Dias-Ferreira E, Cerqueira JJ, Sousa N, Palha JA. Transthyretin influences spatial reference memory. Neurobiol Learn Mem. 2007;88:381–5.

47. Buxbaum JN, Reixach N. Transthyretin: the servant of many masters. Cell Mol Life Sci. 2009;66:3095–101.

48. Costa R, Ferreira-da-Silva F, Saraiva MJ, Cardoso I. Transthyretin protects against A-beta peptide toxicity by proteolytic cleavage of the peptide: a mechanism sensitive to the Kunitz protease inhibitor. PLoS ONE. 2008;3:e2899.

49. Liz MA, Faro CJ, Saraiva MJ, Sousa MM. Transthyretin, a new cryptic protease. J Biol Chem. 2004;279:21431–8.

50. Liz MA, Fleming CE, Nunes AF, Almeida MR, Mar FM, Choe Y, Craik CS, Powers JC, Bogyo M, Sousa MM. Substrate specificity of transthyretin: identification of natural substrates in the nervous system. Biochem J. 2009;419:467–74.

51. Silva CS, Eira J, Ribeiro CA, Oliveira Â, Sousa MM, Cardoso I, Liz MA. Transthyretin neuroprotection in Alzheimer's disease is dependent on proteolysis. Neurobiol Aging. 2017;59:10–4.

52. Alemi M, Gaiteiro C, Ribeiro CA, Santos LM, Gomes JR, Oliveira SM, Couraud PO, Weksler B, Romero I, Saraiva MJ, Cardoso I. Transthyretin participates in beta-amyloid transport from the brain to the liver—involvement of the low-density lipoprotein receptor-related protein 1? Sci Rep. 2016;6:20164.

53. Fleming CE, Saraiva MJ, Sousa MM. Transthyretin enhances nerve regeneration. J Neurochem. 2007;103:831–9.

54. Zawiślak A, Jakimowicz P, McCubrey JA, Rakus D. Neuron-derived transthyretin modulates astrocytic glycolysis in hormone-independent manner. Oncotarget. 2017;8:106625–38.

# 21

# Sex-specific differences in organic anion transporting polypeptide 1a4 (Oatp1a4) functional expression at the blood–brain barrier in Sprague–Dawley rats

Hrvoje Brzica, Wazir Abdullahi, Bianca G. Reilly and Patrick T. Ronaldson[*] (ID)

## Abstract

**Background:** Targeting endogenous blood–brain barrier (BBB) transporters such as organic anion transporting polypeptide 1a4 (Oatp1a4) can facilitate drug delivery for treatment of neurological diseases. Advancement of Oatp targeting for optimization of CNS drug delivery requires characterization of sex-specific differences in BBB expression and/or activity of this transporter.

**Methods:** In this study, we investigated sex differences in Oatp1a4 functional expression at the BBB in adult and prepubertal (i.e., 6-week-old) Sprague–Dawley rats. We also performed castration or ovariectomy surgeries to assess the role of gonadal hormones on Oatp1a4 protein expression and transport activity at the BBB. *Slco1a4* (i.e., the gene encoding Oatp1a4) mRNA expression and Oatp1a4 protein expression in brain microvessels was determined using quantitative real-time PCR and western blot analysis, respectively. Oatp transport function at the BBB was determined via in situ brain perfusion using [$^3$H]taurocholate and [$^3$H]atorvastatin as probe substrates. Data were expressed as mean ± SD and analyzed via one-way ANOVA followed by the post hoc Bonferroni t-test.

**Results:** Our results showed increased brain microvascular *Slco1a4* mRNA and Oatp1a4 protein expression as well as increased brain uptake of [$^3$H]taurocholate and [$^3$H]atorvastatin in female rats as compared to males. Oatp1a4 expression at the BBB was enhanced in castrated male animals but was not affected by ovariectomy in female animals. In prepubertal rats, no sex-specific differences in brain microvascular Oatp1a4 expression were observed. Brain accumulation of [$^3$H]taurocholate in male rats was increased following castration as compared to controls. In contrast, there was no difference in [$^3$H]taurocholate brain uptake between ovariectomized and control female rats.

**Conclusions:** These novel data confirm sex-specific differences in BBB Oatp1a4 functional expression, findings that have profound implications for treatment of CNS diseases. Studies are ongoing to fully characterize molecular pathways that regulate sex differences in Oatp1a4 expression and activity.

**Keywords:** Blood–brain barrier, Drug delivery, Organic anion transporting polypeptides, Sex differences, Transporters

*Correspondence: pronald@email.arizona.edu
Department of Pharmacology, College of Medicine, University of Arizona,
P.O. Box 245050, 1501 N. Campbell Avenue, Tucson, AZ 85724-5050, USA

## Background

Effective pharmacotherapy of neurological diseases requires that drugs permeate the blood–brain barrier (BBB) and attain efficacious concentrations in the central nervous system (CNS). Indeed, current research has significantly advanced our understanding of BBB physiology such that endogenous transporters expressed at the microvascular endothelium have emerged as molecular targets that can be exploited for CNS drug delivery. Transporters that have been identified and characterized at the BBB include members of the solute carrier (SLC) and the adenosine triphosphate (ATP)-binding cassette (ABC) superfamilies of transporter proteins [1, 2]. In most cases, SLC transporters facilitate blood-to-brain transport of drugs. In contrast, ABC family members transport their substrates in the opposite direction (i.e., brain-to-blood) and, therefore, function as efflux transporters [3]. P-glycoprotein (P-gp) is a critical ABC transporter that is expressed at the BBB and is involved in limiting brain penetration of many currently marketed drugs. Many studies have attempted to improve CNS drug delivery by inhibiting transport function of P-gp; however, these strategies have not translated into the clinic due to inhibitor toxicity and poor pharmacokinetics [4–6]. Such observations suggest that direct inhibition of P-gp-mediated transport is not a viable approach for optimization of drug delivery to the brain.

The translational challenges associated with targeting P-gp indicate a need for a change in thought regarding BBB transporters. Our laboratory has proposed that a more rational strategy would be to target SLC transporters. Over the past several years, we have focused our research endeavors on characterizing regulation and functional expression of organic anion-transporting polypeptides (Oatps) [7–10], SLC family members that have several isoforms endogenously expressed at the BBB (i.e., Oatp1a4, Oatp1c1, Oatp2a1) [8, 11–16]. At the rodent BBB, the primary drug-transporting Oatp isoform is Oatp1a4 [8]. This is evidenced by studies in Oatp1a4(−/−) mice where blood-to-brain transport of clinically-relevant Oatp substrates was reduced as compared to wild-type controls [15]. Of particular significance, 3-hydroxy-3-methylglutaryl-coenzyme A (HMG-CoA) reductase inhibitors (i.e., statins) have been shown to be transport substrates for Oatp1a4 [8, 9, 17]. Statins are intriguing compounds for treatment of CNS diseases due to their neuroprotective effects [9, 18, 19]. The human orthologue of Oatp1a4 is OATP1A2, which shows similarities in localization and expression at the brain microvascular endothelium [20, 21]. Of translational significance, OATP1A2 can also transport statins such as atorvastatin and rosuvastatin [22–24].

Critical considerations in development of Oatp1a4/OATP1A2 as a molecular target for CNS drug delivery are biological variables that can modulate expression and/or activity of transporters. Specifically, sex-specific differences in Oatp functional expression must be understood in order to design effective treatment strategies where blood-to-brain drug transport is to be optimized. Indeed, such differences in SLC transporter expression and/or function have been reported in the scientific literature. For example, Cao and colleagues reported reduced expression of monocarboxylate transporter 4 (MCT4), a member of the SLC family, in liver tissue isolated from female Sprague–Dawley rats as compared to their male counterparts [25]. Additionally, this same group observed that ovariectomy caused significant differences in expression of MCT1 and MCT4, indicating a role for sex hormones in regulation of this transporter [25]. In brain tissue, expression of mRNA for organic cation transporter 3 was shown to be higher in male mice as compared to female mice [26, 27]. Several publications have reported sex-specific differences in Oatp1a4 expression in other tissues, albeit with different observations. For example, hepatic expression of Oatp1a4 was reported to be higher in female mice as compared to male mice; however, hepatic expression of this transporter was equal in male and female rats [28–30]. In contrast, Oatp1a4 mRNA and protein expression was observed to be higher in liver tissue from male Sprague–Dawley rats as compared to age-matched females [31]. Similarly, hepatic Oatp1a4 mRNA expression was 67% higher in 42-day-old male Sprague–Dawley rats [32]. This same study did not report any sex-specific differences in Oatp1a4 expression and/or activity in the kidney [32]. At present, there are not any published studies on sex-specific differences in Oatp1a4 functional expression at the BBB or on variability in Oatp-mediated CNS drug delivery between male and female experimental animals.

The goal of this study was to examine Oatp1a4 functional expression at the BBB in female Sprague–Dawley rats and in age-matched male rats. We hypothesize that biologically relevant differences in brain microvascular *Slco1a4* mRNA expression and Oatp1a4 protein expression as well as blood-to-brain transport of established Oatp substrates (i.e., taurocholate, atorvastatin) exist due to variability based on sex. Overall, data derived from this study will provide key information that will inform future work aimed at targeting Oatp-mediated transport for optimization of CNS drug delivery.

## Methods

### Materials

All chemicals utilized in our experiments were purchased from Sigma-Aldrich (St. Louis, MO) unless otherwise stated.

## Animals

Experimental animals were housed under standard 12 h light/12 h dark conditions and provided with food and water ad libitum. Animals were randomly assigned to each treatment group. Male and female Sprague–Dawley rats (200–250 g; 3 months old; Envigo, Denver, CO) were used for our studies. For experiments requiring prepubertal animals, 6-week-old male and female Sprague–Dawley rats (Envigo) were utilized.

## Ovariectomy procedure

Ovariectomy was performed on 6-week-old prepubertal female Sprague–Dawley rats using the dorsal approach as previously described [33]. Briefly, animals were anesthetized (100 mg/kg ketamine, 20 mg/kg xylazine, i.p.) and prepared for surgery. A skin incision was made on each side of an experimental animal in the lumbar region approximately 1 cm lateral to the spinal cord using a sterile surgical blade. A window in the muscular wall was made using surgical scissors and both ovaries were localized and exposed. Following ligation of the ovarian artery, ovarian vein, and uterine horn, the ovaries were removed. The remaining portion of the uterine horn was checked for bleeding and the abdominal wall was closed using 4-0 absorbable surgical thread. The skin was stapled using appropriate skin staplers. Sham operated animals (i.e., controls) underwent the same procedure but without removal of the ovaries.

## Castration procedure

Castrations were performed on 6-week-old prepubertal male Sprague–Dawley rats as previously described [33]. Briefly, animals were anesthetized with ketamine/xylazine and prepared for surgery. Testes were exposed via a transversal incision on the scrotal sac. Each testis was freed and gently excised from the scrotal sac, which enabled access to the deferent duct. The deferent duct was then ligated and both testis with their associated epididymis were removed. The remaining portion of the deferent duct was inspected for bleeding and the scrotal skin was sutured using 4-0 absorbable surgical thread. Sham operated animals (i.e., controls) underwent the same procedure but without testicular removal.

## Microvessel isolation

Microvessel isolation was performed using a protocol developed in our laboratory [10, 34]. Following euthanasia by decapitation, brains were harvested and meninges and choroid plexus were removed. Cerebral hemispheres were homogenized at 3700×g in 5 ml brain microvessel buffer (300 mM mannitol, 5 mM EGTA, 12 mM Tris HCl, pH 7.4) containing protease inhibitor cocktail

(Sigma-Aldrich). At this time, 8 ml 26% (w/v) dextran (MW 75,000; Spectrum Chemical Manufacturing Corporation, Gardena, CA) solution was added to each homogenate sample. Samples were then thoroughly vortexed and centrifuged at 5000×g for 15 min at 4 °C. The supernatant was then aspirated and capillary pellets were resuspended in 5 ml of brain microvessel buffer. Dextran homogenization and centrifugation steps were repeated an additional three times to ensure appropriate quality of microvessels as demonstrated in our recent publication [10]. Following completion of dextran homogenization and centrifugation, the supernatant was aspirated and the microvessel pellet was resuspended in 5 ml of brain microvessel buffer. At this time, samples were homogenized at 3700×g, placed into ultracentrifuge tubes, and centrifuged at 150,000×g for 60 min at 4 °C. Pellets containing total cellular membranes [33] were resuspended in 500 µl of storage buffer (50% brain microvessel isolation buffer; 50% diH$_2$O, v/v) containing protease inhibitor cocktail. Samples were stored at −80 °C until further use. Purity of our microvessel preparations was shown by demonstrating enrichment in platelet endothelial cell adhesion molecule-1 (PECAM-1) as well as reduced expression of neuronal marker proteins (i.e., synaptophysin) [10, 34].

## Western blot analysis

Western blotting was performed as previously described [9, 10] with few modifications. Isolated microvessel membrane samples were quantified for total protein using Bradford reagent (Sigma-Aldrich) and heated at 37 °C for 30 min under reducing conditions (i.e., 2.5% (v/v) 2-mercaptoethanol (Sigma-Aldrich) in 1X Laemmli sample buffer (Bio-Rad, Hercules, CA) for Oatp1a4 detection. Each microvessel sample was derived from brain tissue isolated from a single experimental animal in accordance with our published protocol [34]. Following SDS-PAGE and transfer, polyvinylidene fluoride (PVDF) membranes were incubated overnight at 4 °C with primary antibodies against Oatp1a4 (anti-Oatp2, Santa Cruz Biotechnology, Dallas, TX; 1:1000 dilution) or tubulin (anti-α tubulin, Abcam, Boston, MA; 1:20,000 dilution). Microvessel purity was assessed by incubating PVDF membranes overnight at 4 °C with primary antibodies against platelet endothelial cell adhesion molecule-1 (PECAM-1; anti-CD31, Abcam, 1:100 dilution), glial fibrillary acidic protein (GFAP; anti-GFAP, Abcam; 1:20,000 dilution) or synaptophysin (anti-synaptophysin, Abcam; 1:800,000 dilution). Membranes were washed and incubated with horseradish peroxidase-conjugated anti-rabbit IgG (Jackson ImmunoResearch, 1:40,000 dilution) or anti-mouse IgG (Jackson ImmunoResearch, 1:50,000 dilution) for 60 min at room temperature. Membranes were developed using enhanced chemiluminescence (Super Signal West Pico, Thermo-Fisher). Bands were quantitated using ImageJ software (Wayne Rasband, Research Services Branch, National Institute of Mental Health, Bethesda, MD) and normalized to tubulin.

### Quantitative PCR analysis

Total RNA was extracted from brain microvessels isolated from male and female Sprague–Dawley rats using the Aurum Total RNA extraction kit (Bio-Rad, Hercules, CA). Extracted RNA was treated with amplification grade DNaseI (Bio-Rad) to remove contaminating genomic DNA. The concentration of RNA in each sample was quantified spectrophotometrically by measuring UV absorbance at 260 nm. The iScript reverse transcriptase kit (Bio-Rad) was used to synthesize first-strand cDNA. Primer pairs were prepared by Integrated DNA Technologies (Coralville, IA). Primer sequences for amplification of *Slco1a4* mRNA were as follows: forward primer 5'-GCTTCTTCATAAAAACAGCAGTAA-3', reverse primer 5'-TGCACATGTTAATGCCAACAG-3'. Primers were designed to be complimentary to sequences located on two different exons separated by an intron to avoid amplification of genomic DNA. Quantitative PCR was performed using SYBR green master mix (Bio-Rad) on a CFX96 Touch Real-Time PCR Detection System (Bio-Rad). The quantity of the target gene (i.e., *Slco1a4*) was normalized to GAPDH using the comparative CT method ($\Delta\Delta$CT). Primer sequences for amplification of *GAPDH* mRNA were as previously published by our laboratory [35].

### In situ brain perfusion

Animals were anesthetized (100 mg/kg ketamine, 20 mg/kg xylazine, i.p.) and heparinized (10,000 U/kg, i.p.). Body temperature was maintained at 37 °C using a heating pad. The common carotid arteries were cannulated with silicone tubing connected to a perfusion circuit. The perfusate was an erythrocyte-free modified mammalian Ringer's solution consisting of 117 mM NaCl, 4.7 mM KCl, 0.8 mM $MgSO_4$, 1.2 mM $KH_2PO_4$, 2.5 mM $CaCl_2$, 10 mM D-glucose, 3.9% (w/v) dextran (MW 75,000), and 1.0 g/l bovine serum albumin (type IV), pH 7.4, warmed to 37 °C and continuously oxygenated with 95% $O_2$/5% $CO_2$. Evan's blue dye (55 mg/l) was added to the perfusate to serve as a visual marker of BBB integrity. Perfusion pressure and flow rate were maintained at 95–105 mmHg and 3.1 ml/min, respectively. Both jugular veins were severed to allow for drainage of the perfusate. Using a slow-drive syringe pump (0.5 ml/min per hemisphere; Harvard Apparatus, Holliston, MA), [3H]taurocholate (1.0 µCi/ml; 10 mM total concentration; PerkinElmer, Boston, MA) or [3H]atorvastatin (0.5 µCi/ml; 0.013 µM

total concentration; American Radiolabeled Chemicals, St. Louis, MO) was added to the inflowing perfusate. For inhibition studies, animals were perfused with erythrocyte-free modified mammalian Ringer's solution containing transport inhibitor [i.e., 100 µM estrone-3-sulfate (E3S) or fexofenadine (FEX)] for 10 min prior to perfusion with [3H]taurocholate or [3H]atorvastatin. After perfusion, the rat was decapitated and the brain was removed. Meninges and choroid plexus were excised and cerebral hemispheres were isolated and homogenized. At this time, TS2 tissue solubilizer (1 ml) was added and each sample was allowed to solubilize for 2 days at room temperature. To eliminate chemiluminescence, 100 µl of 30% glacial acetic acid was added, along with 2 ml Optiphase SuperMix liquid scintillation cocktail (PerkinElmer, Boston, MA). Samples were measured for radioactivity on a model 1450 liquid scintillation counter (PerkinElmer).

Results were reported as picomoles of radiolabeled drug per milligram of brain tissue (C; pmol/mg tissue), which is equal to the total amount of radioisotope in the brain ($C_{Brain}$; dpm/mg tissue) divided by the amount of radioisotope in the perfusate ($C_{Perfusate}$; dpm/pmol): $C = C_{Brain}/C_{Perfusate}$. In a previous study using modified Ringer's solution for perfusion, the brain vascular volume in rats was shown to range between 6 and 9 µl/g brain tissue [36]. Since brain tissue was processed immediately after perfusion with radiolabeled substrate, all uptake values required correction for brain vascular volume. This was accomplished by subtracting the average vascular volume (i.e., 8 µl/g brain tissue as calculated from data reported by Takasato and colleagues) from whole-brain uptake data obtained for [3H]taurocholate or [3H] atorvastatin.

### Statistical analysis

Western blot data are reported as mean ± SD of the ratio of Oatp1a4 protein expression to tubulin protein expression where each treatment group consists of microvessel protein samples from six individual animals. These sample sizes were based on the ability to detect a 35% difference between treatment with 20% variability. Quantitative PCR data are reported as mean ± SD where each treatment group consists of microvessel mRNA samples from six individual animals. In situ brain perfusion data are reported as mean ± SD from six individual animals per treatment group. To determine statistical significance between treatment groups, Student's *t*-test was used for unpaired experimental data. When an experiment incorporated more than two treatment groups (i.e., in situ brain perfusion inhibition studies), statistical significance was determined using one-way ANOVA followed by the post hoc multiple-comparison Bonferroni $t$-test. A value of $p < 0.05$ was accepted as statistically significant.

## Results

### Oatp1a4 mRNA and protein expression is increased in brain microvessels isolated from female adult Sprague–Dawley rats

Our laboratory has previously demonstrated that functional expression of Oatp1a4 at the BBB is a critical determinant of blood-to-brain transport of drugs [7, 9]; however, it is unknown if expression and/or activity of this transporter differs between male and female experimental animals. To address this critical pharmacological question, we performed brain microvessel isolations from male and female Sprague–Dawley rats and measured expression of *Slco1a4* mRNA and Oatp1a4 protein. We have confirmed purity of our microvessel samples by demonstrating enrichment of the endothelial cell marker PECAM-1 (Fig. 1). Additionally, we show increased PECAM-1 expression in our microvessel samples as compared to expression of the astrocyte marker glial fibrillary acidic protein (GFAP) and the neuronal marker synaptophysin, which further demonstrates the purity of our microvessel preparations (Fig. 1). Microvessel sample preparations of similar purity were used for all subsequent biochemical experiments performed in this study. We observed increased expression of *Slco1a4* (4.2-fold) in rat brain microvessels isolated from female Sprague–Dawley rats as compared to their male counterparts (Fig. 2a). Similarly, Oatp1a4 protein expression was greater (3.3-fold) in microvessels isolated from female animals as compared to male Sprague–Dawley rats (Fig. 2b). The anti-Oatp2 antibody that was used in

these western blot experiments recognizes an epitope corresponding to amino acids 611–660 on the Oatp1a4 protein sequence. Proper sample loading was confirmed by measurement of tubulin, a protein that polymerizes into microtubules and forms a critical component of the cytoskeleton in eukaryotic cells.

### Brain uptake of Oatp transport substrates are increased in female Sprague–Dawley rats

To determine whether differences in Oatp1a4 expression at the BBB between male and female animals corresponded to altered blood-to-brain transport of Oatp1a4 substrates (i.e., functional changes), the in situ brain perfusion technique was utilized. Brain uptake of [3H]taurocholate, a soluble bile salt and established probe drug for Oatp-mediated transport, was measured in adult male and female Sprague–Dawley rats. We have previously demonstrated that perfusion with [3H]taurocholate provides a unique opportunity to rigorously study differences in BBB uptake transport due to pathophysiological and pharmacological stress [7, 9, 10]. In this study, we are applying this approach to examine differences in Oatp-mediated transport due to biological variability. After a 10 min perfusion, [3H]taurocholate (10 µM) accumulation was significantly greater (2.2-fold) in brain tissue isolated from female Sprague–Dawley rats (Fig. 3a). To confirm that observed changes in [3H]taurocholate brain uptake was associated with changes in Oatp-mediated transport, male and female Sprague–Dawley rats were perfused in the presence and absence of known Oatp transport inhibitors [i.e., estrone-3-sulfate (E3S), fexofenadine (FEX)] for 10 min before perfusion with [3H]taurocholate. E3S significantly decreased [3H]taurocholate accumulation in both sexes (Fig. 3a), suggesting that blood-to-brain transport of taurocholate is an Oatp-dependent process. Similarly, we observed increased accumulation of [3H]atorvastatin (2.2-fold), a currently marketed Oatp transport substrate, in brain tissue extracted from female Sprague–Dawley rats as compared to their male counterparts (Fig. 3b). Both estrone-3-sulfate and fexofenadine decreased brain uptake of [3H] atorvastatin, an observation that indicates involvement of an Oatp-mediated process (Fig. 3b). Using high performance liquid chromatography analysis of inflow and outflow perfusate, we have previously shown that both [3H[taurocholate and [3H]atorvastatin remain intact throughout our perfusion experiments [7, 9].

### There are no differences in Oatp1a4 protein expression in brain microvessels isolated from Male and female prepubertal Sprague–Dawley rats

Since we observed elevated Oatp1a4 protein expression in female rats as compared to male rats, we postulated

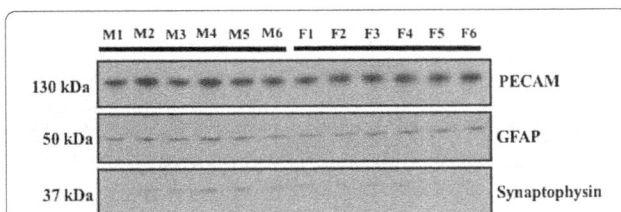

**Fig. 1** Expression of endothelial cell, astrocyte, and neuronal marker proteins in brain microvessels isolated from male and female Sprague–Dawley rats. Western blot analysis shows the presence of a single band corresponding to the endothelial marker platelet endothelial cell adhesion molecule-1 (PECAM-1; also known as CD31) (130 kDa) in male (M1–6) and female (F1–6) experimental animals. While single bands for the astrocyte marker glial fibrillary acidic protein (GFAP) (50 kDa) and the neuronal marker synaptophysin (37 kDa) in samples prepared from male and female animals, their expression was considerably lower as compared to PECAM. These observations emphasize the high purity of the microvessel preparations utilized in all subsequent experiments

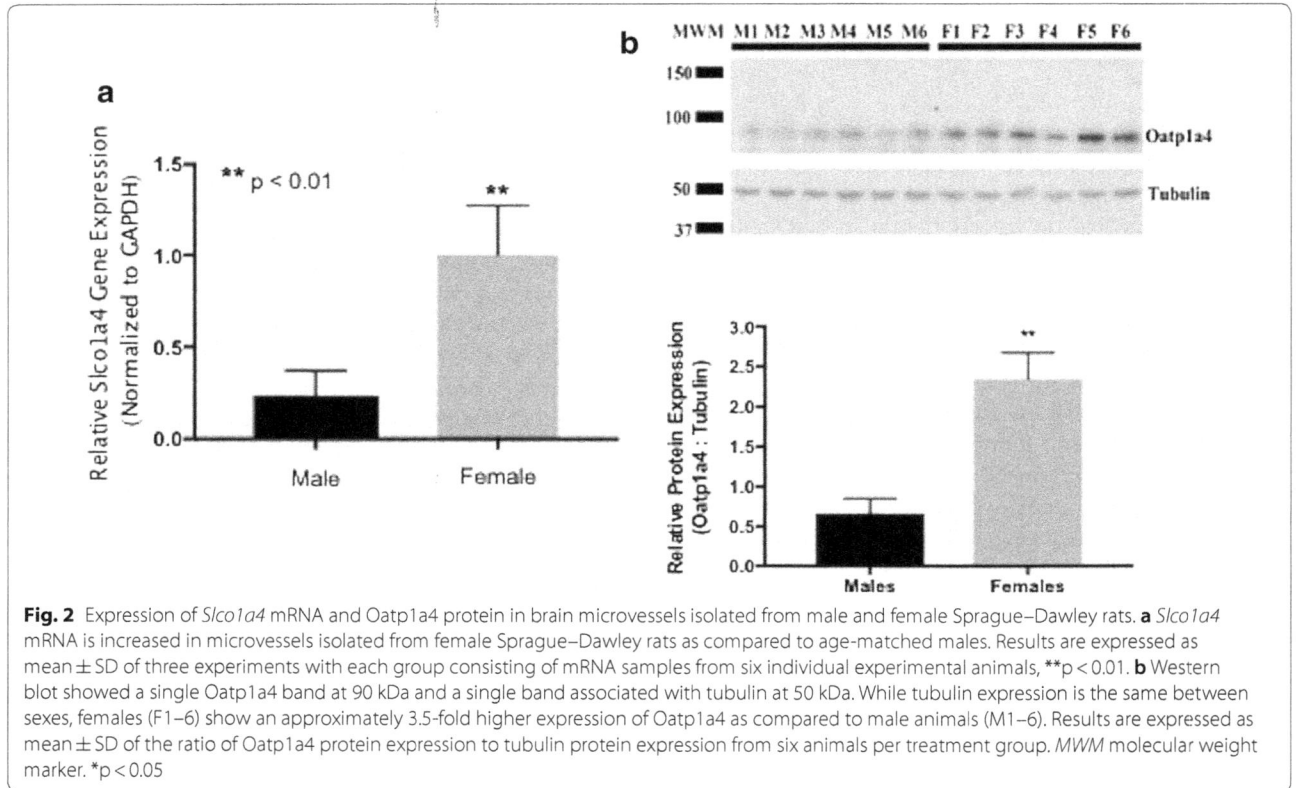

**Fig. 2** Expression of *Slco1a4* mRNA and Oatp1a4 protein in brain microvessels isolated from male and female Sprague–Dawley rats. **a** *Slco1a4* mRNA is increased in microvessels isolated from female Sprague–Dawley rats as compared to age-matched males. Results are expressed as mean ± SD of three experiments with each group consisting of mRNA samples from six individual experimental animals, **p < 0.01. **b** Western blot showed a single Oatp1a4 band at 90 kDa and a single band associated with tubulin at 50 kDa. While tubulin expression is the same between sexes, females (F1–6) show an approximately 3.5-fold higher expression of Oatp1a4 as compared to male animals (M1–6). Results are expressed as mean ± SD of the ratio of Oatp1a4 protein expression to tubulin protein expression from six animals per treatment group. *MWM* molecular weight marker. *p < 0.05

that sex hormones may play a role in regulation of this critical BBB transporter. To address this hypothesis, brain microvessels were isolated from male and female prepubertal rats. These experimental animals were 6 weeks old, an age where gonadal hormones are considerably lower than observed in adult Sprague–Dawley rats [37]. We did not observe a significant difference in Oatp1a4 protein expression in brain microvessels isolated from prepubertal male Sprague–Dawley rats as compared to their female counterparts (Fig. 4). There was also no significant difference in tubulin expression in male and female prepubertal animals, which confirmed equal sample loading.

### Oatp1a4 protein expression in increased in brain microvessels isolated from castrated male Sprague–Dawley rats

To further assess the role of gonadal hormones on regulation of Oatp1a4 expression at the BBB, we castrated prepubertal male Sprague–Dawley rats. These animals were permitted to recover and then were aged 8 weeks (i.e., when gonadal hormones are typically produced). At this time, castrated male rats and age-matched control animals were euthanized and brain microvessels were isolated for western blot analysis. We detected a significant increase in Oatp1a4 protein expression (up

to 6.5-fold) in brain microvessels isolated from castrated males (Fig. 5). Proper sample loading was confirmed by measuring tubulin expression in microvessels isolated from castrated male Sprague–Dawley rats and from control animals. Similarly, we assessed Oatp1a4 protein expression in brain microvessels isolated from ovariectomized female Sprague–Dawley rats and age-matched controls. We observed that ovariectomy did not result in any change in microvascular Oatp1a4 protein expression (Fig. 6).

### Brain uptake of the Oatp transport substrate taurocholate is increased in castrated male Sprague–Dawley rats

Since we observed enhancement of brain microvascular Oatp1a4 expression in castrated male Sprague–Dawley rats, we sought to determine if this increase resulted in modification of Oatp transport activity. Therefore, we used in situ brain perfusion to measure brain uptake of the established Oatp transport substrate [³H]taurocholate in castrated male animals and in age-matched controls. We observed a significant increase in [³H]taurocholate accumulation in brain tissue isolated from castrated male Sprague–Dawley rats, suggesting an increase in Oatp transport activity (Fig. 7a). We also measured [³H]taurocholate uptake in brain tissue derived from

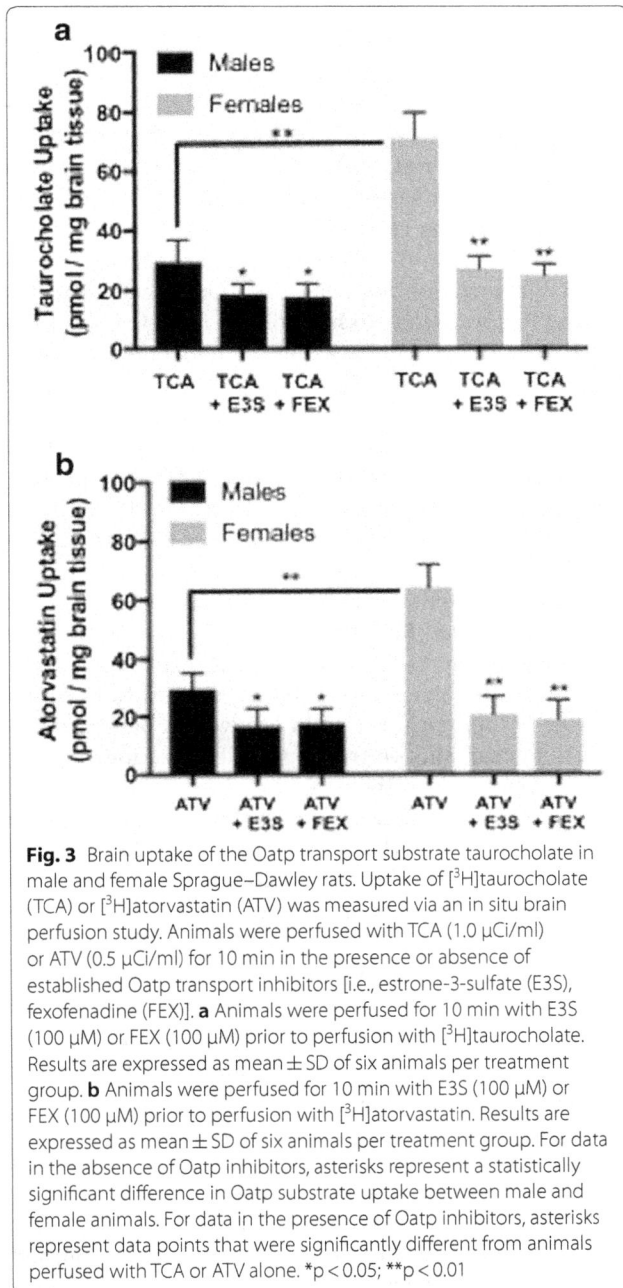

**Fig. 3** Brain uptake of the Oatp transport substrate taurocholate in male and female Sprague–Dawley rats. Uptake of [$^3$H]taurocholate (TCA) or [$^3$H]atorvastatin (ATV) was measured via an in situ brain perfusion study. Animals were perfused with TCA (1.0 µCi/ml) or ATV (0.5 µCi/ml) for 10 min in the presence or absence of established Oatp transport inhibitors [i.e., estrone-3-sulfate (E3S), fexofenadine (FEX)]. **a** Animals were perfused for 10 min with E3S (100 µM) or FEX (100 µM) prior to perfusion with [$^3$H]taurocholate. Results are expressed as mean ± SD of six animals per treatment group. **b** Animals were perfused for 10 min with E3S (100 µM) or FEX (100 µM) prior to perfusion with [$^3$H]atorvastatin. Results are expressed as mean ± SD of six animals per treatment group. For data in the absence of Oatp inhibitors, asterisks represent a statistically significant difference in Oatp substrate uptake between male and female animals. For data in the presence of Oatp inhibitors, asterisks represent data points that were significantly different from animals perfused with TCA or ATV alone. *p < 0.05; **p < 0.01

## Discussion

Sex is a significant determinant in the pathogenesis of multiple neurological diseases. This concept is best exemplified by ischemic stroke where current epidemiological data strongly indicates that stroke severity and post-stroke outcomes are highly dependent on biological variability [38]. Specifically, younger men (i.e., under the age of 45 years) are more likely to experience ischemic stroke with poorer functional recovery as compared to women of the same chronological age [39]. Incidence of stroke in women between 45 and 54 years of age increases, possibly as an effect related to changes in circulating sex hormone levels that are associated with menopause [1, 39]. From the age of 55 years onward, there are no sex differences in stroke incidence until the age of 85 years when women are at an elevated risk for ischemic stroke [39]. Within the past few years, the National Institutes of Health has emphasized the critical requirement to understand biological differences between sexes in an effort to design and develop more effective treatments for neurological diseases including ischemic stroke [40, 41]. Indeed, several studies have been reported in the scientific literature that demonstrate sex-specific differences in neuronal signaling, immune responses, and inflammation following stroke onset [41–45]. Clearly, this knowledge can inform development of new chemical entities that engage molecular targets in brain parenchyma relevant to ischemic stroke; however, such therapies cannot be rendered effective if therapeutic agents are unable to permeate the BBB and achieve efficacious concentrations in the CNS. This pharmacological fact implies a necessity to characterize sex-specific differences in BBB transport mechanisms. To date, there are no published studies examining such differences in endogenous transporter expression and/or function at the BBB. This constitutes an immense knowledge gap in the field. Indeed, understanding sex-specific differences in transporter expression offers an opportunity to provide more efficient brain delivery of neuroprotective agents to all patients afflicted by ischemic stroke.

Over the past several years, our laboratory has been interested in studying BBB transport properties of Oatp1a4, an SLC transporter that can facilitate blood-to-brain transport of multiple currently-marketed drugs [1, 7–10]. While our observations generally agreed with previous studies that reported Oatp1a4 functional expression at the BBB [14, 15, 20, 46], others showed limited, or lack of, expression of this transporter at the BBB [47, 48]. For example, Roberts and colleagues observed weak luminal Oatp1a4 staining by immunofluorescence microscopy and were unable to detect Oatp1a4 protein in microvascular protein fractions by western blotting analysis [47]. While a targeted

ovariectomized female Sprague–Dawley rats and corresponding age-matched controls. In these animals, there was no difference in brain [$^3$H]taurocholate uptake (Fig. 7b). Taken together, these data provide evidence for sex-related differences in Oatp1a4 functional expression at the BBB in Sprague–Dawley rats. Our novel results also suggest that male gonadal hormones may be a critical determinant of BBB expression and/or activity of this critical endogenous uptake transporter.

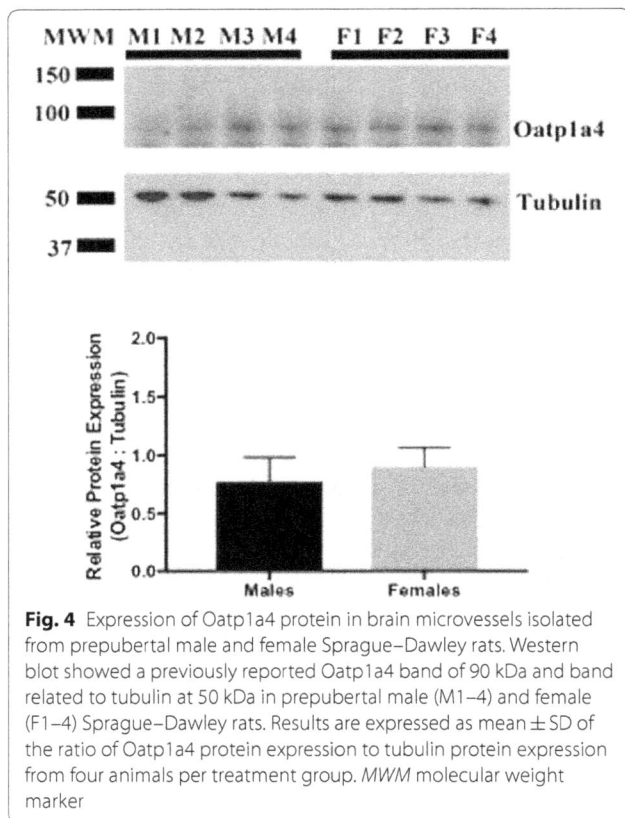

**Fig. 4** Expression of Oatp1a4 protein in brain microvessels isolated from prepubertal male and female Sprague–Dawley rats. Western blot showed a previously reported Oatp1a4 band of 90 kDa and band related to tubulin at 50 kDa in prepubertal male (M1–4) and female (F1–4) Sprague–Dawley rats. Results are expressed as mean ± SD of the ratio of Oatp1a4 protein expression to tubulin protein expression from four animals per treatment group. *MWM* molecular weight marker

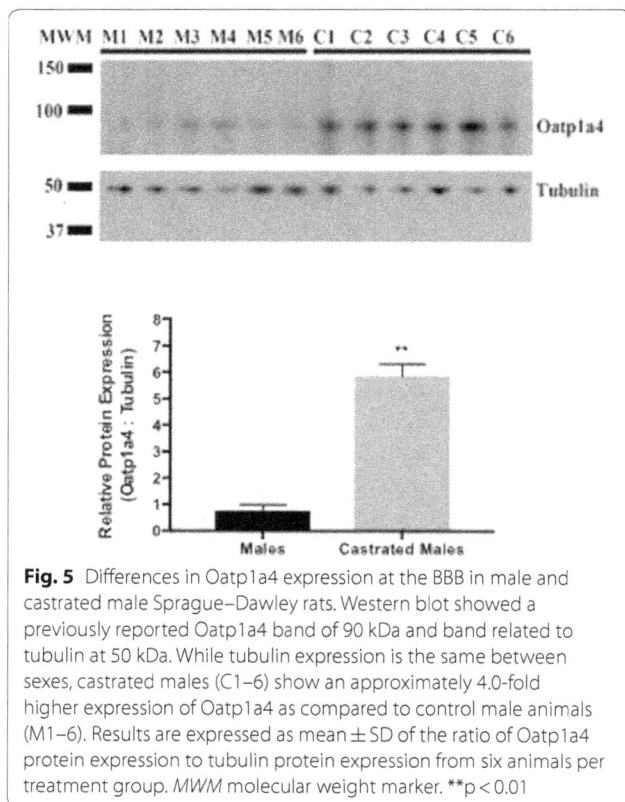

**Fig. 5** Differences in Oatp1a4 expression at the BBB in male and castrated male Sprague–Dawley rats. Western blot showed a previously reported Oatp1a4 band of 90 kDa and band related to tubulin at 50 kDa. While tubulin expression is the same between sexes, castrated males (C1–6) show an approximately 4.0-fold higher expression of Oatp1a4 as compared to control male animals (M1–6). Results are expressed as mean ± SD of the ratio of Oatp1a4 protein expression to tubulin protein expression from six animals per treatment group. *MWM* molecular weight marker. **$p < 0.01$

proteomic quantitative analysis of BBB transporters in male ddy mice showed expression of Oatp1a4 at the brain microvascular endothelium [49], similar studies in rats (i.e., Sprague–Dawley and Wistar) and in non-human primates (i.e., marmosets) of both sexes did not attempt to measure Oatp1a4 expression [48]. This same group used a similar approach in human brain tissue and could not detect expression of OATP1A2 [50, 51]. Indeed, Uchida and colleagues examined brain tissue isolated from males [50] while Shawahna and colleagues studied temporal lobe tissue isolated from females [51]. It is particularly significant that the female tissue specimens examined in the Shawahna study were collected from the brain of individuals with a positive diagnosis of epilepsy. Interestingly, preclinical studies in a rodent model of chronic epilepsy showed decreased protein expression of Oatp1a4 (also known as Oatp2) in brain tissue [52]. Additionally, OATP1A2 protein expression was detected at the luminal membrane of brain microvascular endothelial cells in brain tissue isolated from male and female glioma patients [53]. The conflicting observations on OATP1A2/Oatp1a4 expression indicate a need for detailed preclinical studies to examine the role of biological variability as well as pathophysiological mechanisms on transporter localization, expression, and function at the BBB.

In the present study, we show for the first time that BBB expression of Oatp1a4 is more than threefold higher in female Sprague–Dawley rats as compared to their male counterparts. Such sex-specific differences in Oatp1a4 expression at the brain microvascular endothelium may explain differences between our data and other published studies that have utilized only male experimental animals. We also showed that sex-specific differences in Oatp1a4 protein expression at the BBB corresponds to a measurable enhancement in CNS uptake of the known Oatp transport substrates, taurocholate and atorvastatin, in female Sprague–Dawley rats. While Oatp-mediated transport has been observed in male experimental animals [14, 15, 24], ours is the first study to directly compare differences in BBB transport of two established Oatp transport substrate (i.e., taurocholate, atorvastatin) between male and female experimental animals. Using pharmacological inhibitors of Oatp-mediated transport (i.e., estrone-3-sulfate, fexofenadine), we also demonstrate that differences in taurocholate and atorvastatin brain delivery between male and female animals are primarily due to differences in Oatp-mediated transport. Sex-specific differences in atorvastatin brain uptake are particularly compelling in light of observations indicating that this highly prescribed therapeutic may act as a neuroprotectant in diseases such as Alzheimer's disease [18] and hypoxia/reoxygenation stress [9]. Although other

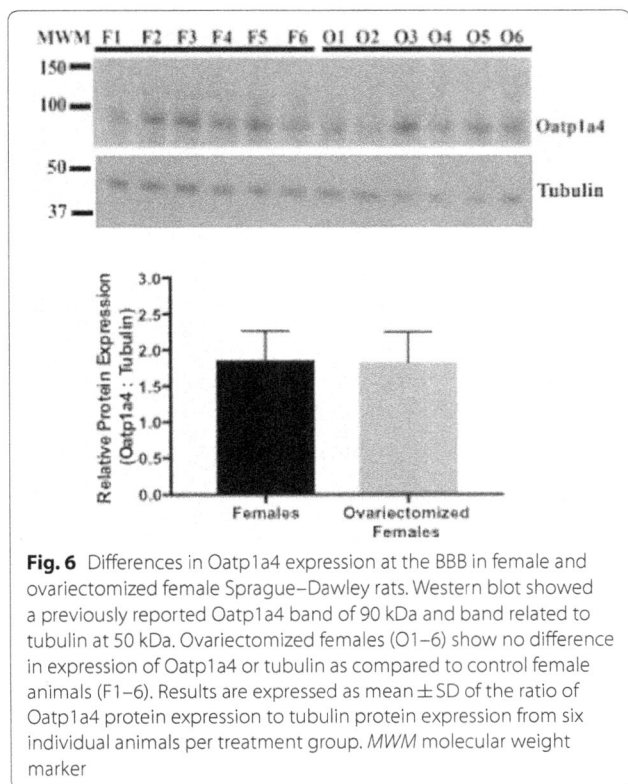

**Fig. 6** Differences in Oatp1a4 expression at the BBB in female and ovariectomized female Sprague–Dawley rats. Western blot showed a previously reported Oatp1a4 band of 90 kDa and band related to tubulin at 50 kDa. Ovariectomized females (O1–6) show no difference in expression of Oatp1a4 or tubulin as compared to control female animals (F1–6). Results are expressed as mean ± SD of the ratio of Oatp1a4 protein expression to tubulin protein expression from six individual animals per treatment group. *MWM* molecular weight marker

Oatp isoforms are expressed at the BBB, their substrate profiles do not include currently marketed drugs. Specifically, Oatp1c1 primarily transports thyroid hormones while Oatp2a1 is a prostaglandin transporter [8]. This renders our new data on Oatp1a4 particularly relevant to pharmacotherapy because it can inform translational studies aimed at improving CNS drug delivery where treatment paradigms are tailored towards an individual patient (i.e., precision medicine).

Additionally, our data demonstrates that functional expression of Oatp1a4 in male Sprague–Dawley rats is upregulated by castration, a unique observation that suggests that this BBB transporter may be repressed by testosterone. Testosterone signaling at the BBB is mediated by androgen receptors, which are well known to be expressed in brain microvascular endothelial cells [54, 55]. The classical model of androgen receptor signaling involves binding of a ligand (i.e., testosterone or its metabolite 5α-dihydrotestosterone) following permeation across the plasma membrane. Once the ligand has bound, androgen receptors undergo a conformational change that causes dissociation of heat shock proteins and translocation of the ligand–receptor complex to the nucleus. Once inside the nucleus, androgen receptor complexes dimerize, bind co-activators, and trigger transcription by binding at androgen response elements in the promoter of target genes [56]. Activated androgen receptors can also interact with caveolae and trigger kinase signaling via pathways such as Src, extracellular signal-regulated protein kinases (ERK), phosphoinositide 3-kinase (PI3K), and Akt [56]. Such non-genomic activity of androgen receptors can lead to regulation of other nuclear receptors, transcription factors, and cytoplasmic signaling events such as intracellular calcium release from the endoplasmic reticulum or mitochondria [56]. Furthermore, these non-genomic actions of androgen receptors may be critical in understanding how testosterone and its metabolites can decrease transporter functional expression at the BBB.

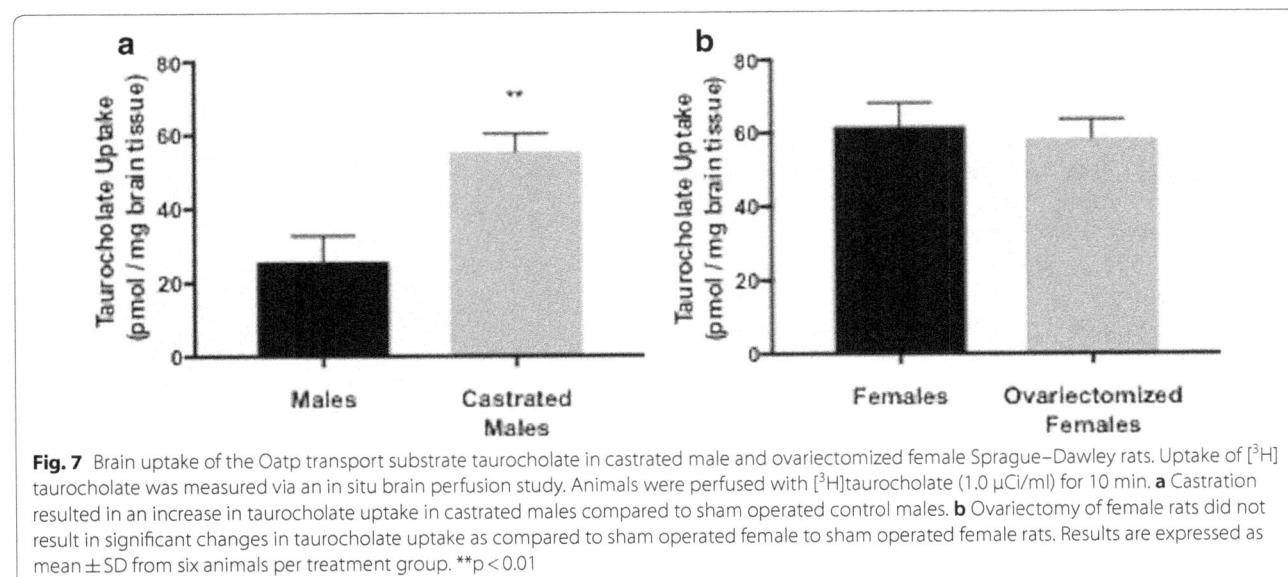

**Fig. 7** Brain uptake of the Oatp transport substrate taurocholate in castrated male and ovariectomized female Sprague–Dawley rats. Uptake of [³H] taurocholate was measured via an in situ brain perfusion study. Animals were perfused with [³H]taurocholate (1.0 µCi/ml) for 10 min. **a** Castration resulted in an increase in taurocholate uptake in castrated males compared to sham operated control males. **b** Ovariectomy of female rats did not result in significant changes in taurocholate uptake as compared to sham operated female to sham operated female rats. Results are expressed as mean ± SD from six animals per treatment group. **p < 0.01

Indeed, repression of SLC transporters in response to testosterone has been reported in other tissues. For example, organic anion transporter 3 (Oat3) expression in the kidney was shown to be elevated in male mice, upregulated following castration, and downregulated in response to testosterone treatment [57]. Similarly, renal expression of Oat2 was lower in adult male rats, increased in castrated males, and decreased following administration of exogenous testosterone [58]. While ours is the first study to provide evidence of SLC transporter repression at the BBB in response to castration, the precise mechanism as to how androgen receptor signaling regulates Oatp isoforms has not been clearly elucidated. Studies are ongoing in our laboratory to determine the complex signaling pathways involved in male sex hormone-mediated transporter repression at the BBB.

## Conclusions

In summary, our novel data show sex-specific differences in Oatp1a4 functional expression at the BBB. Our results indicate that Oatp1a4 expression and transport activity may be repressed at the brain microvascular endothelium in male Sprague–Dawley rats in response to male sex hormones (i.e., testosterone and/or its metabolites). This is the first time that sex-specific differences have been reported for an Oatp isoform at the BBB. Furthermore, these observations are particularly relevant to CNS drug delivery. Since Oatp1a4 has been shown to transport HMG-CoA reductase inhibitors (i.e., statins) such as atorvastatin, and has a similar substrate profile to its human orthologue OATP1A2 [1, 5, 8, 16], these results have considerable pharmacological implications for treatment of CNS diseases. For example, our previous work has shown that atorvastatin has potential to exert neuroprotective effects in the brain [9]; however, sex-specific differences in BBB transport may lead to variable responses to neuroprotective therapies between males and females. Therefore, it is critical to rigorously examine molecular pathways that regulate Oatps at the BBB in order to provide effective pharmacotherapy to all patients via precision medicine approaches. Indeed, studies are ongoing in our laboratory to fully understand sex differences in Oatp1a4 regulation and functional expression at the BBB, work that can inform development of novel therapeutic strategies for treatment of CNS diseases such as ischemic stroke.

## Abbreviations

ABC: ATP-binding cassette; ALK: activin receptor-like kinase; BBB: blood–brain barrier; BMP: bone morphogenetic protein; E3S: estrone-3-sulfate; ERK: extracellular signal-regulated protein kinases; FEX: fexofenadine; GFAP: glial fibrillary acidic protein; H/R: hypoxia–reoxygenation; HMG-CoA: 3-hydroxy-3-methylglutaryl-coenzyme A; MCT: monocarboxylate transporter; Oat: organic anion transporter; Oatp: organic anion transporting polypeptide; PARP: poly-ADP ribose polymerase; PECAM-1: platelet endothelial cell adhesion molecule-1; PI3K: phosphoinositide 3-kinase; P-gp: P-glycoprotein; PVDF: polyvinylidene fluoride; SLC: solute carrier; TGF: transforming growth factor.

## Authors' contributions
Participated in research design: HB, WA, and PTR. Conducted experiments and performed data analysis: HB, WA, BGR, and PTR. Wrote or contributed to the writing of the manuscript: HB and PTR. All authors read and approved the final manuscript.

## Competing interests
The authors declare that they have no competing interests.

## Funding
This work was supported by grants from the National Institutes of Health (R01-NS084941) and the Arizona Biomedical Research Commission (ADHS16-162406) to PTR.

## References
1.  Brzica H, Abdullahi W, Ibbotson K, Ronaldson PT. Role of transporters in central nervous system drug delivery and blood–brain barrier protection: relevance to treatment of stroke. J Cent Nerv Syst Dis. 2017;9:1179573517693802.
2.  Sanchez-Covarrubias L, Slosky LM, Thompson BJ, Davis TP, Ronaldson PT. Transporters at CNS barrier sites: obstacles or opportunities for drug delivery? Curr Pharm Des. 2014;20(10):1422–49.
3.  Stieger B, Gao B. Drug transporters in the central nervous system. Clin Pharmacokinet. 2015;54(3):225–42.
4.  Kalvass JC, Polli JW, Bourdet DL, Feng B, Huang SM, Liu X, et al. Why clinical modulation of efflux transport at the human blood–brain barrier is unlikely: the ITC evidence-based position. Clin Pharmacol Ther. 2013;94(1):80–94.
5.  Abdullahi W, Davis TP, Ronaldson PT. Functional expression of P-glycoprotein and organic anion transporting polypeptides at the blood–brain barrier: understanding transport mechanisms for improved CNS drug delivery? AAPS J. 2017;19(4):931–9.
6.  Eyal S, Hsiao P, Unadkat JD. Drug interactions at the blood–brain barrier: fact or fantasy? Pharmacol Ther. 2009;123(1):80–104.
7.  Ronaldson PT, Finch JD, Demarco KM, Quigley CE, Davis TP. Inflammatory pain signals an increase in functional expression of organic anion transporting polypeptide 1a4 at the blood–brain barrier. J Pharmacol Exp Ther. 2011;336(3):827–39.
8.  Ronaldson PT, Davis TP. Targeted drug delivery to treat pain and cerebral hypoxia. Pharmacol Rev. 2013;65(1):291–314.
9.  Thompson BJ, Sanchez-Covarrubias L, Slosky LM, Zhang Y, Laracuente ML, Ronaldson PT. Hypoxia/reoxygenation stress signals an increase in organic anion transporting polypeptide 1a4 (Oatp1a4) at the blood–brain barrier: relevance to CNS drug delivery. J Cereb Blood Flow Metab. 2014;34(4):699–707.
10.  Abdullahi W, Brzica H, Ibbotson K, Davis TP, Ronaldson PT. Bone morphogenetic protein-9 increases the functional expression of organic anion transporting polypeptide 1a4 at the blood–brain barrier via the activin receptor-like kinase-1 receptor. J Cereb Blood Flow Metab. 2017;37(7):2340–5.
11.  Westholm DE, Salo DR, Viken KJ, Rumbley JN, Anderson GW. The blood–brain barrier thyroxine transporter organic anion-transporting polypeptide 1c1 displays atypical transport kinetics. Endocrinology. 2009;150(11):5153–62.

12. Westholm DE, Stenehjem DD, Rumbley JN, Drewes LR, Anderson GW. Competitive inhibition of organic anion transporting polypeptide 1c1-mediated thyroxine transport by the fenamate class of nonsteroidal antiinflammatory drugs. Endocrinology. 2009;150(2):1025–32.

13. Kis B, Isse T, Snipes JA, Chen L, Yamashita H, Ueta Y, et al. Effects of LPS stimulation on the expression of prostaglandin carriers in the cells of the blood–brain and blood–cerebrospinal fluid barriers. J Appl Physiol. 2006;100(4):1392–9.

14. Dagenais C, Ducharme J, Pollack GM. Uptake and efflux of the peptidic delta-opioid receptor agonist. Neurosci Lett. 2001;301(3):155–8.

15. Ose A, Kusuhara H, Endo C, Tohyama K, Miyajima M, Kitamura S, et al. Functional characterization of mouse organic anion transporting peptide 1a4 in the uptake and efflux of drugs across the blood–brain barrier. Drug Metab Dispos. 2010;38(1):168–76.

16. Hagenbuch B, Meier PJ. Organic anion transporting polypeptides of the OATP/SLC21 family: phylogenetic classification as OATP/SLCO superfamily, new nomenclature and molecular/functional properties. Pflugers Arch. 2004;447(5):653–65.

17. Abbruscato TJ, Davis TP. Protein expression of brain endothelial cell E-cadherin after hypoxia/aglycemia: influence of astrocyte contact. Brain Res. 1999;842(2):277–86.

18. Barone E, Cenini G, Di Domenico F, Martin S, Sultana R, Mancuso C, et al. Long-term high-dose atorvastatin decreases brain oxidative and nitrosative stress in a preclinical model of Alzheimer disease: a novel mechanism of action. Pharmacol Res. 2011;63(3):172–80.

19. Wood WG, Eckert GP, Igbavboa U, Muller WE. Statins and neuroprotection: a prescription to move the field forward. Ann N Y Acad Sci. 2010;1199:69–76.

20. Gao B, Stieger B, Noe B, Fritschy JM, Meier PJ. Localization of the organic anion transporting polypeptide 2 (Oatp2) in capillary endothelium and choroid plexus epithelium of rat brain. J Histochem Cytochem. 1999;47(10):1255–64.

21. Cheng Z, Liu H, Yu N, Wang F, An G, Xu Y, et al. Hydrophilic anti-migraine triptans are substrates for OATP1A2, a transporter expressed at human blood–brain barrier. Xenobiotica. 2012;42(9):880–90.

22. Ho RH, Tirona RG, Leake BF, Glaeser H, Lee W, Lemke CJ, et al. Drug and bile acid transporters in rosuvastatin hepatic uptake: function, expression, and pharmacogenetics. Gastroenterology. 2006;130(6):1793–806.

23. Mandery K, Sticht H, Bujok K, Schmidt I, Fahrmayr C, Balk B, et al. Functional and structural relevance of conserved positively charged lysine residues in organic anion transporting polypeptide 1B3. Mol Pharmacol. 2011;80(3):400–6.

24. Liu H, Yu N, Lu S, Ito S, Zhang X, Prasad B, et al. Solute carrier family of the organic anion-transporting polypeptides 1A2-Madin-Darby Canine Kidney II: a promising in vitro system to understand the role of organic anion-transporting polypeptide 1A2 in blood–brain barrier drug penetration. Drug Metab Dispos. 2015;43(7):1008–18.

25. Cao J, Ng M, Felmlee MA. Sex hormones regulate rat hepatic monocarboxylate transporter expression and membrane trafficking. J Pharm Pharm Sci. 2017;20(1):435–44.

26. Alnouti Y, Petrick JS, Klaassen CD. Tissue distribution and ontogeny of organic cation transporters in mice. Drug Metab Dispos. 2006;34(3):477–82.

27. Cui YJ, Cheng X, Weaver YM, Klaassen CD. Tissue distribution, gender-divergent expression, ontogeny, and chemical induction of multidrug resistance transporter genes (Mdr1a, Mdr1b, Mdr2) in mice. Drug Metab Dispos. 2009;37(1):203–10.

28. Guo GL, Choudhuri S, Klaassen CD. Induction profile of rat organic anion transporting polypeptide 2 (oatp2) by prototypical drug-metabolizing enzyme inducers that activate gene expression through ligand-activated transcription factor pathways. J Pharmacol Exp Ther. 2002;300(1):206–12.

29. Cheng X, Maher J, Chen C, Klaassen CD. Tissue distribution and ontogeny of mouse organic anion transporting polypeptides (Oatps). Drug Metab Dispos. 2005;33(7):1062–73.

30. Klaassen CD, Aleksunes LM. Xenobiotic, bile acid, and cholesterol transporters: function and regulation. Pharmacol Rev. 2010;62(1):1–96.

31. Hou WY, Xu SF, Zhu QN, Lu YF, Cheng XG, Liu J. Age- and sex-related differences of organic anion-transporting polypeptide gene expression in livers of rats. Toxicol Appl Pharmacol. 2014;280(2):370–7.

32. de Zwart L, Scholten M, Monbaliu JG, Annaert PP, Van Houdt JM, Van den Wyngaert I, et al. The ontogeny of drug metabolizing enzymes and transporters in the rat. Reprod Toxicol. 2008;26(3–4):220–30.

33. Brzica H, Breljak D, Krick W, Lovric M, Burckhardt G, Burckhardt BC, et al. The liver and kidney expression of sulfate anion transporter sat-1 in rats exhibits male-dominant gender differences. Pflugers Arch. 2009;457(6):1381–92.

34. Brzica H, Abdullahi W, Reilly BG, Ronaldson PT. A simple and reproducible method to prepare membrane samples from freshly isolated rat brain microvessels. J Vis Exp. 2018. https://doi.org/10.3791/57698.

35. Ibbotson K, Yell J, Ronaldson PT. Nrf2 signaling increases expression of ATP-binding cassette subfamily C mRNA transcripts at the blood–brain barrier following hypoxia–reoxygenation stress. Fluids Barriers CNS. 2017;14(1):6.

36. Takasato Y, Rapoport SI, Smith QR. An in situ brain perfusion technique to study cerebrovascular transport in the rat. Am J Physiol. 1984;247(3 Pt 2):H484–93.

37. Vetter-O'Hagen CS, Spear LP. Hormonal and physical markers of puberty and their relationship to adolescent-typical novelty-directed behavior. Dev Psychobiol. 2012;54(5):523–35.

38. Gibson CL, Attwood L. The impact of gender on stroke pathology and treatment. Neurosci Biobehav Rev. 2016;67:119–24.

39. Benjamin EJ, Blaha MJ, Chiuve SE, Cushman M, Das SR, Deo R, et al. Heart disease and stroke statistics—2017 update: a report from the American Heart Association. Circulation. 2017;135(10):e146–603.

40. Clayton JA, Collins FS. Policy: NIH to balance sex in cell and animal studies. Nature. 2014;509(7500):282–3.

41. Spychala MS, Honarpisheh P, McCullough LD. Sex differences in neuroinflammation and neuroprotection in ischemic stroke. J Neurosci Res. 2017;95(1–2):462–71.

42. Klein SL, Marriott I, Fish EN. Sex-based differences in immune function and responses to vaccination. Trans R Soc Trop Med Hyg. 2015;109(1):9–15.

43. Liu F, Li Z, Li J, Siegel C, Yuan R, McCullough LD. Sex differences in caspase activation after stroke. Stroke. 2009;40(5):1842–8.

44. Manwani B, Bentivegna K, Benashski SE, Venna VR, Xu Y, Arnold AP, et al. Sex differences in ischemic stroke sensitivity are influenced by gonadal hormones, not by sex chromosome complement. J Cereb Blood Flow Metab. 2015;35(2):221–9.

45. Mirza MA, Ritzel R, Xu Y, McCullough LD, Liu F. Sexually dimorphic outcomes and inflammatory responses in hypoxic-ischemic encephalopathy. J Neuroinflammation. 2015;12:32.

46. Harati R, Benech H, Villegier AS, Mabondzo A. P-glycoprotein, breast cancer resistance protein, organic anion transporter 3, and transporting peptide 1a4 during blood–brain barrier maturation: involvement of Wnt/beta-catenin and endothelin-1 signaling. Mol Pharm. 2013;10(5):1566–80.

47. Roberts LM, Black DS, Raman C, Woodford K, Zhou M, Haggerty JE, et al. Subcellular localization of transporters along the rat blood–brain barrier and blood–cerebral-spinal fluid barrier by in vivo biotinylation. Neuroscience. 2008;155(2):423–38.

48. Hoshi Y, Uchida Y, Tachikawa M, Inoue T, Ohtsuki S, Terasaki T. Quantitative atlas of blood–brain barrier transporters, receptors, and tight junction proteins in rats and common marmoset. J Pharm Sci. 2013;102(9):3343–55.

49. Kamiie J, Ohtsuki S, Iwase R, Ohmine K, Katsukura Y, Yanai K, et al. Quantitative atlas of membrane transporter proteins: development and application of a highly sensitive simultaneous LC/MS/MS method combined with novel in silico peptide selection criteria. Pharm Res. 2008;25(6):1469–83.

50. Uchida Y, Ohtsuki S, Katsukura Y, Ikeda C, Suzuki T, Kamiie J, et al. Quantitative targeted absolute proteomics of human blood–brain barrier transporters and receptors. J Neurochem. 2011;117(2):333–45.

51. Shawahna R, Uchida Y, Decleves X, Ohtsuki S, Yousif S, Dauchy S, et al. Transcriptomic and quantitative proteomic analysis of transporters and drug metabolizing enzymes in freshly isolated human brain microvessels. Mol Pharm. 2011;8(4):1332–41.

52. Guo Y, Jiang L. Drug transporters are altered in brain, liver and kidney of rats with chronic epilepsy induced by lithium–pilocarpine. Neurol Res. 2010;32(1):106–12.

53. Bronger H, Konig J, Kopplow K, Steiner HH, Ahmadi R, Herold-Mende C, et al. ABCC drug efflux pumps and organic anion uptake transporters in human gliomas and the blood-tumor barrier. Cancer Res. 2005;65(24):11419–28.

54. Ohtsuki S, Tomi M, Hata T, Nagai Y, Hori S, Mori S, et al. Dominant expression of androgen receptors and their functional regulation of organic anion transporter 3 in rat brain capillary endothelial cells; comparison of gene expression between the blood–brain and –retinal barriers. J Cell Physiol. 2005;204(3):896–900.

55. Papadopoulos D, Scheiner-Bobis G. Dehydroepiandrosterone sulfate augments blood–brain barrier and tight junction protein expression in brain endothelial cells. Biochim Biophys Acta. 2017;1864(8):1382–92.

56. Bennett NC, Gardiner RA, Hooper JD, Johnson DW, Gobe GC. Molecular cell biology of androgen receptor signalling. Int J Biochem Cell Biol. 2010;42(6):813–27.

57. Breljak D, Brzica H, Sweet DH, Anzai N, Sabolic I. Sex-dependent expression of Oat3 (Slc22a8) and Oat1 (Slc22a6) proteins in murine kidneys. Am J Physiol Renal Physiol. 2013;304(8):F1114–26.

58. Ljubojevic M, Balen D, Breljak D, Kusan M, Anzai N, Bahn A, et al. Renal expression of organic anion transporter OAT2 in rats and mice is regulated by sex hormones. Am J Physiol Renal Physiol. 2007;292(1):F361–72.

# 22

# Challenges in cerebrospinal fluid shunting in patients with glioblastoma

Bujung Hong[1*] , Manolis Polemikos[1], Hans E. Heissler[1], Christian Hartmann[2], Makoto Nakamura[1,3] and Joachim K. Krauss[1]

## Abstract

**Background:** Cerebrospinal fluid (CSF) circulation disturbances may occur during the course of disease in patients with glioblastoma. Ventriculoperitoneal shunting has generally been recommended to improve symptoms in glioblastoma patients. Shunt implantation for patients with glioblastoma, however, presents as a complex situation and produces different problems to shunting in other contexts. Information on complications of shunting glioma patients has rarely been the subject of investigation. In this retrospective study, we analysed restropectively the course and outcome of glioblastoma-related CSF circulation disturbances after shunt management in a consecutive series of patients within a period of over a decade.

**Methods:** Thirty of 723 patients with histopathologically-confirmed glioblastoma diagnosed from 2002 to 2016 at the Department of Neurosurgery, Hannover Medical School, underwent shunting for CSF circulation disorders. Treatment history of glioblastoma and all procedures associated with shunt implementation were analyzed. Data on follow-up, time to progression and survival rates were obtained by review of hospital charts and supplemented by phone interviews with the patients, their relations or the primary physicians.

**Results:** Mean age at the time of diagnosis of glioblastoma was 43 years. Five types of CSF circulation disturbances were identified: obstructive hydrocephalus (n = 9), communicating hydrocephalus (n = 15), external hydrocephalus (n = 3), trapped lateral ventricle (n = 1), and expanding fluid collection in the resection cavity (n = 2). All patients showed clinical deterioration. Procedures for CSF diversion were ventriculoperitoneal shunt (n = 21), subduroperitoneal shunt (n = 3), and cystoperitoneal shunt (n = 2). In patients with lower Karnofsky Performance Score (KPS) (< 60), there was a significant improvement of median KPS after shunt implantation (p = 0.019). Shunt revision was necessary in 9 patients (single revision, n = 6; multiple revisions, n = 3) due to catheter obstruction, catheter dislocation, valve defect, and infection. Twenty-eight patients died due to disease progression during a median follow-up time of 88 months. The median overall survival time after diagnosis of glioblastoma was 10.18 months.

**Conclusions:** CSF shunting in glioblastoma patients encounters more challenge and is associated with increased risk of complications, but these can be usually managed by revision surgeries. CSF shunting improves neurological function temporarily, enhances quality of life in most patients although it is not known if survival rate is improved.

**Keywords:** Glioblastoma, Ventriculoperitoneal shunt, Hydrocephalus, Cerebrospinal fluid

*Correspondence: hong.bujung@mh-hannover.de
[1] Department of Neurosurgery, Hannover Medical School, Hannover, Germany
Full list of author information is available at the end of the article

## Background

Glioblastoma still has a dismal prognosis: significantly limiting quality of life and survival of patients suffering from this aggressive tumor [1, 2]. Maximal safe surgical resection followed by adjuvant combined radiochemotherapy is one of the most important factors to improve overall survival of patients [3–5]. Cerebrospinal fluid (CSF) circulation disturbances may occur during the course of disease and reduce a patient's quality of life as well as treatment capability significantly. Neurological deterioration associated with the development of hydrocephalus has been observed in 5–10% of patients with glioblastoma [6–13].

Ventriculoperitoneal shunting has generally been recommended to improve symptoms in glioblastoma patients with CSF circulation disturbances [6–13]. Shunt implantation in patients with glioblastoma, however, presents as a complex situation and produces different problems to shunting in other contexts [14, 15]. Although hydrocephalus is seen in a significant number of patients with glioblastoma, there are only a few studies which have concentrated on outcome of CSF shunting in this fragile group of patients [6, 8–13, 27]. Even more so, information on complications of shunting rarely has been the subject of investigation [11–13, 54].

Against this background, we sought to analyse the course and outcome of glioblastoma-related CSF circulation disturbances after shunt management in a consecutive series of patients within a period of over a decade.

## Methods

For this retrospective study a data base of 723 glioblastoma patients with histopathologically-confirmed glioblastoma diagnosed from 2002 to 2016 at the Department of Neurosurgery, Hannover Medical School, was reviewed. All patients that underwent shunting for CSF circulation disorders were included. Treatment history of glioblastoma, including surgical interventions and postoperative therapy were reviewed. In addition, all procedures associated with shunt implementation, including type of shunt, technical problems, and complications, were analysed. Data on follow-up, time to progression and survival rates were obtained by review of hospital charts and supplemented by phone interviews with the patients, their relations or the primary physicians.

Radiological evaluation of glioblastoma and tumor progression, in general, was made using contrast-enhanced MRI. CSF circulation disturbance was defined as disproportionate enlargement of inner and/or outer CSF spaces within the cranial vault or CSF collections in the resection cavity in postoperative imaging studies associated with the appearance of new clinical symptoms. Follow-up MRIs were obtained regularly at 3 months intervals.

After CSF shunting, all patients had X-ray shuntograms confirming valve settings and the location of catheters.

Microsurgical resection for tumor removal was performed according to standard surgical techniques for tumors not involving eloquent areas of the brain. Depending on tumor localization, neuronavigation, electrophysiological mapping, and/or 5-aminolevulinic acid (5-ALA) were applied intraoperatively [16, 17]. Gross total microsurgical resection was achieved when the neurosurgeon determined that all areas of visible tumor were resected intraoperatively. Resection was defined as subtotal when remnants of tumor were left behind.

Shunt surgery was performed after diagnosis of a clinically-relevant CSF circulation disturbance. Depending on the cause of the CSF circulation disturbance, ventriculoperitoneal, subduroperitoneal, or cystoperitoneal CSF diversion was performed. Programmable valve systems were implanted in 28 patients. While only four patients had a programmable valve (Codman & Shurtleff, Inc. Raynham, USA), in 24 patients, this was combined with implantation of a gravitational anti-siphon device [18]. Two patients received a medium pressure CSF-flow control valve system (Medtronic, Minneapolis, MN, USA). Due to poor accessibility of the ventricle system, a neuronavigation system was used for insertion of the ventricular catheter in three patients [16, 17].

## Statistical methods

Sigma Stat software (version 3.5; Systat Software, Inc. California, USA) was used for statistical analysis. To analyse the differences between groups, Student's $t$ test was used. The survival rate was estimated by the Kaplan–Meier method. Summary data were presented as median. Statistical significance was defined as a probability value less than 0.05. Measures were presented as mean ± standard deviations.

## Results

### Patient characteristics

Overall, 30/723 patients with histopathologically-proven glioblastoma (4.2%) underwent CSF shunting procedures during the study period. Patient characteristics are presented in Table 1. Mean age at the time of diagnosis of glioblastoma was 43 years (range 1 to 79 years). Initial surgical treatment included stereotactic biopsy (n = 7), partial resection (n = 6), subtotal resection (n = 8), and complete resection (n = 9). Two of 7 patients, who had stereotactic biopsy, underwent subsequent surgical resection after confirmation of the histopathological diagnosis of glioblastoma, since tumor location was considered accessible. In 18 patients the infiltrated ependymal wall of the ventricle system was opened during surgical resection.

**Table 1 Demographics and clinical characteristics of glioma patient group**

| Variable | n (%) |
| --- | --- |
| Sex | |
| Male | 20 (66.7) |
| Female | 10 (33.3) |
| Age at diagnosis | |
| <60 | 23 (76.7) |
| ≥60 | 7 (23.3) |
| Number of microsurgical tumor resections prior to shunt implantation | |
| None | 5 (16.7) |
| 1 time | 17 (56.7) |
| 2 times | 3 (10.0) |
| 3 times | 4 (13.3) |
| 4 times | 1 (3.3) |
| Type of CSF circulation disturbance | |
| Obstructive hydrocephalus | 9 (30.0) |
| Communicating hydrocephalus | 15 (50.0) |
| External hydrocephalus | 3 (10.0) |
| Trapped ventricle | 1 (3.3) |
| Expanding CSF collection in resection cavity | 2 (6.7) |
| Type of CSF diversion | |
| Ventriculoperitoneal | 21 (70.0) |
| Subduroperitoneal | 3 (10.0) |
| Cystoperitoneal | 2 (6.7) |
| Combined two catheters | |
| Frontal horn + temporal horn | 2 (6.7) |
| Frontal horn bilateral | 1 (3.3) |
| Expanding cyst + temporal horn | 1 (3.3) |

*CSF* cerebrospinal fluid

## Treatment

After histopathological confirmation of glioblastoma, temozolomide (TMZ) was administered in 14 patients concurrently with radiotherapy according to current standard therapy [19]. One patient received ACNU/VM26 within the NOA-1 protocol [20]. Three children were treated in accordance to HIT-GBM (German Society of Paediatric Oncology and Haematology) treatment protocols. Eighteen patients received conventional-fractionated partial brain radiotherapy with a total dose of 54–60 Gy (single dose, 1.8–2.0 Gy) starting within 6 weeks after initial resection. Eight patients underwent one or more microsurgical resections for recurrent GBM, of whom three patients tumor resection once, 5 patients twice, and 1 patient 3 times.

## CSF circulation problems

Overall, five types of CSF circulation disturbances were identified: obstructive hydrocephalus (n=9) (Fig. 1a), communicating hydrocephalus (n=15) (Fig. 1d), external hydrocephalus (n=3) (Fig. 1g), trapped lateral ventricle (n=1) (Fig. 1j), and expanding CSF collection in the resection cavity (n=2) (Fig. 1m). All patients showed clinical deterioration, mainly due to increase of intracranial pressure, predominantly presenting with headache, drowsiness, psychomotor slowing, hemiparesis, or aphasia.

## Treatment for CSF diversion

In five patients, a rapid symptomatic progression of hydrocephalus, as confirmed in the initial radiological images, was detected, so that a CSF shunt was implanted prior to surgical tumor resection. The other patients had one (n=17) or repeated (n=8) surgical tumor resection prior to shunt implantation. The type of CSF diversion included ventriculoperitoneal (n=21), subduroperitoneal (n=3), and cystoperitoneal shunting (n=2). In four patients, two catheters were inserted in separate intracranial compartments due to combined causes of CSF circulation disturbances. Three patients who underwent subduroperitoneal shunting had previously undergone subdural drainage via a burr hole. Shunting was performed for persistent subdural CSF collection with impaired consciousness or focal neurological signs. Depending on the clinical and radiological findings, the programmable valve was initially set to 6–8 cm $H_2O$ (n=24) for the ProGAV® valve system and to 50–140 mm Hg (n=4) for the Codman® Hakim® valve system. CSF sampling from 11 patients taken at shunt surgery showed no cytological evidence of tumor dissemination.

## Shunt failure and revision surgery

In five patients with programmable valve system, the valve pressure settings were subsequently adjusted due to over- or underdrainage as determined on clinical and radiological findings.

Shunt failure occurred in nine patients. The main symptoms of shunt failure were impairment of consciousness (n=10), cephalgia (n=8), and focal neurological deficits (n=5). Other symptoms included seizures, gait disorder, and aphasia (n=5). In three patients, routine follow-up imaging showed persistent hydrocephalus, and valve malfunction. Neither specific symptoms nor new neurological deficits were evident in these patients.

A total of 16 revision surgeries were performed in 9 (30.0%) adult patients (7 men, 2 women; mean age 55 years) due to various complications (Table 2), of which 11 (68.8%) revision surgeries were performed within the first year after shunt implantation. Overall, three patients (10%) required multiple revision surgeries (2 revision surgeries, n=1; 3 revision surgeries, n=1; 6 revision surgeries, n=1). In three patients, the anti-siphon device

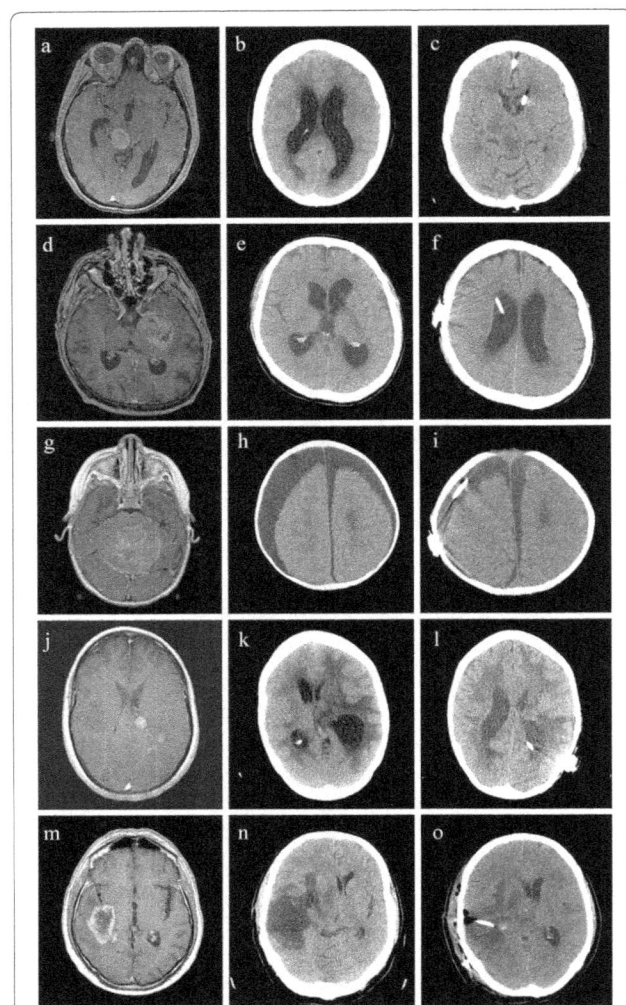

**Fig. 1** Images of glioblastoma patients: left column T1-weighted MR image after administration of gadolinium, centre collumn native CT scan showing CSF circulation disturbances and right collumn postoperative native CT scan after shunt placement. **a** A 41-year-old woman shows a pontomesencephalic glioblastoma in with compression of the aqueduct. **b** Widening of the lateral ventricles due to obstructive hydrocephalus. **c** Reduction of ventricular size after implantation of a ventriculoperitoneal shunt. **d** A 64-year-old man shows a glioblastoma in the left temporomesial lobe. **e** Ventricular enlargement due to communicating hydrocephalus. **f** The intracranial catheter in situ after implantation of a ventriculoperitoneal shunt. **g** A 1-year-old boy shows a midline glioblastoma, which resulted initially in obstructive hydrocephalus. **h** External hydrocephalus with extensive subdural hygroma. **i** After implantation of a subduroperitoneal shunt. **j** A 43-year-old woman shows a glioblastoma in the left parietal lobe/subcortical white matter. **k** Three weeks after tumor resection, CT imaging reveals isolated extension of the left posterior horn with local compression of adjacent structures and midline shift. **l** A shunt catheter in the posterior horn after implantation of a ventriculoperitoneal shunt. **m** A 69-year-old man shows a glioblastoma in the left temporal lobe. **n** A space occupying fluid collection in the resection cavity. **o** The proximal shunt catheter inserted in the resection

was removed over the course of disease. The patient with 6 revision surgeries had delayed shunt malfunction, which occurred approximately 3 years after the time of implantation.

### Outcome

Twenty-two patients temporarily benefitted from shunting with subsequent improvement of consciousness and neurological symptoms. Overall, the median KPS improved significantly from 50 to 70 after shunt implantation ($p = 0.008$ of which, six patients remained stable at a median KPS of 70 at 3 months postoperatively. The other two patients deteriorated further due to tumor progression within a median follow-up time of 5.5 months. When patients were dichotomized in two groups, there was a significant improvement of the median KPS after shunt implantation in those with a lower KPS ($< 60$) prior to shunt implantation ($p = 0.019$), while improvement in those with a higher prior KPS ($\geq 60$) did not reach statistical significance. The follow-up time of all patients ranged from 1 to 138 months with a median of 10 months. Twenty-eight patients died due to disease progression. Two patients were still alive at the time of writing manuscript. The median overall survival (mOS) time after diagnosis of glioblastoma was 10 months (Fig. 2). The two-year survival rate was 23.3%, 3-year survival rate 16.7%, and 5-year survival rate 6.7%.

### Discussion

Despite the development of hydrocephalus and the subsequent need for shunting in patients with glioblastoma is not an uncommon problem, this topic has attracted relatively little attention. Here we show that although shunting may not prolong overall survival, it significantly improves functional performance if only at least temporarily. The fact that there is relatively little information available on this issue most likely is due to circumstances which may have excluded these patients from larger studies or outcomes. Even less information is available on shunt complication during follow-up in this group of patients as summarized in Table 3.

Among the aforementioned types of CSF circulation disturbances, communicating hydrocephalus appears to be the most frequent one. Communicating hydrocephalus may occur due to entry of blood into the CSF spaces during surgery, due to elevated CSF protein, secondary to radiotherapy-induced fibrosis of arachnoid granulations, or to leptomeningeal dissemination of tumor cells [6–9, 21–24]. All these events may finally result in obliteration of the subarachnoid spaces over the surface of the brain with reduction of CSF absorption. Some authors reported a significant correlation between ventricular opening during tumor resection and development

**Table 2** Indications for revision surgery in nine patients with shunt malfunction on 16 occasions

| Indication | n | Type of surgical revision |
|---|---|---|
| Wound dehiscence with pneumocephalus | 1 | Wound revision |
| Delayed fluid collection in resection cavity | 1 | Additional cystoperitoneal shunt implantation |
| Valve and proximal catheter obstruction | 3 | Catheter replacement |
| Proximal catheter obstruction | 1 | Valve and catheter replacement |
| Proximal catheter dislocation | 1 | Reinsertion |
| Distal catheter dislocation | 1 | Reinsertion |
| Valve malfunction | 3 | Valve replacement |
| Delayed trapped ventricle and CSF collection in cavity, valve malfunction | 1 | New implantation of proximal shunt catheters without anti-siphon device |
| Intracerebral abscess | 1 | Removal of ventriculoperitoneal shunt, implantation of external ventricle drainage |
| Delayed trapped ventricle and CSF collection in cavity | 1 | New implantation of proximal catheters |
| Persistent hydrocephalus despite adjustment of programmable valve | 2 | Removal of anti-siphon device |

*CSF* cerebrospinal fluid

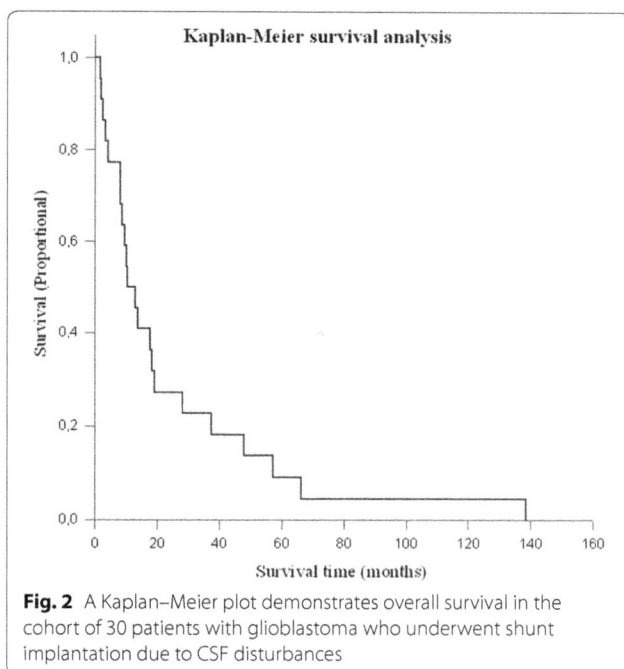

**Fig. 2** A Kaplan–Meier plot demonstrates overall survival in the cohort of 30 patients with glioblastoma who underwent shunt implantation due to CSF disturbances

of hydrocephalus [6, 9, 25], which, however, was not confirmed in other studies [10]. Multiple microsurgical resection for recurrent glioblastoma is likely to prolong survival [26]. However, it is also associated with an increased risk for communicating hydrocephalus [6]. Furthermore, previous radiotherapy increases the production of transforming growth factor-ß (TGF-ß) in cerebral tissues and glioma cells, supporting the transformation of fibroblasts into myofibroblasts, which promotes fibrosis of arachnoid granulations [21, 23].

The second most common type of CSF circulation disturbances in glioblastoma is obstructive hydrocephalus, which is caused by the obstruction of CSF pathways, mostly due to compression of the 3rd or the 4th ventricle, as typically detected in midline, cerebellar, or thalamic glioblastoma [27]. External hydrocephalus, trapped ventricle, and expanding space-occupying fluid collection in the resection cavity are seen more rarely. The pathological mechanism behind the development of external hydrocephalus is not fully understood. Some investigators have suggested that CSF absorption failure by widespread leptomeningeal and subependymal tumor metastases with simultaneous loss of ventricular compliance could be the underlying causes for the CSF collections in the subdural space [9, 28]. Others hypothesized that differential pressure between the ventricles and the subarachnoid spaces would allow CSF to pass from the ventricles to the subarachnoid space, and thus, result in CSF accumulation in the resection cavity or in the subdural space [29, 30]. Trapped ventricles occur typically as a complication of intraventricular hemorrhage [31–33]. Entry of blood in the ventricles during the surgery may result in adhesions and scarring of the ventricular wall, finally sealing off the posterior horn. CSF shunting is the treatment of choice to relieve the rapid ventricular dilatation.

Given the complexity of the development of CSF disturbances and the clinical condition, shunting in glioblastoma patients presents frequent challenges since treatment appears to be associated with increased risks for peri- and intraoperative complications. A higher incidence of shunt complications has been reported in the few studies focussing on this issue. Roth and colleagues have indicated that 8 of 16 glioblastoma patients with

**Table 3 Reported studies of cerebrospinal fluid shunting in patients with glioblastoma**

| Author, year | Frequency, n (%) | Type of CSF circulation disturbance | Shunt complication |
|---|---|---|---|
| Marquardt et al. 2002 [7] | 12/351 malignant gliomas (3.4) | CH (n = 12) | Multiple surgeries due to multiloculated hydrocephalus (n = 1) |
| Inamasu et al. 2003 [8] | 5/50 GBM (10) | CH (n = 5) | None reported |
| Roth et al. 2008 [11] | 16/530 GBM (3) | CH (n = 16) | Infection (n = 6), shunt malfunction (n = 1), overdrainage and hemorrhage (n = 1) |
| Montano et al. 2011 [6] | 11/124 GBM (8.9) | CH (n = 7), OH (n = 2), fluid in resection cavity (n = 2) | None reported |
| de la Fuente et al. 2014 [12] | 41/2433 gliomas WHO grade II–IV (1.7) | CH (n = 41) | Meningitis (n = 5), subdural hematoma (n = 5), haemorrhage (n = 1), infection (n = 6) |
| Fischer et al. 2014 [9] | 11/151 GBM (7.3) | CH (n = 11) | n.a. |
| Esquanazi et al., 2017 [27] | 20/57 thalamic GBM (35) | OH (n = 20) | n.a. |
| Behling et al. 2017 [10] | 13/229 GBM (5.7) | IH (n = 11), EH (n = 2) | n.a. |
| Castro et al. 2017 [13] | 64/841 GBM (7.6) | CH (n = 42), OH (n = 22) | Infection (n = 10), catheter occlusion (n = 1), combined overdrainage, ventriculitis and haemorrhage (n = 1) |

*GBM* glioblastoma; *CH* communicating hydrocephalus; *OH* obstructive hydrocephalus; *IH* internal hydrocephalus; *EH* external hydrocephalus; *CSF* cerebrospinal fluid; *n.a.* not available

ventriculoperitoneal shunts had shunt-related complications, of which 3 patients died due to such complications [11]. De la Fuente analysed 62 patients with supratentorial glioma, of which 41 had glioblastoma. Among these patients, 27% had complications related to ventriculoperitoneal shunts [12]. Further, a more recent study reported that shunt complications required surgical revision in 4 of 12 (33%) high-grade glioma patients with ventriculo-/cystoperitoneal shunts [34]. In our study, shunt failure affected mainly the ventricular catheter and the valve system. Hence, proximal complications appear to be the major causes of shunt dysfunction, whereas abdominal complications do not appear to occur more frequently in glioblastoma. Shunt complications are manifest most frequently within the first year after implantation. Some authors have suggested elevation of CSF protein levels and dissemination of tumor cells to be the causes for proximal obstruction and valve defects [9, 34, 35]. The clinical symptoms of shunt failure in glioblastoma patients are not always readily recognizable, particularly in patients with a lower KPS, impaired consciousness, or pre-existing focal neurological deficits. Regular follow-up CT or MR scans might provide evidence for shunt failure. Cohen et al. [36], however, found no correlation between clinical symptoms and radiological findings of shunt failure.

Shift of anatomical landmarks as a result of perifocal edema, tumor growth, or distention of the resection cavity during the course of treatment can make the implantation of the proximal catheter technically more challenging in some instances [37–40] resulting in a

higher risk for misplaced catheters [34]. In cases of poor accessibility to the ventricular system, neuronavigation is a valuable tool for achieving adequate placement of ventricular catheter [16, 17]. In cases of multiple CSF-filled compartments, insertion of separate catheters or even separate shunt systems is sometimes necessary. Such surgeries need to consider existing scars and previous craniotomies when draining the CSF compartments, thus making shunt surgery more challenging. Interestingly, there are hardly any studies in the literature dealing with the role of multiple intracranial catheters in patients with ventriculoperitoneal shunts.

Radiation and chemotherapy are prone to weaken the immune system [41]. Temozolomid chemotherapy which may induce lymphopenia and myelosuppression has been associated with poor immune surveillance leading to opportunistic infection in patients with malignant glioma [42, 43]. Other alkylating agents, such as Lomustine (CCNU) and PCV (Procarbazine—CCNU—Vincristine) induce predominantly neutropenia which can also increase the risk of infection [44]. Especially the combination of previous surgeries and radiochemotherapy can considerably contribute to wound-healing impairment. Furthermore, prolonged corticosteroid application, immobility, long hospitalisation and advanced age are other unfavorable factors often present in glioblastoma which increase the risk for infection [45, 46]. In some studies, up to 50% of glioblastoma patients with ventriculoperitoneal shunts experienced infection within 2 weeks after surgery [11]. In a recent study, Beez et al. reported 4 revision surgeries due to infection in 12 patients with high grade glioma and ventriculo-/cystoperitoneal shunts [34]. When shunt removal is inevitable, temporary external ventricle drainage is required. Shunt infection may be lethal in such patients [11].

Disease progress is associated with declined physical activity and some patients may be confined to bed for a long time. When patients are mobile, the integration of a gravity-assisted shunt valve can reduce the problem of siphoning and the occurrence of over drainage, and thus avoid posture-related headaches and the risk of subdural hygromas or hematoma [18, 47]. When patients are bedridden, however, gravity-assisted shunt valves should be avoided, since they may carry risk of underdrainage and persistent hydrocephalus [48]. A particular problem arises in such instances when patients are mobile initially but become bedridden in a later stage of the disease as detected in three patients of our series, making additional surgery to remove the gravity-assisted device unavoidable.

Although dissemination of glioblastoma within the ventricular system is well known [49], intraperitoneal metastasis via a ventriculoperitoneal shunt appears to occur very rarely [50–56]. We did not find any evidence of peritoneal seeding in any patient of our series. It has to be mentioned, however, that manifestation of glioblastoma in the abdominal cavity following ventriculoperitoneal shunting has been detected mainly by postmortem autopsy. Nevertheless, thus far, there is no systematic study using appropriate methods to detect metastatic seeding of glioblastoma cells into the peritoneal cavity via a shunt system intra vitam. Thus, the true incidence of intraperitoneal metastasis through shunting remains to be elucidated.

We acknowledge several limitations of our study, particularly related to its retrospective characters. We cannot determine the role of CSF shunt on survival time since the median KPS was quite low indicating a population with poorer prognosis. Furthermore, we did not study systematically the possibility of seeding of glioblastoma cells via the shunt system. In addition, it would have been be interesting to compare outcome between shunted and non-shunted GBM patients in a larger study.

## Conclusions

Different types of CSF circulation disturbances may occur during the course of disease in patients with glioblastoma. Shunting achieved temporary improvement for functional performance in the majority of the patients studied, but it is not known if shunting increases survival rate. Shunt implantation in patients with glioblastoma is more complex and burdened with a higher risk of complications, which, nevertheless, can usually be managed by revision surgery. Careful evaluation of the indication for CSF shunting and close postoperative follow-up is necessary.

## Abbreviations
5-ALA: 5-Aminolevulenic acid; CSF: cerebrospinal fluid; CT: computer tomography; GBM: glioblastoma; HIT-GBM: Hirntumor-Glioblastoma Multiforme; Gy: gray; KPS: Karnofsky Performance Score; mOS: median overall survival; MRI: magnetic resonance imaging; NOA: Neuroonkologische Arbeitsgemeinschaft; PCV: Procarbazine—CCNU—Vincristine; TGF-ß: transforming growth factor-ß; TMZ: temozolomide.

## Authors' contributions
BH collected the data, designed the study, and drafted the manuscripts. MP drafted the manuscripts. HEH performed statistical data analyses. CH collected the data. MN: designed the study. JKK drafted the manuscripts. All authors read and approved the final manuscript.

## Author details
[1] Department of Neurosurgery, Hannover Medical School, Hannover, Germany. [2] Institute for Pathology, Department for Neuropathology, Hannover Medical School, Hannover, Germany. [3] Department of Neurosurgery, Cologne Mehrheim Medical Center, University of Witten/Herdecke, Cologne, Germany.

## Competing interests
The authors declare that they have no competing interests.

## Funding
No funding received from any institution and/or foundation.

## References
1. de Robles P, Fiest KM, Frolkis AD, Pringheim T, Atta C, St Germaine-Smith C, et al. The worldwide incidence and prevalence of primary brain tumors: a systematic review and meta-analysis. Neuro Oncol. 2015;17:776–83.
2. Emmanuel C, Lawson T, Lelotte J, Fomekong E, Vaz G, Renard L, et al. Long-term survival after glioblastoma resection: hope despite poor prognosis factors. J Neurosurg Sci. 2018. https://doi.org/10.23736/S0390-5616.18.04180-2.
3. Stummer W, Picchlmeier U, Meinel T, Wiestler OD, Zanella F, Reulen HJ, et al. Fluorescence-guided surgery with 5-aminolevulinic acid for resection of malignant glioma: a randomised controlled multicentre phase III trial. Lancet Oncol. 2006;7:392–401.
4. Stupp R, Hegi ME, Mason WP, van den Bent MJ, Taphoorn MJ, Janzer RC, et al. Effects of radiotherapy with concomitant and adjuvant temozolomide versus radiotherapy alone on survival in glioblastoma in a

randomised phase III study: 5-year analysis of the EORTC-NCIC trial. Lancet Oncol. 2009;10:459–66.

5. Weller M, Stupp R, Hegi M, Wick W. Individualized targeted therapy for glioblastoma: fact or fiction? Cancer J. 2012;18:40–4.

6. Montano N, D'Alessandris QG, Bianchi F, Lauretti L, Doglietto F, Fernandez E, et al. Communicating hydrocephalus following surgery and adjuvant radiochemotherapy for glioblastoma. J Neurosurg. 2011;115:1126–30.

7. Marquardt G, Setzer M, Lang J, Seifert V. Delayed hydrocephalus after resection of supratentorial malignant gliomas. Acta Neurochir. 2002;144:227–31.

8. Inamasu J, Nakamura Y, Saito R, Kuroshima Y, Mayanagi K, Orii M, et al. Postoperative communicating hydrocephalus in patients with supratentorial malignant glioma. Clin Neurol Neurosurg. 2003;106:9–15.

9. Fischer CM, Neidert MC, Pèus D, Ulrich NH, Regli L, Krayenbühl N, et al. Hydrocephalus after resection and adjuvant radiochemotherapy in patients with glioblastoma. Clin Neurol Neurosurg. 2014;120:27–31.

10. Behling F, Kaltenstadler M, Noell S, Schittenhelm J, Bender B, Eckert F, et al. The prognostic impact of ventricular opening in glioblastoma surgery: a retrospective single center analysis. World Neurosurg. 2017;106:615–24.

11. Roth J, Constatini S, Blumenthal DT, Ram Z. The value of ventriculo-peritoneal shunting in patients with glioblastoma multiforme and ventriculomegaly. Acta Neurochir. 2008;150:41–6.

12. de la Fuente MI, DeAngelis LM. The role of ventriculoperitoneal shunting in patients with supratentorial glioma. Ann Clin Transl Neurol. 2014;1:45–8.

13. Castro BA, Imber BS, Chen R, McDermott MW, Aghi MK. Ventriculoperitoneal shunting for glioblastoma: risk factors, indications, and efficacy. Neurosurgery. 2017;80:421–30.

14. Krauss JK, von Stuckrad-Barre SF. Clinical aspects and biology of normal pressure hydrocephalus. Handb Clin Neurol. 2008;89:887–902.

15. Mirzayan MJ, Luetjens G, Borremans JJ, Regel JP, Krauss JK. Extended long-term (<5 years) outcome of cerebrospinal fluid shunting in idiopathic normal pressure hydrocephalus. Neurosurgery. 2010;67:295–301.

16. Hermann EJ, Polemikos M, Heissler HE, Krauss JK. Shunt surgery in idiopathic intracranial hypertension aided by electromagnetic navigation. Stereotact Funct Neurosurg. 2017;95:26–33.

17. Rodt T, Köppen G, Lorenz M, Majdani O, Leinung M, Bartling S, et al. Placement of intraventricular catheters using flexible electromagnetic navigation and a dynamic reference frame: a new technique. Stereotact Funct Neurosurg. 2007;85:243–8.

18. Sprung C, Schlosser HG, Lemcke J, Meier U, Messing-Jünger M, Trost HA, et al. The adjustable proGAV shunt: a prospective safety and reliability multicenter study. Neurosurgery. 2010;66:465–74.

19. Stupp R, Mason WP, van den Bent NJ, Weller M, Fisher B, Taphoorn MJ, et al. Radiotherapy plus concomitant and adjuvant temozolomide for glioblastoma. N Engl J Med. 2005;352:987–96.

20. Weller M, Müller B, Koch R, Bamberg M, Krauseneck P. Neuro-Oncology Working Group of the German Cancer Society. Neuro-Oncology Working Group 01 trial of nimustine plus teniposide versus nimustine plus cytarabine chemotherapy in addition to involved-field radiotherapy in the first-line treatment of malignant glioma. J Clin Oncol. 2003;21:3276–84.

21. Major O, Szeifert GT, Fazekas I, Vitanovics D, Csonka E, Koscis B, et al. Effect of a single high-dose gamma irradiation on cultured cells in human cerebral arteriovenous malformation. J Neurosurg. 2002;97(5 Suppl):459–63.

22. Perrini P, Scollato A, Cioffi F, Mouchaty H, Conti R, Di Lorenzo N. Radiation leukoencephalopathy associated with moderate hydrocephalus: intracranial pressure monitoring and results of ventriculoperitoneal shunting. Neurol Sci. 2002;23:237–41.

23. Shao C, Prise KM, Folkard M. Signaling factors for irradiated glioma cells induced bystander responses in fibroblasts. Mutat Res. 2008;638:139–45.

24. Dardis C, Milton K, Ashby L, Shapiro W. Leptomeningeal metastases in high-grade adult glioma: development, diagnosis, management, and outcomes in a series of 34 patients. Front Neurol. 2014;5:220.

25. John JK, Robin AM, Pabaney AH, Rammo RA, Schultz LR, Sadry NS, et al. Complications of ventricular entry during craniotomy for brain tumor resection. J Neurosurg. 2017;127:426–32.

26. Hong B, Wiese B, Bremer M, Heissler HE, Heidenreich F, Krauss JK. Multiple microsurgical resections for repeated recurrence of glioblastoma. Am J Clin Oncol. 2013;36:261–8.

27. Esquenazi Y, Moussazadeh N, Link TW, Hovinga KE, Reiner AS, DiStefano NM, et al. Thalamic glioblastoma: clinical presentation, management strategies, and outcome. Neurosurgery. 2017. https://doi.org/10.1093/neuros/nyx349.

28. Arita N, Taneda M, Hayakawa T. Leptomeningeal dissemination of malignant gliomas. Incidence, diagnosis and outcome. Acta Neurochir. 1994;126:84–92.

29. Bulstrode HJ, Natalwala A, Grundy PL. Atypical presentation of delayed communicating hydrocephalus after supratentorial glioma resection with opening of the ventricles. Br J Neurosurg. 2012;26:222–6.

30. Dörner L, Ulmer S, Rohr A, Mehdorn HM, Nabavi A. Space-occupying cyst development in the resection cavity of malignant gliomas following Gliadel® implantation—incidence, therapeutic strategies, and outcome. J Clin Neurosci. 2011;18:347–51.

31. Eller TW, Pasternak JF. Isolated ventricles following intraventricular haemorrhage. J Neurosurg. 1985;62:357–62.

32. Oi S, Abbott R. Loculated ventricles and isolated compartments in hydrocephalus: their pathophysiology and the efficacy of neuroendoscopic surgery. Neurosurg Clin N Am. 2004;15:77–87.

33. Pomeraniec IJ, Ksendzowsky A, Ellis S, Roberts SE, Jane JA Jr. Frequency and long-term follow-up of trapped fourth ventricle following neonatal posthemorrhagic hydrocephalus. J Neurosurg Pediatr. 2016;17:552–7.

34. Beez T, Burgula S, Kamp M, Rapp M, Steiger HJ, Sabel M. Space-occupying tumor bed cysts as a complication of modern treatment for high-grade glioma. World Neurosurg. 2017;104:509–15.

35. Turhan T, Ersahin Y, Dinc M, Mutluer S. Cerebro-spinal fluid shunt revisions, importance of the symptoms and shunt structure. Turk Neurosurg. 2011;21:66–73.

36. Cohen JS, Jamal N, Dawes C, Chamberlain JM, Atabaki SM. Cranial computed tomography utilization for suspected ventriculoperitoneal shunt malfunction in a pediatric emergency department. J Emerg Med. 2014;46:449–55.

37. Wick W, Küker W. Brain edema in neurooncology: radiological assessment and management. Onkologie. 2004;27:261–6.

38. Blystad I, Warntjes JBM, Smedby Ö, Lundberg P, Larsson EM, Tisell A. Quantitative MRI for analysis of peritumoral edema in malignant gliomas. PLoS ONE. 2017;12:e0177135.

39. Yang Z, Zhang Z, Wang X, Hu Y, Lyu Z, Huo L, et al. Intensity-modulated radiotherapy for gliomas: dosimetric effects of changes in gross tumor volume on organs at risk and healthy brain tissue. Onco Targets Ther. 2016;9:3545–54.

40. Vymazal J, Wong ET. Response patterns of recurrent glioblastomas treated with tumor-treating fields. Semin Oncol. 2014;41(6 Suppl):S14–24.

41. Grossman SA, Ye X, Lesser G, Sloan A, Carraway H, Desideri S, et al. Immunosuppression in patients with high-grade gliomas treated with radiation and temozolomide. Clin Cancer Res. 2011;17:5473–80.

42. Sengupta S, Marrinan J, Frishman C, Sampath P. Impact of temozolomide on immune response during malignant glioma chemotherapy. Clin Dev Immunol. 2012;2012:891090.

43. Kizilarslanoglu MC, Aksoy S, Yildrim NO, Ararat E, Sahin I, Altundaq K. Temozolomide-related infections: review of the literature. J BUON. 2011;16:547–50.

44. Thiepold AL, Lemercier S, Franz K, Atta J, Sulzbacher A, Steinbach JP, et al. Prophylactic use of pegfilgrastim in patients treated with a nitrosourea and teniposide for recurrent glioma. Pharmacotherapy. 2014;34:633–42.

45. Dix AR, Brooks WH, Roszman TL, Morford LA. Immune defects observed in patients with primary malignant brain tumors. J Neuroimmunol. 1999;100:216–32.

46. Hughes MA, Parisi M, Grossman S, Kleinberg L. Primary brain tumors treated with steroids and radiotherapy: low CD4 counts and risk of infection. Int J Radiat Oncol Biol Phys. 2005;62:1423–6.

47. Chapman PH, Cosman ER, Arnold MA. The relationship between ventricular fluid pressure and body position in normal subjects with shunts: a telemetric study. Neurosurgery. 1990;26:181–9.

48. Kaestner S, Kruschat T, Nitzsche N, Deinsberger W. Gravitational shunt units may cause under-drainage in bedridden patients. Acta Neurochir. 2009;151:217–21.

49. Onda K, Tanaka R, Takahashi H, Takeda N, Ikuta F. Cerebral glioblastoma with cerebrospinal fluid dissemination: a clinicopathological study of 14 cases examined by complete autopsy. Neurosurgery. 1989;25:533–40.

50. Newton HB, Rosenblum MK, Walker RW. Extraneural metastases of infratentorial glioblastoma multiforme to the peritoneal cavity. Cancer. 1992;69:2149–53.

51. Wakamatsu T, Matsuo T, Kawano S, Teramoto S, Matsumura H. Glioblastoma with extracranial metastasis through ventriculopleural shunt. Case report. J Neurosurg. 1971;34:697–701.

52. Yasuhara T, Tamiya T, Meguro T, Ichikawa T, Sato Y, Date I, et al. Glioblastoma with metastasis to the spleen—case report. Neurol Med Chir. 2003;43:452–6.

53. Matsuyama J, Mori T, Hori S, Nakano T, Yamada A. Gliosarcoma with multiple extracranial metastases. Case report. Neurol Med Chir. 1989;29:938–43.

54. Lin JC, Liu WH, Ma HI. Metastasis of glioblastoma multiforme via ventriculo-peritoneal shunt. J Med Sci. 2012;32:179–82.

55. Fecteau AH, Penn I, Hanto DW. Peritoneal metastasis of intracranial glioblastoma via a ventriculoperitoneal shunt preventing organ retrieval: case report and review of the literature. Clin Transplant. 1998;12:348–50.

56. Kumar R, Jain R, Tandon V. Thalamic glioblastoma with cerebrospinal fluid dissemination in the peritoneal cavity. Pediatr Neurosurg. 1999;31:242–5.

# Permissions

All chapters in this book were first published in FBOC, by BioMed Central; hereby published with permission under the Creative Commons Attribution License or equivalent. Every chapter published in this book has been scrutinized by our experts. Their significance has been extensively debated. The topics covered herein carry significant findings which will fuel the growth of the discipline. They may even be implemented as practical applications or may be referred to as a beginning point for another development.

The contributors of this book come from diverse backgrounds, making this book a truly international effort. This book will bring forth new frontiers with its revolutionizing research information and detailed analysis of the nascent developments around the world.

We would like to thank all the contributing authors for lending their expertise to make the book truly unique. They have played a crucial role in the development of this book. Without their invaluable contributions this book wouldn't have been possible. They have made vital efforts to compile up to date information on the varied aspects of this subject to make this book a valuable addition to the collection of many professionals and students.

This book was conceptualized with the vision of imparting up-to-date information and advanced data in this field. To ensure the same, a matchless editorial board was set up. Every individual on the board went through rigorous rounds of assessment to prove their worth. After which they invested a large part of their time researching and compiling the most relevant data for our readers.

The editorial board has been involved in producing this book since its inception. They have spent rigorous hours researching and exploring the diverse topics which have resulted in the successful publishing of this book. They have passed on their knowledge of decades through this book. To expedite this challenging task, the publisher supported the team at every step. A small team of assistant editors was also appointed to further simplify the editing procedure and attain best results for the readers.

Apart from the editorial board, the designing team has also invested a significant amount of their time in understanding the subject and creating the most relevant covers. They scrutinized every image to scout for the most suitable representation of the subject and create an appropriate cover for the book.

The publishing team has been an ardent support to the editorial, designing and production team. Their endless efforts to recruit the best for this project, has resulted in the accomplishment of this book. They are a veteran in the field of academics and their pool of knowledge is as vast as their experience in printing. Their expertise and guidance has proved useful at every step. Their uncompromising quality standards have made this book an exceptional effort. Their encouragement from time to time has been an inspiration for everyone.

The publisher and the editorial board hope that this book will prove to be a valuable piece of knowledge for researchers, students, practitioners and scholars across the globe.

# List of Contributors

**Camilla Cerutti**
Department of Life, Health and Chemical Sciences, Biomedical Research Network, Open University, Walton Hall, Milton Keynes MK7 6AA, UK
Randall Division of Cell and Molecular Biophysics, King's College London, New Hunt's House, Guy's Campus, London SE1 1UL, UK

**Patricia Soblechero-Martin, David Kingsley Male and Ignacio Andres Romero**
Department of Life, Health and Chemical Sciences, Biomedical Research Network, Open University, Walton Hall, Milton Keynes MK7 6AA, UK

**Dongsheng Wu**
Department of Life, Health and Chemical Sciences, Biomedical Research Network, Open University, Walton Hall, Milton Keynes MK7 6AA, UK
School of Engineering and Materials Science, Queen Mary University of London, Mile End Road, London E1 4NS, UK

**Miguel Alejandro Lopez-Ramirez**
Department of Life, Health and Chemical Sciences, Biomedical Research Network, Open University, Walton Hall, Milton Keynes MK7 6AA, UK
Department of Medicine, University of California, San Diego, La Jolla, CA 92093, USA

**Helga de Vries**
Department of Molecular Cell Biology and Immunology, MS Centre Amsterdam, VU University Medical Centre, Amsterdam, The Netherlands

**Basil Sharrack**
Department of Neuroscience, Sheffield University, 385a Glossop Road, Sheffield S10 2HQ, UK

**Amauri Dalla Corte and Roberto Giugliani**
Post-Graduate Program in Medical Sciences, Universidade Federal do Rio Grande do Sul, Porto Alegre, Brazil
Medical Genetics Service, Hospital de Clínicas de Porto Alegre, Rua Ramiro Barcelos 2350, Porto Alegre, RS 90035-903, Brazil

**Carolina F. M. de Souza and Solanger G. P. Perrone**
Medical Genetics Service, Hospital de Clínicas de Porto Alegre, Rua Ramiro Barcelos 2350, Porto Alegre, RS 90035-903, Brazil

**Maurício Anés**
Medical Physics and Radioprotection Service, Hospital de Clínicas de Porto Alegre, Porto Alegre, Brazil

**Fabio K. Maeda**
Clinical Engineering, Santa Casa de Misericórdia de Porto Alegre, Porto Alegre, Brazil

**Armelle Lokossou and Olivier Balédent**
Image Processing Unit, Amiens University Hospital, Amiens, France

**Leonardo M. Vedolin**
Department of Neuroradiology, DASA Group, São Paulo, Brazil

**Maria Gabriela Longo**
Department of Radiology, Massachusetts General Hospital, Boston, USA

**Monica M. Ferreira**
Anesthesiology Service, Hospital de Clínicas de Porto Alegre, Porto Alegre, Brazil

**Aaron Dadas**
Flocel Inc., Cleveland, OH 44103, USA
The Ohio State University, Columbus, OH, USA

**Jolewis Washington**
Flocel Inc., Cleveland, OH 44103, USA
John Carroll University, University Heights, OH, USA

**Nicola Marchi**
Laboratory of Cerebrovascular Mechanisms of Brain Disorders, Institut de Génomique Fonctionnelle, Université Montpellier, Montpellier, France

**Damir Janigro**
Flocel Inc., Cleveland, OH 44103, USA
Case Western Reserve University, Cleveland, OH, USA

**Mahdi Asgari**
The Interface Group, Institute of Physiology, University of Zurich, Winterthurerstrasse 190, 8057 Zurich, Switzerland
Neuroscience Center Zurich, University of Zurich, Zurich, Switzerland

**Diane A. de Zélicourt**
The Interface Group, Institute of Physiology, University of Zurich, Winterthurerstrasse 190, 8057 Zurich, Switzerland

**Vartan Kurtcuoglu**
The Interface Group, Institute of Physiology, University of Zurich, Winterthurerstrasse 190, 8057 Zurich, Switzerland
Neuroscience Center Zurich, University of Zurich, Zurich, Switzerland
Zurich Center for Integrative Human Physiology, University of Zurich, Zurich, Switzerland

**Petter Holmlund, Sara Qvarlander, Khalid Ambarki and Anders Eklund**
Department of Radiation Sciences, Umeå University, 901 87 Umeå, Sweden

**Elias Johansson, Lars-Owe D. Koskinen and Jan Malm**
Department of Pharmacology and Clinical Neuroscience, Umeå University, 901 87 Umeå, Sweden

**Anders Wåhlin**
Department of Radiation Sciences, Umeå University, 901 87 Umeå, Sweden
Umeå Centre for Functional Brain Imaging, Umeå University, 901 87 Umeå, Sweden

**Martin J. Schmidt, Jessica Hauer, Malgorzata Kolecka and Nele Ondreka**
Department of Veterinary Clinical Sciences, Small Animal Clinic, Justus- Liebig-University, Frankfurter Strasse 108, 35392 Giessen, Germany

**Christoph Rummel and Joachim Roth**
Institute for Veterinary Physiology and Biochemistry, Justus-Liebig-University, Frankfurter Strasse 100, 35392 Giessen, Germany

**Vanessa McClure**
Department of Companion Animal Clinical Studies, Faculty of Veterinary Science, University of Pretoria, Onderstepoort, Pretoria 0110, Republic of South Africa

**Xiaomei Chen**
Department of Pharmaceutical Biosciences, Translational PKPD Research Group, Uppsala University, SE-75124 Uppsala, Sweden
Department of Pharmaceutical Sciences, College of Pharmacy, University of Michigan, Ann Arbor, MI 48109, USA

**Tim Slättengren and Margareta Hammarlund-Udenaes**
Department of Pharmaceutical Biosciences, Translational PKPD Research Group, Uppsala University, SE-75124 Uppsala, Sweden

**Elizabeth C. M. de Lange**
Department of Pharmacology, Leiden Academic Centre for Drug Research, Leiden, The Netherlands

**David E. Smith**
Department of Pharmaceutical Sciences, College of Pharmacy, University of Michigan, Ann Arbor, MI 48109, USA

**Prakash Ambady**
Department of Neurology, Oregon Health and Science University, 3181 SW Sam Jackson Park Road, L603, Portland, OR 97239, USA
Portland Veterans Affairs Medical Center, Portland, OR, USA

**Rongwei Fu**
School of Public Health, Oregon Health and Science University, Portland, OR, USA
Department of Emergency Medicine, Oregon Health and Science University, Portland, OR, USA

**Joao Prola Netto**
Department of Neurology, Oregon Health and Science University, 3181 SW Sam Jackson Park Road, L603, Portland, OR 97239, USA
Department of Radiology, Oregon Health and Science University, Portland, OR, USA

**Cymon Kersch, Jenny Firkins and Nancy D. Doolittle**
Department of Neurology, Oregon Health and Science University, 3181 SW Sam Jackson Park Road, L603, Portland, OR 97239, USA

**Edward A. Neuwelt**
Department of Neurology, Oregon Health and Science University, 3181 SW Sam Jackson Park Road, L603, Portland, OR 97239, USA
Portland Veterans Affairs Medical Center, Portland, OR, USA
Department of Neurosurgery, Oregon Health and Science University, Portland, OR, USA

**Charles P. Schaefer, Margaret E. Tome and Thomas P. Davis**
Department of Pharmacology, University of Arizona, Tucson, AZ 85724, USA

**Kathryn Ibbotson**
Department of Pharmacology and Toxicology, College of Pharmacy, University of Arizona, 1295 N. Martin Avenue, Tucson 85721, AZ, USA

**Joshua Yell and Patrick T. Ronaldson**
Department of Pharmacology, College of Medicine, University of Arizona, 1501 N. Campbell Avenue, Tucson, AZ 85724-5050, USA

**Anuriti Aojula and Hannah Botfield**
Institute of Metabolism and Systems Research, University of Birmingham, Edgbaston, Birmingham B15 2TT, UK
Centre for Endocrinology, Diabetes and Metabolism, Birmingham Health Partners, Birmingham B15 2TH, UK
Neurotrauma, College of Medicine and Dentistry, University of Birmingham, Edgbaston, Birmingham B15 2TT, UK

**James Patterson McAllister II**
Department of Neurosurgery, Division of Pediatric Neurosurgery at the Washington University School of Medicine and the Saint Louis Children's Hospital, St. Louis, MO 63110, USA

**Ana Maria Gonzalez**
Institute of Metabolism and Systems Research, University of Birmingham, Edgbaston, Birmingham B15 2TT, UK
Neurotrauma, College of Medicine and Dentistry, University of Birmingham, Edgbaston, Birmingham B15 2TT, UK

**Osama Abdullah**
Department of Bioengineering, University of Utah, Salt Lake City, UT 84112, USA

**Ann Logan**
Department of Bioengineering, University of Utah, Salt Lake City, UT 84112, USA
Neurotrauma, College of Medicine and Dentistry, University of Birmingham, Edgbaston, Birmingham B15 2TT, UK

**Alexandra Sinclair**
Institute of Metabolism and Systems Research, University of Birmingham, Edgbaston, Birmingham B15 2TT, UK
Centre for Endocrinology, Diabetes and Metabolism, Birmingham Health Partners, Birmingham B15 2TH, UK
Neurotrauma, College of Medicine and Dentistry, University of Birmingham, Edgbaston, Birmingham B15 2TT, UK
Department of Neurology, University Hospitals Birmingham NHS Foundation Trust, Birmingham B15 2TH, UK

**Be'eri Niego, Heidi Ho and Robert L. Medcalf**
Molecular Neurotrauma and Haemostasis, Australian Centre for Blood Diseases, Monash University, Level 4 Burnet Building, 89 Commercial Road, Melbourne 3004, VIC, Australia

**Brad R. S. Broughton**
Cardiovascular and Pulmonary Pharmacology Group, Biomedicine Discovery Institute, Department of Pharmacology, Monash University, Clayton, VIC, Australia

**Christopher G. Sobey**
Vascular Biology and Immunopharmacology Group, Department of Physiology, Anatomy and Microbiology, School of Life Sciences, La Trobe University, Bundoora, VIC, Australia

**Marija Djukic, Ralf Trimmel and Roland Nau**
Department of Geriatrics, Evangelisches Krankenhaus Göttingen-Weende, Göttingen, Germany
Institute of Neuropathology, University Medical Center Göttingen (UMG), Robert-Koch-Strasse 40, 37075 Göttingen, Germany

**Ingelore Nagel and Peter Lange**
Department of Neurology, University Medical Center Göttingen (UMG), Göttingen, Germany

**Annette Spreer**
Department of Neurology, University Medical Center Göttingen (UMG), Göttingen, Germany
Department of Neurology, University Medical Centre Mainz, Mainz, Germany

**Christine Stadelmann**
Institute of Neuropathology, University Medical Center Göttingen (UMG), Robert-Koch-Strasse 40, 37075 Göttingen, Germany

**Ryann M. Fame**
Whitehead Institute for Biomedical Research, Nine Cambridge Center, Cambridge, MA 02142, USA

**Jessica T. Chang and Hazel Sive**
Whitehead Institute for Biomedical Research, Nine Cambridge Center, Cambridge, MA 02142, USA
Massachusetts Institute of Technology, 77 Massachusetts Avenue, Cambridge, MA 02139-4307, USA

**Alex Hong and Nicole A. Aponte-Santiago**
Massachusetts Institute of Technology, 77 Massachusetts Avenue, Cambridge, MA 02139-4307, USA

**Jackson G. DeStefano and Peter C. Searson**
Institute for Nanobiotechnology, Johns Hopkins University, 100 Croft Hall, 3400 North Charles Street, Baltimore, MD 21218, USA
Department of Materials Science and Engineering, Johns Hopkins University, Baltimore, MD 21218, USA

**Zinnia S. Xu**
Institute for Nanobiotechnology, Johns Hopkins University, 100 Croft Hall, 3400 North Charles Street, Baltimore, MD 21218, USA
Department of Biomedical Engineering, Johns Hopkins University, 720 Rutland Avenue, Baltimore, MD 21205, USA

**Ashley J. Williams and Nahom Yimam**
Institute for Nanobiotechnology, Johns Hopkins University, 100 Croft Hall, 3400 North Charles Street, Baltimore, MD 21218, USA

**Marija Djukic and Roland Nau**
Department of Geriatrics, Evangelisches Krankenhaus Göttingen-Weende, Göttingen, Germany
Institute of Neuropathology, University Medical Center Goettingen (UMG), Robert-Koch-Strasse 40, D-37075 Göttingen, Germany

**Annette Spreer**
Department of Neurology, University Medical Center Goettingen (UMG), Göttingen, Germany
Department of Neurology, University Medical Centre Mainz, Mainz, Germany

**Peter Lange**
Department of Neurology, University Medical Center Goettingen (UMG), Göttingen, Germany

**Stephanie Bunkowski**
Institute of Neuropathology, University Medical Center Goettingen (UMG), Robert-Koch-Strasse 40, D-37075 Göttingen, Germany

**Jens Wiltfang**
Department of Psychiatry and Psychotherapy, University Medical Center Goettingen (UMG), Göttingen, Germany
German Center for Neurodegenerative Diseases (DZNE), Georg August University Göttingen, Göttingen, Germany

**Dominique Endres, Evgeniy Perlov, Sabine Hellwig, Bernd L. Fiebich and Ludger Tebartz van Elst**
Section for Experimental Neuropsychiatry, Department of Psychiatry and Psychotherapy, Medical Center-University of Freiburg, Faculty of Medicine, University of Freiburg, Freiburg, Germany

**Daniela Huzly**
Institute for Virology, Medical Center-University of Freiburg, Faculty of Medicine, University of Freiburg, Freiburg, Germany

**Rick Dersch, Oliver Stich, Benjamin Berger, Florian Schuchardt and Tilman Hottenrott**
Department of Neurology and Neurophysiology, Medical Center-University of Freiburg, Faculty of Medicine, University of Freiburg, Freiburg, Germany

**Nils Venhoff**
Department of Rheumatology and Clinical Immunology, Medical Center-University of Freiburg, Faculty of Medicine, University of Freiburg, Freiburg, Germany

**Daniel Erny**
Institute of Neuropathology, Medical Center-University of Freiburg, Faculty of Medicine, University of Freiburg, Freiburg, Germany
Berta-Ottenstein-Programme, Faculty of Medicine, University of Freiburg, Freiburg, Germany

**Daphne M. P. Naessens, Judith de Vos, Ed VanBavel and Erik N. T. P. Bakker**
Department of Biomedical Engineering and Physics, Academic Medical Center, University of Amsterdam, Meibergdreef 9, 1105 AZ Amsterdam, The Netherlands

**Julian Rey and Malisa Sarntinoranont**
Department of Mechanical and Aerospace Engineering, University of Florida, Gainesville, FL 32611, USA

**Young-Jin Kang, Brett A. Johnson, Margaret Coutts, Hillary M. Vo, Xinya Hao, Nida Fatima and Michael J. Neel**
Department of Pathology and Laboratory Medicine, UC Irvine, Irvine, USA
Sue and Bill Gross Stem Cell Research Center, UC Irvine, Irvine, USA

**Maria J. Rivera and Robert J. Sims**
Department of Biological Sciences, California State University, Long Beach, USA

**Edwin S. Monuki**
Department of Pathology and Laboratory Medicine, UC Irvine, Irvine, USA
Sue and Bill Gross Stem Cell Research Center, UC Irvine, Irvine, USA
Department of Developmental and Cell Biology, UC Irvine, Irvine, USA

**Hrvoje Brzica, Wazir Abdullahi, Bianca G. Reilly and Patrick T. Ronaldson**
Department of Pharmacology, College of Medicine, University of Arizona, 1501 N. Campbell Avenue, Tucson, AZ 85724-5050, USA

**Bujung Hong, Manolis Polemikos, Hans E. Heissler and Joachim K. Krauss**
Department of Neurosurgery, Hannover Medical School, Hannover, Germany

**Christian Hartmann**
Institute for Pathology, Department for Neuropathology, Hannover Medical School, Hannover, Germany

**Makoto Nakamura**
Department of Neurosurgery, Hannover Medical School, Hannover, Germany
Department of Neurosurgery, Cologne Mehrheim Medical Center, University of Witten/Herdecke, Cologne, Germany

# Index

www.ingramcontent.com/pod-product-compliance
Lightning Source LLC
Chambersburg PA
CBHW080513200326
41458CB00012B/4186